Clinical Management of
Children with Cochlear Implants

Clinical Management of Children with Cochlear Implants

LAURIE S. EISENBERG, Ph.D.

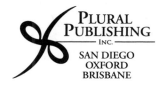

PLURAL
PUBLISHING
INC.

SAN DIEGO
OXFORD
BRISBANE

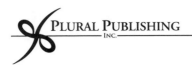

5521 Ruffin Road
San Diego, CA 92123

e-mail: info@pluralpublishing.com
Web site: http://www.pluralpublishing.com

49 Bath Street
Abingdon, Oxfordshire OX14 1EA
United Kingdom

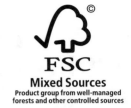

FSC
Mixed Sources
Product group from well-managed
forests and other controlled sources

Cert no. SW-COC-002283
www.fsc.org
© 1996 Forest Stewardship Council

Library of Congress Cataloging-in-Publication Data

Clinical management of children with cochlear implants / [edited by] Laurie S. Eisenberg.
       p. ; cm.
  Includes bibliographical references and index.
  ISBN-13: 978-1-59756-251-5 (alk. paper)
  ISBN-10: 1-59756-251-3 (alk. paper)
  1. Cochlear implants. 2. Deaf children—Rehabilitation. I. Eisenberg, Laurie S.
  [DNLM: 1. Cochlear Implantation. 2. Child. 3. Cochlear Implants. 4. Deafness—
therapy. 5. Infant. WV 274 C6405 2009]
  RF305.C55 2009
  617.8'82—dc22
                                                                    2008052901

Contents

Preface

I was very fortunate to have begun my career as an audiologist at the House Ear Institute (then called the Ear Research Institute) in the mid-1970s during the very early years of clinical research with the single-channel cochlear implant. Interviewed for the position by Norma Norton, a speech-language pathologist and audiologist who worked with William F. House, M.D. on the first cochlear implant clinical program, I was informed that cochlear implants were so controversial that working in this field could ruin my career as an audiologist. This, indeed, was an unsettling start to a career that has now spanned more than 30 years. For 10 years, I participated in the first cochlear implant clinical trials with postlingually and prelingually deaf adults and then with deaf children. I also had the opportunity to work with the first group of auditory brainstem implant patients before leaving the House Ear Institute to pursue my doctorate. Thus, having begun my career as a clinical audiologist on one of the first cochlear implant clinical programs, the editing of a book on the clinical management of children with cochlear implants brings me back to my roots. When working on those early clinical trials, there were no texts or resources on the topic. My colleagues and I had to start from scratch, develop our own materials, and learn as we went along. The primary reason for editing this book is to provide clinicians with a text that can become a useful and practical resource.

Readers of this book will have the advantage of learning from a select group of masters in the field. Highly experienced clinicians and prominent researchers have been solicited to write these chapters. Some authors will be very recognizable; others not as much, particularly those who are practitioners. It is often a fact that those clinicians working in the trenches on a daily basis rarely receive the recognition they so justly deserve. It also is notable that several of the well-known researchers who have written chapters in this book started their careers in the clinic and, thus, have an appreciation for this difficult but often very rewarding endeavor. Other authors are junior investigators who I have no doubt will become part of the next crop of leaders in this field.

The chapters are as diverse as the different disciplines that contribute to pediatric cochlear implantation. The authors come from a variety of professional backgrounds, including neurotology, pediatric otolaryngology, audiology, speech-language pathology, auditory-verbal therapy, clinical psychology, experimental psychology, education of the deaf and hard-of-hearing, and early intervention. Several chapters provide guidance for managing a pediatric implant program, ranging from candidacy, general assessment, medical/surgical aspects, programming the implant processor, and postimplant follow-up. Other chapters address specific areas of assessment, including electrophysiology, vestibular functioning, speech perception, spoken word recognition, speech production, language, intelligence, psychosocial functioning, and quality of life. There are chapters oriented to the child and family, entailing habilitation, education, and parental contributions, with attention to families of low socioeconomic status. Hearing aids, bilateral implants, and auditory brainstem implants also are addressed in individual chapters. Finally, special cases that might be encountered in clinical practice are highlighted, including those with auditory neuropathy, multiple disabilities, and/or developmental delays.

I wish to acknowledge the many individuals with whom I have worked during the early years of cochlear implants. Most notably, I thank William F. House for giving me the opportunity to participate in this special project so early in my career. Other notable people include Norma Norton, Karen Berliner, Margaret Thielemeir, Bill Luxford, Betty Peterson, Karen Iler Kirk, Carolyn Brown, Lisa Tonokawa, Julie Gonzales, Bill Crary, Murray Wexler, Linda Miller, and Norm Tiber. I also wish to recognize those mentors who played a major role in guiding my career as a clinical scientist—Harry Levitt, Arthur Boothroyd, and Don Dirks.

This book could never have come to fruition without the administrative assistance of Barbara Serrano, who has spent many hours interacting with the authors, preparing tables, and helping in the formatting/ editing of the book. Liz Gnerre, our librarian at the House Ear Institute, has been instrumental in accessing difficult to find references upon request. My colleagues, Amy Martinez, Leslie Visser-Dumont, and Dianne Hammes-Ganguly, have been tireless in their proofreading and citation checking for the different drafts that have come across my desk. Lastly, I wish to acknowledge all my colleagues in the Children's Auditory Research and Evaluation (CARE) Center and throughout the House Ear Institute—the place where I started my career as an audiologist and, I hope, the place where I will end it as an audiologist (but not quite yet!).

Laurie S. Eisenberg

Contributors

Paul J. Abbas, Ph.D.
Professor and Chair
Department of Communication Sciences
and Disorders
Department of Otolaryngology
University of Iowa
Iowa City, Iowa
Chapter 7

Sophie E. Ambrose, M.A.
Pediatric Speech-Language Pathologist
Research Associate
Division of Communication and
Auditory Neuroscience
Children's Auditory Research and
Evaluation (CARE) Center
House Ear Institute
Los Angeles, California
Chapter 11

Arthur Boothroyd, Ph.D.
Distinguished Professor Emeritus
City University of New York
New York, New York
Scholar-in-Residence
San Diego State University
San Diego, California
Distinguished Visiting Scientist
House Ear Institute
Los Angeles, California
Chapter 9

Carolyn J. Brown, Ph.D.
Professor
Department of Communication Sciences
and Disorders
Department of Otolaryngology—Head
and Neck Surgery

University of Iowa
Iowa City, Iowa
Chapter 7

Craig A. Buchman, M.D.
Professor and Chief
Division of Otology/Neurotology, and
Skull Base Surgery
Medical Director, W. Paul Briggers
Carolina Children's Communicative
Disorders Program (CCCDP)
Department of Otolaryngology—Head
and Neck Surgery
University of North Carolina at Chapel Hill
Chapel Hill, North Carolina
Chapter 20

Marco Carner, M.D.
Adjunct Professor
Department of Otolaryngology
University of Verona Medical School
Verona, Italy
Chapter 21

Sangsook Choi, Ph.D.
Postdoctoral Research Associate
Department of Speech, Language and
Hearing Sciences
Purdue University
West Lafayette, Indiana
Chapter 10

Patricia M. Chute, Ed.D.
Interim Dean
School of Health Sciences
Mercy College
Dobbs Ferry, New York
Chapter 16

Lilliana Colletti, Ph.D.
Researcher
Department of Otolaryngology
University of Verona Medical School
Verona, Italy
Chapter 21

Vittorio Colletti, M.D.
Professor and Chair
Department of Otolaryngology
University of Verona Medical School
Verona, Italy
Chapter 21

Sharon L. Cushing, M.D.
Resident
Department of Otolaryngology—Head
   and Neck Surgery
University of Toronto
Toronto, Ontario, Canada
Chapter 8

Jean L. DesJardin, Ph.D.
Adjunct Professor
School of Education and Human Services
Canisius College
Buffalo, New York
Chapter 17

Laurie S. Eisenberg, Ph.D.
Scientist III
Division of Communication and
   Auditory Neuroscience
Children's Auditory Research and
   Evaluation (CARE) Center
House Ear Institute
Los Angeles, California
Clinical Professor of Otolaryngology
Member, Neuroscience Graduate Program
University of Southern California
Los Angeles, California
Preface, Chapters 1 and 21

Christine P. Etler, M.A., CCC-A
Research Audiologist

Department of Otolaryngology—Head
   and Neck Surgery
University of Iowa
Iowa City, Iowa
Chapter 7

Jose N. Fayad, M.D.
Associate Professor of Clinical
   Otolaryngology
University of Southern California
Los Angeles, California
Associate
House Clinic
Los Angeles, California
Chief, Section of Otology/Neurotology
St. Vincent Medical Center
Los Angeles, California
Chapter 5

Howard W. Francis, M.D.
Associate Professor
Department of Otolaryngology—Head
   and Neck Surgery
Johns Hopkins University
Baltimore, Maryland
Chapter 14

Brian F. French, Ph.D.
Associate Professor
Washington State University
College of Education
Pullman, Washington
Chapter 10

Sarah Gehlert, Ph.D.
E. Desmond Lee Professor of Racial and
   Ethnic Diversity
Washington University
St. Louis, Missouri
Chapter 18

Dianne M. Hammes-Ganguly, M.A.
Pediatric Speech-Language Pathologist
   and Research Associate
Division of Communication and
   Auditory Neuroscience

Children's Auditory Research and
  Evaluation (CARE) Center
House Ear Institute
Los Angeles, California
Chapter 11

Karen C. Johnson, Ph.D.
Advanced Research Associate
Division of Communication and
  Auditory Neuroscience
Children's Auditory Research and
  Evaluation (CARE) Center
House Ear Institute
Los Angeles, California
Chapters 19 and 21

Karen Iler Kirk, Ph.D., CCC-SLP
Professor
Department of Speech, Language and
  Hearing Sciences
Purdue University
West Lafayette, Indiana
Chapter 10

Liat Kishon-Rabin, Ph.D.
Professor
Department of Communication
  Disorders, Sackler Faculty of Medicine
Tel-Aviv University
Tel-Hashomer, Israel
Chapter 12

John F. Knutson, Ph.D.
Professor
Department of Psychology
University of Iowa
Iowa City, Iowa
Affiliated Scientist
Oregon Social Learning Center
Eugene, Oregon
Chapter 13

Abbie K. Larson, B.A.
Department of Communication Sciences
  and Disorders

University of Iowa
Iowa City, Iowa
Chapter 7

Kathleen M. Lehnert, M.S.
Pediatric Speech-Language Pathologist
Children's Auditory Research and
  Evaluation (CARE) Center
House Ear Institute
Los Angeles, California
Chapter 11

Frank R. Lin, M.D.
Chief Resident
Johns Hopkins Department of
  Otolaryngology—Head and Neck
  Surgery
Baltimore, Maryland
Chapter 14

Ruth Y. Litovsky, Ph.D.
Professor, Communicative Disorders
University of Wisconsin—Madison
Madison, Wisconsin
Chapter 4

William M. Luxford, M.D.
Associate
House Clinic
Los Angeles, California
Clinical Professor of Otolaryngology
University of Southern California
Keck School of Medicine
Los Angeles, California
Chapter 5

Jane Madell, Ph.D.
Director, Hearing and Learning Center
Co-Director, Cochlear Implant Center
The Ear Institute, The New York Eye and
  Ear Infirmary
New York, New York
Professor Clinical Otolaryngology
Albert Einstein College of Medicine
Bronx, New York
Chapter 4

Kristin E. Musser, B.A.
Department of Communication Sciences
    and Disorders
University of Iowa
Iowa City, Iowa
Chapter 7

Mary Ellen Nevins, Ed.D.
National Director
Professional Preparation in Cochlear
    Implants (PPCI)
Tecumseh, MI
Independent Contractor
Children's Hospital of Philadelphia
Philadelphia, Pennsylvania
Chapter 16

John K. Niparko, M.D.
George T. Nager Professor
Director, Division of Otology,
    Neurotology and Skull Base Surgery
Department of Otolaryngology—Head
    and Neck Surgery
Baltimore, Maryland
Chapter 14

Sara N. O'Brien, M.A., CCC-A
Research Audiologist
Department of Otolaryngology—Head
    and Neck Surgery
University of Iowa
Iowa City, Iowa
Chapter 7

**Blake C. Papsin, M.D., M.Sc., FRCSC,
FACS, FAAP**
Cochlear Chair, Auditory Development
Director, Cochlear Implant Program
Staff Otolaryngologist
Associate Scientist, The Research
    Institute
Hospital for Sick Children
Professor of Otolaryngology
The Faculty of Medicine

University of Toronto
Toronto, Ontario, Canada
Chapter 8

Brooke Nicholson Phillips, Au.D.
Pediatric Audiologist
Children's Auditory Research and
    Evaluation (CARE) Center
House Ear Institute
Los Angeles, California
Chapter 2

**Sylvia F. Rotfleisch, M.Sc.A., LSLS
Cert AVT, CCC-A**
HEAR to Talk
Los Angeles, California
Adjunct Faculty
Deaf and Hard-of-Hearing Program
California Lutheran University
Thousand Oaks, California
Chapter 15

Patricia A. Roush, Au.D.
Assistant Professor
Department of Otolaryngology—Head
    and Neck Surgery
Director, Pediatric Audiology
University of North Carolina Hospitals
University of North Carolina at Chapel Hill
Chapel Hill, North Carolina
Chapters 3 and 20

Richard C. Seewald, Ph.D.
Distinguished University Professor
National Centre for Audiology
University of Western Ontario
London, Ontario, Canada
Chapter 3

Osnat Segal, M.A.
Department of Communication
    Disorders, Sackler Faculty of Medicine
Tel-Aviv University
Tel-Hashomer, Israel
Chapter 12

Robert V. Shannon, Ph.D.
Scientist III, Lab Chief, Auditory Implant
    Research Laboratory
Division of Communication and
    Auditory Neuroscience
House Ear Institute
Los Angeles, California
Research Professor of Biomedical
    Engineering and Neuroscience
Member, Neuroscience Graduate Program
University of Southern California
Los Angeles, California
Chapter 21

Casey J. Stach, M.A.
Cochlear Implant Audiologist
Department of Otolaryngology
University of Michigan
Ann Arbor, Michigan
Chapter 6

Carren J. Stika, Ph.D.
Adjunct Faculty
San Diego State University
San Diego, California
Clinical Psychologist
Psychology Consultant
Children's Auditory Research and
    Evaluation (CARE) Center
House Ear Institute
Los Angeles, California
Chapter 13

Dana L. Suskind, M.D.
Associate Professor
Division Otolaryngology
University of Chicago
Chicago, Illinois
Chapter 18

Riki Taitelbaum-Swead, Ph.D.
Department of Communication
    Disorders, Sackler Faculty of Medicine
Tel-Aviv University
Speech and Hearing Center, Chaim
    Sheba Medical Center

Tel-Hashomer, Israel
Chapter 12

Holly F. B. Teagle, Au.D.
Assistant Professor and UNC-CCCDP
    Director
University of North Carolina
Chapel Hill, North Carolina
Chapter 20

Susan Wiley, M.D.
Associate Professor
University of Cincinnati
Cincinnati Children's Hospital Medical
    Center
Division of Developmental and
    Behavioral Pediatrics
Cincinnati, Ohio
Chapter 19

Eric P. Wilkinson, M.D.
Associate
House Clinic
Los Angeles, California
Clinical Assistant Professor of Clinical of
    Otolaryngology
University of Southern California
Los Angeles, California
Chapter 5

Margaret E. Winter, M.S.
Coordinator of Clinical Services
Children's Auditory Research and
    Evaluation (CARE) Center
House Ear Institute
Los Angeles, California
Chapter 2

Carlton J. Zdanski, M.D., FAAP, FACS
Associate Professor
Department of Otolaryngology—Head
    and Neck Surgery
University of North Carolina
Chapel Hill, North Carolina
Chapter 20

Teresa A. Zwolan, Ph.D.
Associate Professor, Director, Cochlear
    Implant Program
Department of Otolaryngology
University of Michigan Medical Center
Ann Arbor, Michigan
Chapter 6

CHAPTER 1

Cochlear Implants in Children: Historical Perspectives and Personal Reflections

Introduction

The cochlear implant is a sensory device that bypasses damaged or missing hair cells in the cochlea and electronically stimulates residual auditory neural elements in ears too impaired to respond effectively to acoustic amplification. There have been numerous upgrades in cochlear implant technology, beginning with fairly crude single-channel and multichannel devices, progressing to today's highly sophisticated, multichannel, digital signal processing systems. All present-day cochlear implants contain both internal and external components (Figure 1–1). The internal components, which are surgically implanted, consist of a stimulator that is seated in the temporal-parietal area and an electrode array that is threaded through the round window into the scala tympani of the cochlea. The externally worn compo-

nents consist of a signal processor, microphone, and a transmitter that sits on the head behind the ear. The acoustic stimulus is picked up by the microphone and transduced to an electrical signal, which undergoes digital signal processing before being delivered to the transmitter. A magnet is placed in both the transmitter and stimulator so that the two components, separated by skin, can be aligned. The electrical signal is transmitted across the skin by radio frequency. Today's external components primarily use a modular behind-the-ear design, that allows flexible placement of components on the head or body, which is particularly important for young children. Although all cochlear implant systems have basic features in common, they differ in how these features are implemented. Important differences exist in electrode design, electronics platform in the implanted stimulator, and signal processing. Signal processing

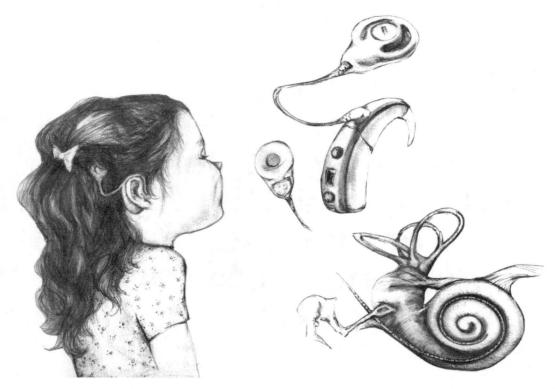

Figure 1–1. Illustration of a cochlear implant as worn by a young child. The internal and external components are shown on the right side of the illustration.

differences include compression algorithms and characteristics of sound coding strategies, such as waveform type, temporal pattern of stimulation (simultaneous versus sequential), and rate of stimulation. Cochlear implant processors also are equipped with multiple memories, enabling the use of different programs.

Advances in implant technology have been accompanied by systematic improvements in performance. The earliest devices yielded benefits in the form of improved lipreading, voice monitoring, awareness of environmental sounds, and closed-set speech understanding. Present technology enables many adults and children to understand speech without visual cues. However, co-chlear implant outcomes are characterized by wide variability for adults and children alike. The ability to reduce this variability has been illusive and remains a goal for implant manufacturers, researchers, and clinicians. It is notable, therefore, that even select children with the early devices (both single-channel and multichannel) achieved some open-set speech recognition (Berliner & Eisenberg, 1987; Berliner, Tonokawa, Dye, & House, 1989; Miyamoto, Osberger, Robbins, Renshaw, Myres, Kessler, & Pope, 1989; Osberger et al., 1991; Staller, Beiter, Brimacombe, Mecklenberg, & Arndt, 1991). Thus, performance with the cochlear implant in children is attributed to more than just implant mechanics and cochlear anatomy; child, family, and intervention factors interact to play important roles in overall performance outcomes.

The purpose of this chapter is to provide the reader with a glimpse of the early days when pediatric cochlear implantation was in its infancy. Germane to the early years, my viewpoint is injected to some extent. As a result, comments and reflections are somewhat exclusive to work occurring in the United States. This chapter sets the stage for subsequent chapters in the book, which provide background and guidance to students learning about the clinical aspects of pediatric cochlear implantation as well as to experienced practitioners seeking a resource when specific clinical questions arise. The chapters in this book cite many pertinent references relevant to pediatric cochlear implantation too numerous to summarize in this one chapter.

This chapter does not lay out a general history of cochlear implants. Interesting chronologies are available that present a broad perspective of the emerging technology. Noteworthy histories have been written by Luxford and Brackmann (1985), House and Berliner (1991), Mecklenburg and Lehnhardt (1991), Clark (2003), and Eisen (2003). Valuable background information, including several of historical significance, also can be found in the following writings: Simmons (1966), the NIH-funded Pittsburgh study (Bilger et al., 1977), proceedings from early conferences on cochlear implants (Merzenich, Schindler, & Sooey, 1974; Parkins & Anderson, 1983; Schindler & Merzenich, 1985), the NIH Consensus Statement, (1995), the American Speech-Language-Hearing Association Technical Report (2004), and a publication by Papsin and Gordon (2007). With regard to pediatric cochlear implantation, the first book published on this topic was edited by Owens and Kessler (1989).

Origins

The event was the West Coast Cochlear Prosthesis Conference at the Asilomar Conference site in Pacific Grove, California. The conference was held in the spring of 1980, and brought together the prominent players in the United States working on all aspects of cochlear implants. Much of the research at the time was being carried out in California and the primary implant centers were the Ear Research Institute (later renamed the House Ear Institute), Stanford University, and the University of California, San Francisco. It was at this conference where William House announced to the cochlear implant scientific and clinical community that he had decided to implant a congenitally deaf child with the House single-channel device in July of that year. A bombshell had been dropped—participants were stunned and appalled. Notably, this was not the first child to be implanted. Claude-Henri Chouard, from Paris, France, had been implanting teens since 1976 (Chouard, Fugain, Meyer, & Lacombe, 1983). However, the first preschool-age child, a 3-year-old deafened by meningitis, would soon be implanted by Dr. House in 1981 (Eisenberg, Berliner, Thielemeir, Kirk, & Tiber, 1983; Eisenberg & House, 1982).

William House made the decision to implant children after evaluating data obtained from postlingually and prelingually deafened adults implanted with the House single-channel system. It was his belief that children with prelingual deafness could benefit much more than adults from the use of this new technology. As stated in House, Berliner, Eisenberg, Edgerton, and Thielemeir, (1981):

The cochlear implant does not take the prelingually deaf adult out of the world of deafness—nor does it significantly alter any style of living, as these patterns have been long established. However, the fact that these patients have accepted sound, and find it useful and enjoyable, has encouraged us to begin looking at the congenitally deaf child, who has not yet established the patterns of living in a deaf world. (p. 461)

There was another important development that preceded the implantation of children—the placement of magnets in the transmitter and receiver (Dormer, Richard, Hough, & Hewett, 1980). Prior to this development, alignment across the skin between the external transmitter and internal receiver was problematic. A number of solutions had been tried previously, including headbands, ear molds, tape, toupee glue, and eye glasses. None of these solutions would have been practical for use with children. Consequently, this small innovation had a major impact on the initiation of implant trials with children (as well as adults) and is still in use today.

The year 1980 was significant not only because it ushered in the era of pediatric cochlear implantation in the United States and incorporated the use of magnets, it also was the year that the United States Food and Drug Administration (FDA) published their regulations for the marketing of medical devices.

United States Food and Drug Administration

The FDA regulations governing medical devices require that a multicenter clinical trial be initiated in order to establish the safety and efficacy of a medical device before it can receive market approval and commercial distribution. The first cochlear implant clinical trial was sponsored by the 3M Company to establish the safety and effectiveness of the House single-channel implant (herein known as the 3M/House cochlear implant) in adults with profound deafness. In November, 1984, this device became the first cochlear implant to receive FDA approval for adults (Berliner, Luxford, & House, 1985b).

The process of bringing a device to market is time consuming, labor intensive, and of high cost to the sponsor of the investigation. The companies that manufacture cochlear implants are required to submit an investigational device exemption (study plan) to the FDA for approval before clinical trials can commence. FDA clinical trials require that investigative sites follow a set protocol. During the first clinical trials, the prerequisite to establishing device efficacy led to the development of new assessment batteries to characterize cochlear implant benefits. These batteries often continued to be used in clinical practice even after a device received FDA approval as a means to determine preimplant candidacy and postimplant benefits. Today many clinics continue to administer a set battery of tests on a regular basis, although resource constraints at many sites often make this difficult to accomplish. Many small clinical centers, however, sometimes have opportunities to participate in newly initiated clinical trials sponsored by the implant manufacturers as technology is being upgraded. Results from these different types of investigations can be found throughout the pediatric implant literature.

Manufacturer-Sponsored Clinical Trials in Children

From 1980 to 1986, pediatric clinical trials with the 3M/House system were undertaken at select coinvestigator sites from around the country to determine the safety and efficacy of this device for deaf children between the ages of 2 and 18 years. Collaborating with William House on this first investigation were otologic surgeons and their teams from around the United States. These included H. Edward Maddox (Houston, Texas), J. V. D. Hough (Oklahoma City, Oklahoma), Richard Miyamoto (Indianapolis, Indiana), Charles Luetje (Kansas City, Missouri), Simon Parisier (New York City, New York), Sam Kinney (Cleveland, Ohio), and Robert Mischke (Denver, Colorado). In helping to guide the children's cochlear implant program, leaders in deaf education and rehabilitation provided input through special conferences. Included were Daniel Ling (McGill University), Arthur Boothroyd (City University of New York), Norman Erber (Glendonald School for Deaf Children), Mary Joe Osberger (Boys Town National Research Hospital), Agnes Ling Phillips (Montreal Oral School for the Deaf), Joanne Subtelny (National Technical Institute for the Deaf), Pat Stone (Tucker-Maxon Oral School), and Julia Davis (University of Iowa).

The children participating in this first clinical trial were, on average, 8 years of age at time of implant, over half were deafened prelingually by meningitis, and the majority communicated by sign language (Berliner, Eisenberg, & House, 1985a). Today it is generally accepted in clinical circles that prelingually deafened children who are implanted at older ages and who communicate exclusively by sign language do not have a high prognosis for developing spoken language with the implant. Such children would not be implanted in a number of implant centers. Despite the characteristics of this first large sample, the results were modestly successful. On average, children demonstrated small but significant improvements on closed-set measures of speech perception as well as on measures of speech production and language relative to their preimplant performance with traditional, high-powered hearing aids (Berliner et al., 1985a).

Pediatric trials with the 3M/House system soon paved the way for investigations with the device pioneered in Australia, the Nucleus 22-Channel system, which commenced toward the end of 1986. Prior to initiating these trials, Cochlear Corporation (the company that marketed the Nucleus 22-Channel implant in the United States) sponsored a colloquium in February, 1986 to debate the important issues that were relevant to cochlear implantation in children (Mecklenburg, 1986). One of the important outcomes of this colloquium was the listing of characteristics thought to determine success with the implant (Northern et al., 1986). Influential characteristics were: (1) postlingual deafeness, (2) prelingual deafness but of short duration, and (3) commitment by the family that their child be trained in oral educational programs. Outcomes from this colloquium were instrumental in designing that company's FDA pediatric clinical trials (Mecklenburg, Demorest, & Staller, 1991). Although the 3M/House device was the first cochlear implant to receive FDA marketing approval in 1984, it was only approved for adults. In 1990, the Nucleus 22-Channel cochlear implant became the first system to receive FDA marketing approval for children 2 years of age and older (Staller, 1991). Two other companies marketing multichannel cochlear implants in the United States subsequently achieved this benchmark—Advanced Bionics in 1997 (Osberger, Fisher, & Murad, 1997) and MED-EL in 2001 (Franz, 2002). The sponsors of these clinical trials demonstrated conclusively that the children with multichannel cochlear implants produced significantly higher performance levels when compared to baseline performance on tests that measured auditory skill development. Of particular significance was the finding that implanted children, as a group, demonstrated open-set speech recognition with multichannel cochlear implants.

An Interesting Controversy

The debate about whether to implant or not implant deaf children was highly contentious during the 1980s, and this dispute continued even into the 1990s. Of course, the team working on the first pediatric trials with the 3M/House single-channel device suffered the brunt of the hostility, both at professional meetings and in print. However, those working on the multichannel implant trials were not immune. Concerns were raised about risks or other issues specific to the child: long-term effects of electrical stimulation, otitis media, skull growth, damage to cochlear structures, and loss of residual hearing.

The scientific community, in particular, was most indignant over the implantation of deaf children, at least with the single-channel system. Succinctly stated by Nelson Kiang during an early international symposium on cochlear implants (Parkins & Anderson, 1983):

> . . . I consider the idea of implanting intracochlear single-channel electrodes in young children to be indefensible at this time . . . (p. 510)

Scientists, as a group, viewed cochlear implants in the context of normal hearing. The relatively low level of auditory functioning produced by the single-channel system clearly did not excite the interest of the scientists. As a group, they deemed it highly unlikely that a device as crude as the single-channel system could provide anything more useful than time-intensity speech cues, which could be obtained with other sensory devices that were less invasive (i.e., high-powered hearing aids, vibrotactile devices).

In contrast, the clinician viewed performance with the implant from the context of deafness, and any small improvement was seen as a positive outcome and of clinical significance. Even gaining an ability to alert to a warning signal, such as an alarm or siren, was considered to be an improvement. Interestingly, these same issues currently are being debated (but with less rancor) for those deaf children identified with developmental delays and/or multiple disabilities, as well as those children who meet criteria for the auditory brainstem implant. That is, even though open-set speech recognition or spoken language may not be achievable with implants in the majority of these children, the question is raised whether benefits outweigh the risks.

During the time when the pediatric 3M/House trials were being initiated, multichannel cochlear implants also were under development. Many believed that the families of these children should wait until a more advanced system was available. However, clinical experience suggested that having some access to sound, even with the single-channel implant, was better than waiting for the multichannel implant because of developmental time windows. Once multichannel implants began FDA clinical trials, these systems became the preferred devices.

There also was debate regarding pediatric cochlear implantation within the clinical implant community itself, as highlighted during a panel discussion at the 10th Anniversary Conference on Cochlear Implants held in 1983 at the University of California, San Francisco (House et al., 1985). For example, there was discussion about the level and type of aural rehabilitation the children received with hearing aids prior to implantation. The point was raised that children not enrolled in strong aural habilitation programs were the very ones being selected for the implant. Had such children been provided with strong auditory training, they might have maximized their use of hearing aids and not have need for an implant. This concern was probably true for some children who went on to receive the implant. However, it is known that not all deaf children succeed using an auditory approach. In fact, some families who sought the implant for their child had been released from auditory-verbal therapy because there was not enough residual hearing to succeed in this type of program. Recall that the majority of children during the first clinical trial were deafened by bacterial meningitis, as this was an era that preceded the meningitis vaccines. Such children essentially had no residual hearing.

Another concern posed by clinicians was the potential damage to cochlear structures caused by an intracochlear electrode. It was felt that damage to the cochlea would preclude use of more technologically advanced systems in the future. During the late 1970s, a group in the United Kingdom, headed by Ellis Douek, began experimenting with an extracochlear electrode that was stationed on the promontory near the round window (Douek, Fourcin, Moore, & Clarke, 1977; Fourcin et al., 1983). The sound processor extracted laryngeal frequency cues and was considered to be a supplement to lipreading. Although never attempted with children, this device created a great deal of interest because it was judged to be the more conservative, less invasive approach. During the panel discussion at the San Francisco meeting, William House addressed the extra-cochlear implant (House et al., 1985):

. . . First of all, I think that the procedure which Mr. Douek is recommending is very definitely an invasive procedure.
We are talking about taking out the ossicles in this child. We are talking *about dropping the ear drum to the promontory. We are talking about altering the middle ear function dramatically. We are talking about asking a child to adjust a device against his promontory, which can sometimes cause pain. We are talking about the problems of the patient being struck on the ear possibly at some time, and therefore causing further damage . . .* (p. 585)

Amazingly, the issue of implanting very young children was not a major concern. During this same panel discussion from the 1983 conference (House, et al., 1985), there was consensus that the earlier the better. In the words of Gerald Loeb, a neuroscientist who surprisingly was on this panel of practitioners:

I'm not much in favor of implanting children between the ages of 5 and 15 given currently available devices, but perhaps paradoxically, I think there are some interesting reasons for implanting children, providing neural prostheses, between the ages of 2 and 5 . . . (p. 577)

Particularly intrigued by the potential of cochlear implants were teachers of the deaf who advocated oral education (e.g., Ling & Nienhuys, 1983). In fact, many pediatric referrals began coming from these oral programs. Of course, once results from the early pediatric implant trials began to show promise, the field began to blossom.

The Deaf World

The highly charged response by individuals from the Deaf World was even more confrontational than the research/clinical debates. This negative reaction persisted even when pediatric implantation was becoming standard clinical practice. Following FDA approval of the first multichannel implant for deaf children, the National Association of the Deaf (NAD) issued a position statement about cochlear implants in children (National Association of the Deaf, 1991). NAD questioned the ethics of cochlear implants in children and the position statement characterized children with implants as human guinea pigs. Furthermore, the position statement suggested that the implant would delay parents' acceptance of their child's deafness, depriving these children of their heritage as part of the Deaf World. Concerns were raised that the FDA did not seek guidance from members of the Deaf World when evaluating the efficacy of cochlear implants.

Even earlier than the release of this NAD position statement, the Greater Los Angeles Council on Deafness and the National Deaf Children's Society of England issued strong statements opposing cochlear implants in children. The weightiest issue raised was whether parents had a right to make the decision of implantation for their child. In response, William House (1986) wrote that it was important for all professionals working in the field of cochlear implants to appreciate the concerns proffered by representatives of the Deaf World. He also countered by suggesting that the Deaf World needed to be sensitive to the wishes of hearing parents in making decisions for their children. It was his hope that the cochlear implant would enable the deaf child to move more easily between hearing and Deaf cultures.

This 1986 publication by William House was followed by a debate in the 1990s between Thomas Balkany and Harlan Lane about Deaf culture versus pediatric cochlear implantation. Dr. Balkany, a well-established implant surgeon, advocated for the cochlear implant. Dr. Lane, a professor from Northeastern University, championed the cause of the Deaf World. The dialogue started with a short article in the *New England Journal of Medicine*, in which Balkany (1993) briefly mentioned the controversy and suggested to leaders of the Deaf World that their negative view may not be in the best interests of children who are deaf and that the majority of deaf children were born to hearing parents. This article was followed by other publications by Balkany and colleagues, in which they highlighted some of the Deaf World's misconceptions about cochlear implants. They then raised the issue about who "owns" the deaf child—the family or the Deaf World (Balkany & Hodges, 1995; Balkany, Hodges, & Goodman, 1996). Lane and Bahan (1998) countered with an article that highlighted the ethical dilemmas involved in pediatric cochlear implantation. In particular, they renounced the belief that deafness is a disability. They went on to describe the Deaf World, detailing the oppression of the Deaf, the pride in their culture and language, and eventual self-determination. The scientific literature about pediatric cochlear implantation then was critically examined, leaving Lane and Bahan underwhelmed by the results. Lane and Behan made the claim that the Deaf World is a viable minority that should be preserved as is the case with all minorities.

The controversy has quieted considerably during the past 10 years, and a growing number of individuals in the Deaf Community are receiving cochlear implants. Despite more general acceptance of the cochlear implant, respect for the culture and language of the Deaf World is an important consideration for all who work in the field of pediatric cochlear implantation.

Evolving Clinical Research

There are important milestones that mark the advancement of pediatric cochlear implantation in terms of clinical assessment and management. As mentioned earlier, the first large-scale investigations on children with cochlear implants involved FDA clinical trials. These multicenter studies were sponsored by the implant manufacturers with the ultimate purpose of bringing these devices to the market place. Essential to the advancement of the field, were those clinical studies that were independent of manufacturer sponsorship. Funded by the National Institutes of Health (NIH), the first studies were intent on: (1) comparing performance outcomes with cochlear implants versus outcomes with hearing aids and tactile devices, and (2) comparing outcomes between single- and multichannel implants. On measures of communication skills, implants were shown to be superior to hearing aids and tactile devices (Geers & Moog, 1994; Miyamoto et al., 1989). Children with multichannel implants achieved greater improvements in speech perception relative to outcomes of children with the single-channel device (Osberger et al., 1991). Of even greater significance was the finding that children with the multichannel system appeared to be developing these skills at a faster rate than children with the single-channel device (Miyamoto, Osberger, Robbins, Myres, Kessler, & Pope, 1992). Speech perception also was shown to improve with increased device use (Fryauf-Bertschy, Tyler, Kelsay, Gantz, & Woodworth, 1997; Miyamoto et al., 1992).

The earliest NIH-funded investigations on pediatric cochlear implantation were conducted at Central Institute for the Deaf (CID) and Indiana University School of Medicine (IUSM). These two investigations commenced in the 1980s and are still ongoing. A more recent multicenter study was initiated in 2002 at Johns Hopkins University. Several important contributions from these three studies are highlighted below.

Central Institute for the Deaf

The research program at CID was directed by Ann Geers and Jean Moog, who contributed a number of innovations to the field of pediatric cochlear implantation. An important innovation involved test development. One of the most well-known tests in use today is the Early Speech Perception Test (ESP) (Moog & Geers, 1990). Because the ESP can be administered to children as young as 2 years, it is used extensively in pediatric implant test protocols. The ESP is a closed-set test designed to assess pattern perception (syllabification and stress), spondaic word identification, and monosyllabic word identification. When first developed, the ESP was found to be very useful in identifying those children who might be considered implant candidates because the test differentiated children who may be "pattern perceivers" from children who may be "spectral perceivers" with their hearing aids. A pattern perceiver was a child who could identify the correct syllabic or stress pattern of words but could not identify the actual word itself. In contrast, a spectral perceiver could identify the actual words. In the early days of pediatric cochlear implantation, it was believed that a child who could only perceive patterns with their hearing aids would benefit from an implant.

In one of the earliest implant studies, Geers and Moog (1994) evaluated performance outcomes as a function of sensory device in children who had profound hearing loss. In the design of the study, triads of children with profound hearing loss were formed and were assessed over a 3-year period. The children in each triad were matched on a number of characteristics, but differed in the use of sensory device: one child in the triad used the Nucleus 22-Channel implant, the second child used the Tactaid, and the third child used hearing aids. As was noted earlier in this chapter, the children with implants obtained higher scores on measures of speech perception when compared to the children with the other sensory devices.

In 2003, Geers and colleagues published a series of papers detailing an in-depth investigation of 8- and 9-year-old children with multichannel implants (for a summary of results see Moog & Geers, 2003). The results demonstrated that children of this age who received an early emphasis on speech and auditory skill development were outperforming those who used sign language on measures of speech perception, speech production, and language. However, children performed equally well on measures of literacy, irrespective of communication mode. It is notable that these studies are continuing and data are being analyzed on these same children who are now in high school (Geers, 2008; Geers, Tobey, & Moog, 2008).

Indiana University School of Medicine

The IUSM group, headed by Richard Miyamoto and Mary Joe Osberger, launched several longitudinal investigations of children with cochlear implants in the 1980s. Similar to the CID studies, the IUSM group designed studies to compare cochlear implants with tactile devices and hearing aids (Miyamoto

et al., 1989; Osberger et al., 1991). One important innovation developed by this group was the comparison of performance outcomes in children with implants to those of hearing aid users with differing degrees of profound hearing loss (Osberger, Maso, & Sam, 1993). The comparison group was classified according to the following categories: hearing loss greater than 110 dB HL (bronze), hearing loss between 101 to 110 dB HL (silver), and losses between 90 to 100 dB HL (gold). This study showed that children with cochlear implants performed comparably to the "silver" hearing aid group in terms of speech intelligibility.

Throughout the years, studies from other implant centers continued to compare children with implants to children who benefited from hearing aids, including the IUSM group. The benchmark for defining implant performance, in terms of degree of hearing loss, has continued to be raised with upgrades in implant technology. In a study conducted by researchers at IUSM and the House Ear Institute, performance outcomes in children with implants were shown to be comparable to children with hearing losses of 78 dB HL on measures of speech recognition (Eisenberg, Kirk, Martinez, Ying, & Miyamoto, 2004). It is expected this benchmark will change in coming years.

Similar to CID, the group at IUSM has been involved in test development for children and several of these tests continue to be in widespread use. The first two measures are the Meaningful Auditory Integration Scale (MAIS) (Robbins, Renshaw, & Berry, 1991) and its companion, the Infant-Toddler: Meaningful Auditory Integration Scale (IT-MAIS) (Zimmerman-Phillips, Robbins, & Osberger, 2000). The MAIS and IT-MAIS use structured parent-interview formats that probe the child's bonding with the sensory device, auditory awareness, and ability to derive meaning from sound in everyday situations. The IT-MAIS also probes the child's vocal behavior. Because of the lack of auditory-based outcome measures for very young children, these two measures remain one of the most used scales with the young pediatric implant population.

The other two widely used tests are the Multisyllabic Lexical Neighborhood Test (MLNT) and Lexical Neighborhood Test (LNT) (Kirk, Pisoni, & Osberger, 1995). Both tests measure open-set word recognition in young children with cochlear implants. Theoretically motivated, MLNT and LNT tap into higher level cognitive/linguistic processes when compared to other traditional measures of speech recognition.

Childhood Development After Cochlear Implantation (CDaCI) Study

The latest endeavor in NIH-funded pediatric implant investigations is the national CDaCI study headed by John Niparko from Johns Hopkins University. This study differs from its predecessors because it involves the collaboration of six implant centers from around the United States that administer an extensive multidimentional protocol and is the first large-scale study to incorporate a normal-hearing control group (Fink et al., 2007). Children were enrolled into the study between 2002 and 2004; the average age of enrollment was 2.2 years.

The intent of the CDaCI study is to generate a multivariate model which identifies factors that both affect and are affected by language development. The domains being tracked are language, speech production, speech recognition, psychosocial development, and quality of life. Data for 3-year outcomes postimplant are in the process of being analyzed at the time of this writing.

However, one early outcome has been the development of a speech recognition cumulative index that represents speech recognition over a period of time across different speech recognition measures as children mature (Wang et al., 2008).

At its completion, one of the important contributions of this study will be the availability of a large database of results. In fact, some investigators not affiliated with the CDaCI study are beginning to adopt parts of the protocol as part of their clinical programs or research projects. It is notable that most of the children enrolled in the CDaCI study originally received only one implant. During the course of the study, greater numbers of children are now receiving a second implant in the opposite ear. With the changing demographics of pediatric cochlear implantation, future large-scale studies will be needed to evaluate children who are bilaterally implanted in infancy.

Final Reflections

Cochlear implantation has become standard clinical practice for children with severe to profound hearing loss. This standard practice could never have come to fruition had results not progressed beyond those first reported in the early clinical trials. The impressive outcomes in communication skill development (open-set speech recognition, intelligible speech, and spoken language) are due to a combination of advances in technology and collaborations among clinicians, scientists, and engineers. The perseverance of the early clinical pioneers cannot be understated, particularly in view of the contemptuous attitudes projected both by the scientific and Deaf communities during the early years. Indeed, it is ironic to observe the growing number of scientists who now devote entire careers to the study of cochlear implants. We have come full circle.

Pediatric cochlear implantation is still a very young field and there is much to learn. The long-term effects of this technology are not known and won't be known for a number of years. Questions raised in the early days of pediatric cochlear implantation are still being asked. What are the potential deleterious effects of electrical stimulation over a life span? How many times will hardware need to be replaced? These questions plus many others remain.

There also is reason to hope that performance outcomes will improve with continuing upgrades in technology and earlier implantation. Children considered to be borderline candidates in terms of their residual hearing may be much more likely to receive cochlear implants, and electric-acoustic stimulation may be implemented in the near future with children who have significant low-frequency residual hearing. Bilateral implantation of infants younger than 12 months probably will become standard practice in the years to come. For those children not able to receive a cochlear implant for anatomical reasons (i.e., those born without an auditory nerve), auditory brainstem implants in this population may become the logical next step. Referrals for mainstream classroom placement are expected to grow as the number of infants receiving auditory implants increases. All-in-the-head devices are envisioned in the future, although challenges concerning microphone placement and size of components (Briggs et al., 2008) make it unlikely that such technology will be available for children for some time to come.

Pediatric cochlear implantation has always been and will continue to be an exciting field of study. It appears that F. Blair Simmons, one of the early pioneers in cochlear implants, was prophetic when in 1985 during the very early days of pediatric cochlear implantation he concluded:

> *... cochlear implants are likely to continue to be part of the selected management of deafness in childhood ... Short of a national mandate to the contrary, implants in children are on the increase. "Thou has seen nothing yet." (Don Quixote).* (p. 63)

Acknowledgments. I am most grateful to Ann Geers, Mary Joe Osberger, and Nancy Fink for their very helpful comments on earlier drafts of this chapter. Special thanks to Tracy L. Williams for her beautiful illustration of a child wearing the cochlear implant and the cochlear implant components (Figure 1–1).

References

American Speech-Language-Hearing Association. (2004, March). *Cochlear implants* [Technical report]. Retrieved August 6, 2008, from http://www.asha.org/docs/html/TR2004-00041.html

Balkany, T. (1993). A brief perspective on cochlear implants. *New England Journal of Medicine, 328,* 281–282.

Balkany, T. J., & Hodges, A. V. (1995). Misleading the deaf community about cochlear implantation in children. *Annals of Otology, Rhinology, and Laryngology, 104*(Suppl. 116), 148–149.

Balkany, T., Hodges, A. V., & Goodman, K. W. (1996). Ethics of cochlear implantation in young children. *Otolaryngology-Head and Neck Surgery, 114,* 748–755.

Berliner, K. I., & Eisenberg, L. S. (1987). Our experience with cochlear implants: Have we erred in our expectations? *American Journal of Otology, 8,* 222–229.

Berliner, K. I., Eisenberg, L. S., & House, W. F. (1985a). The cochlear implant: An auditory prosthesis for the profoundly deaf child. *Ear and Hearing, 6*(Suppl.), 1S–69S.

Berliner, K. I, Luxford, W. M., & House, W. F. (1985b). Cochlear implants: 1981–1985. *American Journal of Otology, 6*, 173–186.

Berliner, K. I., Tonokawa, L. L., Dye, L. M., & House, W. F. (1989). Open-set speech recognition in children with a single-channel cochlear implant. *Ear and Hearing, 10*, 237–242.

Bilger, R. C., Black, F. O., Hopkinson, N. T., Myers, E. N., Payne, J. L., Stenson, N. R., et al. (1977). Evaluation of subjects presently fitted with implanted auditory prostheses. *Annals of Otology, Rhinology, and Laryngology, 86* (Suppl. 38), 3–176.

Briggs, R. J., Eder, H. C., Seligman, P. M., Cowan, R. S., Plant, K. L., Dalton, J., et al. (2008). Initial clinical experience with a totally implantable cochlear implant research device. *Otology and Neurotology, 29*, 114–119.

Chouard, C.-H., Fugain, C., Meyer, B., & Lacombe, H. (1983). Long-term results of the multi-channel cochlear implant. *Annals of the New York Academy of Sciences, 405*, 387–411.

Clark, G. (2003). A history. In G. Clark, *Cochlear implants: Fundamentals and applications* (pp. 1–57). New York: Springer-Verlag.

Dormer, K. T., Richard, G. P., Hough, J. V., & Hewett, T. M (1980). The cochlear implant (auditory prosthesis) utilizing rare earth magnets. *American Journal of Otology, 2*, 22–27.

Douek, E., Fourcin, A. J., Moore, B. C., & Clarke, G. P. (1977). A new approach to the cochlear implant. *Proceedings of the Royal Society of Medicine, 70*, 379–383.

Eisen, M. D. (2003). Djourno, Eyries, and the first implanted electrical neural stimulator to restore hearing. *Otology and Neurotology, 24*, 500–506.

Eisenberg, L. S., Berliner, K. I., Thielemeir, M. A., Kirk, K. I., & Tiber, N. (1983). Cochlear implants in children. *Ear and Hearing, 4*, 41–50.

Eisenberg, L. S., & House, W. F. (1982). Initial experience with the cochlear implant in children. *Annals of Otology, Rhinology, and Laryngology, 91*(Suppl. 91), 67–73.

Eisenberg, L. S., Kirk, K. I., Martinez, A. S., Ying, E. A., & Miyamoto, R. T. (2004). Communica-

tion abilities of children with aided residual hearing: Comparison with cochlear implant users. *Archives of Otolaryngology-Head and Neck Surgery, 130*, 563–569.

Fink, N. E., Wang, N-Y., Visaya, J., Niparko, J. K., Quittner, A., Eisenberg, L. S., Tobey, E. A., & the CDaCI Investigative Team. (2007). Childhood development after cochlear implantation (CDaCI) study: Design and baseline characteristics. *Cochlear Implants International, 8*, 92–116.

Fourcin, A. J., Douek, E. E., Moore, B. C., Rosen, S., Walliker, J. R., Howard, D. M., et al. (1983). Speech perception with promontory stimulation. *Annals of the New York Academy of Sciences, 405*, 280–294.

Franz, D. C. (2002). Pediatric performance with the Med-El Combi 40+ cochlear implant system. *Annals of Otology, Rhinology, and Laryngology, 111*(Suppl. 189), 66–68.

Fryauf-Bertschy, H., Tyler, R. S., Kelsay, D. M., Gantz, B. J., & Woodworth, G. G. (1997). Cochlear implant use by prelingually deafened children: The influences of age at implant and length of device use. *Journal of Speech, Language, and Hearing Research, 40*, 183–199.

Geers, A. (2008, April). *Long-term outcomes of cochlear implantation in early childhood: A mid-term report.* Paper presented at the 10th International Conference on Cochlear Implants and Other Implantable Auditory Technology, San Diego, CA.

Geers, A. E., & Moog, J. S. (1994). Effectiveness of cochlear implants and tactile aids for deaf children: The sensory aids study at Central Institute for the Deaf. *Volta Review, 95*, 1–231.

Geers, A., Tobey, E., & Moog, J. (2008). Long-term outcomes of cochlear implantation in the preschool years: From elementary grades to high school. *International Journal of Audiology, 47*(Suppl. 2), S21–S30.

House W. F. (1986). Opposition to the cochlear implant in deaf children. *American Journal of Otology, 7*, 89–92.

House, W. F., & Berliner, K. I. (1991). Cochlear implants: From idea to clinical practice. In Cooper, H. (Ed.), *Cochlear implants: A practical guide* (pp. 9–33). London: Whurr.

House, W. F., Berliner, K. I., & Eisenberg, L. S. (1983). Experiences with the cochlear implant in preschool children. *Annals of Otology, Rhinology, and Laryngology, 92,* 587–592.

House, W. F., Berliner, K. I., Eisenberg, L. S., Edgerton, B. J., & Thielemeir, M. A. (1981). The cochlear implant: 1980 update. *Acta Otolaryngologica, 91,* 457–462.

House, W. F., Grammatico, L. F., Fugain, C., Loeb, G. E., Douek, E. E., & Simmons, F. B. (1985). Cochlear implants in children: Panel discussion. In R. A. Schindler & M. M. Merzenich (Eds.), *Cochlear implants* (pp. 575–587). New York: Raven Press.

Kirk, K. I., Pisoni, D. B., & Osberger, M. J. (1995). Lexical effects on spoken word recognition by pediatric cochlear implant users. *Ear and Hearing, 16,* 470–481.

Lane, H., & Bahan, B. (1998). Ethics of cochlear implantation in young children: A review and reply from a deaf-world perspective. *Otolaryngology-Head and Neck Surgery, 119,* 297–313.

Ling, D., & Nienhuys, T. G. (1983). The deaf child: Habilitation with and without a cochlear implant. *Annals of Otology, Rhinology, and Laryngology, 92,* 593–598.

Luxford, W. M., & Brackmann, D. E. (1985). The history of cochlear implants. In R. F. Gray (Ed.), *Cochlear implants* (pp. 1–26). San Diego, CA: College-Hill Press.

Mecklenburg, D. J. (Ed.) (1986). Cochlear Implants in Children. *Seminars in Hearing, 7,* 341–440.

Mecklenburg, D. J., Demorest, M. E., & Staller, S. J. (1991). Scope and design of the clinical trial of the Nucleus multichannel cochlear implant in children. *Ear and Hearing, 12* (Suppl. 4), 10S–14S.

Mecklenburg, D., & Lehnhardt, E. (1991). The development of cochlear implants in Europe, Asia and Australia. In H. Cooper (Ed.), *Cochlear implants: A practical guide* (pp. 34–57). London: Whurr.

Merzenich, M. M., Schindler, R. A., & Sooey, F. (Eds.). (1974). *Proceedings of the First International Conference on Electrical Stimulation of the Acoustic Nerve as a Treatment for Profound Sensorineural Deafness in Man.* San Francisco: University of California.

Miyamoto, R. T., Osberger, M. J., Robbins, A. M., Myres, W. A., Kessler, K., & Pope, M. L. (1992). Longitudinal evaluation of communication skills of children with single- or multichannel cochlear implants. *American Journal of Otology, 13,* 215–222.

Miyamoto, R. T., Osberger, M. J., Robbins, A. J., Renshaw, J., Myres, W. A., Kessler, K., et al. (1989). Comparison of sensory aids in deaf children. *Annals of Otology, Rhinology, and Laryngology, 142,* 2–7.

Moog, J. S., & Geers, A. E. (1990). *Early Speech Perception Test of profoundly hearing-impaired children.* St. Louis, MO: Central Institute for the Deaf.

Moog, J. S., & Geers, A. E. (2003). Epilogue: Major findings, conclusion and implications for deaf educations. *Ear and Hearing, 24*(Suppl. 1), 121S–125S.

National Association of the Deaf (NAD). (1991). Report of the task force on childhood cochlear implants. *NAD Broadcaster, 13,* 1.

National Institutes of Health (NIH). (1995, May 15–17). *Cochlear implants in adults and children. NIH consensus statement online, 13*(2), 1–30. Retrieved August 6, 2008, from http://consensus.nih.gov/1995/1995Cochlear Implants100html.htm

Northern, J. L., Black, F. O., Brimacombe, J. A., Cohen, N. L., Eisenberg, L. S., Kuprenas, S. V., et al. (1986). Selection of children for cochlear implantation. In D. J. Mecklenburg (Ed.), Cochlear implants in children. *Seminars in Hearing, 7,* 341–347.

Osberger, M. J., Fisher, L. M., & Murad, C. (1997). Clinical results with the CLARION multi-strategy cochlear implant in children. In G. Clark (Ed.), *Cochlear implants* (pp. 291–296). Bologna, Italy: Monduzzi Editore.

Osberger, M. J., Maso, M., & Sam, L. K. (1993). Speech intelligibility of children with cochlear implants, tactile aids, or hearing aids. *Journal of Speech and Hearing Research, 36,* 186–203.

Osberger, M. J., Robbins, A. M., Miyamoto, R. T., Berry, S. W., Myres, W. A., Kessler, K. S., et al. (1991). Speech perception abilities of children with cochlear implants, tactile aids, or hearing aids. *American Journal of Otology, 12*(Suppl.), 105–115.

Owens, E., & Kessler, D. K. (1989). *Cochlear implants in young deaf children*. Boston: College-Hill Press.

Papsin, B. C., & Gordon, K. A. (2007). Cochlear implants for children with severe-to-profound hearing loss. *New England Journal of Medicine, 357*, 2380-2387.

Parkins, C. W., & Anderson, S. W. (Eds.) (1983). *Cochlear prostheses: An international symposium*. New York: New York Academy of Sciences.

Robbins, A. M., Renshaw, J. J., & Berry, S. W. (1991). Evaluating meaningful auditory integration in profoundly hearing-impaired children. *American Journal of Otology, 12*(Suppl.), 144-150.

Schindler, R. A., & Merzenich, M. M. (Eds.) (1985). *Cochlear implants*. New York: Raven Press.

Simmons, F. B. (1966). Electrical stimulation of the auditory nerve in man. *Archives of Otolaryngology, 84*, 2-54.

Simmons, F. B. (1985). Cochlear implants in young children: Some dilemmas. *Ear and Hearing, 6*, 61-63.

Staller, S. J. (1991). Multichannel cochlear implants in children. *Ear and Hearing, 12*(Suppl. 4), 1S-89S.

Staller, S. J., Beiter, A. L., Brimacombe, J. A., Mecklenberg, D. J., & Arndt, P. (1991). Pediatric performance with the Nucleus 22-channel cochlear implant system. *American Journal of Otology, 12*, 126-136.

Wang, N-Y., Eisenberg, L. S., Johnson, K. C., Fink, N. E, Tobey, E. A., Quittner, A. L., Niparko, J. K., & the CDaCI Investigative Team (2008). Tracking development of speech recognition: Longitudinal data from hierarchical assessments in the Childhood Development after Cochlear Implantation (CDaCI) Study. *Otology and Neurotology, 29*, 240-245.

Zimmerman-Phillips, S., Robbins, A. M., & Osberger, M. J. (2000). Assessing cochlear implant benefit in very young children. *Annals of Otology, Rhinology, and Laryngology, 109* (Suppl. 185), 42-43.

CHAPTER 2

Clinical Management of Cochlear Implants in Children: An Overview

MARGARET E. WINTER
BROOKE NICHOLSON PHILLIPS

Introduction

The cochlear implant is arguably the most important development in the treatment of bilateral sensorineural deafness in history. Although it has unquestionably provided the only avenue through which many deaf children have been able to learn to communicate using spoken language, it is also true that not all deaf children are good candidates for the implant procedure. Determination of candidacy rests largely on the goals of the implant center. Where the goal is audition, with the expectation that many recipients will not necessarily develop spoken language as a primary communication mode, the pool of candidates is wide. Where the goal is development of oral language skills, if not spoken language as a primary communication mode, the pool of candidates is smaller. Yet even with established

goals many centers may have to triage cochlear implant candidates due to center specific constraints that may include staffing and funding issues.

Language, whether spoken or manual, should be the primary aim of any intervention with deaf children. Because more than 90% of deaf children are born into hearing families (Stern, Yueh, Lewis, Norton, & Sie, 2005), it is not surprising that a majority of these families hope their children will be able to communicate using spoken language. Cochlear implants can and do make development of oral language skills possible for many children (Waltzman, Cohen, Green, & Roland, 2002; Geers, Nicholas, & Sedey, 2003; Beadle et al., 2005), but not for all, and for some children provision of cochlear implants and the necessary habilitative follow-up can delay the development of communication skills through a more functional modality. When implant surgery is successful, the vast majority of implant recipients will be able to detect sounds across the speech frequency spectrum at or above normal conversational levels (Papsin & Gordon, 2007). There is, however, no guarantee that any individual will be able to learn to understand speech or develop speech as a primary communication mode. In fact, despite all the appropriate interventions known to produce the best possible outcomes, some recipients do not develop auditory skills sufficient to support the development of oral language. Many factors contribute to linguistic success with cochlear implants. Some of these factors are known and can be assessed, providing valuable information regarding probable outcomes following implantation. Other factors are individual to a given child, and many may not be evident until a child is older especially given that children are now being implanted at and below a year of age.

In the approximately 20 years that children have been receiving multichannel cochlear implants, it has become standard practice for pediatric implant centers to use a team approach in determining candidacy (Beiter, Staller, & Dowell, 1991; Geers et al., 2002; Papsin & Gordon, 2007). The process of selecting children for whom the implant can be expected to provide benefit (which may be defined variously by different centers) is best done with a multidisciplinary approach in which professionals with different areas of expertise can contribute based on their specific knowledge and experience. Working as a team, they can assess the multiple aspects of a child's development, auditory skills, communicative status, and potential for auditory-oral growth. Members of the team may also provide necessary habilitative services postimplant. Part of the assessment must involve working with parents to ensure that they have appropriate expectations and

are well prepared to participate in the habilitative process. Of all the influences known to impact linguistic outcomes, parental involvement and the intervention services parents receive are the most *controllable* factors in how well children will succeed with cochlear implants.

Criteria

The following inclusion criteria are generally accepted by most pediatric cochlear implant centers, and within each category there is room for individual considerations, according to the goals of the implant program and the families with whom they work.

Minimum Age 12 Months, as Approved by the FDA, or Younger Under Certain Circumstances as Determined to Be Safe by Medical Professionals on the Implant Team

If the goal of implantation is primarily the development of spoken language skills, it must be recognized that the best candidates are very young children and those with already established oral language (Nicholas & Geers, 2007; Zwolan et al., 2004). A plethora of studies confirms that early implantation produces the best oral language outcomes, both because of auditory plasticity issues (Sharma, Dorman, & Kral, 2005; Sharma, Dorman, Spahr, & Todd, 2002) and because children who are implanted later are that much further behind in their oral language milestones (Connor, Craig, Raudenbuch, Heavner, & Zwolan, 2006). Children who receive cochlear implants before 2 years of age have been shown to develop speech similar to that of normal-hearing children (Manrique, Cervera-Paz, Huarte & Molina, 2004; Nicholas & Geers, 2007). Because a good outcome from cochlear implantation is generally considered to be oral language development that parallels language development of normally hearing children (that is, a year's growth in a year's time), a child who does not begin to develop oral language until he is four, five, or even seven years of age will likely—under the best of circumstances—always remain at least as many years behind in oral language milestones. Children for whom circumstances are less than ideal are likely to see the age-language gap continue to widen.

Among older children for whom the goal is oral language development, good candidates for implantation are usually those who have already developed at least fundamental oral language skills: children with normal hearing who have lost it due to illness or accident, children with progressive hearing loss (Dowell et al., 2002), and children whose residual hearing is sufficient to derive linguistic benefit from hearing aids but for whom the cochlear implant can be expected to provide better access especially to high-frequency sounds (Osberger, Zimmerman-Phillips, & Koch, 2002). Older children must be given a voice in the decision to implant, as they might be coerced into having surgery but cannot be coerced into using the external equipment consistently. For fearful children and those who do not fully understand how the implant works or who have inappropriate expectations, provision of materials that explain the entire process at a level appropriate to their age and language facility can alleviate many impediments to success. Perhaps the most effective means of enlisting a child's cooperation is to arrange communication with other implanted children their age. Older candidates who are firm in their

refusal to get an implant often return to the clinic with enthusiasm after having been reassured by establishing relationships with other children like themselves.

With the advent of newborn hearing screening and early intervention, children are identified as candidates for cochlear implantation well below 12 months of age (Morton & Nance, 2006). Although implanting children under a year is not recommended under current FDA guidelines, many cochlear implant centers have begun to explore the benefits of implanting children before their first birthday. Emerging research shows the benefits of very early implantation (Coletti et al., 2005; Dettman, Pinder, Briggs, Dowell, & Leigh, 2007; Tait, Raeve, & Nikolopoulos, 2007). A study by Tait et al. (2007) demonstrated the preverbal communication skills of children with cochlear implants not to be significantly different from those of normal hearing peers when cochlear implantation is performed before 12 months of age. Additionally, in a study by Dettman et al. (2007) the rate of receptive and expressive language growth in children implanted under 12 months of age was shown to be significantly greater than the rates of children implanted between 12 to 24 months of age. The identified risks of implantation under a year of age are primarily medical/surgical (James & Papsin, 2004) and the likely benefits of early implantation must be weighed against these risks by the surgeon and other medical personnel. With regard to non-medical candidacy issues, it is imperative that physiologic test results (auditory brainstem and auditory steady state responses, otoacoustic emissions, tympanograms, and acoustic reflexes) be validated with behavioral testing using age-appropriate techniques. There is sufficient documentation (Luxford, Eisenberg, Johnson, & Mahnke, 2004) to indicate that in some cases physiologic test results performed in the first few months of life are not confirmed by later behavioral tests that indicate a greater amount of residual hearing. A test battery approach raises the degree of confidence for the implant team in determining candidacy in younger infants. Although behavioral observation audiometry does not yield threshold information, a lack of any visible response at least strongly suggests that residual hearing is not substantially better than physiologic testing has indicated. visual reinforcement audiometry does yield threshold information in children who are developmentally able to participate (usually >6 months developmental age) and can provide information not only about ear-specific, frequency-specific thresholds but can contribute valuable information about the child's developmental level and auditory behavior as well.

Bilateral Sensorineural Hearing Loss Sufficient in Degree That Detection Levels with Cochlear Implants Are Expected to Be Better Than Those Obtainable with High-Quality Hearing Aids

The dividing line between the degree of hearing loss best addressed with amplification or cochlear implantation has changed over time and undoubtedly will continue to do so as technology improves. Initially, only children with profound loss qualified for cochlear implantation; it is now clear that children with much more residual hearing can obtain greater benefit from cochlear implantation than from hearing aids (Dettman et al., 2004; Gantz et al., 2000). Included among these children are those with asymmetric hearing loss who clearly benefit from a combination of implantation of the poorer ear and hearing aid use on the better ear and children who have displayed a pattern of progressive loss and who receive implants before the progression reaches severe to profound levels.

Benefit from Properly Fitted Amplification Inadequate to Support Continued Auditory/Oral Skill Development

Benefit from hearing aids is usually determined after a 3- to 6-month hearing aid trial, during which the child receives education/therapy geared toward maximizing auditory development. Exceptions to the trial requirement are children whose hearing loss is secondary to meningitis or other conditions where immediate implantation is critical to surgical success. Particularly in infants and very young children who are unable to perform formal speech perception testing to determine hearing aid benefit, early intervention services are a critically important element of candidacy consideration and a close working relationship between the implant center and the providers of these services is essential.

No Medical Contraindications

Certainly, determination of a clear medical contraindication by an experienced surgeon signals the end of consideration of implantation. Where there is a surgical concern rather than a contraindication (Buchman et al., 2004)—for example, a significantly malformed cochlea, or a present but abnormal-appearing auditory nerve—there may be situations in which the entire team weighs in. A child who is otherwise an excellent candidate may be expected to gain significant benefit from an implant, even with surgical concerns, if the surgeon is willing; a child who is a less good candidate because of age, language development, access to services, or parental involvement may not be considered a candidate at all if there are surgical concerns as well.

Implantation of Children with Cognitive Developmental Delays and/or Behavioral Disorders Is Undertaken Only with Carefully Considered, Realistic Expectations

As the minimum age of implantation continues to decrease, more children will receive implants who later are found to have developmental delays or serious behavioral issues that were not apparent in infancy. Implant programs whose criteria preclude implantation of children with such disorders will inevitably find themselves dealing with these issues in some early implanted children anyway, and as diagnoses are made, certain goals may need to be modified. The primary consideration should be the development of functional communication skills and the most expedient and most likely successful routes to establishment of these skills. When considering implantation of older children in whom developmental delays are already determined, communication and education issues should weigh heavily in candidacy decisions. Where cochlear implantation can be expected to enhance communication, it should be undertaken only with a thorough discussion regarding possible and likely outcomes. Where cochlear implantation can be expected to enhance quality of life, though not necessarily oral communication, it is the responsibility of the implant team to direct

parents to focus on communication skills through another modality.

Availability of Appropriate Therapy and Educational Services

Surgical placement of a cochlear implant does not in itself result in improved hearing, nor does even the most appropriate programming of the device provide functional communication skills. These essential first steps to the implant process must be followed by intensive therapy and/or educational services through which the child can learn to identify and understand speech and develop spoken language. Appropriate educational services can be difficult to access in suburban and rural areas where the population of deaf children is small and the population of implanted children is smaller. Difficulties also may arise in urban areas where the focus of education of deaf children has not been auditory/oral. During the candidacy evaluation, it is essential to investigate available services and to begin the process of establishing them if none exist, so that precious time is not wasted following implantation. Extremely resourceful parents may, with good advice and appropriate materials, be able to provide family-based education to their implanted children with good success, but many more families will need to rely on intervention through public or private educational establishments and supplemental speech-language services. An educational specialist on the implant team can be enormously helpful to parents who, new to the issues of childhood deafness, may not know what services to seek out or how to evaluate the quality of those available. Establishing and implementing appropriate intervention plans prior to implantation is critical to success.

Reasonable Expectations on the Part of Parents and Strong Parental Dedication to Participation in the Habilitative Process

Many parents come to the process of implantation with high hopes and not a few misconceptions. An advantage of the cochlear implant team approach is that multiple professionals have the opportunity to use different words to convey the same concepts to families: cochlear implants do not cure deafness or create normal hearing, and children will not begin talking immediately or be able to go forward in their lives successfully without specialized intervention for the foreseeable future. The responsible cochlear implant team sets aside adequate time before, during, and after the evaluations to counsel families regarding reasonable expectations and the importance of family follow-through with the programs and recommendations of educators and therapists. Parents who appear not to understand likely outcomes, or those who appear to assume that the school will provide all the necessary intervention, must be gently but firmly —and repeatedly—reminded that success through cochlear implantation requires no less involvement on their part than learning sign language would have required, and that the process may be a slow and gradual one.

Evaluation

Protocols used to diagnose and treat sensorineural hearing loss vary among clinics. A multidisciplinary approach to assessment of children for cochlear implant candidacy yields the most accurate picture of the "whole" child and family unit. Additional information beyond the audiologic and med-

ical results may or may not preclude a child from receiving a cochlear implant depending on a center's specific criteria. This information is essential for developing a child's individual intervention plan whether or not that plan includes a cochlear implant.

The pediatric cochlear implant team in most centers consists of the surgeon, audiologist, speech-language pathologist, and psychologist. Some centers are able to include an educator or educational specialist; where this is not possible, concerted efforts should be made to include the candidate's teacher in the process. It should be a priority of the implant team to ensure that a child's teachers are aware when an implant is being considered and when it has been provided. Much useful information comes from the observations of the teachers regarding the child and family, pre- as well as postimplant, so the relationship between implant program and educator is a crucial one. Some implant centers also include a social worker on their team to help parents coordinate services and address issues involving family circumstances that may affect outcomes. Counseling and education of families should be ongoing throughout the candidacy process and should come from all members of the team as the individual evaluations progress.

The candidacy evaluation protocols differ among clinics, but generally they cover the following areas.

History

If the child is new to the implant clinic, medical, developmental, and educational history is taken. Some implant programs get to know children and families by administering questionnaires such as the Infant-Toddler Meaningful Auditory Integration Scale (IT-MAIS) (Zimmerman-Phillips, Robbins, & Osberger, 2000) or other appropriate survey tools, and others use one of a number of available tools to begin rating candidacy in a variety of areas such as age, communication mode and proficiency, speech, developmental delays, and support services. This initial visit provides a good opportunity to begin to understand the parents' knowledge of cochlear implants and their expectations should their child receive the device.

Otologic Evaluation

Where possible, imaging (computed tomography and magnetic resonance imaging scans, as required by the surgeon) and other required medical procedures should be arranged before other evaluations are performed. If a child is clearly not a surgical candidate, the focus of the implant team shifts to helping the family establish appropriate services for their child through other avenues.

Audiologic Evaluation

Physiologic assessment data (auditory steady state responses/auditory brainstem responses tympanograms and acoustic reflexes, otoacoustic emissions) are reviewed or obtained as needed. An ear-specific unaided audiogram is performed using age-appropriate testing techniques. Aided testing, including threshold and appropriate speech perception measures, is performed with suitable amplification.

Speech-Language Evaluation

Parent report scales or standardized tests are used to assess the child's communication skills, receptive and expressive oral language facility, and fundamental speech skills. In some cases, results of these evaluations may influence candidacy and in others may influence the kind of educational and therapy services that should be made available to the family currently or after implantation.

Psychological Evaluation

The goal of this assessment is to evaluate whether the child has met general developmental targets and, in older children, to establish a nonverbal IQ score with appropriate tests. The psychological evaluation provides an excellent opportunity for the psychologist to interact both formally and informally with the child. Parents may be encouraged to discuss their expectations and concerns and the psychologist has the opportunity to reiterate basic information about the implant process. The psychologist may identify areas of concern regarding development, behavior, or attention that may or may not affect candidacy, but may certainly require attention when counseling the family about expectations and educational services.

Educational Assessment

Not all implanted children require the same educational placement, but all require the availability of a strong auditory learning environment. Children who have communicated exclusively through manual communication prior to implantation may not be enrolled in a program that will be appropriate after implantation. It is possible that neither an oral nor a sign program will be the best placement initially, but rather an environment where language can be supported and at the same time listening skills can be developed effectively in order to be able to transition the child to a more auditory-oral environment. A majority of implanted children will benefit from one-on-one auditory habilitation therapy. It is not always reasonable to expect the public schools to provide the amount of therapy that will be most beneficial. Supplemental services provided by a therapist or educator outside the school should be arranged where needed.

The results of evaluations performed by each team member are discussed by the entire implant team, and probable benefits of cochlear implantation are weighed against possible risks. Possible risks may be, as examples, not only the standard risks of anesthesia and surgery, but the likelihood that the child may not derive significant benefit from the implant, that parental expectations are unreasonable (and, perhaps, their participation in the habilitation process too unreliable), and/or that appropriate habilitative services are not in place and have no immediate promise of being implemented. In some situations the candidacy decision may be delayed until concerns resolve. The team's findings are discussed with parents and recommendations are made that may or may not include cochlear implantation. In all cases where a child is found not to be a cochlear implant candidate in a facility, the team is obligated to help the family obtain appropriate services that can be expected to lead to the development of language that can support educational, communicative, and social success. For families whose children are found to be candidates for cochlear implantation, counseling regarding expectations will need to continue even after the initial fitting.

Implant Device Choice

The choice of which implant(s) a child will receive varies with different implant centers. Some centers provide only one type of device; in others the team or surgeon may make the selection. In cases where there is a surgical preference for one device over another because of the physiology of a particular child, this preference must of course take precedence over other considerations. Where the choice of device is up to the parents, it is incumbent upon the implant center to assist parents in making an informed decision and to support that decision. It is helpful for parents to have contact with other families of children with cochlear implants of different types, to communicate directly with the manufacturers who often provide a network of contacts for families in this decision-making stage, and to be given access to information that they may read or view repeatedly. Team members should expect to answer the many questions most families have about how each device works, what distinguishes it from the others, the reliability of each device, and future upgrades that are likely to be available, among others. In all cases where the choice is left up to families, it will be important to assure them that their choice is a good one and that their child will do as well with this device as they would have with any of the other choices.

Bilateral Implants

The principle that two ears are better than one, long a foundation of hearing aid fitting in children, has been slow to be applied to cochlear implantation. Research demonstrates the potential benefit of bimodal hearing devices (Holt, Kirk, Eisenberg, Martinez, & Campbell, 2005; Mok, Galvin, Dowell, & McKay, 2007), and most implant programs encourage the use of a hearing aid on the non-implant ear as long as the child tolerates it or is able to express preference for wearing it. Increasingly, families may be offered an implant for one ear or implants for both, and if they opt for bilateral implantation the surgeries may be simultaneous or sequential. An expanding body of research indicates that benefits of bilateral implantation can include better understanding of speech in noise (Peters, Litovsky, Parkinson, & Lake, 2007; Wolfe et al., 2007), better ability to localize (Litovsky et al., 2006), and binaural processing (Gordon, Valero, & Papsin, 2007). In many cases advantages cannot be measured, at least at first, but parental and child reports confirm the subjective benefits of two devices. Depending on the length of time between implants if the surgeries are sequential, the child may always prefer the first implant even as speech perception benefit improves with the second; in some cases speech perception skills in the newer ear never approach those of the first (Galvin, Mok, & Dowell, 2007). Moreover the interval between the first and second implant may affect the development of binaural processing in children (Gordon et al., 2007). Families whose children are not eligible for bilateral implants for reasons of candidacy, choice, or financial coverage should be given reassurance that most of the benefit of cochlear implantation comes from one device which provides access to the sounds of speech and the environment at levels that make it possible to acquire oral language skills. Long before bilateral implantation was an option, thousands of children developed the ability to speak and attend mainstream educational programs with the benefit of one implant. As research and clinical experience support the additional benefits of bilateral implantation, though, it is reasonable to assume that this trend will grow and will eventually become the standard for surgically appropriate candidates.

Mapping

The cochlear implant should provide good audibility of speech sounds without discomfort. At initial stimulation, however, it may be more important for a young child to be comfortable wearing the device and free of fear, even if audibility has not yet been achieved. The combination of new equipment that is usually more cumbersome than hearing aids they are used to plus perception of a stimulus that is undoubtedly different from what they have heard with hearing aids can be overwhelming for children. Children who have heard little or no sound even with hearing aids may not initially perceive the implant stimulus as an auditory one; they may localize the percept or feeling to other areas (in their backs or abdomens). At initial activation behavioral responses most likely do not represent threshold but rather suprathreshold perception, so stimulation levels should be set well below response levels until it is clear that the child can comfortably tolerate higher levels. Often parents are anxious to move forward quickly, but they should be advised that overstimulation at initial mapping can result in an extreme adverse reaction from the child, such that progress is delayed while parents and audiologists struggle to get the equipment back on the child without a negative response.

Well-established techniques and strategies that have produced good results in adults and older children can be used with younger children as well, whenever possible. However, it may be years before a young child can express preferences or make loudness judgments reliably. Physiologic tools such as neural response and electrically evoked acoustic reflex measurements are invaluable in confirming behavioral responses and in setting initial levels for a child who is not yet able to respond well behaviorally (Brown, 2003). Audiologists must be alert to subtle reactions from young children in order to recognize both auditory responses and discomfort. Minimal auditory responses should be reinforced enthusiastically to help the child understand what he is supposed to respond to. Facial stimulation of any sort is not acceptable and whether it results from overall excess stimulation or excess stimulation on a single electrode, it must be eliminated (Cushing, Papsin, & Gordon, 2006).

Multiple program memories are a particular boon to pediatric implant programming, allowing storage of more than one map which helps the child to adapt to gradual increases in current strength without repeated office visits. With very young children necessarily there will be some trial and error in setting mapping levels. Children need some time to learn to listen and initial lack of clear response does not necessarily mean the map is not providing enough access to speech sounds. Similarly, higher current levels are not necessarily better; there may be a point at which a "louder" map produces not necessarily an uncomfortable response but simply a poor one. It is extremely helpful to parents and teachers for the audiologist to clearly note the recommended progression through these memories and what to do if one of the memories produces a negative response. Flexibility of processor technology (volume and sensitivity controls, error messages, alerting signals for battery strength, and communication of the headpiece with the internal device, as examples) allows implementation of features appropriate to the child's age and experience. Implant manufacturers, recognizing the benefits of FM technology, have designed products that are increasingly simple to use with a variety of FM products.

Mapping changes initially will be frequent as the child adapts to the device and can tolerate more current. Once the child is on the road to becoming a functional listener, changes may be based more on his or her increased sophistication of listening skill, ability to make finer discriminations, and ability to express preferences. Children like what they are used to; conversions to new maps or new processing strategies may require an adjustment period of hours or days, and it is usually wise to leave the most used and best loved map stored in one program of the child's processor even as he is encouraged to try the new, in case the new levels or strategy are intolerable and he is unable to return to the office soon.

The importance of parent involvement in the implant process cannot be overemphasized. Parents should be invited to participate in therapy sessions so they can carry over at home principles and activities that facilitate auditory development. Therapists, educators, audiologists, and other providers of services can make materials and resources available to help parents interact effectively with their children and stimulate auditory and language growth. Parents can be made aware of, and encouraged to attend, group meetings in their geographic area where they can interact with other families and learn more about techniques to facilitate language development at home.

Bilingual/English As A Second Language Issues

In many areas, parents of implant recipients may not speak English or may not speak it well. In some cases there is no common language among family members; children in oral programs are taught English at school, children in total communication programs are taught sign and English together, but parents speak a different language and may not sign. It is tempting to insist that parents of implanted children make an effort to learn and speak only English at home, to reinforce what is taught in the child's educational program; the reality is often that limited English-speaking parents under this dictum may cease to talk much to their children at all. Although there is little literature to guide families, common sense suggests that more effective language stimulation is provided when the parents speak to their children in their most fluent language as they narrate daily activities. English can and should be used to teach and reinforce vocabulary and simple concepts and language structures. Levi and colleagues found that among children of non-English-speaking parents, those educated in oral programs developed English skills essentially equal to those from English-speaking families (Levi, Boyett-Solano, Nicholson, & Eisenberg, 2001). Children from non-English-speaking families educated in total communication (TC) programs fared less well than orally educated children and less well than TC children from English-speaking families. Good English language models provided through educational programs appear to strongly influence the development of English language skills in implanted children, even when English is not spoken in the home. Good language models at home in the parents' native language likely are crucial to essential bonding between parents and infants, even as the parents do their best to learn and improve their English skills.

Continued Evaluation

Not only are the parents' observations of their young child's responses at home important, so are the observations of the child's teacher or early intervention specialist, as sometimes parents are hoping for large reactions and do not detect more subtle responses that mark the beginning of auditory awareness. Children who receive cochlear implants acquire auditory and oral skills in the same sequence as normal hearing infants do, and the standard expectation is that their growth will parallel that of normal hearing children. In fact, some children are slower starters than others, and rate of progress may also depend partly on the initial age-language gap and how much auditory/oral experience the child was able to gain with hearing aids prior to implantation. By a year postimplant, good progress would be reflected by auditory/oral growth of approximately one year, continuing at this general rate over time. Because implanted children do not have normal thresholds, are affected by noisy environments, and may already have significant language delay by the time they receive their implants, they cannot be expected to make progress that parallels normal auditory development without intensive intervention. Although this intervention is best provided by a teacher, auditory verbal therapist, or speech-language pathologist experienced in working with oral deaf children, there are multiple sources of information for professionals with less experience in this area. Step-by-step auditory curricula offer guidelines for therapy and regular evaluation of progress. An increasing number of books focus on appropriate activities for implanted children of various ages in both one-on-one and classroom settings.

Comprehensive postimplant assessments by the implant team should be performed on a regular basis and should include evaluations of the child's adjustment to use of the device, growth in auditory skills, growth in speech-language skills, and mapping. Age-appropriate standardized evaluation measures must be used, but with very young children there will be some period of time where standardized measures produce little useful response and parent and teacher reports will be the most informative. Even when standardized measures can be used, flexibility is often required to fully assess a child's progress. A parent may report enthusiastically that the child can make choices, knows colors, and uses 10 spontaneous oral words meaningfully but the child does not demonstrate these skills on standard tests; it is not only useful but reassuring to parents if the clinician invites the parent to interact with their child to elicit these kinds of responses, even if they cannot be scored. Evaluations can be a source of much anxiety for both parents and child, and it is essential that clinicians not view test results in a vacuum or make recommendations based on test results without considering the bigger picture. Individual circumstances vary with children and with their families. A 10-year-old child in an oral program who is five years behind in oral language development and knows no sign language will not be served well by a recommendation to switch to a total communication program, whereas a 7-year-old with the same age-language gap might. A 2-year-old implanted child might have good potential to benefit from auditory verbal therapy but if he or she has two deaf, signing siblings it is likely that sign language will always be a part of this child's communication skills. Speech perception measures together with the speech-language evaluation can provide valuable information regarding the best areas of focus in auditory and speech-language therapy and even the best approaches to educational placement. They can also impact decisions regarding mapping; for example, missing certain sounds (receptively or expressively) during testing

may in some cases be successfully addressed by changes in stimulation levels, gains, and/or processing strategies.

Mapping is usually performed on an annual basis once a child's map has been established and levels are essentially stable, which generally occurs after the first two years or so. Interim mappings should be offered when there are concerns on the part of parents, teachers, or therapists. Although changes in mapping levels, strategies, or features can indeed impact speech and language, it is important not to view mapping as a cure-all for a child's communication issues. Mapping does not address speech production in itself, except insofar as production is affected by perception; that is, to the extent that a child produces incorrectly what he hears incorrectly, there may be mapping changes that will address the production. In a young child it can be difficult to distinguish between what they can discriminate through listening alone and what they can produce, but to the extent possible it is important to make this distinction. Certainly there are implanted children who may have had speech and language delay or learning disabilities that would have impacted their communication skills even had they had normal hearing, so not all speech and language problems can be remedied through mapping. Frequently, what is thought to be a mapping issue is, in fact, an equipment malfunction. Bad microphones, worn cables, and corroded battery contacts can result in a distorted or intermittent signal and are problems that are easily remedied in most cases. Equipment malfunction should be suspected when there is a sudden decrease in performance but may also be the culprit with gradual decline in performance if the equipment is still functioning although incorrectly. Physical health may affect mapping levels; children with otitis media may variously complain that they cannot hear with their implants or sounds are too loud, and mapping will need to be adjusted for the duration of the condition. Families should be encouraged to contact the implant center as soon as any type of equipment or mapping problem is suspected, whether it is a sudden or gradual decrease in the child's responsiveness, decline in speech intelligibility, intolerance to loud sound, evidence of facial stimulation, or any other concern they may have.

Parents will require reassurance as auditory skills develop, especially if progress is less rapid than they would like. One of the most difficult situations the implant team will encounter is the child whose progress is very poor. There is no clear-cut point at which the focus of language-learning should no longer be exclusively auditory/oral, as it will depend on the age of the child and skill level they have achieved. If the child's oral language is clearly not keeping pace with his or her hearing age, though, and before a child is irretrievably far behind in language milestones such that she or he is seriously at risk educationally, consideration should be given to a change of communicative strategy. It is best if this kind of discussion has been ongoing and part of each visit, so that parents will not feel stunned by the suggestion or that lack of auditory/oral progress is a failure on their part, or on their child's part. They may feel this way anyway. But if their understanding from the start has been that cochlear implantation provides a tool to access auditory information, and effective use of this tool will depend on factors known and unknown, they may be more receptive when it is becoming clear that a different communication modality may be in order. A recommendation for a total communication program does not mean that auditory/oral therapy must or should stop; auditory skills may indeed continue to develop with appropriate support,

even as the primary communication mode shifts to one that is more visual.

On the other hand, as some children display such remarkable development of speech and language skills as a result of implantation, it can be tempting to lose appreciation for the fact that they do not hear normally. Simultaneously bilaterally implanted children still have detection thresholds in the range of mild hearing loss in both ears. Sequentially bilaterally implanted children may or may not derive equal benefit from their two implants. Children with only one implant have detection thresholds in the range of mild hearing loss in the better ear and severe or profound hearing loss in the poorer ear. Hearing loss of any degree, no matter how well addressed by technology, interferes with the ability of all persons to understand well in the presence of competing noise and in poor acoustic environments. Classrooms, cafeterias, and multipurpose rooms where assemblies may be held are all noisy places and are all environments in which critical listening skills are often required.

Children with cochlear implants can benefit greatly from FM and other assistive listening technology, just as children with hearing aids do. Often, it is less a matter of "needing" an FM system than it is a matter of enabling a child to do more easily what he already does well, and it can be very helpful to present the option of an FM to parents and child in just this way. A difference between FM use with cochlear implants and FM use with hearing aids is that although it is possible to monitor the FM signal transmitted through the hearing aid by listening to it, it is not possible to listen to the FM signal transmitted through a cochlear implant processor as the user hears it. For this reason, it is usually recommended that children who are unable to report on the quality of the FM signal themselves be provided with this technology via a speaker. Many class-rooms for very young children now use multi-speaker sound field FM systems that benefit all the children in the class, especially including those with attention and learning issues. Portable desktop or pillar-type FM speakers may be useful for situations where the child has limited movement in the classroom and may usually be seated at his desk or move only between desk and a group reading table, for instance. As children become capable of reporting when an FM signal is inconsistent or distorted, it is appropriate to move to a personal FM system. However, even a child who has become a reliable reporter should have FM monitoring strategies incorporated into her education plan.

All the current cochlear implant sound processors are FM-compatible. Depending on the particular processor, the use of personal FM technology may require the purchase of new, device-specific receivers, or cables and interface equipment to attach the same types of receivers that are also used with hearing aids and other implant processors. Device-specific FM equipment may have less signal interference, fewer accessory parts, and a more secure attachment to the speech processor. A disadvantage of device-specific equipment is that not all schools may be enthusiastic about purchasing equipment that does not have a universal application to children with a variety of hearing aids and cochlear implants. Audiologists in a position to recommend or order FM equipment for implant users should take care to look not only at the currently worn implant equipment but at predictable future upgrades as FM equipment that works well with a child's current processor may be incompatible with upgraded processors. As new FM systems are designed, the audiologist should ensure that each is recommended by the implant manufacturers as being known to be effective and problem free with their particular device. If the equipment is purchased by the school, it is incumbent on the school either to employ an audiologist to troubleshoot and maintain equipment or to contract with an outside professional and make the equipment available for fitting, inspection, and troubleshooting as needed. Where multiple professionals are involved in procuring, setting, monitoring and maintaining FM equipment, communication is essential. As implant equipment, FM equipment, and programming software are changed and upgraded over time, different features may be employable and different settings on FM and/or implant equipment advisable.

Children may benefit from FM use not only in school but in the course of outside activities such as in sports, social and service groups, and religious services. Extensive commutes to school and/or therapy sessions are often part of an implanted child's weekly, if not daily, routine. Personal FM systems are often recommended for commuting, especially in cars, to optimize communication and promote auditory skill development. The value of an FM is often defined by its benefit in the classroom yet the need for FM technology outside the classroom is vast. Where the school keeps physical custody of FM equipment purchased for a student's use, families can certainly consider purchase of an FM system for these kinds of activities.

Conclusion

Cochlear implants are an evolving technology, and candidacy criteria, assessment techniques, and approaches to auditory habilitation and facilitation of language continue to be impacted by new research and understanding of long-term outcomes. It is essential to remember that the most important skill children acquire and develop is not hearing per se, but language. To the extent that a cochlear implant can enhance language development, it is an appropriate and remarkable device, and indeed a majority of good candidates for cochlear implantation are successful in developing functional oral language skills. Some children whose primary communication mode is not oral may develop enough auditory/oral skill to function comfortably in the hearing world even as they communicate with friends and in school through sign. There may always be a segment of the implant population that is unable to use the information from the cochlear implant to develop oral skills. The benefit of a comprehensive team approach is not only the determination of candidacy but the assistance they can provide to families after this determination is made, to maximize the benefit of implantation and to support development of communication skills through whatever modality makes for communicative, educational, and social success.

References

Beadle, E. A., McKinley, D. J., Niklopulos, T. P., Brough, J., O'Donoghue, G. M., & Archbold, S. M. (2005). Long-term functional outcomes and academic occupational status in implanted children after 10 to 14 years of implant use. *Otology and Neurotology, 26*, 1152–1160.

Beiter, A. L., Staller, S. J., & Dowell, R. C. (1991). Evaluation and device programming in children. *Ear and Hearing, 12*, 25–33.

Brown, C. J. (2003). Clinical uses of electrically evoked auditory nerve and brainstem responses. *Current Opinion in Otolaryngology-Head and Neck Surgery, 11*, 383–387.

Buchman, C. A., Copeland, B. J., Yu, K. K., Brown, C. J., Carrasco, V. N., & Pillsbury, H. C. (2004). Cochlear implantation in children with congenital inner ear malformations. *Laryngoscope, 114*, 309–316.

Colletti, V., Carner, M., Miorelli, V., Guida, M., Colletti, L., & Fiorino, F. G. (2005). Cochlear implantation at under 12 months: Report on 10 patients. *Laryngoscope, 115*, 445–449.

Connor, C. M., Craig, H. K., Raudenbuch, S. W., Heavner, K., & Zwolan, T. A. (2006). The age at which deaf children receive cochlear implants and their vocabulary and speech production growth: Is there added value for early implantation? *Ear and Hearing, 27*, 628–644.

Cushing, S. L., Papsin, B. C., & Gordon, K. A. (2006). Incidence and characteristics of facial nerve stimulation in children with cochlear implants. *Laryngoscope, 116*, 1787–1791.

Dettman, S. J., D'Costa, W. A., Dowell, R. C., Winton, E. J., Hill, K. L., & Williams, S. S. (2004). Cochlear implants for children with significant residual hearing. *Archives of Otolaryngology-Head and Neck Surgery, 130*, 612–618.

Dettman, S. J., Pinder, D., Briggs, R. J., Dowell, R. C., & Leigh, J. R. (2007). Communication development in children who receive the cochlear implant younger than 12 months: Risks versus benefits. *Ear and Hearing, 28*(Suppl. 2), 11–18.

Dowell, R. C., Dettman, S. J., Hill, K., Winton, E., Barker, E. J., & Clark, G. M. (2002). Speech perception outcomes in older children who use multichannel cochlear implants: Older is not always poorer. *Annals of Otology, Rhinology, and Laryngology, 111*(Suppl. 189), 97–101.

Galvin, K. L., Mok, M., & Dowell, R. C. (2007). Perceptual benefit and functional outcomes for children using sequential bilateral cochlear implants. *Ear and Hearing, 28*, 470–482.

Gantz, B. J., Rubenstein, J. T., Tyler, R. S., Teagle, H. F., Cohen, N. L., Waltzman, S. B., et al. (2000). Long-term results of cochlear implants in children with residual hearing. *Annals of Otology, Rhinology, and Laryngology, 109* (Suppl. 185), 33–36.

Geers, A., Brenner, C., Nicholas, J., Uchanski, R., Tye-Murray, N., & Tobey, E. (2002). Rehabilitation factors contributing to implant benefit in children. *Annals of Otology, Rhinology, and Laryngology, 111*(Suppl. 189), 127–130.

Geers, A. E., Nicholas, J., & Sedey, A. L. (2003). Language skills of children with early cochlear implantation. *Ear and Hearing, 24*(Suppl. 1), 46–58.

Gordon, K. A., Valero, J., & Papsin, B. C. (2007). Auditory brainstem activity in children with 9–30 months of bilateral cochlear implant use. *Hearing Research, 233*, 97–107.

Holt, R. F., Kirk, K. I., Eisenberg, L. S., Martinez, A. S., & Campbell W. (2005). Spoken word recognition in children with residual hearing using cochlear implants and hearing aids in opposite ears. *Ear and Hearing, 26*(Suppl. 4), 82–91.

James, A. L., & Papsin, B. C. (2004). Cochlear implant surgery at 12 months of age and younger. *Laryngoscope, 114*, 2191–2195.

Levi, A. V., Boyett-Solano, J., Nicholson, B., & Eisenberg, L. S. (2001). Multilingualism and children with cochlear implants. *Hearing Review, 8*, 44–49.

Litovsky, R. Y., Johnstone, P. M. Goder, S., Agrawai, S., Parkinson, A., Peters, R., et al. (2006). Bilateral cochlear implants in children: Localization acuity measured with minimum audible angle. *Ear and Hearing, 27*, 43–59.

Luxford, W. M., Eisenberg, L. S., Johnson, K. C., & Mahnke, E. M. (2004). Cochlear implantation in infants younger than 12 months. In R. T. Miyamoto (Ed.), *Proceedings of the 8th International Cochlear Implant Conference. International Congress Series, Vol. 1273* (pp. 376–379). Netherlands: Elsevier.

Manrique, M., Cervera-Paz, F. J., Huarte, A., & Molina, M. (2004). Advantages of cochlear implantation in prelingual deaf children before 2 years of age when compared with later implantation. *Laryngoscope, 114*, 1462–1469.

Mok, M., Galvin, K. L., Dowell, R. C., & McKay, C. M. (2007). Spatial unmasking and binaural advantage for children with normal hearing, a cochlear implant and a hearing aid, and bilateral implants. *Audiology and Neurotology, 12*, 295–306.

Morton, C. C., & Nance, W. E. (2006). Newborn hearing screening—a silent revolution. *New England Journal of Medicine, 354*, 2151–2164.

Nicholas, J. G., & Geers, A. E. (2007). Will they catch up? The role of age at cochlear implantation in the spoken language development of children with severe to profound hearing loss. *Journal of Speech, Language, and Hearing Research, 50*, 1048–1062.

Osberger, M. J., Zimmerman-Phillips, S., & Koch, D. B. (2002). Cochlear implant candidacy and performance trends in children. *Annals of Otology, Rhinology, and Laryngology, 111*(Suppl. 189), 62–65.

Papsin, B. C., & Gordon, K. A. (2007). Cochlear implants for children with severe-to-profound hearing loss. *New England Journal of Medicine, 357*, 2380–2387.

Peters, B. R., Litovsky, R., Parkinson, M., & Lake, J. (2007). Importance of age and postimplantation experience on speech perception measures in children with sequential bilateral cochlear implants. *Otology and Neurotology, 28*, 649–657.

Sharma, A., Dorman, M. F., & Kral, A. (2005). The influence of a sensitive period on central auditory development in children with unilateral and bilateral cochlear implants. *Hearing Research, 203*, 134–143.

Sharma, A., Dorman, M., Spahr, A., & Todd, N. W. (2002). Early cochlear implantation in children allows normal development of central auditory pathways. *Annals of Otology, Rhinology, and Laryngology, 111*(Suppl. 189), 38–41.

Stern, R. E., Yueh, B., Lewis, C., Norton, S., & Sie, K. C. (2005). Recent epidemiology of pediatric cochlear implantation in the United States: Disparity among children of different ethnicity and socioeconomic status. *Laryngoscope, 115*, 125–131.

Tait, M., De Raeve, L., & Nikolopoulos, T. P. (2007) Deaf children with cochlear implants before age of 1 year: Comparison of preverbal communication with normal hearing children. *International Journal of Pediatric Otorhinolaryngology, 71*, 1605–1611.

Waltzman, S. B., Cohen, N. L., Green, J., & Roland, J. T., Jr. (2002). Long-tern effects of cochlear implants in children. *Otolaryngology-Head and Neck Surgery, 126*, 505–511.

Wolfe, J., Baker, S., Caraway, T., Kasulis, H., Mears, A., Smith, J., et al. (2007). 1-year post activation results for sequentially implanted bilateral cochlear implant users. *Otology and Neurotology*, *28*, 589–596.

Zimmerman-Phillips S., Robbins A. M., Osberger, M. J. (2000). Assessing cochlear implant benefit in very young children. *Annals of Otology, Rhinology, and Laryngology*, *109* (Suppl. 185), 42–43.

Zwolan, T. A., Ashbaugh, H. K., Alarfaj, A., Kileny, P. R., Arts, H. A., El-Kashlan, H. K., & Telian, S. A. (2004) Pediatric cochlear implant patient performance as a function of age at implantation. *Otology and Neurotology*, *25*, 112–120.

CHAPTER 3

Acoustic Amplification for Infants and Children: Selection, Fitting, and Management

PATRICIA A. ROUSH
RICHARD C. SEEWALD

Introduction

Over the past 20 years important advances have occurred in the evaluation and treatment of hearing loss in children. Infants are now screened prior to hospital discharge and many are fitted with hearing aids during the first weeks of life. Many of those unable to benefit from acoustic amplification receive cochlear implants by 1 year of age, and some are able to achieve speech, language, and academic milestones on par with their hearing peers. Better tools are now available for screening and evaluation of children with hearing loss, and improvements in hearing aid, FM, and cochlear implant technologies are making it possible for children with severe and profound hear-

ing loss to access spoken language in ways considered impossible only a few years ago.

Cochlear implantation was once limited to children with "little or no residual hearing," but improvements in today's implants combined with changes in candidacy have resulted in children and adults with substantial residual hearing being considered for implantation. Furthermore, as greater benefits have been observed, cochlear implantation is being considered for children at younger ages. These changes present many challenges for the pediatric audiologist: accurate assessment of hearing is needed in the first weeks of life; acoustic amplification must be fitted earlier than ever before; and the benefits of amplification must be determined as soon as possible to ensure the greatest access to spoken language. To accomplish these goals in the first few months of life requires the application of evidence-based hearing assessment and hearing aid fitting protocols combined with knowledge of expected outcomes for both hearing aids and cochlear implants in children with varying degrees of hearing loss. In this chapter we describe protocols for the selection and fitting of hearing instruments in infants and young children with emphasis on the needs of those with severe-to-profound hearing loss.

The Importance of a Systematic Approach

At one time, hearing aid evaluation prior to cochlear implantation consisted of little more than a relatively simple electroacoustic analysis of high gain, linear, analog hearing instruments followed by the measurement of aided detection thresholds in sound field. As many children considered for cochlear implantation had little or no residual auditory capacity, audiologists on cochlear implant teams were not required to have extensive knowledge of pediatric hearing aid fitting and evaluation procedures. However, as criteria for cochlear implantation have broadened to include younger children with more useable residual hearing, it has become important to recognize that there may be several different technologies or strategies that may be considered for a given child including: bilateral cochlear implants, bimodal hearing (i.e., a cochlear implant in one ear and a hearing aid in the other), and frequency compression hearing aids. Consequently, audiologists who participate in determining candidacy for cochlear implantation and other hearing technologies must apply current pediatric amplification

guidelines to ensure the most beneficial intervention.

Several guidelines for evidenced-based practice are now available to pediatric audiologists (American Academy of Audiology Pediatric Amplification Guidelines, 2004; The College of Audiologists and Speech-Language Pathologists of Ontario, Preferred Practice Guideline for the Prescription of Hearing Aids to Children, 2002; Ontario Infant Hearing Program Provision of Amplification Protocol and Guidelines, 2007; Pediatric Working Group of the Conference on Amplification for Children with Auditory Deficits, 1996; and Guidelines for the Fitting, Verification and Evaluation of Digital Signal Processing Hearing Aids within a Children's Hearing Aid Service, University of Manchester, England, 2005).

Limitations of Aided Sound Field Testing

Despite the availability of guidelines for pediatric hearing aid fitting, a survey by Bamford and colleagues indicated that only 20% of audiologists use probe microphone measures when fitting hearing aids to children. Indeed, most pediatric audiologists continue to use sound-field aided threshold measures to verify the electroacoustic performance of hearing instruments for young infants (Bamford et al., 2001). Unfortunately, there are many disadvantages associated with this approach. The limitations of sound field aided threshold measurements for use in hearing aid fitting have been described by numerous investigators (Hawkins, Montgomery, Prosek, & Walden 1987; Seewald, Moodie, Sinclair, & Cornelisse, 1996; Seewald, Moodie, Sinclair, & Scollie, 1999; Stelmachowicz & Lewis, 1988).

Some of the limitations and sources of invalidity associated with sound-field aided threshold testing include: (1) test-retest reliability (Hawkins et al., 1987); (2) the inability to obtain reliable behavioral thresholds on infants under six months of age or those with developmental delays who can't be tested using behavioral audiometry; and (3) the interactions between the low-level frequency specific signals typically used in aided threshold testing and the compression circuits in today's hearing aids, resulting in overestimation of the gain provided by an instrument for conversational speech (Seewald et al., 1999). Another significant limitation is that the sound field procedures do not provide accurate estimates of the aided audibility of soft, average, and loud speech or the real-ear saturation response of the hearing aid, a significant limitation when attempting to provide audibility for a wide range of speech inputs at safe and comfortable levels for an infant.

Prescriptive Fitting Methods

Current pediatric amplification protocols emphasize the need to use an *evidence-based* prescriptive hearing aid approach to determine the recommended levels for amplified speech and the target limits for hearing instrument output as a function of frequency. Prescriptive procedures can be classified according to: (a) evidence-based *generic* prescriptive algorithms such as the DSL[*mi*/o] version 5.1 (Scollie et al., 2005) and the NAL-NL1 algorithm (Dillon, 1999), and (b) manufacturer-specific proprietary algorithms. The manufacturer-specific *proprietary* algorithms are those developed by the manufacturer for use with their hearing instruments. Some manufacturers have chosen not to develop their own proprietary algorithm for fitting children and have instead chosen to incorporate the DSL or NAL prescriptive algorithms into their fitting software. However, these generic algorithms may have been adapted by the manufacturer to account for the unique characteristics (e.g., compression kneepoint) of their hearing instruments.

Several investigators have compared proprietary prescriptive algorithms for use with adults. Keidser, Brew, and Beck (2003), for example, found a 10-dB variation in the amount of gain prescribed by NAL-NL1, DSL[i/o] and four proprietary algorithms for the same audiogram. A more recent study examined behind-the-ear (BTE) hearing aids from six major manufacturers programmed using their 'default' fitting procedure (Mueller, Bentler, & Wu, 2008). For some manufacturers this was a generic fitting formula whereas others applied their own proprietary prescriptive method. The OSPL90 was measured at the default program settings with all special features deactivated. Results for a flat 50 dB HL hearing loss indicated maximum output values ranging from 90 to 109 dB.

Most recently, at the National Centre for Audiology in Canada, Seewald and colleagues (Seewald, Mills, Bagatto, Scollie, & Moodie, 2008) compared five different manufacturer's implementation of the same prescriptive method for varying degrees of hearing loss using BTE instruments frequently used with the pediatric population. Using average real-ear-to-coupler difference (RECD) values for a 6-month-old infant, nine audiograms ranging from mild to profound were used to program the hearing aid and simulated real-ear measurements (S-REM) were measured. Seewald and colleagues found that for the same hearing loss the recommended gain for average speech inputs varied by as much as 21 dB, whereas the prescribed output limiting levels varied by as much as 30 dB across the manufacturer-specific algorithms. Such a wide variation among the electroacoustic characteristics prescribed by current manufacturer specific algorithms is clearly unacceptable for infant hearing aid fitting and underscores the need for a comprehensive set of speech-based real-ear measures to ensure the provision of appropriate gain and output limiting.

A Clinical Protocol

Many of the current pediatric amplification guidelines incorporate components of the Desired Sensation Level (DSL) method for pediatric hearing instrument fitting (Bagatto et al., 2005; Cornelisse, Seewald, & Jamieson, 1995; Scollie et al., 2005; Seewald, 1995). Building on innovative approaches to pediatric hearing aid fitting from the 1970s (Erber, 1973; Gengel, Pascoe, & Shore, 1971; Ross, 1975) the research program in pediatric hearing aid fitting at the National Centre for Audiology in Canada has, for over 20 years, conducted research to develop the DSL method for the fitting of amplification in children. This approach considers the unique needs of infants and young children, and it advocates the use of a systematic, evidence-based approach that accounts for an infant's external ear acoustics at the assessment, selection, and verification stages, as well as measurement of hearing aid output limiting. At one time the DSL method was cumbersome and required the use of look-up tables to select and fit the amplification characteristics of a hearing aid; however, many of the newer versions of manufacturer fitting software systems and real-ear measurement systems incorporate the DSL method into their software resulting in

improved ease and efficiency for the pediatric audiologist.

The process of selecting and fitting hearing aids for infants and young children should be viewed as a "continuum of care," with steps that include:

- accurate assessment of hearing thresholds and evaluation of ear canal acoustics
- selection of appropriate hearing instruments
- device programming
- electroacoustic verification using an evidence-based prescriptive algorithm designed for use with infants and children
- hearing aid orientation for the family
- validation measures.

Audiometric Assessment

For infants and young children, the determination of hearing thresholds provides the foundation for hearing aid fitting. If hearing thresholds used in hearing instrument fitting are inaccurate, the quality of the hearing aid fitting will suffer. Although estimation of hearing thresholds for adults and older children is accomplished using behavioral audiometric procedures, for infants under 6 months of age, assessment using objective methods such as the auditory brainstem response (ABR) or auditory steady-state response (ASSR) is required.

ABR evaluation using frequency-specific test stimuli (e.g., tone bursts) is essential for obtaining frequency-specific estimates of hearing thresholds (Gorga et al., 2006; Stapells, 2000). Considering the variability known to occur for different audiometric configurations, frequency-specific ABR measures are needed to estimate thresholds for hearing instrument fitting. This involves, minimally, an estimate of thresholds for a low and high frequency region prior to initiating hearing instrument fitting. Ideally, threshold estimates should be obtained for 500, 1000, 2000, and 4000 Hz. Audiologists who perform diagnostic ABR evaluations on infants, following referrals from newborn hearing screening, must have the ability to obtain frequency-specific thresholds using tone burst stimuli or to make referrals to a center where these specialized diagnostic procedures can be provided. Although an abnormal response using click stimuli may confirm the presence of hearing loss, frequency-specific ABR is needed before hearing aid fitting can be initiated. When hearing loss is evident, based on air-conducted test results, ABR assessment should also be completed using bone-conducted stimuli to determine if the hearing loss is conductive or sensorineural.

Several factors must be considered prior to estimating behavioral thresholds from ABR for use in hearing instrument fitting. First, it must be remembered that behavioral audiometry is referenced to a normative dB HL scale whereas threshold estimations obtained from ABR are referenced in dB normalized HL (nHL). Once the ABR threshold (nHL) has been obtained, a "correction factor" must be applied to the nHL value to obtain an estimated behavioral threshold (HL). The correction value applied will vary depending on the frequency of the test signal and the specific protocol used. Unfortunately, there is currently no standardized calibration protocol used by equipment manufacturers, and thus calibration procedures vary widely. Furthermore, when entering threshold data into hearing aid verification equipment, some systems require the audiologist to apply the appropriate correction value to the ABR threshold and enter "HL" values whereas others allow the audiologist to enter in "nHL" values and use published

corrections to convert "nHL" to HL values. It is essential that the audiologist performing the ABR be aware of the calibration procedures used for their measurement system and that the appropriate values in "nHL" or estimated "HL" be provided to the audiologist performing the hearing instrument fitting. The reader is referred to Bagatto et al. (2005) for a comprehensive review of factors that must be considered when estimating behavioral thresholds from electrophysiologic tests.

When the ABR is absent or grossly abnormal it is essential that click-evoked ABR testing at a high intensity level be completed using both condensation and rarefaction stimuli in order to rule out auditory neuropathy spectrum disorder (ANSD) (Rance, 2005). The use of alternating polarity clicks alone will likely result in an incorrect diagnosis of profound hearing loss for infants with ANSD. ASSR is a newer electrophysiologic procedure being used in some clinics in addition to ABR during the comprehensive assessment. Although several investigations have shown that both ABR and ASSR provide accurate frequency specific threshold information (Gorga et al., 2006; Johnson & Brown, 2005; Rance & Rickards, 2002), few studies are available using ASSR on infants with hearing loss and, at this time, there is no way to determine if an infant has ANSD if only ASSR is used. Clinicians who perform comprehensive evaluation of hearing loss in infants should stay current with the latest research on ASSR and other methods of evaluating hearing loss in infants.

Infants who have no response for ABR at maximal intensity levels are likely to have at least a severe hearing loss; however, the absence of a response does not necessarily mean that the infant has no residual hearing. Some infants with a "no response ABR" will have residual hearing, particularly in the low frequencies, and may benefit from appropriately fitted acoustic amplification while undergoing further evaluation to determine candidacy for cochlear implantation. Optimal amplification of residual low-frequency hearing will, at a minimum, allow the young infant to have an awareness of environmental sounds and to have access to the low frequency components of their own voice and the speech of caregivers. Furthermore, detection of middle ear pathology in the very young infant is challenging, and the presence of undetected middle ear fluid at the time of the ABR in cases of severe sensorineural hearing loss may also result in an infant with some residual hearing having an absent ABR (Gravel & Hood, 1998).

When no response is obtained from ABR at the maximum intensity levels of the equipment, it is difficult to estimate behavioral thresholds. For example, when an ABR threshold is obtained at 90 dB nHL at 500 Hz and a correction factor of 25 dB is subtracted, the estimated behavioral threshold is 65 dB HL. However, if the maximum intensity level at 500 Hz is 90 dB nHL and no response is obtained at that frequency, it is difficult to be certain of the infant's behavioral threshold for that frequency. The actual threshold may be at 65 dB HL or the child could have no residual hearing at all for that frequency. For high-frequency tone bursts the correction factor to be applied is usually smaller, on the order of 5 dB. For example, if a child has a response of 90 dB nHL for a 4000-Hz tone burst and a 5 dB correction value is applied, the estimated behavioral threshold is 85 dB HL. As described in the previous example, if the child has no response to a 4000 Hz tone burst at 90 dB nHL, the child's actual behavioral threshold could range from 85 dB HL to greater than 110 dB HL. Thus, in cases of a "no response ABR," a reasonable approach would be to provide an estimated threshold at a level that is slightly poorer than the

minimal response estimate. In the examples noted above we would estimate thresholds for purposes of the initial hearing aid fitting to be approximately 75 dB HL for the low frequencies and 95 dB HL for the high frequencies. Once behavioral audiometric thresholds are obtained, the hearing aids can be readjusted as needed.

Electrophysiologic techniques provide reasonable estimates of behavioral hearing thresholds, but behavioral audiometric measures such as visual reinforcement audiometry (VRA) remain the gold standard for infant hearing assessment. Once an infant is sitting up and has reasonable head control, behavioral audiometry using VRA should be attempted. As with other developmental indices, some infants will perform reliably for VRA measures at a younger developmental age than others. However, most infants should successfully perform the VRA procedure by 6 to 8 months developmental age (Widen, 1990; Widen et al., 2000). For a comprehensive clinical VRA protocol see Gravel (2000).

Recently we reviewed data from the first 70 infants with bilateral sensory hearing loss fitted with hearing aids following referral from newborn hearing screening in our pediatric hearing program at the University of North Carolina. For those infants the median age at ABR testing was 2.6 months, the median age at hearing aid fitting was 3.9 months, and the median age when a frequency-specific behavioral audiogram was available for each ear (250 to 4000 Hz) was 8.5 months. Thus, frequency-specific estimates of hearing thresholds obtained from ABR allowed us to fit most infants with hearing aids at least four months earlier than would have been possible had we waited for thresholds from behavioral testing with visual reinforcement audiometry. It is important to remember, however, that physiologic measures provide an *estimate* of behavioral thresholds and that actual measurement of hearing threshold levels should be completed as soon as possible to ensure accuracy in adjusting the hearing instruments. Furthermore, a complete audiogram obtained using VRA will provide the audiologist with additional information regarding the audiometric configuration. Infants who are already accustomed to wearing hearing aids will tolerate the use of insert earphones attached to their custom earmolds more readily than if standard foam inserts are used. This allows us to obtain frequency- and ear-specific audiometric thresholds as early as possible. When updated hearing thresholds are obtained, the hearing instruments are re-adjusted to provide the best match to prescriptive targets for both gain and output limiting.

Evaluation of Ear Canal Acoustics

Once estimates of behavioral hearing thresholds are available, it is important to account for differences in the size and shape of the infant's ear canal. The ear canal of an infant is significantly smaller than that of an average adult, and sound levels measured in the ear canal of an infant can be as much as 20 dB higher than the same sound in the ear of an adult (Scollie, Seewald, Cornelisse, & Jenstad, 1998; Seewald & Scollie, 1999). In addition, there is significant variability in the acoustic properties among different infants and for the same infant over time (Bagatto, Scollie, Seewald, Moodie, & Hoover, 2002). These differences must be accounted for to ensure audibility and safety during the hearing aid fitting. Differences in the size and shape of adult ears are accounted for during actual "real-ear measurements."

Although conventional real-ear measurements are feasible for adults and older children, they are not easily accomplished on infants or small children due to the need to remain still during the measurement procedure. For this reason, a substitute procedure called the real-ear-to-coupler difference (RECD) measurement (Moodie, Seewald, & Sinclair, 1994) is recommended. To measure the RECD, the sound of a known intensity is measured in a 2-cc coupler and subsequently the same signal is introduced via an insert earphone attached to a foam tip or the child's custom earmold. A probe microphone is placed in the infant's ear canal and the SPL at the child's eardrum is measured (Figure 3–1). The difference between the sound in the coupler and the sound in the child's ear is "the real-ear-to-coupler difference" (Figure 3–2). Once this variable has been measured for an infant, the remainder of the hearing aid adjustments and verification can be completed within a hearing aid test box and without the cooperation of the infant. The RECD measurement is relatively easy to perform in young infants and takes less than a minute for each ear. If the infant is too active or noisy to complete the RECD measurement for both ears, it is possible to obtain the measurement for one ear and enter those values for use with the other ear (Munro, 2005). This procedural modification assumes no significant differences in the size and shape of the other ear. If the RECD measurement cannot be completed for either ear, predicted values based on normative data can be used until the necessary cooperation from the child is obtained (Bagatto et al., 2002; Seewald et al., 1999).

Because of the variability among infants even at the same age, the goal should be to perform the actual RECD measurement whenever possible. Due to the rapid ear canal growth in infants during the first year of life, it is often necessary to complete the RECD measure whenever a new set of earmolds is needed. Once the RECD measurement has

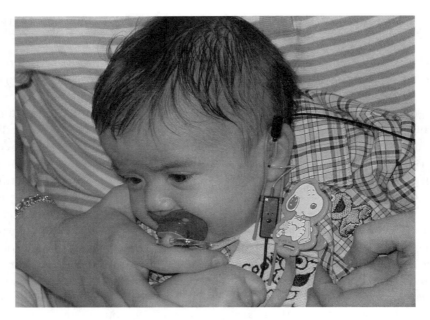

Figure 3–1. Infant with probe tube assembly for RECD measurement.

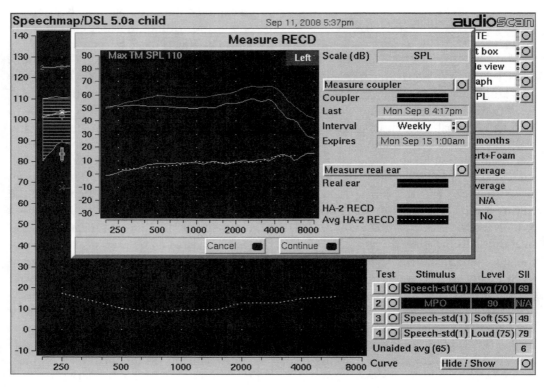

Figure 3–2. Graphic display of the results of a Real-Ear-to-Coupler Difference (RECD) measurement, in dB, as a function of frequency.

been completed, the values are stored in the verification system and used in subsequent stages of the fitting process to accurately predict how the hearing instrument will perform when fitted to the infant.

An example of an audiogram for an infant with hearing threshold estimates obtained from electrophysiologic testing is shown in Figure 3–3. The "+" symbols correspond to the lowest observable response on the ABR in dB nHL, the appropriate correction values are applied and subtracted from the dB nHL value to obtain the infant's estimated hearing threshold in dB HL, indicated by the open circles. Recall that the correction values used depend on the type of calibration used in the ABR system.

In Figure 3–4, the same audiogram has been converted to dB SPL (ear canal level) and displayed in an "SPLogram" format. At the bottom of the graph, the lowest levels of sound a person with normal hearing can detect are shown as a function of frequency. Note that for this infant with hearing loss, higher intensities are required before sound can be detected. Also note that greater intensities are required for detection of the higher frequencies compared to the levels needed for the lower frequencies. The levels of unamplified conversational speech are also shown relative to the

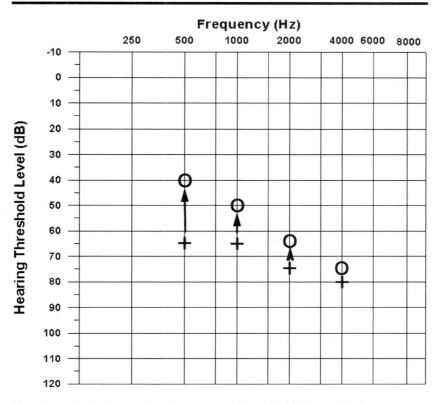

Figure 3–3. Estimated audiogram in dB eHL (O) from ABR measurements obtained in dB nHL(+).

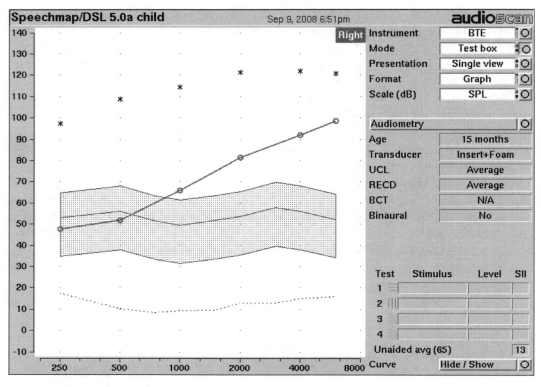

Figure 3–4. Audiogram from Figure 3–3 converted into dB SPL in the ear canal shown in SPLogram format. In addition to the child's thresholds, the long-term spectrum of conversational speech is shown (*shaded area*).

infant's hearing thresholds. Note that average conversational speech lies above this infant's thresholds in the lower frequencies, but falls below the thresholds in the higher frequencies. In this case it can be predicted that the infant will hear the lower pitch sounds of speech—vowel sounds, for example, but would be unable to detect many of the higher pitch sounds, such as voiceless consonants, without amplification. Once a prescriptive formula is selected, target levels are displayed for average conversational speech and for maximum hearing instrument output. Target values for average speech, the maximum output response of a hearing aid, and the amplified speech spectrum are shown in Figure 3-5. The latest version of the DSL prescriptive algorithm (DSL[*mi*/o] version 5.1; Scollie et al., 2005) also provides target levels for soft and loud conversational speech inputs.

Hearing Instrument Selection and Fitting

Preselection Considerations

Selecting hearing instruments for infants and young children requires consideration of their unique needs. Prior to ordering a hearing aid several factors must be consid-

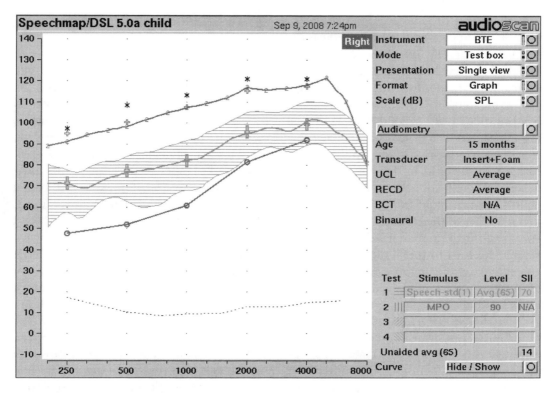

Figure 3–5. Electroacoustic verification measures plotted in ear canal SPL as a function of frequency (Hz). Variables shown include, from bottom to top, average normal hearing levels, the child's thresholds, the targets (*crosses*) for and measured amplified spectrum of average conversational speech (*shaded area*), as well as the targets for and measured output limiting levels across frequencies.

ered including: size, style, safety features and electroacoustic characteristics. Assuming the electroacoustic characteristics are appropriate, small, behind-the-ear instruments with soft earmolds are preferred. There are many reasons why in-the-ear (ITE) style hearing aids are not appropriate for infants and young children, including the need to re-case hearing aids as the child grows, lack of FM compatibility, safety issues related to the hard acrylic casing in the ear canal, and the inability to use a loaner instrument when the child's hearing aid is in need of repair.

Safety features, including tamper resistant battery doors and a mechanism to limit the child's access to the volume control, should be considered depending on the age of the child. Tamper resistant doors must function in a way that prevents the infant from gaining access to the battery while allowing the hearing instrument to be easily turned on and off during insertion or removal from the infant's ear. Ease of operation for the battery door is especially important for infants who will be in a daycare setting with multiple caregivers. Protection of the volume control mechanism requires careful thought when providing amplification for infants. Although care is taken to adjust the hearing instrument using prescriptive formulas, there are times when a family may return home following a visit to the audiology clinic only to find that the infant is reacting negatively to loud sounds or that the instrument has excessive feedback that was not obvious prior to the family's departure from the clinic. In these instances and in cases where feedback occurs prior to the child's next earmold fitting, it is useful for parents to have the option of reducing the volume control on a short-term basis until they can return to the audiology clinic for corrective action. In previous generations of hearing instruments this was accomplished using a volume control cover; however, in newer hearing instruments it is possible to deactivate the volume control. Although this may be a useful feature in certain situations, when working with infants it is necessary to prevent the child from changing the volume control setting while allowing parents access.

Electroacoustic flexibility also is a key consideration when selecting hearing instruments whereas because it is often necessary to proceed with limited information regarding the degree and configuration of hearing loss. In addition, some infants will have progressive hearing loss and will require adjustments to the hearing aid to provide additional gain. Furthermore, as the ear canal grows during the first several months of life, the RECD will decrease resulting in the need for a greater amount of gain than was required at the time of the initial hearing aid fitting. Finally, the hearing aid selected for a child should be sufficiently flexible to meet their changing listening needs as they grow and include features such as telecoils, FM compatibility, and an option to include multiple programs.

Hearing Instrument Programming

When using the manufacturer's software to program the electroacoustic performance of a hearing instrument, audiologists must make many decisions on which features to activate for a given child. Decisions must be made regarding choice of signal processing, feedback management, noise reduction strategies, and number of programs to include. The specific needs of infants and young children are different than those of adults. Although adults are able to judge when a feature is detrimental in a given listening situation, a young child is unable to control the selective use of these features. In addition, the listening behaviors and requirements of infants and toddlers are significantly different from those of older children and adults (Pittman, Stelmachowicz, Lewis, & Hoover, 2003; Stelmachowicz, Pittman, Hoover, & Lewis, 2001). For example, the importance of "overhearing speech" to the communication development of infants and young children makes a hearing instrument with an omnidirectional microphone the best choice for infants and young children in most listening situations. For this reason, whereas many hearing instruments have multiple programs, including some that sample sound in the environment and automatically switch between directional and omindirectional modes, a single, basic omnidirectional program is preferred during the initial stage of hearing instrument fitting for infants.

Toddlers whose families are using FM in the home environment may require a hearing aid that starts up in a program with both the FM microphone and the hearing aid microphone active and a second basic program with the FM deactivated for use at times when the FM transmitter is turned off. This type of program will eliminate the possibility of the child receiving an unwanted

FM signal and any interference that may occur from the FM receiver searching for an FM signal when the transmitter is off. School-aged children who are able to make decisions regarding their specific listening needs and are able to change programs in their hearing aids effectively may require multiple programs such as an FM and microphone setting, a program for "quiet" listening without FM that uses an omnidirectional microphone, a program that uses directional microphone technology and noise reduction, and a telephone program. Once programs have been selected, it is critical that electroacoustic verification of hearing instrument performance is completed to be certain that each program is functioning appropriately. It is important that the audiologist communicate with the family and the child to determine settings that are appropriate for their specific needs and that these needs are addressed periodically as the child grows.

When feedback management is required, it should be accomplished using algorithms that reduce feedback with minimal reduction in the high-frequency gain of the instrument.

Electroacoustic Verification

The goal of the verification stage in hearing instrument fitting is to determine if the performance characteristics of the hearing instrument match those specified by the selected evidence-based prescriptive algorithm (i.e., DSL, NAL). As previously discussed this is accomplished by using conventional real-ear probe microphone measures for older children and adults and by using a substitute procedure that incorporates the RECD measurement for infants and young children. Once the RECD has been measured, hearing thresholds have been entered into the verification system and the prescriptive formula has been specified, the hearing instrument is placed in a test chamber and attached to the hearing instrument coupler.

Newer verification systems use speech or speechlike signals to test the performance of current hearing instruments that use advanced digital processing. A recording of average conversational speech is delivered into the test chamber and the measured speech output, as amplified by the hearing instrument, is displayed on the screen. This allows comparison of the hearing instrument's actual performance to target levels. Next, a high level signal is delivered into the test chamber and the appropriateness of the maximum hearing instrument output can be evaluated against the prescribed target values. Any required modifications to performance can then be made using the programming capabilities of the manufacturer's fitting software. Finally, this approach to verification can be used to confirm the performance of the hearing instrument for average conversational speech as well as for soft and loud speech inputs to the hearing instrument. Once the audiologist has verified that the hearing instrument is performing appropriately, the settings are saved to memory.

Case Studies

The following two cases illustrate the importance of hearing aid verification at the time of hearing aid fitting and at follow-up visits, as well as the need for appropriate management after the fitting of acoustic amplification.

Case #1 is a child who failed her newborn hearing screen and a subsequent rescreening at one month of age. Frequency-specific ABR testing was completed at

2 months of age and she was diagnosed with severe bilateral sensorineural hearing loss. At 2½ months of age she returned for RECD measures and fitting of hearing aids matched to DSL targets verified using simulated real-ear measures. She was immediately enrolled in early intervention and received weekly home visits by a teacher of the deaf and hard of hearing; supplemental services were provided by a speech-language pathologist. RECD measures were repeated at the time of each earmold re-make. Behavioral audiometry was completed at 7 to 8 months of age using VRA with insert earphones and a complete audiogram for each ear was obtained for 250 to 4000 Hz. She returned to our clinic for hearing evaluation and verification of hearing aid function every 3 months. At 1 year of age a personal FM system was fitted and the family used it regularly during daily activities. Now at 4 years of age she uses speech as her primary mode of communication and recent speech-language evaluation scores were age appropriate. Her aided speech recognition threshold in sound field is 20 dB HL and her aided word recognition score for monosyllabic words at a conversational level is 88%. Her current audiogram and electroacoustic verification measures of hearing aid performance are shown in Figures 3–6 and 3–7, respectively. As shown in Figure 3–7, we successfully

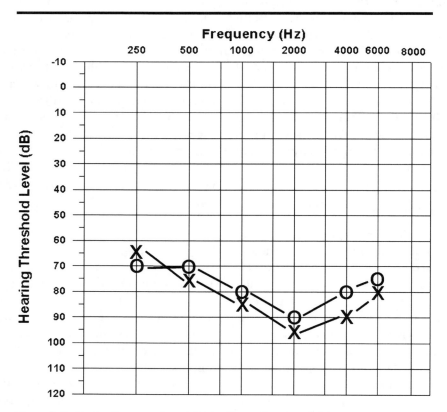

Figure 3–6. Audiogram for child in Case Study #1. Measures are plotted in dB HL.

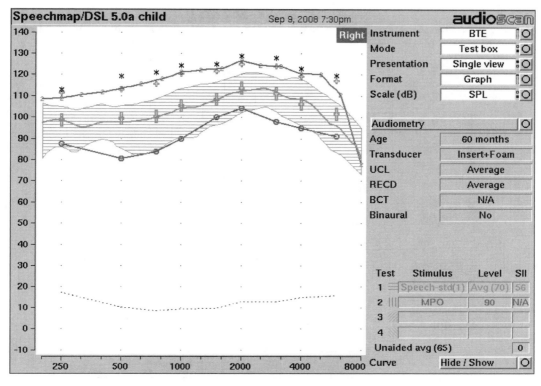

Figure 3–7. Verification measures for Case Study #1. Measures are plotted in dB SPL in the ear canal.

accomplished an appropriate match to the prescribed targets for both amplified conversational speech and output limiting. Based on these measures it can be predicted that conversational speech will be audible to this child across a broad range of frequencies.

The second child (Case #2) also was identified with hearing loss following a failed newborn hearing screen and subsequent re-screening a month after birth. Diagnostic ABR testing was completed and he was found to have a severe bilateral sensorineural hearing loss. He was fitted with binaural hearing aids at another clinic at 4 months of age, and subsequently enrolled in the state early intervention program with weekly

home visits by a teacher of the deaf and hard of hearing. At 2 years of age the child was referred for cochlear implant evaluation by his teacher due to lack of progress with communication goals. At the time of the evaluation his parents reported that he was not using any words expressively, and although their preference was for spoken language, he had acquired no speech and was communicating primarily through gestures. Behavioral audiometry using VRA confirmed a severe, bilateral sensorineural hearing loss (Figure 3–8). Prior to formal cochlear implant evaluation, the electroacoustic performance of his hearing aids was evaluated using simulated real-ear measures

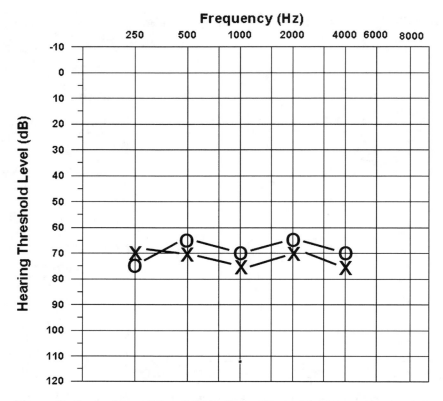

Figure 3–8. Audiogram for child in Case Study #2. Measures are plotted in dB HL.

with DSL targets for gain and output. As shown in Figure 3-9, this child's hearing aids delivered amplified speech well below target levels, and consequently provide limited audibility of speech in the mid frequencies and essentially no audibility for the low- or high-frequency components of speech. Figure 3-9 also shows that the output limiting characteristics for the child's hearing aids were below DSL targets by as much as 25 dB. In fact, the measured output limiting level at 250 Hz fell well below the child's threshold of detection for that frequency, ensuring inaudibility of all sounds in that frequency region. In this case the potential benefits derived from early identi-

fication and fitting were lost due to inappropriate hearing aid fitting. Regrettably, such cases are not unusual in our experience.

Although both of these children were identified with hearing loss at birth and received regular home-based intervention, their outcomes are significantly different. The child illustrated in Case #2 received suboptimal amplification and, consequently, missed the opportunity to develop speech and language on a normal trajectory. Although the audibility of speech does not ensure that spoken language will develop at a normal rate, lack of audibility, as shown in Case #2 makes poor communication development a certainty.

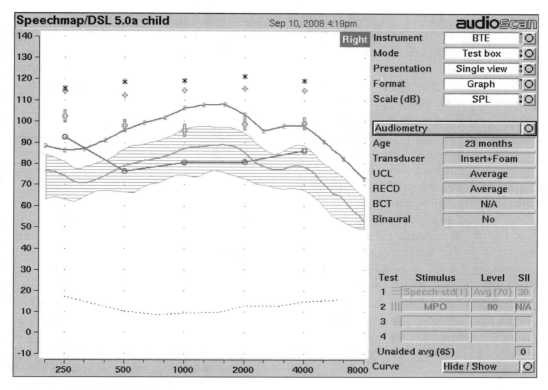

Figure 3–9. Verification measures for Case Study #2. Measures are plotted in dB SPL in the ear canal.

Hearing Aid Orientation

Sufficient time must be allotted during the hearing instrument fitting to provide a comprehensive orientation to the care and use of the instruments. Family members need practice inserting and removing the hearing aids and instruction regarding maintenance of the hearing aids and earmolds, warranty information, and troubleshooting techniques. Our "care kit" includes a listening stethoset, battery tester, air blower, dehumidifier, and retention strap. Families of infants and toddlers must be informed of the need for frequent earmold replacements as their child grows. In our experience it is not unusual for an infant fitted with hearing

aids at 2 months of age to require six to eight sets of earmolds in the first year. Finally, families must be encouraged to pursue full-time hearing aid use and active participation in early intervention services.

There are many practical issues that need to be considered. Families must understand that infants can learn to remove their hearing aids and, once removed, put them in their mouths. Although this may not be a significant concern at 2 to 3 months of age, many families report problems with removal of hearing aids beginning at 4 to 5 months of age. Options for retaining the instruments include retention straps and double-sided tape. If these techniques are unsuccessful another option families have found to be successful on a short-term basis is the use of a lightweight cap that ties under the chin. This is not a permanent solution but one that can be effective in cases where the parents, despite their best efforts, are unable to keep the hearing aids in place. This short-term strategy combined with persistence by the family will likely result in full-time hearing aid use within the first few weeks.

Time spent educating the family about hearing aid retention, troubleshooting, repair, and follow-up, will not only help them get off to a good start, but it will reduce the number of phone calls to the audiologist during the first few weeks after hearing instrument fitting. A return appointment should be scheduled 3 to 4 weeks following the initial fitting. During that visit the audiologist can answer questions, check on the progress of early intervention services, and discuss the infant's auditory behavior and benefits of amplification.

Validation Measures

Validation measures are used to determine if the amplification characteristics are providing the infant or young child with access to auditory information that is sufficient to achieve communication goals. For older children this can be accomplished with open-set aided speech recognition testing using recorded word or sentence materials. Although the tools available to obtain reliable outcome measures for young children are limited, closed-set speech recognition tests such as the Early Speech Perception test (Moog & Geers, 1990) may be useful in the assessment of emerging skills. For a comprehensive review of this topic the reader is referred to the chapters in this volume dedicated to assessment of speech perception (Arthur Boothroyd) and spoken word recognition (Karen Iler Kirk and colleagues). In addition to performing devel-

opmentally appropriate speech perception measures the pediatric audiologist should communicate regularly with the child's early intervention providers so that adjustments or changes in technology are made in a timely manner.

Other Considerations

FM Systems

The benefits of personal FM systems for improving speech recognition in noise have been known for many years (Fabry, 1994; Hawkins, 1984). Even so, FM technology continues to be underused. When effectively applied, FM can significantly improve access to acoustic information for children with hearing loss. Indeed, studies have shown that FM technology can improve the signal-to-noise ratio in the classroom by as much as 10 to 20 dB (Crandell & Smaldino, 2000, 2001). It is imperative, therefore, that any child with bilateral hearing loss be provided access to personal FM for use in the classroom and other settings.

In years past FM systems were large, bulky, body-worn devices used primarily in the educational setting. Improvements in design and reduction in size have made it possible for FM systems to be considered for use by parents and other caregivers in the home environment. Many families are now electing to use personal FM to improve the signal-to-noise ratio during day-to-day activities in the car, the grocery store, or on the playground.

In an effort to evaluate benefit from personal FM in the home environment, Moeller and colleagues evaluated language outcomes for two groups of preschool-aged children with mild to severe hearing loss (Moeller, Donaghy, Beauchaine, Lewis, & Stelmachowicz, 1996). One group used FM combined with their hearing aids at home and the other group used hearing aids alone. Although language scores for the FM group were not significantly different, some of the children in the FM group made unusual gains in language acquisition during the course of the study. Furthermore, parents and children in the study reported that FM systems were beneficial in a variety of specific listening environments. Practical issues regarding FM system use were also evaluated. Challenges included the cumbersome nature of body-worn devices and problems associated with electromagnetic interference. Fortunately, FM technology has improved significantly since this study was conducted and many of the problems reported have been eliminated.

Today, the options for FM use include: (1) fully integrated receivers incorporated into the design of the hearing aid; (2) dedicated receivers that can be attached to a specific make and model of hearing aid; and (3) universal receivers that can be used with many different models and coupled using a small "audio shoe" that provides an interface between the hearing aid and the FM receiver.

In our experience, a good time to introduce FM systems is around the first birthday when the child begins to walk and when there is increasing distance between the parent and child. It is preferable to establish full-time hearing aid use prior to the introduction of FM. Families need to understand the importance of frequent device monitoring and troubleshooting in environments where FM systems will be used, and the need to activate both the hearing aid microphone and the transmitter.

New and Future Technologies

Frequency Compression

For many years concerns have been raised regarding the limited ability of hearing aids to provide audibility of high-frequency speech sounds and the resulting negative effect on children's speech production and language abilities (Boothroyd & Medwetsky, 1992; Moeller et al., 2007a, 2007b; Stelmachowicz et al., 2001). Recently, Stelmachowicz and colleagues (Stelmachowicz, Pittman, Hoover, Lewis, & Moeller, 2004) evaluated the phonological development of two groups of infants with hearing loss compared to a group of infants with normal hearing. They found marked delays in the acquisition of all phonemes for the infants with hearing loss, with the longest delays occurring for fricatives. This was true even for children amplified before 12 months of age. Stelmachowicz et al. (2004) concluded that the bandwidth of current behind-the-ear hearing aids is inadequate to accurately represent the high-frequency sounds of speech, particularly for female speakers.

A variety of different frequency lowering strategies have been used over the years in an effort to provide greater access to high-frequency information including: time varying whole-band frequency transposition; time varying whole-band frequency transposition of a pass-band centered on a high-frequency peak; and time-varying proportional frequency compression. Recently, a strategy using high-frequency nonlinear frequency compression has been implemented and is now available for clinical use (Scollie, Bagatto, Seewald, & Johnson, 2008; Glista, et al., under review; Scollie, et al., under review). The strategy is showing promise and may be beneficial for some children; however, there is a need for further research involving larger groups of children with varying degree and configuration of hearing loss. Audiologists who recommend amplification and cochlear implantation should stay current on these and other options available for children hearing loss.

Conclusion

In 2006, Dr. Mark Ross, an audiologist with hearing loss whose pioneering work formed the basis of what we now call the Desired Sensation Level (DSL) prescriptive formula, received a cochlear implant after many years of hearing aid use. Dr. Ross carefully chronicled his experience with the implant process, including the preimplant evaluation and postimplant follow up. In an article that appeared in *Hearing Loss Magazine* (Ross, 2007) he wrote: "The organized and careful follow-up testing that is done for people receiving cochlear implants does raise a question about the relative absence of such care for people wearing hearing aids . . . " (p. 28). We concur with Dr. Ross. In our experience it is not unusual for children identified at birth with significant residual hearing to be referred for cochlear implantation as toddlers due to "lack of progress" from acoustic amplification. Yet, evaluation of their hearing aids often reveals settings that are inadequate for the perception of speech even at conversational levels. We recognize that there are many factors that affect outcomes for children with hearing loss including age at identification, age at hearing aid fitting, consistency of hearing aid use, and, for some, additional disabilities. But in many cases, outcomes might have been better had optimally fitted acoustic amplification been available from the initial hearing aid fitting.

As pediatric audiologists, our goal should be to provide the best possible access to sound for every child diagnosed with hearing loss. Accurate diagnostic procedures combined with the application of evidence-based protocols for pediatric hearing aid selection and fitting will ensure that cochlear implantation is reserved for children unable to benefit from hearing aid use, whereas those with sufficient residual hearing receive optimal benefit from acoustic amplification.

References

American Academy of Audiology. (2004). Pediatric Amplification Guidelines. *Audiology Today, 16,* 46–53.

Bagatto, M., Moodie, S., Scollie, S., Seewald, R., Moodie, S., Pumford, J., et al. (2005). Clinical protocols for hearing instrument fitting in the Desired Sensation Level Method. *Trends in Amplification, 9,* 199–226.

Bagatto, M. P., Scollie, S. D., Moodie, K. S., & Hoover, B. M. (2002). Real-ear-to-coupler difference predictions as a function of age for two different coupling procedures. *Journal of the American Academy of Audiology, 13,* 407–415.

Bamford, J., Beresford, D., Mencher, G., DeVoe, S., Owen, V., & Davis, A. (2001). Provision and fitting of new technology hearing aids: Implications from a survey of some "good practice services" in UK and USA. In R. C. Seewald & J. S. Gravel (Eds.), *A sound foundation through early amplification: Proceedings of the Second International Conference* (pp. 213–219). Stäfa, Switzerland: Phonak AG.

Boothroyd, A., & Medwetsky, M. (1992). Spectral distribution of /s/ and the frequency response of hearing aids. *Ear and Hearing, 13*(3), 150–157.

College of Audiologists and Speech-Language Pathologists of Ontario. (2002). *Preferred practice guideline for the prescription of hearing aids to children.* Retrieved July 25, 2008, from: http://www.caslpo.com/Portals/0/ppg/preshearingaidschild.pdf

Cornelisse, L. E., Seewald, R. C., & Jamieson, D. G. (1995). The input/output formula: A theoretical approach to the fitting of personal amplification devices. *Journal of the Acoustical Society of America, 97,* 1854–1864.

Crandell, C., & Smaldino, J. (2000). Room acoustics for listeners with normal hearing and hearing impaired. In M. Valente., R. Roeser, & H. Hosford-Dunn (Eds.), *Audiology: Treatment strategies* (pp. 601–638). New York: Thieme Medical.

Crandell, C., & Smaldino, J. (2001). Improving classroom acoustics: Utilizing hearing assistive technology and communication strategies in the educational setting. *Volta Review, 101,* 47–62.

Dillon, H. (1999). NAL-NL1: A new prescriptive fitting procedure for non-linear hearing aids. *Hearing Journal, 52,* 10–16.

Erber, N. P. (1973). Body-baffle and real-ear effects in the selection of hearing aids for deaf children. *Journal of Speech and Hearing Disorders, 38,* 224–231.

Fabry, D. A. (1994). Noise reduction with FM systems in FM/EM mode. *Ear and Hearing, 15,* 82–86.

Gengel, R. W., Pascoe, D., & Shore, I. (1971). A frequency-response procedure for evaluating and selecting hearing aids for severely hearing impaired children. *Journal of Speech and Hearing Disorders, 36,* 341–353.

Glista, D., Scollie, S., Bagatto, M., Seewald, R., & Johnson, A. (manuscript submitted for publication). *Evaluation of nonlinear frequency compression II: Clinical outcomes.*

Gorga, M. P., Johnson, T. A., Kaminski, J. R., Beauchaine, K. L., Garner, C. A., & Neely, S. T. (2006). Using a combination of click- and tone burst-evoked auditory brainstem response measurements to estimate pure-tone thresholds. *Ear and Hearing, 27,* 60–74.

Gravel, J. S. (2000). Audiologic assessment for the fitting of hearing instruments: Big challenges from tiny ears. In R. C. Seewald (Ed.), *A sound foundation through early amplification: Proceedings of the First International Conference* (pp. 33–54). Stäfa, Switzerland: Phonak AG.

Gravel, J., & Hood, L. (1998). Pediatric audiologic assessment. In F. E. Musiek & W. F. Rintelmann (Eds.), *Contemporary perspectives in hearing assessment* (pp. 305–326). Boston: Allyn and Bacon.

Guidelines for the Fitting, Verification and Evaluation of Digital Signal Processing Hearing Aids within a Children's Hearing Aid Service. (2005). *Modernising children's hearing aid services programme* (pp. 1–3). UK: University of Manchester, School of Psychological Services Retrieved August 1, 2008, from: http://www.psych-sci.manchester.ac.uk/mchas/guidelines/fittingguidelines.doc

Hawkins, D. B. (1984). Comparisons of speech recognition in noise by mildly-to-moderately hearing impaired children using hearing aids and FM systems. *Journal of Speech and Hearing Disorders, 49,* 409–418.

Hawkins, D. B., Montgomery, A. A., Prosek, R. A., & Walden, B. E. (1987). Examination of two issues concerning functional gain measurements. *Journal of Speech and Hearing Research, 52,* 56–63.

Johnson, T. A., & Brown, C. J. (2005). Threshold prediction using the auditory steady-state response and the tone burst auditory brainstem response: A within-subject comparison. *Ear and Hearing, 26,* 559–576.

Keidser, G., Brew, C., & Peck, A. (2003). Proprietary fitting algorithms compared with one another and with generic formulas. *Hearing Journal, 56,* 28–38.

Moeller, M. P., Donaghy, K. F., Beauchaine, K. L., Lewis, D. E., & Stelmachowicz, P. G. (1996). Longitudinal study of FM system use in nonacademic settings: Effects on language development. *Ear and Hearing, 17,* 28–41.

Moeller, M. P., Hoover, B., Putman, C., Arbataitis, K., Bohnenkamp, G., Peterson, B., et al. (2007a). Vocalizations of infants with hearing loss compared with infants with normal hearing: Part I—Phonetic development. *Ear and Hearing, 28,* 605–627.

Moeller, M. P., Hoover, B., Putman, C., Arbataitis, K., Bohnenkamp, G., Peterson, B., et al. (2007b). Vocalizations of infants with hearing loss compared with infants with normal hearing: Part II—Transition to words. *Ear and Hearing, 28,* 628–642.

Moodie, L. S., Seewald, R. C., & Sinclair, S. T. (1994). Procedure for predicting real-ear hearing aid performance in young children. *American Journal of Audiology, 3,* 23–31.

Moog J. S., & Geers, A. E. (1990). *Early Speech Perception Test.* St. Louis, MO: Central Institute for the Deaf.

Mueller, H. G., Bentler, R. A. , & Wu, Y-H. (2008). Prescribing maximum hearing aid output: Differences among manufacturers found. *Hearing Journal, 61,* 30–36.

Munro, K. J. (2005). Update on RECD measures in children. In R. C. Seewald & J. M. Bamford (Eds.), *A sound foundation through early amplification: Proceedings of the Third International Conference* (pp. 71–89). Stäfa, Switzerland: Phonak AG.

Ontario Infant Hearing Program Provision of Amplification Protocol and Guidelines. (2007). Ministry of Children and Youth Services, Ontario, Canada. Retrieved July 25, 2008 from http://www.mountsinai.on.ca/care/infant-hearing-program/documents/amplification_revision_2007_006.pdf

Pediatric Working Group of the Conference on Amplification for Children with Auditory Deficits. (1996). Amplification for infants and children with hearing loss. *American Journal of Audiology, 5*, 53–68.

Pittman, A. L., Stelmachowicz, P. G., Lewis, D. E., & Hoover, B. M. (2003). Spectral characteristics of speech at the ear: Implications for amplification in children. *Journal of Speech, Language, and Hearing Research, 46*, 649–657.

Rance, G. (2005). Auditory neuropathy and its perceptual consequences. *Trends in Amplification, 9*, 1–43.

Rance, G., & Rickards, F. (2002). Prediction of hearing thresholds in infants using auditory steady-state evoked potentials. *Journal of the American Academy of Audiology, 13*, 236–245.

Ross, M. (1975). Hearing aid selection for preverbal hearing-impaired children. In M. C. Pollack (Ed.), *Amplification for the hearing-impaired* (pp. 207–242). New York: Grune and Stratton.

Ross, M. (2007, March/April). Reflections on my cochlear implant: Part one. *Hearing Loss Magazine*, pp. 24–28.

Scollie, S. D., Bagatto, M. P., Seewald, R. C., & Johnson, A. (2008). Multichannel nonlinear frequency compression: A new technology for children with hearing loss. In R.C. Seewald (Ed.), *A sound foundation through early amplification: Proceedings of an International Conference*. Stäfa, Switzerland: Phonak AG.

Scollie, S., Parsa, V., Glista, D., Bagatto, M., Wirtzfeld, M., & Seewald, R. (manuscript submitted for publication). *Evaluation of non-linear frequency compression I: Fitting rationale*.

Scollie, S. D., Seewald, R. C., Cornelisse, L. E., & Jenstad, L. M. (1998). Validity and repeatability of level-independent HL to SPL transforms. *Ear and Hearing, 19*, 407–413.

Scollie, S., Seewald, R., Cornelisse, L., Moodie, L., Bagatto, M., Laurnagaray, Beaulac, S., & Pumford, J. (2005). The Desired Sensation Level multistage input/output algorithm. *Trends in Amplification, 9*, 159–197.

Seewald, R. C. (1995). The desired sensation level (DSL) method for hearing aid fitting in infants and children. *Phonak Focus, 20*. Stäfa, Switzerland: Phonak AG.

Seewald, R. C., Mills, J., Bagatto, M., Scollie, S., & Moodie, S. (2008). A comparison of manufacturer-specific prescriptive procedures for infants. *Hearing Journal, 61*, 26–33.

Seewald, R. C., Moodie, K. S., Sinclair, S. T., & Cornelisse, L. E. (1996). Traditional and theoretical approaches to selecting amplification for infants and young children. In F. H. Bess, J. S. Gravel, & A. M. Tharpe (Eds.), *Amplification for children with auditory deficits* (pp. 161–192). Nashville, TN: Bill Wilkerson Center Press.

Seewald, R. C, Moodie, K. S., Sinclair, S. T., & Scollie, S. D. (1999). Predictive validity of a procedure for pediatric hearing instrument fitting. *American Journal of Audiology, 8*, 143–152.

Seewald, R. C., & Scollie, S. D. (1999). Infants are not average adults: Implications for audiometric testing. *Hearing Journal, 52*, 64–72.

Stapells, D. R. (2000). Frequency-specific evoked potential audiometry in infants. In R.C. Seewald (Ed.), *A sound foundation through early amplification: Proceedings of an International Conference* (pp. 13–31). Stäfa, Switzerland: Phonak AG.

Stelmachowicz, P. G., & Lewis D. E. (1988). Some theoretical considerations concerning the relation between functional gain and insertion gain. *Journal of Speech and Hearing Research, 31*, 491–496.

Stelmachowicz, P. G., Pittman, A. L., Hoover, B. M., & Lewis, D. E. (2001). Effect of stimulus bandwidth on the perception of /s/ in normal- and hearing-impaired children and adults. *Journal of the Acoustical Society of America, 110*, 2183–2190.

Stelmachowicz, P. G., Pittman, A. L., Hoover, B. M., Lewis,D. E., & Moeller, M. P. (2004). The importance of high-frequency audibility in the speech and language development of children with hearing loss. *Archives of Otolaryngology-Head and Neck Surgery*, *130*, 556–562.

Widen, J. E. (1990). Behavioral screening of high-risk infants using visual reinforcement audiometry. *Seminars in Hearing*, *11*(4), 342–356.

Widen, J. E., Folsom, R. C., Cone-Wesson, B., Carty, L., Dunnell, J. J., Koebsell, K., et al. (2000). Identification of neonatal hearing impairment: Hearing status at 8–12 months corrected age using a visual reinforcement audiometry protocol. *Ear and Hearing*, *21*, 471–487.

CHAPTER 4

Bilateral Cochlear Implants in Children

RUTH Y. LITOVSKY
JANE MADELL

Introduction

Our ability to operate in an auditory environment depends on the extent to which the auditory system is able to perform certain functions, such as determination of **what** is being communicated, and **where** that sound is coming from (Blauert, 1997; Bronkhorst, 2000). These functions in turn depend on the ability of the listener's auditory system to capture and relay directional cues, suppress echoes in reverberant environments, and to group or segregate sounds based on relevant features (Blauert, 1997; Yost, 1997). These functions are highly relevant to children whose lives revolve around spending many hours every day in noisy environments, including classrooms, recreation areas and common eating areas, to name a few (Litovsky, 2005). People with normal hearing sometimes struggle in these situations as well, but they are equipped with basic auditory mechanisms that make

it easier to do so (Blauert, 1997; Hawley, Litovksy, & Culling, 2004). Hearing-impaired people, and cochlear implant users in particular, have a much more challenging mission before them. In this chapter we review basic auditory mechanisms that are involved in binaural hearing, the potential advantages that persons with bilateral hearing might gain, outcomes measures in children with bilateral hearing, and suggestions for bilateral mapping approaches in children who use bilateral cochlear implants.

Defining Binaural Hearing

Acoustics

Binaural hearing comes from the ability of an individual's brain to integrate inputs from the two ears and to utilize acoustic cues that are not present when a single ear is stimulated. However, the mere stimulation of both ears does not mean that by necessity binaural information is available, or that the brain is able to process the incoming binaural cues. In order for binaural hearing to occur, there are obligatory steps along the way. First, the cues themselves must be captured by the listener's anatomical structures. Second, the listener's auditory system must be equipped with functional neural mechanisms that are specifically tuned to binaural stimuli. In addition to these steps, there is the issue of listeners' experiences and expectations, as well as the attentional and cognitive constructs that can vary greatly among individuals. The latter is an area that is often mentioned anecdotally but not well understood.

In the field of audiology, definition of binaural hearing can be challenging because numerous variables limit and/or alter the extent to which binaural cues are preserved by amplification systems and subsequently processed by the auditory system. For example, in persons with hearing impairment who are aided by hearing aids and/or cochlear implants, the directional characteristics and signal processing strategies of the devices alter acoustic cues prior to the arrival of those cues at the auditory system. In addition, limited access to auditory information, also referred to by some as auditory deprivation, can alter the ability of the binaural system to process binaural cues.

Binaural hearing in real-world environments typically can occur when sounds reach the ears from particular locations in space. Due to the fact that the head has a spherical shape, on either side of which the ears are placed, several binaural cues arise. Interaural differences in time (ITDs) occur because any sound that is closer to one of the two ears will reach the closer ear first,

and by the time it arrives at the farther ear there will be a naturally occurring time delay. Each location in space around the head will create a different ITD value. For instance, a sound that is at 90° to the right will create an ITD of about 700 microseconds (less than 1/1000 of a second); a sound that is directly in front will have an ITD equal to zero. ITDs are particularly relevant for stimuli that have low-frequency carriers (<1500 Hz). ITDs also are perceived from stimuli that have high-frequency carriers whose amplitude is modulated. Interaural level differences (ILDs) occur because a sound that is closer to one of the two ears reaches the nearer ear with greater intensity. The head acts as an "acoustic shadow" or "block" that physically interferes with sound waves as they travel around the head. The reduction of intensity of sound waves reaching the ear from the opposite side of the head is particularly relevant to high-frequency stimuli (>2500 Hz). Examples of low- and high-frequency stimuli with ITD and ILD cues are shown in Figure 4–1.

In addition to binaural cues that require two ears, some cues also exist that can be captured with a single ear. Due to the unique anatomical shape of the ear, a listener is able to determine whether sounds arrive from different elevations (up versus down), and also whether sounds that have the same angle on the horizontal plane are in front versus behind. This occurs because the ear acts like a filter; for each location the "filter" lets in more energy at certain frequencies than others. The end result is that listeners can use a set of spectral cues to localize sounds in elevation and front/back. These cues are reduced, if at all available, to people whose amplification systems (hearing aids or cochlear implants) have microphones placed above the ear, rather than inside the ear canal.

Cues for Localizing Sounds in Space

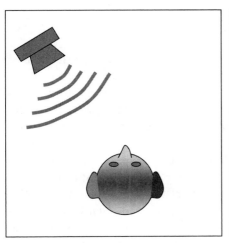 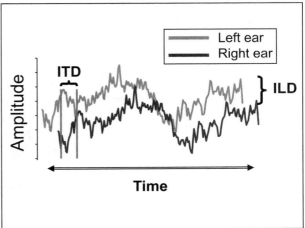

Figure 4–1. As sounds reach the head from a particular location in space, binaural cues are created due to differences in the arrival of the sound at the two ears. Differences include interaural time (ITD) and interaural level (ILD). In this schematic, sounds arrive first in the left ear, and have greater intensity in that ear.

Anatomy and Physiology

Once stimuli are encoded by the cochlea and the auditory nerve, they initially synapse in the cochlear nucleus. Projections from the cochlear nucleus feed into two parallel binaural systems, one that encodes ITDs primarily at low frequencies (medial superior olive; MSO), and one that encodes ILDs, primarily at high frequencies (lateral superior olive; LSO). Inputs from the MSO and LSO then recombine at higher brain centers to form a complete set of cues that represent sound source direction. Neurons at these higher centers are able to perform many of the important functions that enable mammals to initiate behaviors in the environments ultimately resulting in the ability to localize sounds, segregate speech and noise, detect sound motion, and suppres echoes. An area with growing interest is one that focuses on the extent to which binaural hearing utilizing ITD and ILD cues can be achieved by persons who are deaf and use bilateral cochlear implants. There is evidence to suggest that sensitivity to ITDs and ILDs can be achieved when research processors are precisely used to control the relative timing and level between pairs of electrodes in the two ears. However, the extent to which the binaural sensitivity is within the range of that seen in persons who do not have hearing loss remains to be seen. It also must be noted that the need for conducting these studies using research processors arises from the fact that today's speech processors are not designed to work in coordination or under dual-processing schemes. Rather, they were designed as monaural processors intended for single-ear usage. Their ability to preserve binaural cues and provide for the arrival of those cues at the auditory system is greatly limited by the way they are engineered.

Perception

Sound Localization

One of the hallmarks of binaural hearing is the ability of two-eared listeners to localize sounds. Demonstration of these effects is often carried out experimentally by removal of certain cues that are thought to be important, and then by measuring the effect of the cue removal on listeners' performance. A straight-forward example of the utility of binaural hearing comes from experiments in which stimuli are presented to a single ear of normal-hearing listeners. Although it is feasible to conduct testing in free-field and plug an ear, this is an unnatural condition that does not accurately mimic total deafness in the plugged ear and hence is not truly monaural. An alternate approach is to utilize virtual acoustic space (VAS) stimuli whereby directional cues are measured with a microphone placed at the entrance to the ear canal and presented over headphones, thus reproducing free-field listening. This approach enables direct control over stimuli reaching each ear and provides a means of simulating single-ear deafness. Using this approach several studies have demonstrated that the absence of binaural hearing leads to severe degradation in sound localization abilities of persons with normal hearing. Monaural spectral and level cues, although present, are simply not sufficient to enable listeners to perform the same functions that they are able to under binaural conditions (e.g., Hawley et al., 2004; Macpherson & Middle-

brooks, 2002; for review see Middlebrooks & Green, 1991).

Source Segregation

The availability of hearing in both ears also serves the important function of enabling listeners to understand speech in the presence of competing background speech and/or noise. One effect, known as the *better ear effect*, occurs when competing sounds arrive at the ears from different spatial locations such that the signal-to-masker ratio is higher at one ear than at the other ear. An example of this scenario can be seen in Figure 4-2. If both ears are operational, then when speech arrives from the listener's left side, a noise that is on the right will produce less interference than a noise that also arrives from the left. When the speech and noise are spatially separated, the speech effectively has a better signal-to-noise ratio (SNR) in the left ear. Although there are conditions under which having a nonfunctional ear would effectively improve the SNR for speech in the hearing ear, overall, in complex auditory environments there are numerous circumstances under which having two operational ears maximizes listeners' abilities to segregate speech from competing noise. It is noteworthy that even in absence of spatial separation there is an added benefit of having two operational ears due to *binaural summation*, whereby the auditory system can potentially obtain two "looks" at the signal, and to thus extract more information than with a single "look" alone. These two effects (better ear and binaural summation) are due to redundancy of information.

Binaural mechanisms per se can also be invoked to facilitate source segregation. In persons with normal acoustic hearing ITDs and ILDs play an important role (Culling, Hawley, & Litovsky, 2004). By utilizing the

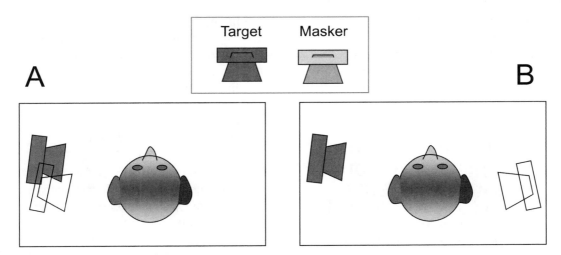

Figure 4–2. Schematic diagram illustrating examples of speech-in-noise configurations. The listener is facing front, with target speech on the left. In panel **A**, the noise source is also on the left, whereas in panel **B** the noise source is on the right, 180° apart from the target.

ITD/ILD circuitry described above, there are effects that can maximize understanding of speech in noise, such as binaural unmasking. When studied over headphones, a signal that is presented to both ears with no interaural differences will be correlated across the ears. If a signal and noise are both highly correlated, and perceived to be in the center of the head, then the audibility of the signal will be reduced. However, the signal can be more easily heard if the phase of the signal in one ear is inverted, which will decorrelate the signal in the two ears. The effect of "interaural decorrelation" can be extended to speech understanding in noisy situations, when the speech and noise arrive from different locations and vary in the extent and type of decorrelation (Akeroyd & Summerfield, 2000; Durlach & Colburn, 1978). The use of interaural correlation information is a critical aspect of listeners' ability to extract speech from noisy backgrounds. More important, it can be achieved in absence of low-frequency ITD information.

Cochlear Implants

Cochlear implants (CI) are used widely to provide hearing to persons with severe-to-profound hearing loss, in particular, when there is little or no benefit from amplification. Adults and children alike can use sound provided by CIs to interpret incoming speech signals. The success rate today is high, such that most adult users understand and communicate with minimal lip reading, especially in quiet listening environments. In addition, many children can learn in mainstream environments and communicate with their hearing peers. However, there is variation in the success of CI use. In part, this is because CI users encounter difficulty when understanding speech in noisy environments, and struggle to find additional vehicles for communication to augment their social interactions and to function in the work place. For children, the same issues apply in learning environments, such as classrooms, which are typically robust with noise, reverberation, and competing signals. In addition, most CI users report that they cannot locate the position of sound sources, and that all sounds appear to come from inside or behind their ear.

Bilateral Cochlear Implants: Potential Advantages and Suggested Clinical Measures

Because of the difficulties that limit the ability of adults and children to orient in the environment and to function easily in complex acoustic spaces, efforts are being made to improve the audibility and intelligibility of speech signals that occur in noise. One approach used in a growing number of clinics, which can help with both speech intelligibility and sound localization, is provision of bilateral CIs (BI-CIs), that is, implantation of both ears. To date, several thousand individuals have been implanted bilaterally worldwide, either in sequential procedures (the two ears are activated months or years apart), or simultaneously (both ears are implanted in a single surgery and activated at the same time). There appears to be a growing recommendation for BI-CIs, and it is important that candidate patients be educated about the potential outcomes with BI-CIs. We adhere to the term *bilateral* rather than *binaural* because the former refers to having two functional ears. The term *binaural*, however, refers to having bilateral hearing plus an additional guarantee that there is an obligatory mechanism for coordination between the inputs arriving at the two ears. These terms are differentiated from one another here because in

persons with BI-CIs the two processors (separate ones attached to each ear) work independently. This is unlike the normal auditory system, whereby the two ears work in synchrony.

General Findings in Adults

In a deaf person fitted with BI-CIs, bilateral hearing occurs because each ear receives a signal, and the brain can generally compare overall differences between the ears in sound level (van Hoesel, 2004). Some gross differences in timing of sounds between the ears might also occur (van Hoesel, 2004). Overall, bilateral hearing plus some minimal binaural hearing can most likely offer BI-CI users some advantages compared to using a single CI. Similar to what has been shown in adults with normal hearing, the ability to localize sounds with two versus one CI has been a widely used measure to demonstrate the potential benefits of bilateral CIs. In the real world, one would want to know about benefits in situations that are similar to the acoustic environments encountered in the work place, in social situations, recreational sport activities, and everyday activities such as crossing the street in traffic. Although these issues have not been directly addressed, numerous studies have documented significant benefits attributed to the use of two CIs compared with one CI in adults, in controlled laboratory environments (Grantham, Ashmead, Ricketts, Labadie, & Haynes, 2007; Litovsky et al., 2004; Neuman, Haravon, Sislian, & Waltzman, 2007; Schleich, Nopp, & D'Haese, 2004; van Hoesel & Tyler, 2003; Verschuur, Lutman, Ramsden, Greenham & O'Driscoll, 2005). For example, when adults are asked to identify the location of sound sources positioned in the horizontal plane, localization errors measured as root-mean-square (RMS) error, typically average 20 to 30° in bilateral listening modes and 50 to 60° when a single CI is used. In this context it is important to recognize that, other than anecdotal reports from patients, little is known about documented benefits in more realistic, complex and challenging listening environments. For children, the issue of sound localization also translates directly to everyday situations, including the need to monitor multiple ongoing sound sources in classrooms, playground situations, and sports activities; safety becomes an issue when the need arises to avoid moving objects, crossing a busy street, and so forth.

Studies with adults also have shown that speech understanding in the presence of competing speech or noise can be significantly better when both CIs are used compared to single-CI conditions. However, the magnitude and type of advantage seen across patients are not universal. Although most patients are able to benefit from the head shadow effect, the size of effect varies from 1 to 2 dB in some subjects to over 20 dB in others. In addition, a relatively small number of BI-CI users show benefits that require binaural processing, such as the "squelch effect" and binaural summation (Nopp et al., 2004; Schleich et al. 2004; van Hoesel, 2004). Variability in performance of CI users extends much beyond bilateral studies and is indeed a commonly reported finding for measures of monaural abilities (e.g., Henry & Turner, 2003; Skinner, Holden, Demorest, & Holden, 1995; Zeng , 2004).

Studies in Children

Recent studies by Litovsky and colleagues have documented improved sound localization precision in children with bilateral implants, in controlled laboratory settings that are relatively quiet. These studies focused on children's ability to identify source locations when using either a single CI or both CIs together, and suggest that, overall, children are better able to discriminate between source locations when using both CIs than when using a single CI alone. The approaches for obtaining these measures are different for children ages 4 years and older (Litovsky, Johnstone, & Godar, 2006a; Litovsky et al., 2006b) and in children who are 1 to 3 years of age (Grieco-Calub, Litovsky, & Werner, 2008). The approaches used by Litovsky and colleagues have been implemented in children who are deemed by their parents and audiologists to be successful users of their CIs, whose primary and dominant mode of communication is auditory-oral, and who do not have known developmental delays or diagnoses other than hearing loss. That is not to say that the approaches are not relevant to children with other modes of communication or who have additional diagnoses, but the conclusions that can be drawn from this work are for now only relevant to the populations studied.

When measuring spatial hearing in children, the question of interest is typically: *how well can a child identify where a sound source is coming from?* For children with normal hearing this ability is present in a rudimentary form at birth. Newborn infants orient toward the direction of auditory stimuli within hours after birth. The head-orienting response is a reflexive behavior that enables the infant to bring visual targets into view, and to integrate auditory and visual information. Reflexive behaviors such as head turns have been used for decades to investigate how accurately young infants can discriminate between sounds that are presented from their right versus left (e.g., Clifton, Morrongiello, Kulig, & Dowd,

1981; Muir & Field, 1979; for review see Litovsky & Ashmead, 1997). Most notable is the fact that spatial hearing acuity emerges during the first few years of life, such that the smallest angle of source location displacement from center (midline) at which left versus right can be discriminated decreases significantly with increased age. This measure of spatial acuity is known as the minimum audible angle (MAA) threshold, which decreases from >30° at a few months of age to 5° at 18 months of age and 1 to 2° at 5 years of age (Litovsky, 1997; for review see Litovsky & Ashmead, 1997). This acuity emerges as the child experiences auditory stimuli in the environment, as the head grows in size, and as the brain matures with ongoing stimulation. In children who are born deaf and who receive CIs in order to be able to hear, spatial hearing abilities emerge at different rates and are unlikely to be governed by the same set of interactions between brain maturity and auditory experience. In the next section, MAA data from children who use CIs are presented and interpreted.

MAA in Pediatric CI Users

Studies in the Litovsky lab with children who use CIs began by using the MAA task because the first group of children to be tested had received two CIs in sequential procedures, some years apart. These children had to undergo a long period of adjustment to listening with both ears and integrating the information, and at first it was clear that they were not quite sure as to what it meant to *localize sounds*. MAA is a good task on which initially to test children who have had little exposure to binaural hearing because it only requires that a child be able to discriminate between two options, left or right. Using interactive computer programs with music and puzzles for reinforce-

ment, children can be tested for numerous hours per day. The MAA task thus provided a good way to determine whether simple sound localization abilities can emerge in these children, despite the absence of auditory stimulation during infancy, and the absence of bilateral stimulation during early childhood. Some children were tested while using a single CI, either with or without a hearing aid in the nonimplanted ear. Of those, there were children who returned to the lab for follow-up testing after receiving a second CI.

Setup for MAA. The test is conducted in a large sound booth. The child is seated facing loudspeakers that are at a distance of at least 1 meter from the head. The speakers are arranged in a semicircular array in the frontal hemifield. In a research booth, multiple speakers are positioned at angles spanning 2° to 90°, at matched locations on the right and left. A computer program is used to implement an adaptive tracking algorithm whereby the side (left or right) is randomly chosen and the angle of the sound is varied from trial to trial, depending on the listeners' performance. In that case, when the child is able to discriminate left from right, the angle is automatically decreased. When the child is not able to discriminate left from right, the angle is increased. If an elaborate multispeaker array is difficult to set up in a clinical setting, then a portable setup, one that utilizes speakers on moveable stands may be considered. Testing is conducted for fixed angles, with a fixed number of trials per angle. Testing commences with speakers at large angles (e.g., ±60°). Within a block of trials, the sound is presented to the right or left speaker in random order. If the child is able to discriminate >75% correct, the speakers are moved to a smaller angle. As such, a psychometric function is obtained that provides a measure of the child's ability to discriminate left versus right at numerous angles, and the MAA is determined mathematically by computing the smallest angle at which the child is consistently above chance, that is ~70.9% correct (see Levitt, 1971). In the likely event that testing was not conducted at an angle that yields exactly that value, threshold is estimated by interpolating between angles that were tested at which performance was above and below 70.9% correct.

Children ages ≥4 years are tested using interactive computer games, whereby the child responds on each trial by pressing buttons on a mouse or keyboard, or by responding verbally and/or pointing (in which case the experimenter enters the responses into the computer). Thus, the child engages with the computer's request for a response regarding the location of a sound. Throughout the test, pieces of a puzzle are filled in and/or musical clips are used to engage and motivate the child to participate.

A recent trend in the field of cochlear implants is to provide bilateral CIs to very young children. The Litovsky lab has recently begun to investigate outcomes in these children with regard to both spatial hearing abilities and language acquisition. With regard to spatial hearing, children between the ages of 1 and 3.5 years are being tested using a method known as the observer-based psychophysical procedure (OBPP) developed by Dr. Lynne Werner (formerly Olsho) at the University of Washington, Seattle (Olsho, Koch, Carter, Halpin, & Spetner, 1988; Olsho, Koch, Haplin, & Carter, 1987). The OBPP method commonly is used in infant psychoacoustics and has proven to be accurate in determining auditory sensitivity. Rather than requiring overt head turns as is the case in visual reinforcement audiometry, in the OBPP approach subtle behaviors are used as indicators that the listener perceived there to be a change in the stimulus. In the Litovsky lab the procedure was modified slightly so that localization acuity could be assessed. On each trial, an observer, who is located in the observation room and unaware of the stimulus location, watches the toddler's behavior via video feed. The observer signals the computer to randomly present a stimulus on the right or left when the child is quiet and looking forward (with the aid of the research assistant in the booth). After the stimulus presentation, the observer makes a "blind" decision regarding the stimulus location (right or left) by watching the child's responses (e.g., head turn, eye widening, and shift in gaze). If the observer selects the correct side of presentation, the child's response is reinforced by the activation of a video on the side of stimulus presentation. Intensive training of observers is required for reliable observation to take place. This method is powerful in particular for young listeners for whom changes in the stimulus parameters may be perceived to be subtle and ambiguous. The OBPP has thus been used to evaluate right-left discrimination and to measure MAAs in young children who receive either one or two CIs (Grieco-Calub et al., 2008).

Parameters of Interest and Issues to Consider for the MAA Test

Angular Displacement of the Source Locations from Center. These can vary from 2° to 90° in each hemifield. The test starts out with a large displacement (as large as the sound booth enables, ideally at least 60°).

Stimulus Type. Although we have attempted to use noise stimuli, these appear to be difficult for the children to attend to on a spatial hearing task. Thus, we recommend using brief speech stimuli such as spondees or other brief utterances.

Listening Mode. Testing is conducted for bilateral listening, as well as with the ear that received the first CI. If time allows, testing with the ear that has the hearing aid or that received the second CI is conducted as well. If the MAA is larger under the unilateral listening mode condition compared with the bilateral condition, then a bilateral benefit is deemed to have occurred.

Sound Level Fixed or Varying. If testing is conducted with the overall sound pressure level fixed from trial to trial, it is likely that the child will be able to use overall monaural level cues to perform the task. To minimize the availability of monaural level cues, we recommend that the overall level be roved, that is, randomized from trial to trial, over a range of at least 8 dB.

Head Position. The child's head should be centered at the onset of each trial. If the child is moving the head or not looking straight ahead, then the trial should not be counted.

Results from MAA Studies. Results from studies using the MAA test (Litovsky et al., 2006a, 2006b) suggest that:

1. Considering children who received sequential bilateral CIs, who were between the ages of 4 and 16 years when tested, the majority (>70%) had MAA thresholds ≤20°, and the majority of those (77%) performed better when using both CIs than when using a single CI. Thus, a significant benefit was found for use of sequential CIs when localization acuity was measured. Average MAA data are shown in Figure 4–3 (left).
2. Performance was significantly better (i.e., MAA thresholds are smaller) in children who used sequential bilateral

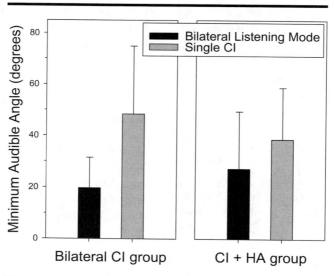

Figure 4–3. Average thresholds for minimum audible angle are compared for the children with two CIs (*left*) and with one CI and one HA (*right*). Dark bars show data collected when two ears were used, and light bars show data when a single ear was used.

CIs than children who use a single CI and a hearing aid (HA) in the other ear, when both groups were tested while using either bilateral CIs or CI+HA. The results from the CI+HA group are shown in Figure 4–3 (right) as well. However, within the group of children who used CI+HA there was large variability. While some of the children performed as well as the best-performing bilaterally implanted children, other children were unable to perform tasks that bilaterally implanted children are able to perform. We are of the opinion that fitting of a HA in the nonimplanted ear should be accompanied by rigorous testing to determine what types of benefits the HA might be providing to each individual child.

3. Performance improved significantly as a function of experience with bilateral CIs. When tested over a 3- to 24-month period following activation of the second CI, the children demonstrated improvements, such that reduction in MAA thresholds ranged from 20 to 60°. In addition there were children who were unable to perform the task at the onset of testing, that is, at 3 months after bilateral activation, but whose thresholds dropped to 10 to 20° within 12 to 24 months of bilateral activation. On average, much of the improvement occurs in the first 12 months following bilateral activation. Although, some children, in particular those who were unilaterally implanted for 5 to 8 years prior to bilateral activation, required up to 24 months of bilateral experience in order to perform well on the task, and then reached MAA thresholds 10 to 20°.

4. Considering children who were 2 years old by the time they received bilateral CIs, the first study (Grieco-Calub et al., 2008) compared MAA thresholds in children who had normal hearing with those who received either bilateral CIs ($n = 10$) or a single CI ($n = 8$), using the OBPP approach described above. None of the children with a single CI were able to perform the task at any angle. Of the children with bilateral CIs, three had MAA thresholds within normal limits, two were able to perform the task with some difficulty (MAA ~40°) and the others could not perform the task. What differentiates the children from one another is the number of months with bilateral listening experience; ≥12 months in the children who were within normal limits and 6 to 12 months in the children who had difficulty or were unable to perform the task. These findings suggest that early bilateral implantation might provide at least some children with sound localization acuity that is age-appropriate for normal hearing children. In addition, auditory experience plays an important role in the acquisition of this ability.

Sound Localization in Pediatric CI Users

The MAA task was selected because it is relatively easy to use with children of all ages, and also with children for whom the concept of a sound being perceived to be coming from a particular location may be difficult. However, we are also interested in the extent to which localization of sounds in a more complex and realistic situation are possible in children who are born deaf and who learn to localize with bilateral CIs. Sound localization abilities are measured in the Litovsky lab using a 15-loudspeaker array, with speakers positioned in the horizontal plane in 10°-increments, at a distance of 1.2 meters from the center of the listener's head. Interactive computerized "listening games" similar to those used in the MAA task are used here as well. To date, those data have not been published, although they have been presented (Grieco, Godar, Johnstone, Yu, & Litovsky, 2007) and submitted for publication (Grieco-Calub & Litovsky, submitted). Results from the first group of 18 children tested on the sound localization task suggest that the root mean square (RMS) error in localizing sounds is significantly smaller when the children are using their bilateral CIs than when they use a single CI, and within the same group of children, RMS error is smaller than it had been prior to implantation and activation of the second CI. Localization abilities vary, however, within this group, such that some children's error rates (around 28°) are as low as average error rates reported in adults whose onset of deafness was at age ≥15. In

other children performance with bilateral CIs is hardly distinguishable from their performance with a single CI, that is, no bilateral benefit on sound localization in a multi-loudspeaker array test situation. Furthermore, there is a range of performance within the group of children whose performance is best on the MAA task, such that some children with low MAA thresholds also are good localizers, whereas others are poor localizers. These data are shown in Figure 4–4. In other words, being able to discriminate left versus right hemifields for the presence of a sound source does not necessarily mean that the ability to identify source location in a multi-speaker array also is present. In addition, more difficult tasks such as locating sources in the presence of competing sounds, that is, more realistic environments needs to be understood in

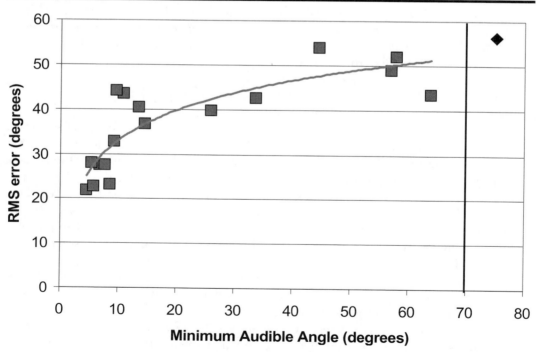

Figure 4–4. Relationship between MAA thresholds and root mean square (RMS) error from localization measures in 18 children who use bilateral cochlear implants.

the context of bilateral CIs and their potential benefit.

In summary, although, the MAA task is useful for measuring localization acuity across hemifields, it is not a direct measure of spatial hearing per se. On the other hand, whereas the localization task is an excellent tool for measuring the existence of a spatial map and evaluation of performance in more realistic environments, it is not easily measured in children younger than age 4 years. In older children with sequential bilateral CIs sound localization can be measured, but performance is variable. Anecdotally, the older children who received their second CI at age 8 to 12 years reported that the concept of determining "where" sounds were coming from was difficult. Despite knowing that objects have a spatial visual component, they seemed to struggle with the idea that the same objects also have a spatial component. Future studies with the children who received bilateral CIs by age 2.5 years (MAA data from above) and who have long-term experience with their CIs will help us to better understand the impact of early bilateral implantation on the emergence of sound localization skills and on the extent to which these children perform in a manner that is similar to their normal-hearing peers.

Understanding Speech in Noise and Spatial Release from Masking

A hallmark of binaural hearing is the ability to understand what one person is saying in the presence of competing speech or noise, a phenomenon that has been long known as the "cocktail party problem" (Cherry, 1953). Many studies with normal-hearing adults have demonstrated the benefits arising from having two ears versus one ear on

tasks that require the listener to segregate sounds. There are numerous auditory cues that are quite helpful for source segregation, such as differences in the fundamental frequencies between the target and competing sounds and momentary dips in the amplitude of the competing speech or noise, due to fluctuations in the envelope (especially when there is a single competing sound). However, when binaural hearing is available, spatial cues add an important and effective means of segregating sources, especially when the target and competing sounds are similar and easily confused with one another. Figure 4–5 depicts a situation in which a listener sitting in a room is presented with target speech from front and competing sounds either from front or from the side. The ability to hear the target speech can be significantly better when the competitor is at the side than in front due to a phenomenon known as spatial release from masking (SRM). SRM is the advantage gained from the spatial separation of targets and maskers (competitors); it can be quantified as change in percent correct under conditions of spatial coincidence versus spatial separation, or as change in speech reception thresholds (SRT) under those conditions. SRM is particularly large when the competitor is similar to the target and few other cues are available; thus, the listener must rely on spatial cues in order to segregate the target from the competitor. SRM also is particularly large when the competitor consists of multiple talkers as would occur in a realistic complex auditory environment (Bronkhorst, 2000; Hawley et al., 2004). For example, SRM can be as high as a 12-dB difference in SRTs under binaural conditions when multiple competitors are present and the competitors and target speech are identical talkers. SRM can be as low as 1- to 2-dB difference in SRT under monaural conditions when a single talker is

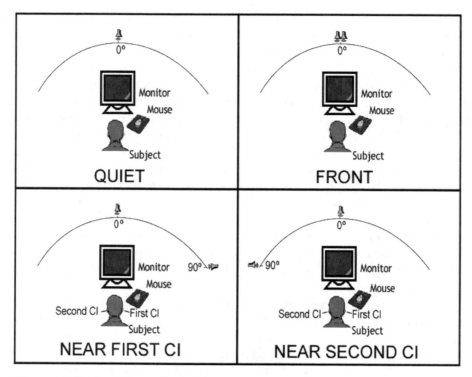

Figure 4–5. Spatial configurations are shown for the speech (*front*) and competing speech (none in quiet; front; 90 deg near first or second CI on right or left).

present and is easily distinguishable from the target voice. The advantage gained in this situation is reduced, however, in the presence of reverberation, whereby the binaural cues are smeared and thus the locations of the target and competitors are not easily distinguishable (Lavandier & Culling, 2007; Lee & Shinn-Cunningham, 2008). The literature on the cocktail party problem and the benefits of binaural hearing has a 60-year history and has grown remarkably in the past 10 years (see Bronkhorst, 2000; Durlach et al, 2003; Hawley et al., 2004; Yost, 1997).

The ability of children with normal hearing to hear in complex environments has been studied more intensively in recent years. Studies from the Litovsky lab have

attempted to simulate realistic complex auditory environments such as those used in the studies with adults (Garadat & Litovsky, 2007; Johnstone & Litovsky, 2006; Litovsky, 2005). By ages 3 to 4 years, children show SRM on the order of 5- to 9-dB difference in SRT, even when the target and competing talkers are of a different sex and easily recognizable from one another, suggesting that the advantage of spatial cues for source segregation is present early in life. In children ages 6 to 7 years, the effects of type of competitor have been studied, and it has been found that SRM is larger when speech or time-reversed speech are used, rather than speech-shaped noise (Johnstone & Litovsky, 2006; Litovsky, 2005).

In persons who are deaf and use CIs, the advantage of binaural hearing for source segregation has been studied in recent years, particularly in adults. The approach is somewhat different than that used in normal-hearing persons because quantification of binaural benefit must take into consideration which ear is active and which is inactive as well as the side of the head from which the competing sound is placed relative to the active/inactive ear. The terms that have been adopted to depict advantages from bilateral activation in the literature include the following:

Head Shadow: If both ears are functional the listener can selectively attend to the ear with the more favorable SNR (i.e., the ear opposite to the noise source) to maximize speech recognition performance (as compared with the unfavorable situation where only the ear with the poorer SNR is functional).

Binaural Squelch: If there is functional input from both ears, the auditory system potentially can combine the information to form a better central representation than that available with only monaural input. The Squelch effect occurs when a noisy source is added near the ear with the better SNR, but improvement in performance occurs nonetheless. Binaural cues are utilized in centrally mediated source segregation mechanisms that can significantly improve speech understanding.

Binaural Summation: Also known as "binaural redundancy" is thought to occur when speech and noise originate from the same location. Binaural redundancy refers to the auditory system's ability to centrally combine and derive benefit from duplicate

representations of the same signal to the two ears. Hearing threshold improves for binaural versus monaural presentation to normal ears, resulting in increased perceptual loudness.

These three benefits have been reported in numerous adult users of bilateral CIs (e.g., Litovsky, Parkinson, Arcaroli, & Sammeth, 2006c; Schleich et al., 2004; Tyler, Dunn, Witt, & Noble, 2007; van Hoesel & Tyler, 2003). The largest benefit is that of head shadow, because it only requires the use of two "good ears" and not necessarily the availability of binaural hearing per se. In some BI-CI users there is also binaural squelch, although the effect size is generally smaller and not found in many users.

In children who use CIs, few studies have been conducted that investigate the effects of bilateral stimulation on speech understanding in the presence of competitors and the extent to which they also show SRM. Litovsky and colleagues have applied their approaches with normal-hearing children to the BI-CI children and children who use CI and a hearing aid (HA) in the other ear. These measures have been made using the CRISP test (Litovsky, 2005), in which a computerized interactive game engages the child and presents speech stimuli in quiet, or in the presence of competitors. Older children are tested with spondees and younger children with a set of words appropriate for ages 2.5 years and older. On each trial, a spondee (e.g., cowboy, hotdog, ice cream) is heard from a loudspeaker in front, while the child views four pictures on the computer monitor, and the child decides which of the pictures matches the speech sound. SRTs are measured by adaptively varying the level of the speech, while holding constant the level of the competing sound (we recommend two-talker speech). Performance is measured in quiet, and also with competing speech whose location varied (front, 90° on the right or left). These configurations can be seen in Figure 4–5 (Litovsky et al., 2006a, 2006b; Peters, Litovsky, Parkinson & Lake, 2007). Our interest lies in comparing SRTs under monaural and bilateral listening modes. Average results from 20 children (10 BI-CI and 10 CI+HA) are shown in Figure 4-6 from a condition in which the competing speech was placed on the side of the head near the second-implanted ear, or near the HA. BI-CI children show average release from masking of 5 dB, within the expected range for normal-hearing children. In contrast, CI+HA children have average values of 1.8 dB, suggesting that, on this task, the HA in the second ear is not as beneficial as the CI in the second ear. In fact, for 4 of 10 children with CI+HA, performance is worse (bilateral disadvantage) when the HA is activated, compared with listening monaurally with only the CI. An important difference between BI-CI children and those using CI+HA arises when comparing their performance with a single (first) CI and with both ears activated. Figure 4–7 shows average bilateral advantage, or the difference in SRTs between the unilateral (first CI) and bilateral modes. The bilateral listening mode produced a reduction in SRTs (positive advantage) with two devices compared with a single device more clearly and significantly in the BI-CI group than in the CI+HA group. A number of individuals in the CI+HA group had a bilateral disruption evidenced by increased SRTs with the addition of the HA. Overall, these findings suggest that children with bilateral CIs show greater improvement from a second CI than do children who wear a HA in the opposite ear. It is important to note that this finding is based on the CRISP-Spondee closed-set test, but has not been confirmed for other measures of speech intelligibility. Results from children in the BI-CI group are consistent though with prior reports of bilateral advantages in adults with BI-CIs (Gantz et al., 2002; Litovsky et al., 2004, 2006c; Muller, Schon, & Helms, 2002; Schleich et al., 2004; van Hoesel, 2004).

An issue that is important to consider, and for which little is known to date, is the importance of age at which the second implant is activated, and whether activation of the two ears at different times, sometimes years apart, has significant long-term effects. These effects could be manifested in the child's ability to use information presented to the second ear, or to combine information from the two ears. Although this question is still under investigation, Peters et al., (2007) recently reported that children who are younger when they receive the second CI achieve higher open-set speech perception scores in the second ear than children who are older when they receive the second CI. In this study, 30 children participated who received the second CI between the ages of 3 and 13 years, received their first implant before 5 years of

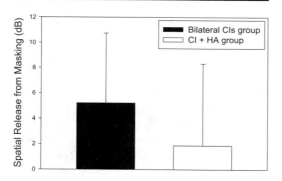

Figure 4–6. Average values for spatial release from masking, in speech intelligibility, are compared for the groups of children who used either bilateral CIs (*dark bar*) or one CI and one HA.

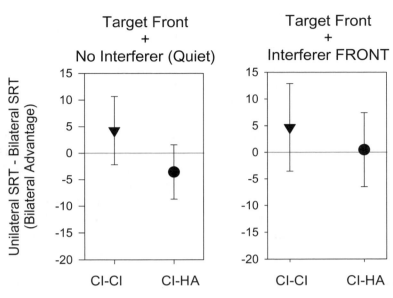

Figure 4–7. Average advantages from bilateral stimulation are compared for the groups of children with CI+CI and CI+HA, for conditions in which the speech was presented in quiet (*left panel*), and when the competing speech was also presented, in front (*right panel*). Differences in SRTs between monaural and bilateral conditions are shown; values above the line indicate lower SRTs (better performance) in the bilateral mode.

age, and had acquired speech perception capabilities with the first device. Children were divided into the following three age groups on the basis of age at time of second ear implantation: 3 to 5 years, 5.1 to 8 years and 8.1 to 13 years. Speech perception in quiet was assessed with the Multisyllabic Lexical Neighborhood Test (MLNT) (Kirk, Pisoni, & Osberger, 1995) for the 3- to 5-year-olds, the Lexical Neighborhood Test (LNT) (Kirk et al., 1995) for the two older groups, and the Hearing In Noise Test for Children (HINT-C) (Nilson, Soli, & Sullivan, 2004) in quiet for the 8- to13-year-olds. In addition, the CRISP test (e.g., Litovsky et al., 2006a, 2006b) was administered. Testing was conducted prior to the second surgery, and at 3, 6, and 12 months following activation of

the second implant. In quiet, open-set speech perception was acquired in the second ear relatively quickly after activation (within 6 months). However, children younger than 8 years acquired this level more rapidly and reached a higher level of speech perception ability at 12 months following activation than did older children. Performance with the second ear for the 8- to 13-year-olds remained poorer than that of the first ear (44 vs. 89%). However, measures with the CRISP test showed that speech intelligibility for spondees in noise was significantly better under bilateral conditions than with either ear alone for all age groups. This bilateral advantage was greatest when interfering stimuli were directed toward the first implanted ear, indicating that the head shadow effect was the most effective mechanism, as is widely found in adults with BI-CIs. Further research obviously is necessary before definitive conclusions can be drawn regarding the effectiveness of sequential bilateral cochlear implantation in children of various ages and gaps between the two implantations. Finally, there are limitations in currently available implant arrays and speech processors which place constraints on the extent to which users are able to receive binaural stimulation per se. Among these are current spread and interaction of stimulation amongst electrodes, lack of obligatory coordination between right- and left-ear processors, lack of fine structure in the signal, and temporal smearing of the signals. Because we do not have control over these features at the moment, the clinician can attempt to optimize the use of binaural hearing by developing methods for conducting bilateral mapping that would optimize coordination of inputs arriving at the two ears on a frequency-by-frequency basis. The next section addresses this important issue of bilateral mapping approaches that are currently in use in some clinics in the United States that are involved in daily mapping of children who are fitted with bilateral CIs.

Criteria for Bilateral Cochlear Implants in Children

Impact of Degree of Hearing Loss on CI Criteria

Given the discussion earlier in this chapter regarding the benefits arising from binaural hearing, it is important to consider ways in which children with severe and profound hearing loss also are expected to benefit from binaural hearing if appropriately fit with available technology. Although fitting of hearing aids binaurally has been the "standard of care" for many years, bilateral fitting of CIs in children is a more recent clinical trend. This trend is growing and becoming more extensive across implant centers such that many consider bilateral implantation to be "routine." This trend is in part due to the changing criteria for cochlear implantation. Although the Food and Drug Administration (FDA) criteria continue to recommend that children with profound hearing loss receive a cochlear implant at 12 to 24 months, children who are older than 24 months and who have severe-to-profound hearing loss also are eligible for implantation. Some implant centers thus choose to provide implants to young children who have appreciable residual hearing. This contrasts with past clinical approaches whereby children were not considered candidates for implantation unless both ears had little or no residual hearing. In addition, some CI centers are now evaluating each ear separately and making separate candidacy recommendations for each ear, the primary consideration being the degree of hearing loss in each ear. If both ears meet the criteria for implantation, consideration by many centers is given to bilateral cochlear implants. If only one ear meets the criteria for implantation, monaural implantation is more typically considered.

Ability to Use a Hearing Aid Successfully

A critical factor in determining candidacy for cochlear implantation is the inability of the child to use amplification successfully. The definition of "successful" is variable, however. We consider successful use of amplification as the ability to hear sufficiently well to develop speech and language and being able to learn in a mainstream classroom environment. This requires hearing at sufficiently soft levels throughout the frequency range that is necessary for speech understanding using audition. Our definition of "sufficiently soft levels," therefore, is the ability to hear at 20 to 30 dB HL throughout the frequency range that includes 4000 Hz. The higher frequency is included because this information may be essential for perception of critical phonemic information, which is essential for language development. Examples include high-frequency information required for perception of pluralization and possessives. Due to the need to hear at high frequencies some CI centers are considering implantation for children who hear well with hearing aids in the low or mid frequencies but do not hear at sufficiently soft levels in the high frequencies. Children who do not meet CI criteria include those who are able to use a hearing aid successfully, who hear high frequencies at soft levels, and for older children, those who have developed good speech perception through the use of a hearing aid.

As mentioned above, an approach that is becoming more commonly used in centers across the United States is one in which a child who is a candidate for implantation in each ear independently is considered a candidate for bilateral implantation. Because there can sometimes be a fine line between what is considered successful use of a hearing aid and the need to move on to an implant for unsuccessful users of hearing aids, these decisions are carefully made. For children who seem to hear well in some situations (such as hearing loud speech in quiet) but have problems in other situations (e.g., hearing soft speech or speech in noise), the decision can be especially difficult. Unfortunately, the answer is not always clear and clinicians often rely on their experience with other patients in helping to make recommendations.

Binaural Benefit

In young children the extent to which binaural benefit can be evaluated and quantified is not fully understood. However, there are some approaches that clinics should consider taking as part of the decision-making process when BI-CI is under consideration. One of the necessary steps, in the opinion of the authors of this chapter, is the assessment of potential benefit from bilateral stimulation. As such, children are evaluated with each ear separately and then with bilateral stimulation. The child is first assessed for improved gain received with technology, and as soon as the child is capable of the task, speech perception testing should be included while using their currently fitted technology (such as, for instance, bilateral HAs). A child who has received a single CI is tested using the implant in one ear and (if worn) the HA in the unimplanted ear; results are compared with results from testing that is conducted while using the CI alone. A number of researchers have demonstrated that children who do not receive benefit from a HA alone in one ear, may receive binaural benefit using a HA in one ear and a CI in the opposite ear. (Ching, Incerti, & Hill, 2004; Ching, Psarros, Hill, Dillon, & Incerti, 2001; Madell, 2008; Madell, Sislian, & Hoffman, 2004). In the clinic, if speech perception is improved in the bilateral condition compared with the unilateral condition, we consider there to be a binaural benefit. Furthermore, if performance does not decrease in the bilateral condition, that is, if there is no binaural disruption, the child is still considered to be a candidate for bilateral implantation. Finally, little is known about expected outcomes from BI-CI in children based on preimplant performance. It is important to recognize that some children demonstrate a reduction in performance when listening with a CI and an HA. Although this is not common, it merits consideration as it leaves open questions regarding treatment of these children. In addition, there exist children who demonstrate a decrease in bilateral performance with HAs but perform well once bilateral implants are provided. It is possible that electrical stimulation from CIs is significantly different than the acoustic stimulation provided by HAs, and that the HA is unable to provide usable input to the child; hence, the input that is provided simply adds noise and results in disruption.

Simultaneous Versus Sequential Implantation

Simultaneous implantation is the term used when CIs are placed in each ear during one surgery. In sequential implantation, CIs are placed in separate surgeries. The decision as to whether a child who is a candidate for BI-CI should be implanted sequentially or simultaneously varies across clinics. Today there does not appear a particular standard of care nor an agreed upon protocol for making these determinations. Hence, the child's surgeon, audiologist and family must work as a team to arrive at a decision that is best suited for that child and the family. Simultaneous BI-CI is most common in children who have had meningitis as, after meningitis, the cochlea can ossify quickly and if implantation does not occur prior to the ossification it may be very difficult to insert the implant successfully. Simultaneous BI-CI also is considered by a number of clinics when both ears are implant candidates; the child receives very limited HA benefit, and there are no medical, financial

or other reasons that raise concern. Sequential BI-CI may be considered for several reasons: (1) When there is medical concern about risk from anesthesia due to a more extended surgery time for placing two devices during one surgery, (2) When a child has been wearing an implant for some time and the family makes the decision to consider a second implant, and (3) When a child who has been using HAs is ready for implant surgery and there is concern about giving up both ears at the same time. Even if it is determined that a child would benefit from BI-CIs, there are considerations if the child has relied on HAs and is accustomed to hearing through those devices. That is, it could be a very traumatic experience for the child to be left with no access to sound for 3 to 4 weeks while the incisions heal, and then have a period of time when the child will not be hearing well while learning to use implants. Most children who have used HAs will be more comfortable having one HA with which to hear while learning to use a CI. Thus, for a child who is used to hearing with HAs, it may be best to proceed with a CI in one ear. If the child shows signs of hearing well with the CI, a second surgery can be considered.

Vestibular Evaluation

There has been some concern that patients implanted bilaterally may demonstrate vestibular problems. It is not unusual for patients with hearing loss to have reduced vestibular functioning. This may be a unilateral or bilateral problem. Some patients demonstrate problems with dizziness and balance after surgery but, in most cases, the problem is minor and resolves itself quickly. Children who are undergoing continued development and whose auditory system and nervous systems have unique adaptive components, otherwise known as "developmental plasticity," appear frequently to resolve vestibular problems more quickly than adults. Many CI centers include a vestibular assessment as part of the evaluation process for BI-CI and may elect not to implant bilaterally if vestibular problems appear to be a concern.

Evaluation Protocol

Audiologic Evaluation. The first step in the evaluation protocol is obtaining hearing thresholds with and without auditory sensory technology. Unaided thresholds are obtained to confirm degree of hearing loss. Patients are then tested with technology. Thresholds with technology should be obtained for each ear separately and bilaterally. At this point it will be possible to tell if the HAs are providing sufficient gain—if the child is able to hear soft speech (20 to 30 dB HL) with HAs throughout the frequency range. If not, either the HA settings can be modified or, if that is not possible, additional HAs with more gain can be tried. For many patients with severe and profound hearing loss it will not be possible to find HAs that provide sufficient gain to allow the child to hear at sufficiently soft levels, especially in the high frequencies.

Once the best HAs for an individual child are identified, word recognition testing should be administered. The specific test used will vary depending on the child's age and auditory capabilities. The standard at the current time is to test at 60 dB SPL (50 dB HL). If a child performs well at normal conversation, testing should be performed at soft conversation (45 dB SPL [35 dB HL]) and at normal conversation at +5 SNR (Madell, 2008). Alternatively, important information about auditory performance in different listening situations in quiet and noise can be obtained using the CRISP test, as described above (Litovsky, 2005; Litovsky et al., 2006b). A child who demonstrates good

speech perception (70% or better) at average and soft conversational levels in quiet and in the presence of competing noise is not a candidate for implantation. However, if a child has difficulty understanding speech at soft levels or in competing noise the child is a candidate for implantation.

Speech-Language-Functional Listening Evaluation. If a child meets the audiologic criteria for implantation the child should receive a speech-language-functional listening evaluation to assess current skills, to determine how the child is using audition, and to assist in planning therapy after receiving implantation. Results from this evaluation will be used to track progress post CI surgery.

Educational Consultation. A consultation with a teacher of the deaf and hard of hearing can be very helpful in determining if the child is in an appropriate educational setting and receiving all the necessary services. If not, the educational consultant can work with the family and school to plan for changes in services and for therapy after implantation.

Social Work Consultation. Many families benefit from meeting with a social worker to discuss feelings about hearing loss, receiving a cochlear implant, and concerns about the future. The social worker can assist in helping assure the team members that families have realistic expectations for implantation. Older children and teens will benefit from the opportunity to talk with a social worker to discuss feelings about surgery, expectations, and concerns about living with hearing loss.

Otologic Evaluation. Children being considered for a CI will have an otologic evaluation to determine medical eligibility for surgery. Important components of the evaluation include, radiological testing (computed tomography and/or magnetic resonance imaging), and counseling to help the family understand what is involved in surgery.

Team Discussion. After all evaluations are completed, members of the CI team meet to determine if a child is a good candidate for the CI. All evaluations are reviewed. Any concerns are discussed and a recommendation is made. The team may recommend that the child have an extended HA trial, pre-CI therapy, or changes in school placement prior to receiving a first or second CI, or may recommend that CI surgery be scheduled. Once a child is implanted, and initial programming is completed, therapy is scheduled to assist the child in learning to use the CI optimally.

Learning to Listen with Two CIs

Children who receive simultaneous CIs will usually start by wearing both full time. As they become good listeners, it is important to evaluate performance with each ear separately. If auditory development is the same in each ear, the child will continue to use BI-CI full time. If the child is performing more poorly with one ear, it may be useful to do some listening practice with the poorer ear alone for a couple of hours each day in the attempt to improve skills in that ear.

Children who receive sequential CIs within a few months of each other usually are treated as if the implants were simultaneous. Children who receive CIs more than a few months apart may need assistance in learning to hear with the second ear. If, after a short time, performance in the second ear is not as good as that of the first ear, it may be useful to do some listening practice with the poorer ear alone for a couple

of hours each day in the attempt to improve skills in that ear. We frequently recommend that the child wear the two implants for most of the day, and all the time they are in school or in other critical listening situations, but that they wear the new implant alone during after school hours to try and build skills in the second ear. The length of time this takes will differ from child to child.

Conclusions

In this chapter we reviewed some of the concepts relating to binaural hearing and how it might be achieved by a normal auditory system. We discussed research to date which suggests that some of the abilities that are achieved by persons with a normal auditory system are also observed in persons who are deaf and who use bilateral cochlear implants. Of course, there are limitations to the benefits provided by bilateral cochlear implants, and there is a reason for using the term bilateral as opposed to binaural. The limitations occur both at the level of the hardware, which limits the extent to which information arriving at the two ears can be coordinated, and at the level of the auditory system of persons with severe-to-profound hearing loss. This chapter focused on outcomes measures in children with bilateral hearing, and although these measures have been informative regarding benefits of bilateral implantation, future work should be conducted to look at nonauditory measures as well. These include language and speech development, cognition, and general abilities that are known to be important for integration into mainstreamed educational environments. Finally, some preliminary suggestions for bilateral mapping approaches in children who use bilateral cochlear implants are made in this chapter.

Research in this area is lacking and should be conducted to determine best approaches for fitting, mapping, and providing rehabilitation to this growing population.

References

Akeroyd, M. A., & Summerfield, A. Q. (2000). Integration of monaural and binaural evidence of vowel formants. *Journal of the Acoustical Society of America, 107*, 3394-3406.

Blauert, J. (1997). *Spatial hearing*. Cambridge, MA: MIT Press.

Bronkhorst, A. W. (2000). The cocktail-party phemonenon: A review of research on speech intelligibility in multiple-talker conditions. *Acta Acoustica, 86*, 117-128.

Cherry, E. C. (1953). Some experiments on the recognition of speech, with one and two ears. *Journal of the Acoustical Society of America, 25*, 975-979.

Ching, T. Y., Incerti, P., & Hill, M. (2004). Binaural benefits for adults who use hearing aids and cochlear implants in opposite ears. *Ear and Hearing, 25*, 9-21.

Ching, T. Y., Psarros, C., Hill, M., Dillon, H., & Incerti, P. (2001). Should children who use cochlear implants wear hearing aids in the opposite ear? *Ear and Hearing, 22*, 365-380.

Clifton, R. K., Morrongiello, B. A., Kulig, J. W., & Dowd, J. M. (1981). Newborns' orientation toward sound: Possible implications for cortical development. *Child Development, 52*, 833-838.

Culling, J. F., Hawley, M. L., & Litovsky, R.Y. (2004). The role of head-induced interaural time and level differences in the speech reception threshold for multiple interfering sound sources. *Journal of the Acoustical Society of America, 116*, 1057-1065.

Durlach, N., & Colburn, H. (1978). Binaural phenomena. In E. Carterette & M. Friedman (Eds.), *Handbook of perception. Volume IV: Hearing* (pp. 365-466). New York: Academic Press.

Durlach, N. I., Mason, C. R., Shinn-Cunningham, B. G., Arbogast, T. L., Colburn, H. S., & Kidd, G., Jr. (2003). Informational masking: Counteracting the effects of stimulus uncertainty by decreasing target-masker similarity. *Journal of the Acoustical Society of America, 114*, 368-379.

Gantz, B. J., Tyler, R. S., Rubinstein, J. T., Wolaver, A., Lowder, M., Abbas, P., et al. (2002). Binaural cochlear implants placed during the same operation. *Otology and Neurotology, 23*, 169-180.

Garadat, S., & Litovsky, R. Y. (2007). Speech intelligibility in free field: Spatial unmasking in preschool children. *Journal of the Acoustical Society of America, 121*, 1047-1055.

Grantham, D. W., Ashmead, D. H., Ricketts, T. A., Labadie, R. F., & Haynes, D. S. (2007). Horizontal-plane localization of noise and speech signals by postlingually deafened adults fitted with bilateral cochlear implants. *Ear and Hearing, 28*, 524-541.

Grieco, T., Godar, S., Johnstone, P. M., Yu, G., & Litovsky, R. Y. (2007). *Emergence of localization abilities in children with sequential bilateral cochlear implants*. Oral Presentation at the Meeting of the Association for Research in Otolaryngology.

Grieco-Calub, T., & Litovsky, R. Y. (submitted). Sound localization abilities in children with normal hearing and with bilateral cochlear implants. *Ear and Hearing*.

Grieco-Calub, T. M., Litovsky, R. Y., & Werner, L. A. (2008). Using the observer-based psychophysical procedure to assess localization acuity in toddlers who use bilateral cochlear implants. *Otology and Neurotology, 29*, 235-239.

Hawley, M. L., Litovsky, R. Y., & Culling, J. F. (2004). The benefit of binaural hearing in a cocktail party: Effect of location and type of interferer. *Journal of the Acoustical Society of America, 115*, 833-843.

Henry, B. A., & Turner, C. W. (2003). The resolution of complex spectral patterns by cochlear implant and normal-hearing listeners. *Journal of the Acoustical Society of America, 113*, 2861-2873.

Johnstone, P. M., & Litovsky, R. Y. (2006). Effect of masker type and age on speech intelligibility and spatial release from masking in children and adults. *Journal of the Acoustical Society of America, 120,* 2177-2189.

Kirk, K. I., Pisoni, D. B., & Osberger, M. J. (1995). Lexical effects of spoken word recognition by pediatric cochlear implant users. *Ear and Hearing, 16,* 470-481.

Lavandier, M., & Culling, J. F. (2007). Speech segregation in rooms: Effects of reverberation on both target and interferer. *Journal of the Acoustical Society of America, 122,* 1713.

Lee, A. K., & Shinn-Cunningham, B. G. (2008). Effects of reverberant spatial cues on attention-dependent object formation. *Journal of the Association for Research in Otolaryngology, 9,* 150-160.

Levitt, H. (1971). Transformed up-down methods in psychoacoustics. *Journal of the Acoustical Society of America, 49,* 467-477.

Litovsky, R. Y. (1997) Developmental changes in the precedence effects: Estimates of minimum audible angle. *Journal of the Acoustical Society of America, 102,* 1739-1745.

Litovsky, R. Y. (2005). Speech intelligibility and spatial release from masking in young children. *Journal of the Acoustical Society of America, 117,* 3091-3099.

Litovsky, R., & Ashmead, D. (1997). Developmental aspects of binaural and spatial hearing. In R. H. Gilkey & T. R. Anderson, (Eds.), *Binaural and spatial hearing* (pp. 571-592). Hillsdale, NJ: Lawrence Earlbaum Associates.

Litovsky, R. Y., Johnstone, P. M., & Godar, S. P. (2006a). Benefits of bilateral cochlear implants and/or hearing aids in children. *International Journal of Audiology, 45*(Suppl. 1), 78-91.

Litovsky, R. Y., Johnstone, P. M., Godar, S., Agrawal, S., Parkinson, A., Peters, R., et al. (2006b). Bilateral cochlear implants in children: Localization acuity measured with minimum audible angle. *Ear and Hearing, 27,* 43-59.

Litovsky, R. Y., Parkinson, A., Arcaroli, J., Peters, R., Lake, J., Johnstone, P., et al. (2004). Bilateral cochlear implants in adults and children. *Archives of Otolaryngology-Head and Neck Surgery, 130,* 648-655.

Litovsky, R. Y., Parkinson, A., Arcaroli, J., & Sammeth, C. (2006c). Simultaneous bilateral cochlear implantation in adults: A multicenter clinical study. *Ear and Hearing, 27,* 714-731.

Macpherson, E. A., & Middlebrooks, J. C. (2002). Listener weighting of cues for lateral angle: The duplex theory of sound localization revisited. *Journal of the Acoustical Society of America, 111,* 2219-2236.

Madell, J. R. (2008). Evaluation of speech perception in infants and young children. In J. R. Madell & C. Flexer (Eds.), *Pediatric audiology: Evaluation, management, and technology* (pp. 89-105). New York: Thieme.

Madell, J. R., Sislian, N., & Hoffman, R. (2004). Speech perception for cochlear implant patients using hearing aids on the unimplanted ear. In R. Miyamoto (Ed.), *Cochlear implants* (pp 223-226). San Diego, CA: Elsevier.

Middlebrooks, J. C., & Green, D. M. (1991). Sound localization by human listeners. *Annual Review of Psychology, 42,* 135-159.

Muir, D., & Field, J. (1979). Newborn infants orient to sounds. *Child Development, 50,* 431-436.

Müller, J., Schön, F., & Helms, J. (2002). Speech understanding in quiet and noise in bilateral users of the MED-EL COMBI 40/40+ cochlear implant system. *Ear and Hearing, 23,* 198-206.

Neuman, A. C., Haravon, A., Sislian, N., & Waltzman, S. B. (2007). Sound-direction identification with bilateral cochlear implants. *Ear and Hearing, 28,* 73-82.

Nilsson, M., Soli, S. D., & Sullivan, J. A. (1994). Development of the hearing in noise test for the measurement of speech reception thresholds in quiet and in noise. *Journal of the Acoustical Society of America, 95,* 1085-1099.

Nopp, P., Schleich, P., & D'Haese, P. (2004). Sound localization in bilateral users of MED-EL COMBI 40/40+ cochlear implants. *Ear and Hearing, 25,* 205-214.

Olsho, L. W., Koch, E. G., Carter, E. A., Halpin, C. F. & Spetner, N. B. (1988). Pure-tone sensitivity of human infants. *Journal of the Acoustical Society of America, 84,* 1316-1324.

Olsho, L. W., Koch, E. G., Haplin, C. F., & Carter, E. A. (1987). An observer-based psychoacoustic procedure for use with young infants. *Developmental Psychology, 23,* 627-640.

Peters, B. R., Litovsky, R. Y., Parkinson, A., & Lake, J. (2007). Importance of age and post-implantation experience on performance in children with sequential bilateral cochlear implants. *Otology and Neurotology, 28,* 649-657.

Schleich, P., Nopp, P., & D'Haese, P. (2004). Head shadow, squelch, and summation effects in bilateral users of the MED-EL COMBI 40/40 cochlear implant. *Ear and Hearing, 25,* 197-204.

Skinner, M. W., Holden, L. K., Demorest, M. E., & Holden, T. A. (1995). Use of test-retest measures to evaluate performance stability in adults with cochlear implants. *Ear and Hearing, 16,* 187-197.

Tyler, R. S., Dunn, C. C., Witt, S. A., & Noble, W. G. (2007). Speech perception and localization with adults with bilateral sequential cochlear implants. *Ear and Hearing, 28*(Suppl. 2), 86S-90S.

van Hoesel, R. J. (2004). Exploring the benefits of bilateral cochlear implants. *Audiology and Neurotology, 9,* 234-246.

van Hoesel, R. J., & Tyler, R. S. (2003). Speech perception, localization, and lateralization with bilateral cochlear implants. *Journal of the Acoustical Society of America, 113,* 1617-1630.

Verschuur, C. A., Lutman, M. E., Ramsden, R., Greenham, P., & O'Driscoll, M. (2005). Auditory localization abilities in bilateral cochlear implant recipients. *Otology and Neurotology, 26,* 965-971.

Yost, W. A. (1997). The cocktail party problem: Forty years later. In R. H. Gilkey & T. R. Anderson (Eds.), *Binaural and spatial hearing* (pp. 329-348). Hillsdale, NJ: Lawrence Earlbaum Associates.

Zeng, F. G. (2004). Trends in cochlear implants. *Trends in Amplification, 8,* 1-34.

CHAPTER 5

Pediatric Cochlear Implantation: Surgical Aspects

ERIC P. WILKINSON
JOSE N. FAYAD
WILLIAM M. LUXFORD

Introduction

Cochlear implantation (CI) represents a triumph of bioengineering. Prior to the development of this technology, options for rehabilitation of patients with severe-to-profound hearing loss were extremely limited. Currently available devices have evolved significantly from the original single-channel implants: multichannel cochlear implantation is now the standard.

The surgical technique for CI has undergone evolution from its initial, large incisions and scalp flaps, to minimally invasive skin incisions with small "minimastoidectomy" and small wells for the devices. These changes in technique have gone hand-in-hand with decreasing size of the internal processors and coils themselves.

In this chapter, we explore the history, indications, contraindications, preoperative assessment, and surgical techniques of cochlear implantation. We discuss possible intraoperative pitfalls and difficult situations that may arise, and discuss surgical nuances of implantation in special populations.

History of Cochlear Implantation

In 1957, French researchers André Djourno and Charles Eyriès, with the help of Danielle Kayser, provided the first detailed description of the effects of directly stimulating the auditory nerve in a human subject (Clark, Tong, & Patrick, 1990; Djourno & Eyriès, 1957). Otologic surgery saw great advances in the 1960s that helped usher in the era of microsurgery of the inner ear, including electrode implantation. Perhaps the most critical development was the introduction of the operating microscope to otologic surgery (Smyth, 1979). This development made it possible to work on the level of the cochlea with extreme accuracy and made the implantation of small electrodes possible.

With the operating microscope a reality, an approach to the cochlea via the mastoid was the next necessity. Dr. William F. House at the House Ear Clinic implanted several experimental devices in deaf volunteers in the early 1960s. However, initial devices were rejected due to rejection of the electrode insulation material (House & Urban, 1973). Blair Simmons at Stanford University reported studies in 1965 and 1966 in which multiple electrodes were implanted into the modiolus of the cochlea in a patient with profound hearing loss (Simmons, 1966).

The first portable implant system in an adult was implanted in 1972 at the House Ear Clinic (House & Urban, 1973). In 1980, children began to be implanted with single-channel devices (Eisenberg, Berliner, Thielemeir, Kirk, & Tiber, 1983; Eisenberg & House, 1982). The United States Food and Drug Administration (FDA) formally approved the marketing of the 3M/House cochlear implant for adults in November 1984 (Clark et al., 1990).

In the same year, Clark and colleagues in Australia were busy at work on what would become the Nucleus-22 implant, and initial U.S. studies were performed at the University of Iowa and New York University (Cohen, Waltzman, & Shapiro, 1985; Lowder, 2004). This work would eventually spawn the Cochlear Corporation, and the Nucleus-22 multichannel cochlear implant would be approved one year later (Clark et al., 1977; Clark et al., 1990; Patrick & Clark, 1991).

Initially, this approval was only for adults with profound hearing loss, but in 1990, approval was widened to include children over 2 years of age, and in 1995, criteria were again broadened to include adults with severe hearing loss and reduced speech discrimination scores. Advanced Bionics received FDA approval for its Clarion device in 1997 (Schindler, Kessler, & Haggerty, 1993). In 1998 the Cochlear Nucleus 24 was approved for use in ages 12 months and older (Lowder, 2004).

Cochlear implant technology has benefited greatly from improved signal processing techniques and the progressive miniaturization of the processors themselves. Many of these developments have occurred in the last decade.

Indications

Indications for cochlear implantation have undergone changes since originally being approved by the FDA. The indications gradually have become more inclusive of patients with severe hearing loss.

In the early 1980s, patients considered candidates for CI included postlingually deafened adults without any residual aidable hearing. In their best aided condition, candidates needed to have speech discrimination no better than 30% and a speech detection threshold no less than 70 dB SPL, though some investigators felt that patients should have no open-set word understanding (Luxford, 1989). A 6-month trial with binaural amplification was mandatory. Original screening also included psychological assessment.

Researchers learned that a better gauge of sentence understanding was needed, with and without the presence of background noise. This led to the development of the Hearing-In-Noise Test, or HINT (Nilsson, Soli, & Sullivan, 1994). At the House Ear Clinic, the HINT test is one of the primary measures used to determine candidacy for cochlear implantation with the Cochlear Nucleus Freedom and Advanced Bionics Hi-Res 90K devices (Tables 5-1 and 5-2). The current preoperative assessment protocol is discussed below in the audiologic evaluation section.

Pediatric candidates for cochlear implantation must have bilateral, severe to profound sensorineural hearing loss with a pure-tone average of 90 dB HL in the better ear. A number of genetic and nongenetic causes of sensorineural hearing loss may render a child a candidate for a cochlear implant. Absence of a gap junction protein *connexin 26* represents the most common cause of hereditary nonsyndromic hearing loss (Gurtler & Lalwani, 2002). Syndromic causes of hearing loss include CHARGE association (Lanson, Green, Roland, Jr., Lalwani, & Waltzman, 2007), Waardenburg syndrome, Usher and Pendred syndromes, and Alport syndrome. Developmental factors associated with hearing loss include extended neonatal intensive care unit stays, hyperbilirubinemia, and prematurity. Ototoxic antibiotics and meningitis are among the acquired causes of hearing loss. The reader is referred to more thorough discussions on the etiology and evaluation of pediatric hearing loss (Morzaria, Westerberg, & Kozak, 2004, 2005).

Auditory neuropathy or dyssynchrony is a condition in which otoacoustic emissions are present, but there is an absent auditory brainstem response. These patients may be candidates for cochlear implants (Mason, De Michele, Stevens, Ruth, & Hashisaki, 2003; Peterson et al., 2003), but the best time to implant may be difficult to determine, as some patients experience spontaneous resynchronization and are able to use traditional amplification (Raveh, Buller, Badrana, & Attias, 2007). The reader is referred to Chapter 20 on auditory neuropathy in this text for further discussion.

Implantation may be performed as young as 12 months, though in certain studies younger patients have been implanted and the lower age limit has been challenged

---

TABLE 5–1. Current Implant Candidacy Criteria for Cochlear Nucleus Freedom Device

- Bilateral severe to profound sensorineural hearing loss (SNHL)
- Pre-op hearing-in-noise test (HINT) sentences ≤50% in the ear to be implanted and ≤60% in the opposite ear *or* binaurally aided
- Pre- or Postlinguistic onset of hearing loss

TABLE 5–2. Current Implant Candidacy for Advanced Bionics Hi-Res 90K Device

- Bilateral severe to profound SNHL (70 dB HL or greater)
- Pre-op hearing-in-noise test (HINT) Sentences of ≤50%
- Postlingual onset of hearing loss

(Miyamoto, Houston, & Bergeson, 2005). The patient must receive no significant benefit from hearing aids and have no medical contraindications. Typically, a 3- to 6-month trial with binaural amplification and intensive auditory training must be completed to ensure that hearing aids cannot provide the same level of benefit as an implant.

Perhaps equally as important as audiologic criteria are appropriate motivation, psychological fitness, and willingness to participate in postactivation programming. Patients (when feasible) as well as parents must have appropriate expectations and there must be appropriate support in the home and school environments.

Preoperative Evaluation

Audiologic Evaluation

Patients being evaluated for suitability for CI should undergo a full audiometric evaluation to determine if they meet the indications required by the FDA and the manufacturer, as well as any additional criteria required by the implant center. The reader is referred to other chapters in this book for more in-depth descriptions of the audiologic evaluation.

Medical Evaluation

As cochlear implantation is an elective procedure, patients under consideration for CI must be medically suitable for general anesthesia. They should be free from comorbid conditions that would place them at risk during the administration of general anesthesia. A complete medical history and physical examination should be performed, with a complete review of systems. A careful history of chronic ear disease should be obtained, and if necessary, staging of the implant procedure should be considered. This is discussed in a separate section of this chapter.

Cognitive factors should also be considered. If a patient would not reliably use their device, or if there are questions as to the mental capacity of the patient, careful discussion and consideration should be undertaken with the patient's family and caregivers.

Although not a contraindication to cochlear implantation, immune deficiencies such as immunoglobulin deficiencies and diabetes mellitus require more vigilance on the part of the cochlear implant team. Treatable immune deficiencies should be addressed prior to implantation, and diabetic blood sugar control should be optimized. All other medical problems should be optimally controlled prior to undergoing this elective surgical procedure (Odabasi, Mobley, Bolanos, Hodges, & Balkany, 2000).

Radiologic Evaluation

High-resolution computed tomography (CT) of the temporal bone is performed in all cases to identify partial or complete ossification of the scala tympani, soft tissue obliteration of the scala, congenital inner ear malformation, and the position of surgical landmarks (Frau, Luxford, Lo, Berliner, & Telischi, 1994; Seidman, Chute, & Parisier, 1994; Wiet, Pyle, O'Connor, Russell, & Schramm, 1990; Woolley, Oser, Lusk, & Bahadori, 1997). Complete agenesis of the cochlea (Michel aplasia) is an absolute contraindication to cochlear implantation, whereas an abnormal cochlear nerve or cochlear aperture is a relative contraindication to cochlear implant placement, and implant candidacy is dependent on preoperative testing and other imaging testing, including magnetic resonance imaging (MRI—see section below). Implantation in inner ear malformations is discussed later in this chapter.

Partial cochlear ossification or fibrosis is not a contraindication for CI, but these cases may require higher output power on the electrodes. Severe obliterative ossification may preclude electrode placement (Figure 5–1).

Although CT traditionally has been used for preoperative imaging, and remains the widespread standard, MR imaging may be used to evaluate a patient preoperatively (Harnsberger, Dart, Parkin, Smoker, & Osborn, 1987; Klein et al., 1992). Some centers are advocating the use of primary MRI as an evaluation tool for all pediatric patients with hearing loss (Adunka et al., 2006; Parry, Booth, & Roland, 2005). Parasagittal images through the internal auditory canal (IAC) may reveal the presence or absence of a cochlear nerve, particularly in cases where CT scanning suggests a narrow IAC (Figure 5–2) or a small cochlear aperture. The use of MRI alone instead of CT imaging remains controversial.

Certain patients in whom atlantoaxial instability is a concern require preoperative flexion-extension radiographs of the cervical spine. Manipulation of the neck in these patients, particularly lateral rotation, occurs during CI surgery and excessive manipulation could result in cervical spine injury.

Promontory Stimulation

Promontory stimulation was regularly performed in the past, but is no longer regularly performed by most teams (Spies, Snik, Mens, & van den Broek, 1993). A positive response is a perception of sound from stimulation of the cochlear promontory or round window membrane. Promontory stimulation may still be performed in selected cases where question has arisen to the viability of the cochlear nerve or in other situations where the success of a successful stimulation may be in doubt. In patients with auditory neuropathy, particularly in adults, some teams have proposed that promontory stimulation may help to determine

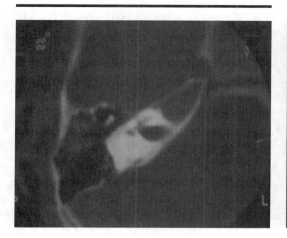

Figure 5–1. Axial computed tomography of the temporal bone reveals severe labyrinthine ossification.

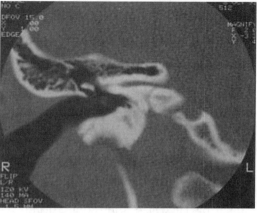

Figure 5–2. Coronal computed tomography of the temporal bone reveals a narrow internal auditory canal.

which patients will receive more benefit from their device (Mason et al., 2003).

The use of intraoperative promontory stimulation with electrically evoked auditory brainstem recording (EABR) has been used in patients with suspected auditory neuropathy and for perioperative correlation with implant performance. This has been done particularly in children who cannot tolerate preoperative awake promontory stimulation or who are not old enough to indicate the perception of sound (Miyamoto & Brown, 1987). In this subset of patients, EABR performed in the operating room both pre- and postimplantation may indicate which patients have stimulable synchronous auditory nerve activity. This may prove to be valuable in deciding which patients with suspected auditory neuropathy/dyssynchrony would benefit from cochlear implantation (Kileny, Zwolan, Boerst, & Telian, 1997).

Device Selection

In the United States, three manufacturers produce cochlear implants for human use: Cochlear Corporation, Advanced Bionics Corporation, and MED-EL Corporation. Each of these manufacturers has specific FDA indications for the use of their particular device. The specific choice of an implant may depend on the age of the patient, hearing thresholds, patient preference, and availability of a particular device to the implant center. There are other manufacturers of cochlear implants, and availability of implant technology outside of the United States depends on regional factors.

All current cochlear implants have a similar package size, and require drilling of a "well," or depression, in the bone of the skull to accommodate the internal proces-

sor. Future cochlear implants may incorporate flat internal processors that do not require drilling of a well.

How Cochlear Implants Function

In contrast to traditional hearing aids that amplify acoustic energy and deliver it to the external ear, cochlear implants process sound and convert it into electrical energy for subsequent delivery to the auditory nerve. The implanted electrode is positioned via the scala tympani of the cochlea, near the osseous spiral lamina and the spiral ganglion. By stimulating the spiral ganglion, diseased or absent cochlear hair cells are bypassed and sound may be relayed to the auditory nerve and subsequently to the cerebral cortex.

The external components of a cochlear implant consist of the microphone, the speech processor, and the external transmitter coil. The internal components include the internal coil, the internal receiver-stimulator, and the electrode.

The microphone of the CI receives analog sound from the external environment and sends it to the speech processor, which converts the sound into a digital signal. The signal is filtered into separate frequency bands that are sent to the appropriate tonotopic regions in the cochlea that correspond to those frequencies. The external processor also amplifies the sounds and compresses the sound based on settings determined at activation of the implant. Frequently, there is a narrow dynamic range of electrical stimulation that the patient tolerates, and the sound must be compressed into this range.

The digital electric signal is then sent by radiofrequency transmission from the external coil through the skin to an internal coil, where the signal is received and sent to the internal receiver-stimulator. The signal is then decoded and sent to the implant electrode array in the cochlea.

A number of sound and speech-processing algorithms may be used to process sound before it is sent to the internal receiver-stimulator. Although each cochlear implant manufacturer has developed signal processing algorithms that are specific to their particular systems, these algorithms generally process the temporal and spectral cues of the incoming speech signal. Cochlear implant manufacturers continue to develop new processing strategies, particularly with the goal of improving open-set speech recognition and music perception (Rubinstein, 2004; Rubinstein & Hong, 2003).

Standard Implantation Procedure

Once a patient has undergone a proper medical, audiologic, and radiologic evaluation, and has been found to be a suitable candidate for implantation, surgery may be undertaken. The standard cochlear implantation procedure for a patient with a normally developed, patent cochlea is described here.

Informed consent is obtained from the patient, including a discussion about possible intraoperative and postoperative complications. Potential complications include postoperative nausea and vomiting, postoperative taste disturbances, the potential for wound infection, as well as hardware-related failure, possible implant extrusion, and nonstimulation. The possibility of facial nerve injury also is discussed. At the House Ear Clinic, a standardized operative consent document is used that outlines the risks of the procedure, and the patient signs this document along with the operative consent

indicating that they comprehend and accept the risks inherent to the procedure (see Appendix 5–A).

One preoperative dose of antibiotic is administered to cover skin bacterial flora. This is typically cefazolin, or in the case of a penicillin-allergic patient, clindamycin or vancomycin. The patient is brought to the operating room, and general endotracheal anesthesia is administered. For infants under the age of 12 months and for young children, pediatric anesthesia principles are followed, including the use of calibrated intravenous infusion systems to provide accurate fluid replacement. Proper sizing of blood pressure cuffs and other monitoring equipment must be ensured. In small children, care is taken during the draping procedure to ensure that the head does not rotate excessively to the contralateral side. A rolled towel or pad may be used to stabilize the head.

Needle monitoring electrodes are placed in the ipsilateral face and attached to the facial nerve monitor (NIM-Response 2.0, Medtronic Xomed, Jacksonville, FL), and proper function of the facial nerve monitor is confirmed. The postauricular region is generously shaved, including the skin over the internal processor and coil. The patient is then prepared with povidone-iodine soap and paint, and draped for the procedure.

A skin incision is designed in the postauricular region, just behind the postauricular sulcus and extending superior to the auricle, curving first anteriorly and then posteriorly in an "S" pattern. A minimally invasive incision is defined as less than 6 cm in length. The positions of the external processor as well as the internal processor are marked on the patient using the manufacturer's template. A drop of methylene blue on a 20-gauge needle may be used to mark the proposed position of the well on the musculopericranium and skull using a transcutaneous puncture (Figure 5–3A).

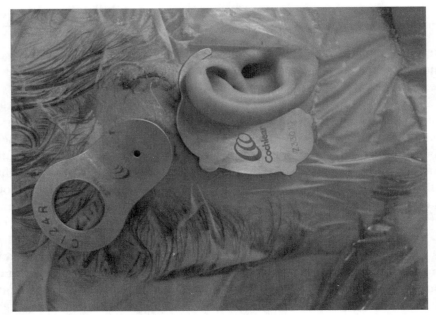

A

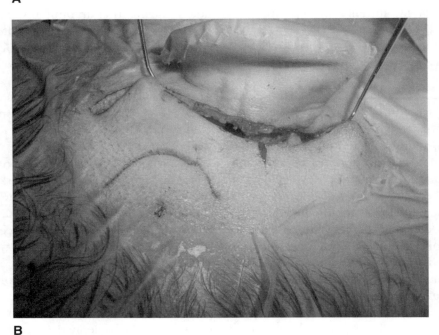

B

Figure 5–3. **A.** The device templates are used to mark the positions of the external speech processor and the position of the internal receiver-stimulator and internal coil. Methylene blue is instilled via the hole in the marker for the receiver-stimulator to mark its position on the musculopericranium and the cranium itself. **B.** The full-length incision is shown. More recently, the most inferior 3 to 4 cm of the incision is not incised. Methylene blue may be seen marking the position of the internal receiver-stimulator.

The incision is infiltrated with local anesthetic with epinephrine. Skin flaps are then elevated both anteriorly and posteriorly (Figure 5–3B). A musculopericranial flap is then elevated, using the previously placed dot of methylene blue dye as a marker for the correct position of the well. An anteriorly based flap is elevated up to the level of the posterior canal wall, cribriform area, and spine of Henle (Figure 5–4). A self-retaining retractor is placed in the wound.

Cortical mastoidectomy is then performed, taking care to leave an overhanging ledge of bone on the tegmen mastoideum as well as the region lateral to the sigmoid sinus for retention of the electrodes. The antrum is opened and the fossa incudis is identified. The facial recess is then opened with successively smaller diamond burrs. The facial nerve is skeletonized as needed to "saucerize" and fully open the facial recess. The incudostapedial

joint, cochlear promontory, and round window niche are identified. A sponge is then placed into the mastoid.

The well and trough for the implant are drilled, using the templates included in the specific device instrument tray. The wound is then extensively irrigated to remove bone dust.

Cochleostomy is perfomed using a 1.5-mm or 1-mm diamond burr. If the facial recess is particularly narrow, a drill that only rotates at the distal diamond ball may be employed, to avoid heat injury to the facial nerve caused by a rotating drill shaft. In all cases, copious irrigation should be applied through the suction-irrigator to reduce any transmission of heat to the facial nerve.

Once the cochleostomy has been performed, the device is inserted under the skin and musculopericranium, and the internal receiver-stimulator is placed into the drilled well. Depending on the device chosen, there

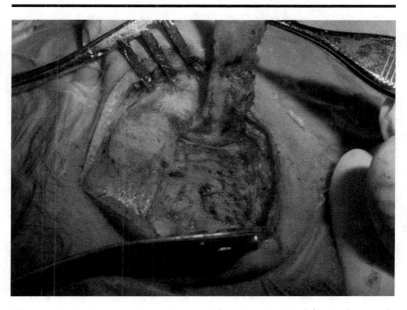

Figure 5–4. A musculopericranial flap is elevated from the position of the internal receiver-stimulator to the cribriform area of the mastoid.

may be a ground electrode to be placed deep to the temporalis muscle. The stimulating electrode is then placed into the scala tympani via the cochleostomy using the technique recommended by the manufacturer. In the advance-off stylet technique, the stiffening wire (stylet) is removed as the electrode is inserted into the cochlea. Some authors have used hyaluronic acid (Roland, Magardino, Go, & Hillman, 1995) or other lubricants to reduce insertional trauma and the inflammation associated with implantation (Figure 5–5).

Once the device is placed, the musculopericranium is closed over the implant and the more superficial muscle and skin are closed in layers (Figures 5–6 and 5–7). Suture fixation of the device to surrounding

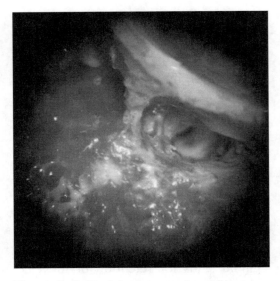

Figure 5–5. Facial recess and cochleostomy are shown.

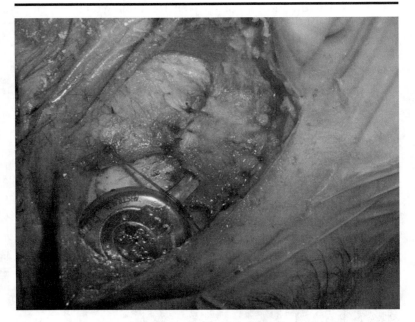

Figure 5–6. The musculopericranial flap is closed over the implant electrodes. The internal receiver-stimulator may be placed deep or superficial to the pericranium, depending on the age of the patient and the scalp thickness.

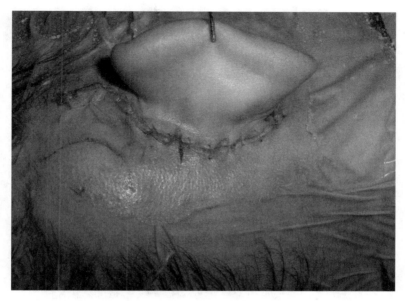

Figure 5–7. Closed incision.

bone or periosteum is performed as dictated by surgeon preference. Intraoperative telemetry is employed at some centers to verify the presence of electrode waveforms and proper electrode impedances. Flouroscopy or plain radiographic images may also be taken to verify the placement of the implant electrode in the cochlea. A standard mastoid pressure dressing is applied for one day postoperatively.

Special Situations

Anatomic Difficulties

Implantation of Developmental Abnormalities

Contraindications to CI include cochlear aplasia (Michel aplasia) and cochlear nerve aplasia. However, implants in patients with inner ear malformations have been performed and shown to be successful in many recipients (Buchman, Joy, Hodges, Telischi, & Balkany, 2004b; Ito, Sakota, Kato, Hazama, & Enomoto, 1999; Loundon et al., 2005; Miyamoto, Robbins, Myres, & Pope, 1986; Papsin, 2005).

In a study by Buchman and colleagues, 28 pediatric cochlear implant patients with known inner ear malformations were implanted. Patients with Mondini malformation (incompletely partitioned cochlea, enlarged vestibular aqueduct (EVA), and a dilated vestibule) as well as those with an isolated EVA (Figure 5–8) or partial semicircular canal aplasia were found to have relatively good levels of speech perception. However, patients with cochlear hypoplasia, total semicircular canal aplasia, isolated incomplete partition, or common cavity malformation demonstrated lower levels of performance (Buchman et al., 2004a).

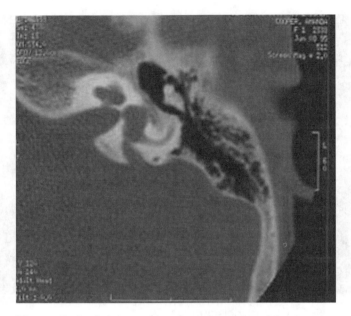

Figure 5–8. Axial computed tomography of the temporal bone reveals enlargement of the vestibular aqueduct.

A study by Papsin (2005) showed that abnormal middle ear anatomy and cerebral spinal fluid (CSF) gusher occur with greater frequency in this patient population, and showed similar decreased cochlear implant performance findings.

When an increased risk of CSF gusher is suspected, the surgeon should be prepared to remove the incus and pack the middle ear and eustachian tube. Lumbar drainage may be needed, but this is rare (Wootten, Backous, & Haynes, 2006).

Postmeningitic Patients

Early Implantation in Labyrinthitis Ossificans

In postmeningitic patients, cochlear ossification may occur within months of infection (Axon, Temple, Saeed, & Ramsden,

1998). CI may be attempted in this group of patients within this time interval if preoperative assessment is reliably completed and the patient is determined to be an appropriate candidate. CT may not reliably show cochlear ossification in this group of patients, and cochlear patency on high resolution tomography is not always predictive of operative findings. Presence or absence of ossification in the lateral semicircular canal may be more predictive of cochlear patency (Young, Hughes, Byrd, & Darling, 2000). If patients with a history of meningitis undergo cochlear ossification, implantation may still be attempted. A discussion of implantation in the setting of cochlear ossification follows.

Cochlear Ossification

Preoperative evaluation of CI patients with high-resolution CT may identify patients in whom cochlear ossification has taken place. Preoperative counseling of the patient and family is essential in this situation to ensure appropriate expectations about electrode placement and the implications of a partial electrode deployment.

In ossified cochleas, an orderly approach should be taken to cochleostomy and placement of the device. The ledge of bone over the round window niche should be drilled away to reveal the round window membrane. If the membrane and scala tympani appear ossified, an initial attempt at cochleostomy may be made in the standard position, but more drilling may need to be performed to traverse the ossified segment. Smaller drills, such as stapes drills, may be necessary in this situation. Care should be taken to prevent heat injury to the facial nerve from the rotating drill shaft.

Scala vestibuli placement is an alternative when the scala tympani is extensively ossified, preventing placement of the elec-trode array via the standard route (Kiefer, Weber, Pfennigdorff, & von Ilberg, 2000; Steenerson, Gary, & Wynens, 1990). Cochleostomy should be widened to allow placement of the electrode into the scala vestibuli (Figure 5–9).

A split-electrode technique may be employed in certain cases. Two electrodes, one 11 mm in length and one 10 mm in length are combined on the same receiver-stimulator. Two cochleostomies are drilled, one in the standard position on the basal turn and one on the second turn anterior to the oval window and caudal to the cochleariform process. The two electrodes are then deployed separately into the cochleostomies (Bredberg et al., 1997; Lenarz et al., 2001; Millar, Hillman, & Shelton, 2005).

Radical cochleostomy may be performed should none of the above methods prove to be viable (Gantz, McCabe, & Tyler, 1988). In this case, a radical mastoidectomy is performed and the eustachian tube obliterated

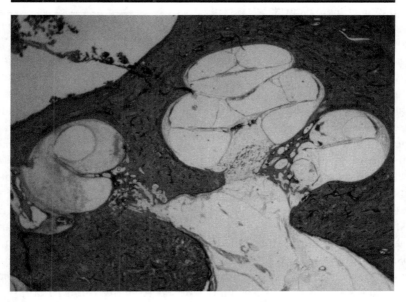

Figure 5–9. Histopathologic section of the temporal bone shows placement of the cochlear implant electrode in the scala vestibuli.

after the removal of all mucosa from the middle ear. The external auditory canal is oversewn. A tympanic neurectomy may be performed to reduce pain on stimulation of the cochlea. A 22- to 24-mm trough is drilled after the first and part of the second cochlear turn. The electrode is then coiled around the modiolus. Fascia and bone are used to secure the implant in position.

A canal closure technique may be used in cases of severe cochlear ossification, to stage the procedure, or cases in which poor anatomy precludes a standard facial recess approach to the cochlea. This is discussed below in the section on CI surgery in chronic otitis media.

Implantation in Chronic Otitis Media

As cochlear implantation introduces a foreign body into the middle and inner ear as well as the contiguous musculopericranium and skull, ears affected by chronic suppurative otitis media (CSOM) carry a risk of inoculating the device and surrounding tissue with colonized bacteria. *Pseudomonas aeruginosa* and other gram-negative bacteria may be found in ears with CSOM.

Most authors concur that a staged approach should be taken when planning to implant ears with CSOM. Generally, this requires the removal of all epithelium from the ear canal, middle ear, and mastoid. A modified Rambo technique is used to close the ear canal with or without obliteration of the mastoid, depending on the clinical situation. After sufficient time for healing of the cavity and confirmation that no infection persists, a second stage follows at which time the implant is placed. The interval between stages may vary (El Kashlan, Arts, & Telian, 2003).

In children with recurrent otitis media (ROM), Fayad (Fayad, Tabaee, Micheletto, & Parisier, 2003a) showed that cochlear implantation may be performed either concomitantly or following myringotomy and tube placement. A history of recurrent otitis media does not preclude an ear from being a candidate for cochlear implantation. Aggressive treatment of otitis media after CI should be undertaken to prevent complications.

Auditory Neuropathy

Patients with absent ABR and present otoacoustic emissions, termed auditory neuropathy or auditory dyssynchrony, may be implanted. In one study, CI performance did not vary between a group of 10 patients with auditory neuropathy who were implanted and a matched group of patients with standard CI indications (Peterson et al., 2003). Clinicians should evaluate these patients fully to determine whether there are any treatable underlying neurologic causes for their auditory nerve dysfunction.

Vestibular Hypofunction and CI

Cochlear implantation has been shown to cause vestibular hypofunction as measured by caloric testing (Buchman et al., 2004b). In Buchman's study, approximately 10% of children were found to experience a significant unilateral vestibular loss from CI. However, despite the presence of a unilateral vestibular loss, these patients were not symptomatic when measured on several vestibular tests. In addition, the risk of bilateral vestibular loss from simultaneous CI in children is estimated to be substantially less than 5%. For those who experience measurable losses, adaptive mechanisms are proposed to allow them to compensate (Fina et al., 2003) Preoperative vestibular hypofunction may influence the surgeon to choose one ear over the other for CI.

Very Young Patients

As newborn hearing screening continues to expand, increasing numbers of infants with hearing loss are potential candidates for CI. Implantation in the United States is currently approved for patients as young as 12 months, but some patients have been implanted earlier than that in selected studies (James & Papsin, 2004; Miyamoto et al., 2005).

Concerns raised about the implantation of very young patients include the immaturity of the temporal bone and the increased risk of general anesthesia, particularly in those patients younger than 6 months of age (Young, 2002). Additionally, there are concerns about the difficulty of achieving a proper amplification trial with conventional hearing aids in patients younger than 6 months, in whom only objective measures of hearing thresholds have been obtained. These patients are too young to be assessed with behavioral tests, and CI teams must rely on caregivers' feedback.

Anatomic concerns have been assuaged as patients as young as 4 months have been found to have adequately developed facial recess anatomy for the placement of cochlear implant electrodes (Colletti et al., 2005). Very early implantation may facilitate the development of key central auditory pathways critical to the development of speech and language. Patients implanted between 12 months to 2 years have been shown to acquire language that is nearly equivalent to children with normal hearing (Manrique, Cervera-Paz, Huarte, & Molina, 2004).

Bilateral Implantation

CI may be performed on both ears either simultaneously or sequentially (Gantz et al., 2002; Litovsky et al., 2006a; Litovsky, Parkinson, Arcaroli, & Sammeth, 2006b; Tyler et al., 2002a). Bilateral CI patients appear to perform better on sound localization tests and benefit from the "head shadow" effect. In the situation where noise is placed on one side of the CI user's head, the CI contralateral to the noise is shadowed and provides better speech understanding. However, the speech understanding scores may be only marginally improved. In one study, the speech understanding gain was 8% (Laszig et al., 2004).

Critics of bilateral implantation argue that the incremental gains achieved by implantation of both ears are not large enough to justify the added cost and use of health care resources (Cohen, 2004). Despite these criticisms, bilateral CIs are becoming standard clinical practice.

When performing bilateral cochlear implantation, blood loss must be kept to a minimum. The total blood volume in an infant is 70 cc/kg, and no more than 5 to 10% of the blood volume should be lost during the procedure, based on the initial hematocrit (Gross, 1983). In a 10-kg infant, this represents 35 to 70 cc of blood loss. For smaller children, the figures are even lower. Care must be taken to avoid injuring the sigmoid sinus or other large veins. If the blood loss is significant, surgery on the second side must be delayed.

Relation of Histopathology to Performance

CI electrode placement results in varying degrees of trauma to the cochlear turns and neural elements. Typically, the basal turn undergoes fibrosis around the electrode, and this fibrosis may extend to the middle cochlear turn (Figures 5–10A and 5–10B).

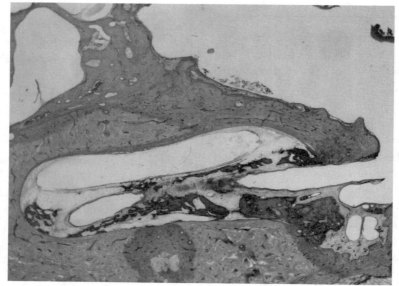

A

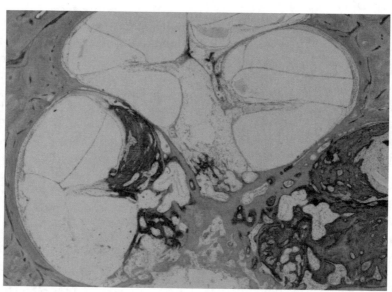

B

Figure 5–10. A. Histopathologic section of the temporal bone showing fibrosis in the cochlear basal turn associated with implantation. **B.** Fibrosis extends to the middle turn of the cochlea.

Fibrosis is usually found along the path of the electrode, and rarely extends beyond the tip of the electrode. In certain temporal bones, there is a mixture of fibrosis and new bone formation which is usually related to the trauma of preparation of the cochleostomy and the trauma of electrode insertion. It is believed that the trauma to the endosteal layer is responsible for the new bone formation. This new bone formation is sometimes extensive in the proximal basal turn of the cochlea (Fayad et al., 1991). However, despite degeneration of the peripheral processes in this area, there are remaining spiral ganglion cells in Rosenthal's canal (Figure 5–11).

More recently, Fayad et al. have used software to reconstruct our temporal bones with implants. They were able to quantify the amount of fibrosis and ossification in each one of these bones. Except for a small number of bones, the most extensive reaction to the presence of the electrode is usu-

ally in the first few millimeters of the basal turn of the cochlea (Makarem, Linthicum, Balaraman, & Fayad, 2008). Correlations between the amount of new tissue formation and the preservation of neural elements were not shown to be statistically significant (Li, Somdas, Eddington, & Nadol, Jr., 2007). In a more recent study, a significant inverse relationship was found between new tissue formation in segment I (basal turn) of the cochlea and the number of spiral ganglion cells; however, no significant relationship was found between these two variables for the rest of the cochlea (Makarem et al., 2008).

Fewer surviving spiral ganglion cells than previously thought are necessary to achieve adequate CI device performance. Attempts have been made to correlate the residual count of spiral ganglion cells in the cochlea to speech understanding performance with cochlear implants. A recent study by Fayad and Linthicum (2006) evaluated

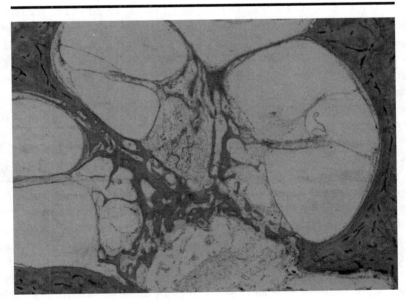

Figure 5–11. The osseous spiral lamina shows degeneration of dendritic cells but relative preservation of spiral ganglion cells.

temporal bone specimens from patients who underwent cochlear implantation. In this study, 14 bones were examined for the presence of spiral ganglion cells and the patient's cochlear implant performance was correlated with the cell counts. Ganglion cell count was generally not related to performance, whereas segment III (mid-apical turn) showed significant negative correlations to speech discrimination scores for words and sentences. Based on this study, performance variability of cochlear implants cannot be explained on the basis of spiral ganglion cell survival. Factors other than spiral ganglion cell counts must also be considered (Khan et al., 2005).

Minor and Major Complications

One minor complication of cochlear implantation is facial nerve stimulation. In one study on adult CI recipients, the incidence of facial nerve stimulation was shown to be 14% (Bigelow et al., 1998). Typically, facial nerve stimulation may be eliminated through electrode reprogramming. Another minor complication is a local wound infection that resolves with oral or intravenous antibiotics. In one study, minor complications occurred in 32% of CI patients and all were managed successfully (Postelmans, Cleffken, & Stokroos, 2007).

Major complications of cochlear implantation include flap necrosis, implant exposure, and interval device malfunction requiring reimplantation. One study estimated major complications occurred in 3.6 percent of their pediatric and adult CI population (Postelmans et al., 2007).

In patients who undergo revision surgery for reimplantation, audiologic performance in the majority of children reaches their prerevision clinical performance (Fayad, Baino, & Parisier, 2004; Fayad et al., 2006; Migirov, Taitelbaum-Swead, Hildesheimer, & Kronenberg, 2007). A recent study of 952 pediatric CI recipients showed a revision rate of 11.2%. The majority of the cases requiring revision were so-called "hard failure" cases where device malfunction was confirmed prior to revision surgery. All of these patients had a sudden loss of sound percepts, and 88% of these patients had a failure of communication (lock) between the external and internal processors. This study also found that the majority of patients return to their pre-revision functional level, though the return to that level of functioning may take up to a year (Cullen, Fayad, Luxford, & Buchman, 2008).

Facial nerve paralysis is another major complication that may occur after cochlear implantation. In a study by Fayad, Wanna, Micheletto, and Parisier (2003b) of 705 patients who underwent CI, the incidence of facial nerve paresis or paralysis was 0.71%. In all cases, facial nerve weakness was delayed and the weakness eventually resolved to normal function. Theorized causes of delayed facial weakness include thermal injury to the facial nerve during the facial recess approach and viral reactivation.

Meningitis—Occurrence and Prevention

In June 2002, the Centers for Disease Control (CDC) received reports of bacterial meningitis in patients who had received cochlear implants. In a study of 4,264 children under the age of 6 years who had undergone CI, 26 patients with bacterial meningitis were identified. This group of patients had a 30 times higher risk of *S.*

pneumoniae bacterial meningitis than the general population. Patients with meningitis were more likely to have had an implant electrode with a perimodiolar positioning device ("positioner"). As a result, the CDC issued guidelines for the vaccination of all children and adults scheduled to undergo CI.

Current immunization recommendations include the use of polyvalent pneumococcal for all patients scheduled to undergo cochlear implantation. The CDC recommends that children up to age 60 months receive the 7-valent pneumococcal conjugate vaccine (PCV-7, Prevnar). Patients over the age of 24 months should receive a single dose of the pneumococcal polysaccharide 23-valent vaccine (PPV-23, Pneumovax). See (http://www.cdc.gov/mmwr/preview/mmwrhtml/m2e731a1.htm).

Future Evolution of Cochlear Implantation

Short Electrode "Hybrid" Implants and Implantation with Residual Hearing

Since the early 2000s, an FDA clinical trial has been underway to examine the usefulness of cochlear implantation in adult patients with residual low-frequency hearing. This device, termed the "hybrid" cochlear implant, uses a shorter electrode (Gantz, Turner, & Gfeller, 2006).

Although the electrode is shorter, it stimulates the basal region of the cochlea and hence the high-frequency tonotopic region. By avoiding insertional trauma to the cochlear apex, lower frequency information may be preserved. In this technique, a "soft" insertion technique is used, in which

excessive trauma to the basal turn of the cochlea is avoided, and the round window is used for insertion of the device. For hearing preservation to be attempted, insertional trauma must be minimized. Implantation via the round window membrane may decrease this trauma (Adunka et al., 2004).

The theorized advantage of such devices is to benefit patients with significant low-frequency residual hearing, who have lost perception in the speech frequency range and, hence, have low speech discrimination scores. Patients implanted with a hybrid cochlear implant essentially use a hearing aid and a cochlear implant in the same ear (Gantz, Turner, Gfeller, & Lowder, 2005).

Experimental electrodes notwithstanding, some centers routinely implant patients who have residual hearing with standard cochlear implants, enabling these patients to benefit from both the CI and a hearing aid (Tyler et al., 2002b). Although the longer electrode may cause trauma to the apex of the cochlea, some reports of hearing preservation have been presented (James et al., 2005).

Totally Implantable CI

The recent advent of behind-the-ear speech processor technology for cochlear implantation has resulted in the modification of the surgical technique to ensure that the internal processor and coil are both posterior to the position of the external processor such that the external processor does not exert pressure on the skin over the internal device. This technique is performed in an attempt to avoid wound breakdown and implant exposure. Despite this precaution, the use of the external magnet does cause some irritation of the skin overlying the internal coil, and infrequently may result in flap necrosis.

In addition, current implant technology requires both frequent recharging of the external processor as well as the need to surgically remove the internal coil magnet in the event that a magnetic resonance imaging (MRI) scan is required. Research is progressing on a totally implantable cochlear implant device that would not require the use of an external processor and magnet. This would enable the patient to undergo MRI scanning, as well as avoid the use of an external processor. Periodic charging of the device would occur transcutaneously, using a charging module (Cohen, 2004). This technology would also require the implantation of a microphone (Maniglia et al., 1999). A small number of patients have undergone implantation with a device that includes an internal microphone on the internal processor, so called "invisible hearing" (Briggs et al., 2008). It is not expected, however, that a totally implanted device would be attempted in children for a number of years.

Evidence-Based Medicine and Cost-Benefit Analysis

With the rising costs of medical technology, any new device or treatment must be evaluated as to its benefit to the patient. Increasingly, governmental and private payers are demanding that advancing technologies be studied to verify that there is an appropriate cost-benefit ratio and that the patient's quality-of-life be appropriately enhanced. Several studies have addressed the cost versus benefit of cochlear implants and have shown their cost-effectiveness (Cheng & Niparko, 1999; Cheng et al., 2000; Sach, O'Neill, Whynes, Archbold, & O'Donoghue, 2003).

Summary

Cochlear implantation has undergone major advances since its introduction. Devices continue to become smaller, more technologically complex, and implanted through smaller incisions. Candidacy criteria have also expanded, and children as young as 12 months of age are currently candidates for CI, with some patients younger than a year being implanted on study protocols.

With proper preoperative evaluation, and properly executed surgical protocols, CI is very safe and cost effective. Complications can be minimized by adherence to proper surgical principles.

References

Adunka, O., Unkelbach, M. H., Mack, M., Hambek, M., Gstoettner, W., & Kiefer, J. (2004). Cochlear implantation via the round window membrane minimizes trauma to cochlear structures: A histologically controlled insertion study. *Acta Oto-Laryngolica, 124*, 807–812.

Adunka, O. F., Roush, P. A., Teagle, H. F., Brown, C. J., Zdanski, C. J., Jewells, V., et al. (2006). Internal auditory canal morphology in children with cochlear nerve deficiency. *Otology and Neurotology, 27*, 793–801.

Axon, P. R., Temple, R. H., Saeed, S. R., & Ramsden, R. T. (1998). Cochlear ossification after meningitis. *American Journal of Otology, 19*, 724–729.

Bigelow, D. C., Kay, D. J., Rafter, K. O., Montes, M., Knox, G. W., & Yousem, D. M. (1998). Facial nerve stimulation from cochlear implants. *American Journal of Otology, 19*, 163–169.

Bredberg, G., Lindstrom, B., Lopponen, H., Skarzynski, H., Hyodo, M., & Sato, H. (1997). Electrodes for ossified cochleas. *American Journal of Otology, 18*(Suppl. 6), S42–S43.

Briggs, R. J., Eder, H. C., Seligman, P. M., Cowan, R. S., Plant, K. L., Dalton, J., et al. (2008). Initial clinical experience with a totally implantable cochlear implant research device. *Otology and Neurotology*, *29*, 114–119.

Buchman, C. A., Copeland, B. J., Yu, K. K., Brown, C. J., Carrasco, V. N., & Pillsbury, H. C., 3rd. (2004a). Cochlear implantation in children with congenital inner ear malformations. *Laryngoscope*, *114*, 309–316.

Buchman, C. A., Joy, J., Hodges, A., Telischi, F. F., & Balkany, T. J. (2004b). Vestibular effects of cochlear implantation. *Laryngoscope*, *114*(Suppl. 103), 1–22.

Cheng, A. K., & Niparko, J. K. (1999). Cost-utility of the cochlear implant in adults: A meta-analysis. *Archives of Otolaryngology-Head and Neck Surgery*, *125*, 1214–1218.

Cheng, A. K., Rubin, H. R., Powe, N. R., Mellon, N. K., Francis, H. W., & Niparko, J. K. (2000). Cost-utility analysis of the cochlear implant in children. *Journal of the American Medical Association*, *284*, 850–856.

Clark, G. M., Tong, Y. C., Black, R., Forster, I. C., Patrick, J. F., & Dewhurst, D. J. (1977). A multiple electrode cochlear implant. *Journal of Laryngology and Otology*, *91*, 935–945.

Clark, G. M., Tong, Y. C., & Patrick, J. F. (Eds.). (1990). History of the cochlear implant. In *Cochlear prostheses* (pp. 1–5). Edinburgh: Churchill Livingstone.

Cohen, N. L. (2004). Cochlear implant candidacy and surgical considerations. *Audiology and Neuro-otology*, *9*, 197–202.

Cohen, N. L, Waltzman, S. B., & Shapiro, W. H. (1985). Clinical trials with a 22-channel cochlear prosthesis. *Laryngoscope*, *95*, 1448–1454.

Colletti, V., Carner, M., Miorelli, V., Guida, M., Colletti, L., & Fiorino, F. G. (2005). Cochlear implantation at under 12 months: Report on 10 patients. *Laryngoscope*, *115*, 445–449.

Cullen, R. D., Fayad, J. N., Luxford, W. M., & Buchman, C. A. (2008). Revision cochlear implant surgery in children. *Otology and Neurotology*, *29*, 214–220.

Djourno, A., & Eyries, C. (1957). Prosthese auditive par excitation electrique a sistance du nerf sensorial a l'aide d'un bobinage inclus a demeure [Auditory prostesis by means of a distant electrical stimulation of the sensory nerve with the use of an indwelt coiling]. *La Presse Medicale*, *35*, 1417.

Eisenberg, L. S., Berliner, K. I., Thielemeir, M. A., Kirk, K. I., & Tiber, N. (1983). Cochlear implants in children. *Ear and Hearing*, *4*, 41–50.

Eisenberg, L. S., & House, W. F. (1982). Initial experience with the cochlear implant in children. *Annals of Otology, Rhinology, and Laryngology*, *91*(Suppl. 91), 67–73.

El-Kashlan, H. K., Arts, H. A., & Telian, S. A. (2003). External auditory canal closure in cochlear implant surgery. *Otology and Neurotology*, *24*, 404–408.

Fayad, J. N., Baino, T., & Parisier, S. C. (2004). Revision cochlear implant surgery: Causes and outcome. *Otolaryngology-Head and Neck Surgery*, *131*, 429–432.

Fayad, J. N., Eisenberg, L. S., Gillinger, M., Winter, M., Martinez, A. S., & Luxford, W. M. (2006). Clinical performance of children following revision surgery for a cochlear implant. *Otolaryngology-Head and Neck Surgery*, *134*, 379–384.

Fayad, J. N., & Linthicum, F. H., Jr. (2006). Multichannel cochlear implants: Relation of histopathology to performance. *Laryngoscope*, *116*, 1310–1320.

Fayad, J., Linthicum, F. H., Jr., Otto, S. R., Galey, F. R., & House, W. F. (1991). Cochlear implants: Histopathologic findings related to performance in 16 human temporal bones. *Annals of Otology, Rhinology, and Laryngology*, *100*, 807–811.

Fayad, J. N., Tabaee, A., Micheletto, J. N., & Parisier, S. C. (2003a). Cochlear implantation in children with otitis media. *Laryngoscope*, *113*, 1224–1227.

Fayad, J. N., Wanna, G. B., Micheletto, J. N., & Parisier, S. C. (2003b). Facial nerve paralysis following cochlear implant surgery. *Laryngoscope*, *113*, 1344–1346.

Fina, M., Skinner, M., Goebel, J. A., Piccirillo, J. F., Neely, J. G., & Black, O. (2003). Vestibular dysfunction after cochlear implantation. *Otology and Neurotology*, *24*, 234–242.

Frau, G. N., Luxford, W. M., Lo, W. W., Berliner, K. I., & Telischi, F. F. (1994). High-resolution computed tomography in evaluation of cochlear patency in implant candidates: A comparison with surgical findings. *Journal of Laryngology and Otology, 108,* 743–748.

Gantz, B. J., McCabe, B. F., & Tyler, R. S. (1988). Use of multichannel cochlear implants in obstructed and obliterated cochleas. *Otolaryngology-Head and Neck Surgery, 98,* 72–81.

Gantz, B. J., Turner, C., & Gfeller, K. E. (2006). Acoustic plus electric speech processing: Preliminary results of a multicenter clinical trial of the Iowa/Nucleus hybrid implant. *Audiology and Neuro-otology, 11*(Suppl. 1), 63–68.

Gantz, B. J., Turner, C., Gfeller, K. E., & Lowder, M. W. (2005). Preservation of hearing in cochlear implant surgery: Advantages of combined electrical and acoustical speech processing. *Laryngoscope, 115,* 796–802.

Gantz, B. J., Tyler, R. S., Rubinstein, J. T., Wolaver, A., Lowder, M., Abbas, P., Brown, C., Hughes, M., & Preece, J. P. (2002). Binaural cochlear implants placed during the same operation. *Otology and Neurotology, 23,* 169–180.

Gross, J. B. (1983). Estimating allowable blood loss: Correcting for dilution. *Anesthesiology, 58,* 277–280.

Gurtler, N., & Lalwani, A. K. (2002). Etiology of syndromic and nonsyndromic sensorineural hearing loss. *Otolaryngologic Clinics of North America, 35,* 891–908.

Harnsberger, H. R., Dart, D. J., Parkin, J. L., Smoker, W. R., & Osborn, A. G. (1987). Cochlear implant candidates: Assessment with CT and MR imaging. *Radiology, 164,* 53–57.

House, W. F., & Urban, J. (1973) Long term results of electrode implantation and electronic stimulation of the cochlea in man. *Annals of Otology, Rhinology, and Laryngology, 82,* 504–517.

Ito, J., Sakota, T., Kato, H., Hazama, M., & Enomoto, M. (1999). Surgical considerations regarding cochlear implantation in the congenitally malformed cochlea. *Otolaryngology-Head and Neck Surgery, 121,* 495–498.

James, A. L., & Papsin, B. C. (2004). Cochlear implant surgery at 12 months of age or younger. *Laryngoscope, 114,* 2191–2195.

James, C., Albegger, K., Battmer, R., Burdo, S., Deggouj, N., Deguine, O., et al. (2005). Preservation of residual hearing with cochlear implantation: How and why. *Acta Oto-Laryngolica, 125,* 481–491.

Khan, A. M., Handzel, O., Burgess, B. J., Damian, D., Eddington, D. K., & Nadol, J. B., Jr. (2005). Is word recognition correlated with the number of surviving spiral ganglion cells and electrode insertion depth in human subjects with cochlear implants? *Laryngoscope, 115,* 672–677.

Kiefer, J., Weber, A., Pfennigdorff, T., & von Ilberg, C. (2000). Scala vestibuli insertion in cochlear implantation: A valuable alternative for cases with obstructed scala tympani. *ORL: Journal for Oto-rhino-laryngology and Its Related Specialties, 62,* 251–256.

Kileny, P. R., Zwolan, T. A., Boerst, A., & Telian, S. A. (1997). Electrically evoked auditory potentials: Current clinical applications in children with cochlear implants. *American Journal of Otology, 18*(Suppl. 6), S90–S92.

Klein, H. M., Bohndorf, K., Hermes, H., Schutz, W. F., Gunther, R. W., & Schlondorff, G. (1992). Computed tomography and magnetic resonance imaging in the preoperative work-up for cochlear implantation. *European Journal of Radiolology, 15,* 89–92.

Lanson, B. G., Green, J. E., Roland, J. T., Jr., Lalwani, A. K., & Waltzman, S. B. (2007). Cochlear implantation in Children with CHARGE syndrome: Therapeutic decisions and outcomes. *Laryngoscope, 117,* 1260–1266.

Laszig, R., Aschendorff, A., Stecker, M., Muller-Deile, J., Maune, S., Dillier, N., et al. (2004). Benefits of bilateral electrical stimulation with the nucleus cochlear implant in adults: 6-month postoperative results. *Otology and Neurotology, 25,* 958–968.

Lenarz, T., Lesinski-Schiedat, A., Weber, B. P., Issing, P. R., Frohne, C., Buchner, A., et al. (2001). The nucleus double array cochlear implant: A new concept for the obliterated cochlea. *Otology and Neurotology, 22,* 24–32.

Li, P. M., Somdas, M. A., Eddington, D. K., & Nadol, J. B., Jr. (2007). Analysis of intracochlear new bone and fibrous tissue formation in human subjects with cochlear implants. *Annals of Otology, Rhinology, and Laryngology, 116,* 731–738.

Litovsky, R. Y., Johnstone, P. M., Godar, S., Agrawal, S., Parkinson, A., Peters, R., et al. (2006a). Bilateral cochlear implants in children: Localization acuity measured with minimum audible angle. *Ear and Hearing, 27*, 43–59.

Litovsky, R., Parkinson, A., Arcaroli, J., & Sammeth, C. (2006b). Simultaneous bilateral cochlear implantation in adults: A multicenter clinical study. *Ear and Hearing, 27*, 714–731.

Loundon, N., Rouillon, I., Munier, N., Marlin, S., Roger, G., & Garabedian, E. N. (2005). Cochlear implantation in children with internal ear malformations. *Otology and Neurotology, 26*, 668–673.

Lowder, M. W. Personal interview, 2-17-2004.

Luxford, W. M. (1989). Cochlear implant indications. *American Journal of Otology, 10*, 95–98.

Makarem, A., Linthicum, F. H., Jr., Balaraman, S., & Fayad, J. N. (2008, April). *Histopathological assessment of fibrosis and new bone formation in implanted human temporal bones using 3-D reconstruction.* Presented at 10th International Conference on Cochlear Implants and Other Implantable Auditory Technologies. San Diego, CA.

Maniglia, A. J., Abbass, H., Azar, T., Kane, M., Amantia, P., Garverick, S., et al. (1999). The middle ear bioelectronic microphone for a totally implantable cochlear hearing device for profound and total hearing loss. *American Journal of Otology, 20*, 602–611.

Manrique, M., Cervera-Paz, F. J., Huarte, A., & Molina, M. (2004). Advantages of cochlear implantation in prelingual deaf children before 2 years of age when compared with later implantation. *Laryngoscope, 114*, 1462–1469.

Mason, J. C., De Michele, A., Stevens, C., Ruth, R. A., & Hashisaki, G. T. (2003). Cochlear implantation in patients with auditory neuropathy of varied etiologies. *Laryngoscope, 113*, 45–49.

Migirov, L., Taitelbaum-Swead, R., Hildesheimer, M., & Kronenberg, J. (2007). Revision surgeries in cochlear implant patients: A review of 45 cases. *European Archives of Oto-Rhino-Laryngology, 264*, 3–7.

Millar, D. A., Hillman, T. A., & Shelton, C. (2005). Implantation of the ossified cochlea: Management with the split electrode array. *Laryngoscope, 115*, 2155–2160.

Miyamoto, R. T., & Brown, D. D. (1987). Electrically evoked brainstem responses in cochlear implant recipients. *Otolaryngology-Head and Neck Surgery, 96*, 34–38.

Miyamoto, R. T., Houston, D. M., & Bergeson, T. (2005). Cochlear implantation in deaf infants. *Laryngoscope, 115*, 1376–1380.

Miyamoto, R. T., Robbins, A. J., Myres, W. A., & Pope, M. L. (1986). Cochlear implantation in the Mondini inner ear malformation. *American Journal of Otology, 7*, 258–261.

Morzaria, S., Westerberg, B. D., & Kozak, F. K. (2004). Systematic review of the etiology of bilateral sensorineural hearing loss in children. *International Journal of Pediatric Otorhinolaryngology, 68*, 1193–1198.

Morzaria, S., Westerberg, B. D., & Kozak, F. K. (2005). Evidence-based algorithm for the evaluation of a child with bilateral sensorineural hearing loss. *Journal of Otolaryngology, 34*, 297–303.

Nilsson, M., Soli, S. D., & Sullivan, J. A. (1994). Development of the Hearing in Noise Test for the measurement of speech reception thresholds in quiet and in noise. *Journal of the Acoustical Society of America, 95*, 1085–1099.

Odabasi, O., Mobley, S. R., Bolanos, R. A., Hodges, A., & Balkany, T. (2000). Cochlear implantation in patients with compromised healing. *Otolaryngology-Head and Neck Surgery, 123*, 738–741.

Papsin, B. C. (2005). Cochlear implantation in children with anomalous cochleovestibular anatomy. *Laryngoscope, 115*(Suppl. 106), 1–26.

Parry, D. A., Booth, T., & Roland, P. S. (2005). Advantages of magnetic resonance imaging over computed tomography in preoperative evaluation of pediatric cochlear implant candidates. *Otology and Neurotology, 26*, 976–982.

Patrick, J. F., & Clark, G. M. (1991). The Nucleus 22-channel cochlear implant system. *Ear and Hearing, 12*(Suppl. 4), 3–9.

Peterson, A., Shallop, J., Driscoll, C., Breneman, A., Babb, J., Stoeckel, R., et al. (2003). Outcomes of cochlear implantation in children with auditory neuropathy. *Journal of the American Academy of Audiology, 14,* 188-201.

Postelmans, J. T., Cleffken, B., & Stokroos, R. J. (2007). Post-operative complications of cochlear implantation in adults and children: Five years' experience in Maastricht. *Journal of Laryngology and Otology, 121,* 318-323.

Raveh, E., Buller, N., Badrana, O., & Attias, J. (2007). Auditory neuropathy: Clinical characteristics and therapeutic approach. *American Journal of Otolaryngology, 28,* 302-308.

Roland, J. T., Jr., Magardino, T. M., Go, J. T., & Hillman, D. E. (1995). Effects of glycerin, hyaluronic acid, and hydroxypropyl methylcellulose on the spiral ganglion of the guinea pig cochlea. *Annals of Otology, Rhinology, and Laryngology, 104*(Suppl.166), 64-68.

Rubinstein, J. T. (2004). How cochlear implants encode speech. *Current Opinion in Otolaryngology-Head and Neck Surgery, 12,* 444-448.

Rubinstein, J. T., & Hong, R. (2003). Signal coding in cochlear implants: Exploiting stochastic effects of electrical stimulation. *Annals of Otology, Rhinology, and Laryngology 112* (Suppl. 191), 14-19.

Sach, T., O'Neill, C., Whynes, D. K., Archbold, S. M., & O'Donoghue, G. M. (2003). Evidence of improving cost-effectiveness of pediatric cochlear implantation. *International Journal of Technology Assessment in Health Care, 19,* 421-431.

Schindler, R. A., Kessler, D. K., & Haggerty, H. S. (1993). Clarion cochlear implant: Phase I investigational results. *American Journal of Otology, 14,* 263-272.

Seidman, D. A., Chute, P. M., & Parisier, S. (1994). Temporal bone imaging for cochlear implantation. *Laryngoscope, 104,* 562-565.

Simmons, F. B. (1966). Electrical stimulation of the auditory nerve in man. *Archives of Otolaryngology, 84,* 2-54.

Smyth, G. D. (1979). Microsurgery in otology and laryngology: A review of developments during the past thirty years. *Journal of Microsurgery, 1,* 72-76.

Spies, T. H., Snik, A. F., Mens, L. H., & van den Broek, B. P. (1993). Preoperative electrical stimulation for cochlear implant selection. The use of ear canal electrodes versus transtympanic electrodes. *Acta Otolaryngologica, 113,* 579-584.

Steenerson, R. L., Gary, L. B., & Wynens, M. S. (1990). Scala vestibuli cochlear implantation for labyrinthine ossification. *American Journal of Otology, 11,* 360-363.

Tyler, R. S., Gantz, B. J., Rubinstein, J. T., Wilson, B. S., Parkinson, A. J., Wolaver, A., et al. (2002a). Three-month results with bilateral cochlear implants. *Ear and Hearing, 23*(Suppl. 1), 80-89.

Tyler, R. S., Parkinson, A. J., Wilson, B. S., Witt, S., Preece, J. P., & Noble, W. (2002b). Patients utilizing a hearing aid and a cochlear implant: Speech perception and localization. *Ear and Hearing, 23,* 98-105.

Wiet, R. J., Pyle, G. M., O'Connor, C. A., Russell, E., & Schramm, D. R. (1990). Computed tomography: How accurate a predictor for cochlear implantation? *Laryngoscope, 100,* 687-692.

Woolley, A. L., Oser, A. B., Lusk, R. P., & Bahadori, R. S. (1997). Preoperative temporal bone computed tomography scan and its use in evaluating the pediatric cochlear implant candidate. *Laryngoscope, 107,* 1100-1106.

Wootten, C. T., Backous, D. D., & Haynes, D. S. (2006). Management of cerebrospinal fluid leakage from cochleostomy during cochlear implant surgery. *Laryngoscope, 116,* 2055-2059.

Young, N. M. (2002). Infant cochlear implantation and anesthetic risk. *Annals of Otology, Rhinology, and Laryngology, 111*(Suppl. 189), 49-51.

Young, N. M., Hughes, C. A., Byrd, S. E., & Darling, C. (2000). Postmeningitic ossification in pediatric cochlear implantation. *Otolaryngology-Head and Neck Surgery, 122,* 183-188.

APPENDIX 5–A.
House Ear Clinic Cochlear Implant Consent Document

CONSENT FOR IMPLANTATION OF WIRE INTO THE COCHLEA AND PLACEMENT OF
AN INDUCTION COIL UNDER THE SKIN BEHIND THE EAR

PATIENT:
PROCEDURE:

I hereby request and authorize Dr. _____ and Dr. _____ as
the operating surgeon(s), to perform upon me an operation for the purpose of implanting wire (electrodes) into the cochlea (inner ear) and the placement of an implanted
induction coil {a small coil of wire wound around a core and imbedded in an insulated
substance), and such further operations, tests and diagnostic procedures which in the
judgment of my physicians may become necessary during or immediately after the presently
contemplated surgery.

Also, I understand there will be hearing evaluations and rehabilitation training beginning
approximately one or two months after surgery and continuing periodically thereafter.

I understand that I, or my third party payor (health insurance. Medicare, or other), must
provide payment for the device and all procedures.

RISK AND COMPLICATIONS OF SURGERY

I understand that the procedure consists essentially of the mastoid operation (operation
on the bone and air cells behind the ear); the placement of wire (electrodes) into the
cochlea (hearing part of the inner ear} and the placement of an induction coil under the
skin behind the ear. The risks are those generally associated with a mastoid operation, plus
those associated with the implantation of electrodes and an induction coil.

Due to the nature of medical research, I understand that the outcome of my case cannot
be predicted with certainty. As a result, should some unforeseen injury result from the
cochlear implant, decisions concerning compensation and medical treatment for that
injury will be made on an individual basis. Should I wish the device removed, I understand that I will be responsible for the surgical costs.

RISK OF MASTOID SURGERY

Infection: The risk of infection is quite small but, should it occur, it would require treatment and could cause the operation to fail.

Facial Paralysis: This is a remote possibility but should it happen, the eye on the side
of surgery would fail to close and the mouth would pull over to the side opposite to the
surgery and further treatment would be required.

Fluid Drainage: Spinal fluid drainage may occur following implant surgery. It is more common in patients with malformation of the inner ear. Bed rest is the usual treatment. Revision surgery is rare.

Meningitis: The risk of meningitis is very rare. However, when present, it can cause serious consequences. Meningitis is an infection of the lining of the surface of the brain. Early symptoms of meningitis include fever, irritability, lethargy and loss of appetite in infants and young children. Older children and adults may also manifest headaches, stiff neck, nausea, vomiting, and confusion or alteration in consciousness. Physicians are encouraged to consider a diagnosis of meningitis in cochlear implant patients when such symptoms exist and to begin appropriate treatment as soon as possible. We recommend preoperative immunization against meningitis. For a copy of the current immunization recommendation sheet, please ask our office staff.

Anesthetic Risks: General anesthesia is required. Complications are rare, but can be serious. You may discuss these with the anesthesiologist if desired.

RISK OF THE IMPLANTATION OF ELECTRODES AND INDUCTION COIL

There is the risk that the device, once implanted, may not work for me. In addition, the implanted wire may break or the induction coil may fail and cause irritation, cause complication or may malfunction in a way totally unanticipated at this time. The length of operation and reliability of each component part is unknown.

The induction coils may contain permanent magnets to assist with the proper alignment of the internal and external coils. I understand that the effects of long-term implantation of permanent magnets are unknown.

I understand that even if totally successful, the cochlear implant will not produce a normal sensation of sound. It may allow me to experience sound in the environment and to have distorted sensations of speech sounds.

RISK OF STIMULATION OF THE HEARING NERVE BY ELECTRIC CURRENTS

I understand that after a period of healing, an external signal processor that is connected by a wire to an external induction coil that is worn over the implanted induction coil behind the ear will be supplied to me. This signal processor causes an electric current to be produced, which constantly goes into the inner ear and stimulates the nerve endings of the hearing nerve during the entire time the device is worn.

The long-term effect of the constant electrical current put out by the implant on the nervous tissue or any other tissue is unknown.

We will not fully understand the results of this constant stimulation by electric currents close to the brain until many patients have used these devices for 70 or more years.

The long-term effect of the constant electrical current put out by the implant on the nervous tissue or any other tissue is unknown.

We will not fully understand the results of this constant stimulation by electric currents close to the brain until many patients have used these devices for 70 or more years.

RISK OF DEVICE BECOMING OUTDATED

I understand the implanted device and the external signal processor device are under constant development and improvement. When a new development is made in the signal processor, or a new electrode system is developed, I understand I am financially responsible for the additional expenses of the devices, costs of the surgery and any additional rehabilitation costs involved as I desire to have these new improvements.

AVAILABLE ALTERNATIVES

I understand that a major consideration in deciding whether I should undergo this surgical procedure is whether an alternative noninvasive treatment is available. The two possibilities are hearing aids and vibrotactile devices.

CONFIDENTIALITY

All patient information will be treated as confidential. Any data published in scientific journals will be pooled summary data without patient identification. Specific data on an individual patient will be published only with specific written permission of that patient or his/her legal representative.

I consent to the presence of other physicians and technicians in the operating room, who may have no direct connection with my case, for educational purposes.

I have read and understand the terms of this consent. I have been given adequate time and have discussed the above material and consent form with those whom I feel may be of benefit in my understanding of the above.

Signature of Patient: _____

Signature of Patient's Spouse or Guardian: _____

Witness: _____   Date: _____

CHAPTER 6

Programming Pediatric Cochlear Implant Systems

TERESA A. ZWOLAN
CASEY J. STACH

Introduction

Setting the parameters of a child's cochlear implant speech processor can be one of the most challenging aspects of postoperative patient management. The importance of properly setting the speech processor cannot be underestimated—inaccurate mapping can result in months or years of poor hearing by a child, and may prevent the child from meeting his or her full potential for success with a cochlear implant.

In many ways, the procedures used to obtain responses from a child for a speech processor program are similar to the procedures used to obtain an audiogram. The implant clinician must be prepared, however, to hold the child's attention long enough to obtain numerous threshold measurements (more than with a typical audiogram), and also will need to determine when mapping stimuli are "comfortable," "loud but comfortable," or "uncomfortable." The measurements used in testing are important as they will determine how well the child hears from that point on until his or her next mapping appointment. Fortunately, objective measurement tools can be used by cli-

nicians to verify or supplement behavioral responses. Such measures are particularly useful with very young children or with children who have other health issues in addition to their deafness.

This chapter aims to provide an overview of the procedures used to program children's speech processors. Being able to program speech processors of pediatric cochlear implant recipients is a highly specialized skill that requires a great deal of training. In order to map speech processors, one must possess a strong understanding of pediatric audiology. Additionally, the implant audiologist should have a strong understanding of the device and the associated programming software.

Preparations for Programming

Preparations for mapping appointments begin with audiologic testing performed prior to the child receiving a cochlear implant. Such testing provides the child and his family with opportunities to become familiar with the audiologist and the learning to listen tasks that are necessary to obtain a preoperative audiogram or a post-operative speech processor map. Prior to device activation, the audiologist and patient should establish a rapport that facilitates ready to listen behaviors.

Test Procedures

A child who is less than approximately 18 months of age should be comfortable participating in behavioral observation audiometry (BOA) or visual reinforcement audiometry (VRA), whereas older children should be comfortable participating in conditioned play audiometry (CPA) and/or traditional response testing (Diefendorf, 2002). If the audiologist is not able to obtain reliable behavioral responses from the child prior to device activation, he or she may want to consider scheduling the child for additional appointments to work on this prior to device activation. Additionally, the audiologist may want to instruct the child's parents or teachers regarding things they can do at home or at school to facilitate the child's ability to provide a conditioned response to sound. If the child is not able to hear test stimuli, it is recommended that the other senses, such as vision or touch, be used as a tool for teaching the conditioned response. This can be accomplished during audiometric testing using the bone oscillator or at home using various toys that vibrate or light up. The importance of early establishment of such a response to mapping stimuli and speech will facilitate greater success in postoperative mapping sessions.

Counseling Prior to Activation

Prior to device activation, parents and the child should possess a clear understanding of the tasks that will be involved in the mapping sessions. If the parents are allowed to remain in the room during testing (or if you choose to have them assist with testing), they need to understand the importance of not providing the child with any type of visual or behavioral cue that may indicate to the child that a signal was presented. Additionally, a frank discussion should take place with the parents regarding any behavior modification techniques that may be used to facilitate continued participation by the child in the mapping session. Parents and audiologists should agree about topics such as use of "time out" behavioral modification techniques (Bean & Roberts, 1981), type and frequency of rewards given for responses, and appropriateness of participation by the parent in the test session. An open discussion regarding why it is important for the child to actively participate in the sessions is recommended. In our clinic, many families drive several hours to attend an appointment that was scheduled months in advance. It is unfortunate when mapping appointments are terminated early due to inappropriate behavior by the child as this may mean that the family must wait several weeks for another appointment to map the speech processor. Thus, an ineffective session could mean that the child's speech processor map may be less than optimal for an unnecessary amount of time.

One additional step that may be taken to prepare the child for mapping of the speech processor is utilization of the external equipment prior to device activation. A child's resistance to wearing the speech processor and headset could waste valuable time during the activation appointment. One way parents can facilitate device use is to have the child continue wearing a hearing aid up until the time of device activation, even if the child receives little or no benefit from the aid. Additionally, one may want to consider providing the parents with an unmapped speech processor with instructions to have the child wear it regularly until the device is activated. Doing so can provide the child with time to adjust to the physical presence of the speech processor and may reduce the negative influence that resistance to wearing the device may have on the activation appointment.

Device Activation

In most clinics, activation of the speech processor occurs 2 to 6 weeks after surgery. This allows for healing of the incision and reduction of swelling around the area of the receiver. In our clinic, all patients have a transorbital view x-ray taken of the temporal bone immediately prior to device activation. An example of such an x-ray is provided in Figure 6-1. The x-ray is viewed by the audiologist prior to beginning mapping and provides important verification of proper device placement. Such an x-ray also can be used to identify potential problems with electrode placement, such as a fold-over of the electrode array (Figure 6-2) or partial insertion of the electrode array (Figure 6-3), and provides important base-

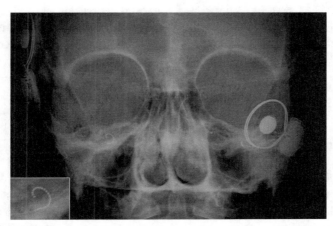

Figure 6–1. An example of a normal plain film x-ray taken postoperatively prior to activation.

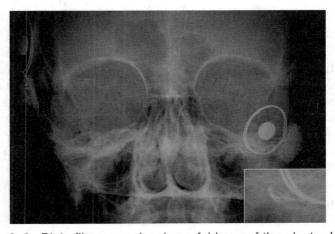

Figure 6–2. Plain film x-ray showing a foldover of the electrode array.

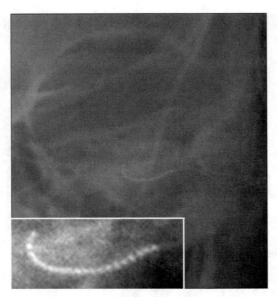

Figure 6–3. Plain film x-ray showing a partial insertion of the electrode array.

line information for later comparison if concerns arise regarding device placement or stability.

After the x-ray has been viewed, the audiologist provides the child and his or her family with instructions regarding what will take place during the mapping session. First, the area surrounding the incision is checked to ensure adequate healing. If there are any concerns about the incision, the child should be seen by the surgeon as soon as possible. Next, the device is interfaced with the computer and the coil is attached to the child's head, and the strength of the magnet is checked to make certain it is appropriate for the child. Use of a magnet that is too strong could result in tenderness, swelling, rejection of the device by the child, or, in more severe cases, development of a sore and possible infection. Use of a magnet that is too weak could prevent retention of the coil on the child's head. The magnet should demonstrate adequate pull but should not be so tight that it leaves a firm impression

of the coil on the child's head following its removal. Because the thickness of the skin overlying the receiver can change during the first few weeks of device use, the audiologist should continue to check the incision at subsequent appointments.

Speech Processor Mapping

Step 1: Check Equipment

Every programming session should begin with a check of the patient's equipment, even the first day of device use. This check should include a listening check of the microphone, visual inspection of all cables and parts, and recognition of the processor by the computer software.

Step 2: Telemetry

All three types of currently available devices provide the audiologist with the ability to send information to the implant and to receive information back from the implant about the device status. This is referred to as telemetry. With the Nucleus device, testing should always begin with administration of the implant test, which determines impedances for all available electrodes in four different modes of stimulation: common ground, Monopolar 1, Monopolar 2, and Monopolar 1 + 2. Such testing identifies short or open-circuit electrodes that can be "flagged," preventing their inclusion in subsequent maps.

The Advanced Bionics device features continuous bidirectional telemetry that allows electrode impedances to be determined during each fitting. Electrodes with impedances that fall outside the range of normal (5 to 150 KOhm) are automatically disabled and are excluded from the patient's map.

In the MED-EL device, a special coil is used to perform telemetry testing. Once all of the electrodes are tested, a printout of the actual impedance values is provided for review. MED-EL recommends that electrodes with impedances outside the range of normal be deactivated.

Impedance testing is essential and should be performed prior to each mapping appointment. Such testing provides information regarding voltage compliance—the ability of the electrode to deliver sufficient voltage to generate the requested current level. Voltage compliance levels are visible on the programming screens of Nucleus devices (Nucleus 24 and beyond) and with all MED-EL devices. When mapping, the audiologist will want to avoid setting comfort levels above the voltage compliance lines as stimulation at such a level could result in delivery of a distorted signal. With the Advanced Bionics devices (90K and beyond), the software automatically adjusts the pulse width of the signal in order to remain within voltage compliance. Early versions of Nucleus and Advanced Bionics devices (such as the Nucleus 22 and the Clarion CI) do not have telemetry capabilities.

Step 3: Psychophysical Testing

Once the equipment has been connected and telemetry measures have been made, psychophysical testing can begin. First, the clinician should determine the parameters that will be used to create the initial program for the speech processor. The specific map parameters will depend on the type and model of the internal device and also will be influenced by the make and model of the speech processor in use by the patient. In our clinic, map parameters with proven success in adults are used as a starting point with children, unless there is a specific reason to use different settings. Default parameters used with contemporary devices in our facility are provided in Table 6–1.

The specific tasks that will be performed during the appointment will depend on the type of internal and external device used by the child. Such measures may include determination of threshold (the softest level of sound that can be heard), C level (a level that is loud but comfortable), or M level (a level of sound that is considered to be "most" comfortable). Such measurements can be obtained using either behavioral or objective test procedures, or obtained using a combination of behavioral and objective procedures.

TABLE 6–1. Default Parameters Used with Contemporary Devices in Our Facility

Nucleus

Strategy—ACE

Rate—900 Hz

Pulse width—25

Mode—MP1+2

Maxima—8

ADRO

Advanced Bionics

Strategy—Hi-Res-S or Hi-Res-P

IDR—60

Filters—Extended Low Pulse Width—18

MED-EL

Strategy—CIS+ or FSP (Opus) AGC:3:1
Frequency Bands: Logarithmic F_s

Reprinted with permission from *Otology and Neurotology* (from Zwolan et al., 2008).

It should be noted that psychophysical responses to the implant will vary greatly from child to child. For example, children with abnormal or ossified cochleae demonstrate higher psychophysical responses than children with normal cochleae (Zwolan, O'Sullivan, Fink, & Niparko, 2008). Thus, it is essential that individual measurements be obtained for each child.

Threshold Testing

Threshold is the softest level of sound perceived by the child. This measure is important even if it does not need to be noted for creation of the speech processor program. With children, the clinician will want to begin the first day of psychophysical testing by delivering a stimulus that is believed to be below the child's threshold of hearing. Testing often begins with an apical or middle electrode in order to avoid stimulation of a basal electrode that may elicit an uncomfortable sound or may not be fully inserted into the cochlea. The clinician conservatively increases the loudness of the test signal until it is noted that the child has heard a sound. Children with an established, conditioned response to sound can be instructed to respond when they first hear a very soft sound. Younger children are unable to provide such feedback. Therefore, the child should be observed closely until a response to sound is noted by the audiologist. This is usually signified by a change in behavior, such as a head turn, eye raise, crying, laughing, cessation of sucking, change in breathing, or a change in eye gaze. Once the audiologist is certain that the child is hearing the signal, he or she should work with the child to develop a conditioned response to sound. Such conditioning usually is performed above threshold at a comfortable listening level where a clear response has been obtained. Once it has

been determined that the child understands the listening task, the level of stimulation can be decreased and threshold can be determined using a traditional descending/ascending method. If the child's device requires notation of the threshold (T), the T should be set to the softest level of stimulation where the child consistently responded to sound. It is often believed that responses provided on the first day are actually suprathreshold. Thus, one may want to consider setting the thresholds a set number of units below the level that elicited a clear response.

Threshold testing is then repeated on several different electrodes. In order to obtain as much information as possible, it is recommended that testing be distributed among electrodes located in different areas of the array. For example, in the Nucleus device, threshold testing may begin with electrode 20, followed by electrodes 5, 15, and 10. If the child loses interest in the task and no longer provides reliable responses, the threshold values that have been obtained can be interpolated for creation of threshold information for the initial "Day 1" map. Presently, threshold information is set automatically by the software for speech processor programs for the MED-EL and Advanced Bionics devices.

Setting "Comfortable" or "Most Comfortable" Listening Levels

Once threshold information has been obtained, the clinician will need to determine the upper level of stimulation for the speech processor program. For Nucleus devices, this is defined as a sound that is "loud but comfortable"—referred to as the C level. Devices manufactured by Advanced Bionics and MED-EL, on the other hand, define the upper level of stimulation as a sound that is "most comfortable—the level where you would find speech most comfortable." This is often referred to as the "M" level.

The audiologist should exercise caution when assessing the upper level of stimulation, particularly during the activation appointment, as even small increases in stimulation can result in delivery of a stimulus that is too loud or uncomfortable. If the child has a negative reaction to sound, he or she may become fearful of wearing the device. Thus, we recommend that T and C or M levels initially be set conservatively with children as doing so will facilitate early device use as the child gradually acclimates to sound.

C and M levels can be obtained from the child in several different ways. In our clinic, when making the program on the first day of device activation, the child is asked to sit quietly and interact with the clinician while stimuli are presented at levels that gradually increase in loudness above the previously determined thresholds (Zwolan & Griffin, 2005). For example, if it has been determined that electrode #15 has a threshold of 150 units, the clinician presents approximately 3 stimuli at a level of 155. If the child appears comfortable, the clinician will present 3 additional stimuli at a level of 160 clinical units. Such increases in stimulation will continue until the child indicates that sound is uncomfortable and/or until a dynamic range (C/M level minus T level) of approximately 25 units has been reached. Several of the electrodes located in different areas of the array will be tested in this manner, and then values will be interpolated to create the first speech processor map. A sweep of the electrodes will then be performed (subsequent presentation of a single stimulus at each electrode's C/M level) at 80% and 100% of the C/M level and the child's reaction to sound will be monitored. If the child has a negative reaction to sound (crying, rapid eye blinking, frowning) with stimulation of

any of the electrodes, the C/M level of the electrode is reduced and the sweep is performed again. Live voice testing of the map should only be performed once it has been determined that all of the C/M levels included in the speech processor map are comfortable for the child when sweep testing has been performed at 100% of the C/M level.

Another option for setting of the C/M levels is to use a procedure referred to as "streamlining." In this procedure, the C/M levels are increased as a group, rather than for each individual electrode. When the clinician begins with streamlined testing, all of the C/M levels are set to be one unit above the threshold level for each individual electrode (referred to as "hug T profile" in the Cochlear programming software). Streamlining is selected in the software, and the map is set to be "live," beginning with the limited dynamic range (DR) of 1 clinical unit. The sensitivity and volume of the map are gradually increased from 0 and 0, respectively, to a setting of approximately 5 and 8 for volume and sensitivity. The map is activated for speech and C/M levels are gradually increased for all of the electrodes in small steps (i.e., 1–5 units) as the clinician introduces speech and watches the child's reaction to sound. The level of stimulation is stopped once a DR of 25 units has been achieved or when the child demonstrates a clear and comfortable response to the auditory signal. The C/M levels are decreased if the child negatively reacts to sound.

If the C/M levels have not been obtained using the streamlined approach, but instead have been determined on an electrode by electrode basis, introduction of speech should follow the procedures similar to those described above for the streamlining procedure. The primary difference is that the DR is not increased globally across the array. Rather, testing begins with the previously determined dynamic range and the volume and sensitivity of the map are gradually increased as the child's response to sound is monitored. Ideally, the child should be comfortable when listening to speech presented at an average conversation level when the device is set to a recommended use setting (such as a volume of 5 and a sensitivity of 10 to 12 for a Nucleus device). Average "C" and "M" levels obtained for children with normal and abnormal cochlae who use Nucleus, Advanced Bionics, and MED-EL devices (Zwolan et al., 2008) are provided in Table 6–2A and 6–2B. These values were obtained as part of a longitudinal study of 188 children enrolled in the childhood Development after Cochlear Implant (CDaCI) study (Fink et al., 2007).

Once it has been determined that the child is comfortable when listening to speech, the clinician should present the child with sounds that exceed average levels (such as clapping, singing, and tapping). The child's reaction should be closely monitored to ensure that the child is comfortable when such sounds are presented. If a negative response has been elicited, the C/M levels should be reduced.

Objective Measures for Speech Processor Mapping

There are several objective electrophysiologic measures that can be used to assess device integrity and to aid in speech processor mapping. These procedures include electrically evoked auditory brainstem response (EABR) (Brown, Abbas, Fryauf-Bertschy, Kelsay, & Gantz, 1994; Kileny, 1991; Shallop, Beiter, Goin, & Mischke, 1990; Shallop, VanDyke, Goin, & Mischke, 1991), elicited acoustic reflex threshold (EART) (Battmer, Laszig, & Lehnhardt, 1990; Gordon, Papsin, & Harrison, 2004; Jerger, Oliver, & Chmiel, 1988), Neural Response

Telemetry (NRT) (Brown, Abbas, & Gantz, 1990; Battmer et al., 2004), and Neural Response Imaging (NRI) (Caner, Olgun, Gültekin, & Balaban, 2007). Nucleus's NRT, Advanced Bionic's NRI, and MED-EL's ART provide the clinician with the ability to measure the electrically evoked compound action potential (ECAP) to aid in setting T and C/M levels in these devices. These measures are noninvasive, can be acquired in awake patients, and do not require the use of evoked potential averaging equipment (Shapiro, 2006). These measurements are available as part of commercial programming software and can be particularly helpful with difficult to test or very young patients. In most clinics, objective measures are used as a rough guide to supplement information obtained using the behavioral programming techniques described previously. Additional information regarding the use of objective measures to map speech processors can be found in Abbas, Brown, and Etler (2006).

Presenting Live Speech

Once it has been determined that the speech processor program is comfortable for the child, the audiologist can evaluate audibility of various speech signals using the Ling 6 Sound test (Ling, 1976, 1989). This test consists of presentation of six different phonemes that broadly represent the speech spectrum from 250 to 8000 Hz: [m], [ah], [oo], [ee], [sh], and [s]. The sounds are presented using live voice at a comfortable listening level. Ability of the child to detect, recognize, or repeat the sounds when using hearing alone indicates good access to sound across the frequency range important for understanding speech. If, for example, the child is able to detect or repeat all of the Ling sounds except /s/ and /sh/,

TABLE 6–2A. Mean C/M levels in nC and clinical units for Advanced Bionics, Nucleus and MED-EL devices obtained on subjects with **normal cochleae** at device activation and 6, 12, and 24 months postactivation.

	Advanced Bionics	Nucleus	MED-EL
Activation			
Number of Ss	50	95	26
Mean (Clinical Units)	135	169	339
Mean (nC)	10.62	9.27	9.05
Minimum	6.25	2.43	2.66
Maximum	19.73	23.41	13.63
S.D.	2.80	3.58	3.10
6 months			
Number of Ss	48	92	26
Mean (Clinical Units)	206	201	750
Mean (nC)	16.11	16.66	20.04
Minimum (nC)	8.27	8.39	6.68
Maximum (nC)	24.98	53.84	30.83
S.D.	3.80	7.03	4.80
12 months			
Number of Ss	45	93	22
Mean (Clinical Units)	219	207	845
Mean (nC)	17.15	18.43	22.57
Minimum (nC)	8.27	8.21	7.44
Maximum (nC)	30.25	64.52	37.47
S.D.	4.21	9.18	6.60
24 months			
Number of Ss	47	87	25
Mean (Clinical Units)	224	207	917
Mean (nC)	17.49	18.39	24.48
Minimum	8.79	6.37	8.42
Maximum	28.07	58.89	74.84
S.D.	4.00	8.34	12.34

The clinical unit measurements assume different pulse widths for each device: Advanced Bionics assumes a CII device with pulse width of 10.8, Nucleus assumes a pulse width of 25, and the MED-EL measurement assumes a pulse width of 26.7.

Reprinted with permission from *Otology and Neurotology* (from Zwolan et al., 2008).

TABLE 6–2B. Mean C/M levels in nC and clinical units for Advanced Bionics, Nucleus and MED-EL devices obtained on subjects with **abnormal cochleae** at device activation and 6, 12, and 24 months postactivation.

	Advanced Bionics	Nucleus	MED-EL
Activation			
Number of Ss	10	6	3
Mean (Clinical Units)	128	171	351
Mean (nC)	10.00	9.71	9.38
Minimum	5.86	8.02	8.85
Maximum	14.55	35.17	10.05
S.D.	2.90	9.24	.609
6 months			
Number of Ss	9	6	3
Mean (Clinical Units)	217	243	818
Mean (nC)	16.99	35.35	21.84
Minimum (nC)	8.67	11.71	18.61
Maximum (nC)	26.64	55.85	26.43
S.D.	5.77	14.82	4.08
12 months			
Number of Ss	9	6	3
Mean (Clinical Units)	237	238 (pw = 50)	857
Mean (nC)	18.54	47.93	22.69
Minimum (nC)	8.83	11.94	20.48
Maximum (nC)	37.93	79.07	26.43
S.D.	8.55	28.96	3.25
24 months			
Number of Ss	9	4	3
Mean (Clinical Units)	235	237 (pw = 50)	835
Mean (nC)	18.38	46.42	22.29
Minimum	6.01	11.03	16.04
Maximum	37.70	85.59	26.86
S.D.	9.41	33.76	5.60

Reprinted with permission from *Otology and Neurotology* (from Zwolan et al., 2008).

this may indicate that the T or C/M values in the basal end of the array need to be increased to improve the child's perception of these sounds.

Importantly, parents should be instructed to assess the child's ability to detect, recognize, or repeat all of the Ling sounds each morning. Doing so will enable them to monitor the child's perception of speech, and will help the parents identify possible problems with the speech processor. Inability of the child to perceive such sounds may indicate trouble with the equipment or a change in hearing that requires remapping of the speech processor.

With older children and adults, C/M levels can be refined further using loudness balancing. With loudness balancing, stimuli are presented to adjacent electrodes at the C/M level. The patient is asked to indicate if the sounds are equal in loudness or if one of the sounds is louder or softer than the others. The C/M levels are adjusted until the patient indicates that all of the C/M levels across the array are equal in loudness. It should be noted that this is a difficult task, even for postlingually deafened adults, because the stimuli being compared often differ greatly in pitch. Thus, loudness balancing primarily is performed with older children and adults. Loudness balancing should only be performed if the recipient is able to provide reliable responses for this task.

Downloading Maps to the Speech Processor

Once the audiologist has determined that a program is appropriate for the child, the audiologist will need to determine the settings of the programs that will be downloaded to the speech processor. The number of programs will depend on the number of locations available in the speech processor, and on the preference of the clinician. Speech processors currently in use have between one and four program locations.

The goal of the activation appointment is to introduce the child to sound, and to introduce the parents to the equipment. Because they will be returning for a second appointment within 1 to 2 days, we usually load a single program onto the speech processor when the device is first turned on. This can be performed by loading the same program into all available program locations or loading a single program into the processor. Loading a single program simplifies the amount of instructions provided to the parents and minimizes the amount of change that may occur with sound for the child during the first few days of device use.

In our clinic, multiple programs are loaded onto the processor following the second appointment. During the first few weeks or months of device use, recipients often demonstrate gradual increases in C/M levels as they acclimate to sound. Thus, at the end of the second appointment, the child is provided with programs with subsequent increases in C/M levels of about 3 to 5 units. This enables the parent to gradually increase the amount of sound being provided to the child without having to return to the implant center. During subsequent appointments, time is spent reviewing care, use, and troubleshooting of the device and its accessories and on provision of instructions regarding when to increase, decrease, or change the speech processor program.

Counseling

During early programming appointments, parents should be provided with information regarding the types of behaviors one expects from a child who has just received a cochlear implant. If the child has no experience with sound, auditory development with the implant will be similar to that of a newborn baby despite the child's advanced chronological age. The child will not only need time to adjust to sound, but will require time before he or she is able to overtly indicate that he or she is hearing sound. It will take even more time before the parents are able to tell that their child is able to identify or respond to words, such as their name.

The sound received with the implant will likely sound different than the sounds the child previously heard if he or she used a hearing aid. If the child had a progressive hearing loss, their progress may be faster than that of a younger child with limited hearing prior to implantation. Parents of postlingually deafened children need to be informed that it will take time for their child to understand speech through their implant, and that such children may demonstrate an early digression of performance, followed by gradual increases in speech recognition skills as they adjust to the sounds provided by the implant.

Use of a Hearing Aid on the Contralateral Ear

Cochlear implant professionals provide a variety of recommendations to cochlear implant recipients regarding use of a contralateral hearing aid in conjunction with a cochlear implant. Some professionals will recommend continued hearing aid use following cochlear implantation whereas others may recommend cessation of hearing aid use for brief or prolonged periods of time following device activation (Zwolan, 2005). In many clinics, such recommendations are made on a case by case basis. Factors one should consider when making reommendations regarding continued hearing aid use include the amount of benefit the patient receives from the hearing aid in the non-implanted ear, appropriateness of the hearing aid, and the willingness of the recipient to use the implant alone as well as his or her willingness to use the hearing aid once it is reintroduced.

There are several possible advantages to using a hearing aid in conjunction with a cochlear implant. Such advantages include improved speech perception in quiet, improved speech perception in noise, enhanced ability to localize sound (Tyler et al., 2002), and continued stimulation of the ear contralateral to the cochlear implant (Ching, Psarro, Hill, Dillon, & Incerti, 2001; Zwolan, 2005). This last point may be particularly important if the recipient is going to be considered a future candidate for bilateral cochlear implants.

If the child uses a hearing aid in the contralateral ear, the hearing aid should be removed during psychophysical testing. Once an adequate map has been created, the child's response to sound should be evaluated using the implant alone, and then reevaluated while the child uses the hearing aid and cochlear implant. In some cases, the volume of the map may need to be adjusted following introduction of the hearing aid.

If a child routinely uses a hearing aid on the contralateral ear, clinicians should be aware that a drop in performance may be due to a drop in performance of the aided ear (rather than due to a drop in performance of the implanted ear). Additionally, one should keep in mind that changes in hearing in the nonimplanted ear may necessitate reprogramming of the implanted ear. Thus, annual performance evaluations should include examination of implant alone, hearing aid alone, and hearing aid plus implant combined conditions when a child regularly uses both devices.

Scheduling Follow-up Appointments

In our clinic, the activation appointments are usually scheduled on two consecutive days. The duration of each appointment will vary depending on the age of the child, but typically lasts either 1 or 2 hours. Subsequent programming appointments occur approximately 2, 4, 8, and 12 weeks postactivation and 6 and 12 months postactivation and last about 1 hour each. Of course, this schedule is modified if the audiologist feels fewer or more appointments are necessary. During these appointments, the audiologist continues to obtain threshold information for some or all of the electrodes and refines the settings for the upper level of stimulation (C/M levels). The procedure used to obtain responses for the child will depend on his or her age. With young children, testing usually progresses from BOA to VRA to CPA within the first year of device use. Examples of typical changes of T, C, and M levels over time for the first year of device use are provided in Tables 6–2A and 6–2B.

During subsequent appointments, the suitability of C/M levels should be determined. The child's response to sound field stimuli should be tested regularly to ensure adequate detection. Second, parents and teacher should be asked about the child's response to sound at home and at school.

The amount of change noted for T and C/M levels over time will vary from patient to patient. Recent research has indicated that changes in the psychophysical measures of C/M may depend on other variables, such as the mapping procedure used by the implant center or audiologist, cochlear anatomy, and type of internal device (Zwolan et al., 2008). Other factors also may influence such measurements, including the patient's perception of loudness and nerve survival in the cochlea.

During subsequent programming appointments, the clinician should teach the child to provide feedback regarding loudness of the test signal. All of the implant manufacturers provide laminated picture cards that can be used to teach children the concept of soft, comfortable, and loud. It is recommended that such training begin early and be part of all subsequent mapping appointments as doing so will facilitate a greater understanding of sound. This in turn will facilitate improved mapping as the child ages.

Use of a "Test Assistant"

Children who are less than 4 years of age at the time of their appointment often require greater guidance during mapping sessions than older children. In our clinic, children who are less than 4 years of age are scheduled with the managing audiologist and an assistant. This assistant can be another audiologist, an audiology technician, a speech-language pathologist, a student, or, on occasion, the parent. The lead audiologist controls delivery of the test stimulus via the computer software while the assistant sits close to the child and assists the child with the listening task, observes the child closely during testing, and provides feedback to the managing audiologist regarding the child's responses to sound. The assistant also controls the type of toys used in the test setting, and informs the audiologist of any negative reactions to sound (such as facial nerve stimulation, eye blinking, etc). Test assistants are particularly helpful when one must rely on BOA, VRA, or CPA to obtain responses from the child. Once the child is old enough to provide a reliable conditioned response without direct oversight from a closely seated adult, he or she can be scheduled with a single audiologist.

Sound Field Verification of Mapping

Sound field measurements should be performed regularly to verify the suitability of the map on the processor. Such testing typically involves assessment of detection skills for frequencies ranging from 250 to 4000 Hz with either narrowband noise (NBN) or warble tone (WT) signals while the processor is set to a typical use setting. Most cochlear implant recipients demonstrate NBN or WT thresholds ranging from 10 to 40 dB HL on the sound field audiogram. Speech detection thresholds (SDT) are often slightly lower and range from 0 to 30 dB HL and should be in good agreement with the soundfield thresholds. If NBN or WT thresholds exceed 40 dB HL, the audiologist should check the settings of the processor, troubleshoot all external equipment, and consider remapping the processor to increase the audibility of the signals.

Sound field testing should be performed anytime the child demonstrates a questionable response to speech. In our clinic, soundfield testing is typically performed every six months in conjunction with the child's six-month mapping appointment. Speech perception testing is performed annually following the first year of cochlear implant use.

Speech Perception Testing

Current technology has made it possible for many profoundly deaf children with implants to develop receptive and expressive language skills comparable to the skills obtained by children with normal hearing. This is only possible, however, if the child is provided with an appropriate and effective map. Speech perception testing is an important part of follow up that verifies the appropriateness and effectiveness of the speech processor map. Such testing additionally helps identify problems with external and internal equipment, and enables a comparison over time to determine if the child is making appropriate progress with the device. With all children, such testing should be performed annually or more often if there are concerns about the integrity of the internal device. Other procedures that provide information about progress include feedback from the parents and teachers and the results of the speech and language evaluation.

Such testing should include a hierarchy of tests that evaluate several different aspects of speech perception. This will range from the simple skill of sound detection to the more complex levels of speech recognition. Additionally, the results of speech perception testing can be evaluated in conjunction with the results of speech and language evaluation to determine if the child is making adequate progress with his or her device. Speech perception tests commonly used with children in our clinic are provided in Table 6–3.

Special Considerations When Mapping

In some instances, the etiology of a child's hearing loss can affect the child's progress with the device and can make mapping of the device particularly challenging. It has been reported that some children with cochlear anomalies demonstrate higher current level requirements to hear with a cochlear implant than children who present with normal cochleae (Zwolan et al., 2008). With such children, the map parameter of pulse width may need to be increased to facilitate detection of sound. Presentation of signals at such high levels of stimulation may result in voltage compliance issues and also may result in stimulation of the facial nerve. If facial nerve stimulation is present with electrical stimulation, the level of the stimulation should be reduced or the problem electrode should be removed from the patient's map. Additionally, high stimulation levels and wider pulse widths may have an effect on battery life that may prohibit some patients from wearing a behind-the-ear style speech processor.

TABLE 6–3. Brief Descriptions of Speech Perception Tests Commonly Used with Children in Our Clinic

Ling Six Sound Test (Ling, 1976, 1989):

This informal test was developed by Daniel Ling as a procedure to quickly determine if a child can detect sounds that lie within the speech spectrum of hearing. Frequent administration of this test helps parents, professionals, and teachers monitor cochlear implant function and possible changes in hearing. It is usually performed live voice with the presenter asking the child to detect or identify the following six sounds: /m/, /oo/, /ah/, /ee/, /sh/, and /s/. The level of difficulty of the task can be varied depending on the skills of the child and can include detection, discrimination, identification, or comprehension.

Early Speech Perception Test (ESP) (Moog & Geers, 1990):

The *standard version* was designed to obtain accurate information about the progression of speech discrimination skills in children with profound hearing loss. Test stimuli include 36 words presented in an auditory-only condition (three subsets of 12). The format involves a closed-set, picture identification task. Each item is randomly presented twice. The first subtest includes a total of 12 words that fall into one of three categories: one, two, or three syllable words. In the first subtest, the child receives pattern credit if he or she chooses any word within the correct syllable pattern category and word credit if it is the correct word. The second subtest contains 12 spondees and the third subtest contains 12 monosyllabic words (i.e., assessing the word % correct score for these two subtests). For each subtest, the child is presented with a card containing pictures of all 12 possible words and is asked to point to the correct picture. The material can be presented live voice or a recording. Minimum age for this test is 6 years.

The *low verbal version* was designed to estimate speech perception abilities in very young children (2 years and up) with limited verbal abilities. The number of choices in the closed-set is smaller (4 versus 12) than in the standard version, and all three levels of the low verbal version use objects (toys) instead of pictures. Similar to the standard version, stimuli for the first level include words that vary in number of syllables or stress pattern. The second level contains only spondaic words, and the third level contains only monosyllabic words. The material can be presented via live voice or a recording. Minimum age for this test is 2 years or when vocabulary has been acquired.

Meaningful Auditory Integration Scale (MAIS) (Robbins, Renshaw, & Berry, 1991):

This questionnaire assesses a child's meaningful listening skills in every day situations. There are 10 questions scored on a scale of 0 to 4 (0 = never to 4 = always). Parental response to client administered questions is sought to determine the child's history with their hearing device. Minimum age for this test is 2 years. For children younger than 2 years the Infant-Toddler Meaningful Auditory Integration Scale (IT-MAIS) has been developed.

Word Intelligibility by Picture Identification (WIPI) Test (Ross & Lerman, 1970):

This test was designed to evaluate the child's ability to perceive words. Stimuli consist of four lists of 25 single-syllable words with similar vowels but different consonants. Carrier phrase: "Show me . . . " is used to present stimuli. Format is a closed-set containing six possible picture stimuli. Minimum age for administration is 5–6 years for children with moderate hearing loss and 7–8 years for children with severe to profound hearing losses.

continues

TABLE 6–3. *continued*

Northwestern University-Children's Perception of Speech (NU-CHIPS) Test (Elliot & Katz, 1980):

This test assesses word recognition abilities in children. Stimuli consist of monosyllabic words. Stimuli are presented in a closed-set containing four different pictures. Presentation can be live voice or a recording. Minimum age requirement is an age equivalency of 2.5 years on the Peabody Picture Vocabulary Test.

PBK-50 Word List (Haskins, 1949):

Stimuli consist of three lists of 50 monosyllabic words. Each response is scored for word and phoneme accuracy. Format is open-set. Presentation can be live-voice or a recording. Minimum age is 6 years. This test was not specifically designed for children with hearing loss.

Bamford-Kowal-Bench Sentences (BKB) (Bench, Kowal, & Bamford, 1979):

This test assesses speech recognition at a sentence level. Stimuli consist of key words in sentences, which are used to derive a percent-correct score. Format is open-set. Presentation is either recorded or monitored-live-voice. Minimum age is 6 years.

Glendonald Auditory Screening Procedure (GASP) (Erber, 1982):

This test was designed to assess a child's open-set speech recognition abilities using both words and sentences that are familiar. Stimuli consist of 3 lists of 12 words and 2 lists of 10 sentences. Sentences are in the form of questions. Presentation is via monitored-live voice.

Lexical Neighborhood Test (LNT) (Kirk, Pisoni, & Osberger, 1995):

This test was designed to assess a child's open-set speech recognition abilities using monosyllabic words. Stimuli consist of 50 words presented either monitored-live-voice or via a recording. The test contains lexically "easy" words (those high in frequency of occurrence but phonemically dissimilar to other words) and lexically "hard" words (those low in frequency of occurrence but phonemically similar to other words).

Multi Syllabic Lexical Neighborhood Test (MLNT) (Kirk, Pisoni, & Osberger, 1995):

This test was designed to assess a child's open-set speech recognition abilities using multi-syllabic words. Stimuli consist of 24 words presented either monitored-live-voice or via a recording. The test contains lexically "easy" words (those high in frequency of occurrence but phonemically dissimilar to other words) and lexically "hard" words (those low in frequency of occurrence but phonemically similar to other words).

Hearing-In-Noise Test for Children (HINT-C) (Nilsson, Soli, & Gelnett, 1996):

The children's version of the Hearing-In-Noise Test was designed to assess a child's open-set speech recognition abilities for children ages 6–12 years. This test is designed to be given with a signal to noise ratio. Most implant programs present these sentences in quiet, and as the child progresses, noise is introduced.

Additionally, it has been reported that children with abnormal cochleae (Buchman et al., 2004; Eisenman, Ashbaugh, Zwolan, Arts, & Telian, 2001) and children with cochlear ossification (El-Kashlan, Ashbaugh, Zwolan, & Telian, 2003) demonstrate poorer post-implant speech recognition skills than children with normal cochleae. If the anomaly is identified preoperatively, the parents should be counseled that their child's outcome may be poorer than average and that their child may require more appointments to optimize the map on the speech processor.

of detection thresholds in a sound field and examination of speech perception and speech and language skills over time. Such testing is essential as it provides the clinician with important information regarding the child's performance with the device, verifies the appropriateness of the map in the speech processor, and provides the clinician with important information regarding function of the internal and external device. Such monitoring of the map, and monitoring of performance with the map, is an essential part of implant patient follow-up that implant recipients likely will require throughout their lifetime.

Summary and Conclusions

Setting the parameters of a child's speech processor is a complicated task. Performing mapping with children requires skills in the areas of pediatric audiology, pediatric behavior management, electrophysiologic testing, and psychophysical assessment of hearing. Thus, speech processor mapping can be one of the most challenging aspects of post-operative patient care. The importance of properly setting the speech processor cannot be underestimated—inaccurate mapping can result in months or years of inadequate hearing by a child. Speech processor mapping is a dynamic process that has changed greatly over the past several years; such mapping will continue to change as technologic advancements in internal and external equipment are made. It is the responsibility of the implant audiologist to remain knowledgeable about changes and advances in cochlear implant technology in order to provide patients with the best possible care.

Along with mapping comes the responsibility of measuring performance with the device. Such testing includes evaluation

References

Abbas, P. J., Brown, C. J., & Etler, C. P. (2006). Electrophysiology and device telemetry. In S. B. Waltzman & J. T. Roland, Jr. (Eds.), *Cochlear implants* (2nd ed., pp. 96–109). New York: Thieme.

Battmer, R. D., Dillier, N., Lai, W. K., Weber, B. P., Brown, C., Gantz, B. J., et al. (2004). Evaluation of the neural response telemetry (NRT) capabilities of the nucleus research platform 8: Initial results from the NRT trial. *International Journal of Audiology, 43*(Suppl. 1), 10–50.

Battmer, R. D., Laszig, R., & Lehnhardt, E. (1990). Electrically elicited stapedius reflex in cochlear implant patients. *Ear and Hearing, 11,* 370–374.

Bean, A. W., & Roberts, M. W. (1981). The effect of time-out release contingencies on changes in child noncompliance. *Journal of Abnormal Child Psychology, 9,* 95–105.

Bench, J., Kowal, A., & Bamford, J. (1979). The BKB (Bamford-Kowal-Bench) sentence lists for partially-hearing children. *British Journal of Audiology, 13,* 108–112.

Brown, C. J., Abbas, P. J., Fryauf-Bertschy, H., Kelsay, D., & Gantz, B. J. (1994). Intraoperative and postoperative electrically evoked auditory brain stem responses in nucleus cochlear implant users: Implications for the fitting process. *Ear and Hearing, 15,* 168–176.

Brown, C. J., Abbas, P. J., & Gantz, B. (1990). Electrically evoked whole-nerve action potentials: Data from human cochlear implant users. *Journal of the Acoustical Society of America, 88,* 1385–1391.

Buchman, C. A., Copeland, B. J., Yu, K. K., Brown, C. J., Carrasco, V. N., & Pillsbury, H. C., III. (2004). Cochlear implantation in children with congenital inner ear malformations. *Laryngoscope, 114,* 309–316.

Caner, G., Olgun, L., Gültekin, G., & Balaban, M. (2007). Optimizing fitting in children using objective measures such as neural response imaging and electrically evoked stapedius reflex threshold. *Otology and Neurotology, 28,* 637–640.

Ching, T. Y., Psarros, C., Hill, M., Dillon, H. & Incerti, P. (2001). Should children who use cochlear implants wear hearing aids in the opposite ear? *Ear and Hearing, 22,* 365–380.

Diefendorf, A. O. (2002). Detection and assessment of hearing loss in infants and children. In. J. Katz (Ed.), *Handbook of clinical audiology* (5th ed., pp. 469–480). Philadelphia: Lippincott Williams and Wilkins.

Eisenman, D., Ashbaugh, C. A., Zwolan, T. A., Arts, H. A., & Telian, S. A. (2001). Implantation of the malformed cochlea. *Otology and Neurotology, 22,* 834–841.

El-Kashlan, H. K., Ashbaugh, C., Zwolan, T., & Telian, S. A. (2003). Cochlear implantation in prelingually deaf children with ossified cochleae. *Otology and Neurotology, 24,* 596–600.

Elliot, L. L., & Katz, D. (1980). *Northwestern University-Children's Perception of Speech (NU-CHIPS) test.* St. Louis, MO: Auditec.

Erber, N. P. (1982). *Auditory training.* Washington, DC: A. G. Bell Association for the Deaf.

Fink, N. E., Wang, N. Y., Visaya, J., Niparko, J. K., Quittner, A., Eisenberg, L. S., Tobey, E. A., & CDaCI Investigative Team. (2007). Childhood Development after Cochlear Implantation (CDaCI) study: Design and baseline charac-

teristics. *Cochlear Implants International, 8,* 92–116.

Gordon, K., Papsin, B. C., & Harrison, R. V. (2004). Programming cochlear implant stimulation levels in infants and children with a combination of objective measures. *International Journal of Audiology, 43*(Suppl. 1), 28–32.

Haskins, H. (1949). *A phonetically balanced test of speech discrimination for children.* Unpublished master's thesis, Northwestern University, Evanston, IL.

Jerger, J., Oliver, T. A., & Chmiel, R. A. (1988). Prediction of dynamic range from stapedius reflex in cochlear implant patients. *Ear and Hearing, 9,* 4–8.

Kileny, P. R. (1991). Use of electrophysiologic measures in the management of children with cochlear implants: Brainstem, middle latency, and cognitive (P300) responses. *American Journal of Otology, 12*(Suppl.), 37–42; discussion 43–47.

Kirk, K. I., Pisoni, D. B., & Osberger, M. J. (1995). Lexical effects on spoken word recognition by pediatric cochlear implant users. *Ear and Hearing, 16,* 470–481.

Ling, D. (1976). *Speech and the hearing-impaired child: Theory and practice.* Washington, DC: Alexander Graham Bell Association for the Deaf.

Ling, D. (1989). *Foundations of spoken language for the hearing-impaired child.* Washington, DC: Alexander Graham Bell Association for the Deaf.

Moog, J., & Geers, A. (1990). *Early speech perception test (ESP) for profoundly hearing-impaired children.* St. Louis, MO: Central Institute for the Deaf.

Nilsson, M., Soli, S., & Gelnett, D. (1996). *Development and norming of the hearing-in-noise test for children (HINT-C).* House Ear Institute internal report.

Robbins, A. M., Renshaw, J. J., & Berry, S. W. (1991). Evaluating meaningful auditory integration in profoundly hearing-impaired children. *American Journal of Otology, 12*(Suppl.), 144–150.

Ross, M., & Lerman, J. (1970). A picture identification test for hearing-impaired children.

Journal of Speech and Hearing Research, 13, 44-53.

Shallop, J. K., Beiter, A. L., Goin, D. W., & Mischke, R. E. (1990). Electrically evoked auditory brainstem responses (EABR) and middle latency responses (EMLR) obtained from patients with the Nucleus multichannel cochlear implant. *Ear and Hearing, 11*, 5-15.

Shallop, J. K., VanDyke, L., Goin, D. W., & Mischke, R. E. (1991). Prediction of behavioral threshold and comfort values for Nucleus 22-channel implant patients from electrical auditory brain stem response test results. *Annals of Otology, Rhinology, and Laryngology, 100*, 896-898.

Shapiro, W. (2006). Device programming. In S. B. Waltzman & J. T. Roland, Jr. (Eds.), *Cochlear implants* (2nd ed., pp. 135-145). New York: Thieme.

Tyler, R. S., Parkinson, A. J., Wilson, B. S., Witt, S., Preece, J. P., & Noble, W. (2002). Patients utilizing a hearing aid and a cochlear implant: Speech perception and localization. *Ear and Hearing, 23*, 98-105.

Zwolan, T. (2005, January/February). Hearing aid use in conjunction with a cochlear implant. *Hearing Loss Magazine, 26*, 26-28.

Zwolan, T., & Griffin, B. (2005). How we do it: Tips for programming the speech processor of an 18-month-old. *Cochlear Implants International, 6*, 169-177.

Zwolan, T., O'Sullivan, M. B., Fink, N. E., Niparko, J. K., & CDaCI Investigative Team. (2008). Electric charge requirements of pediatric cochlear implant recipients enrolled in the Childhood Development after Cochlear Implant Study. *Otology and Neurotology, 29*, 143-148.

CHAPTER 7

Electrically Evoked Auditory Potentials: Clinical Applications

CAROLYN J. BROWN
PAUL J. ABBAS
CHRISTINE P. ETLER
ABBIE K. LARSON
KRISTIN E. MUSSER
SARA N. O'BRIEN

Introduction

The first studies describing auditory evoked potentials measured from human subjects were published in the late 1960s and early 1970s (e.g., Jewett, Romano, & Williston, 1970; Sohmer & Feinmesser, 1967; Yoshie, Ohashi, & Suzuki, 1968). Over the course of the next decade, a great deal of research was published that described techniques for measuring these gross neural potentials and defined some of the basic clinical applications for this technology. Today, auditory evoked potentials are widely used to assess hearing in children or individuals who are unable to be tested using standard behavioral techniques. They also are used as a tool for assessing auditory function during surgical procedures affecting the skull base, and to help diagnose pathologic conditions affecting the auditory pathways within the brainstem.

Another major technologic advance to affect the otolaryngology community during 1980s was the introduction of cochlear implants (CI) as a potential treatment for individuals with profound, bilateral sensorineural hearing loss. In the early years, CI technology was relatively crude and performance with CIs varied widely; however, it quickly became apparent that these devices could provide significant benefit to many profoundly hearing-impaired individuals who were not able to benefit from the conventional forms of amplification available at the time. Although early studies focused on postlingually deafened adults, it soon became apparent that congenitally deaf children could also benefit from cochlear implantation. These children presented special challenges for the audiologists who worked with them and their families. Typically, they had little or no experience with audition; many had severely limited communication skills and their age alone made testing using traditional behaviorally based measures difficult. As a result, researchers from several different laboratories began to focus on identifying ways in which electrically evoked auditory potentials might be used to facilitate the programming process or to help determine which individuals might benefit most from the device.

Early attempts at recording electrically evoked auditory potentials were only moderately successful. One challenge confronting investigators at that time was that commercial instrumentation used for measuring acoustically evoked auditory potentials was not designed to deal with the stimulus artifact inherent to electrical stimulation. Early studies with experimental animals demonstrated several sources of contamination, such as the electrical stimulus artifact or non-auditory myogenic or vestibular activity (Black, Clark, Sheperd, O'Leary, & Walters, 1983; Dobie & Kimm, 1980; Smith & Simmons, 1983). As methods for minimizing artifact contamination improved, a number of different research groups reported successful recordings of the electrically evoked auditory brainstem responses (EABR) from CI users (Abbas & Brown, 1988, 1991; Game, Gibson, & Pauka, 1987; Miyamoto & Brown, 1987; van den Honert & Stypulkowski, 1986). Several studies (e.g., Brown, Abbas, Fryauf-Bertschy, Kelsey, & Gantz, 1994; Mason et al., 1993b; Shallop, VanDyke, Goin, & Mischke, 1991) reported the relationship (or lack thereof) between measures of EABR latency and/or thresholds and performance on tests of speech recognition as well as the levels needed to program the speech processor of the Nucleus CI. Although it was at least theoretically possible that EABR thresholds could be used to program the speech processor of these early CIs, enthusiasm about doing so was never particularly high within the clinical community. This was primarily a reflection of the fact that the EABR, like its acoustic counterpart, is very small in amplitude and easily affected by muscle artifact. As a result, sedation often was required in order to allow clean repeatable EABRs to be recorded efficiently from pediatric CI users. Additionally, the process of recording the EABR proved to be time consuming, effectively limiting the number of electrodes that could be evaluated within a single recording session. Because of these practical limitations, at most clinics, EABR recordings were made, if at all, only in the operating room at the time of surgery. Few centers ever recorded the EABR postoperatively and if they did, it was not done for the purpose of programming the speech processor of the CI but because there was some serious concern about device failure.

In 1990, a technique for recording the electrically evoked compound action potential (ECAP) from an intracochlear electrode in Ineraid CI users was first described (Brown, Abbas, & Gantz, 1990). Although no longer marketed, the Ineraid CI system was unique in that there were no implanted electronics and a percutaneous connector was used to couple the externally worn speech processor with the electrodes in the cochlea. This design allowed an electrically isolated, differential recording amplifier to be directly connected to the intracochlear electrodes. The close proximity of the stimulation and recording electrodes resulted in significant problems with artifact contamination, but Brown et al. (1990) developed a technique for reliably extracting the ECAP from the stimulus artifact.

The ECAP was (and continues to be) the most direct measure of the response of the auditory nerve to electrical stimulation that can be measured in clinical settings. It has several advantages over the EABR. First, the proximity of the recording electrode to the stimulable neural elements results in responses that are as much as an order of magnitude larger than those recorded using surface electrodes. Additionally, because the recording electrode is seated in the temporal bone rather than on the scalp, contamination of the neural response by muscle artifact is greatly reduced. In fact, the ECAP could be measured from these patients without sedation. Moreover, the fact that it was generated peripherally meant that ECAPs would not be affected by development, attention or other cognitive factors, making it an ideal tool for pediatric applications. However, because children were not typically considered to be candidates for the Ineraid device, ECAPs remained primarily a research tool for several years.

In 1998, Cochlear Corporation introduced the Nucleus CI24M cochlear implant. This CI system was unique in that it was equipped with reverse telemetry capabilities that made it possible to record the ECAP from individuals who used CIs without a percutaneous connector. The system developed by Cochlear Corporation to record the ECAP was called Neural Response Telemetry (NRT) and for the first time it became possible to record neural activity from the auditory nerve of a pediatric CI user. Recognizing the potential clinical significance that this technology had, particularly for very young children, the other

major CI manufacturers soon followed suit. Advanced Bionics Corporation introduced Neural Response Imaging (NRI) software in 2001. More recently, MED-EL introduced Auditory Response Telemetry (ART). All of these neural response telemetry systems include software to control the stimulation and recording parameters as well as methods for minimizing stimulus artifact, averaging, filtering, and analyzing the recorded waveforms.

Over the next decade, research describing characteristics and applications of ECAPs expanded. The ECAP was used to study in more detail how electrical impulses provided by a CI are coded at the level of the auditory nerve (Wilson, Finley, Lawson, & Zerbi, 1997). Many reports explored the relationship between individuals' ECAP thresholds and the psychophysical measures used to program the speech processor (Brown et al., 1994, 2000; Cullington, 2000; Gordon, Ebinger, Gilden & Shapiro, 2002; Hughes, Brown, Abbas, Wolaver, & Gervais, 2000; Mason, Cope, Garnham, O'Donoghue & Gibbin, 2001; Mason et al., 1993a, 1993b; Shallop, Beiter, Goin, & Mischke, 1990; Shallop, et al., 1991; Thai-Van et al., 2001). The body of research published during this era had a direct impact on clinical practice. However, recently there has been recognition of the fact that these responses, although robust and easy to record in clinical settings, have limitations. The primary limitations arise from the very peripheral nature of the responses themselves. They do not reflect the impact of neural processing at more central levels within the auditory system. Additionally, recording the ECAP requires the use of very simple, low rate pulsatile stimuli and such stimuli are not representative of the kinds of stimulus patterns that are typically produced by the CI. These realizations have led to a resurgence of interest in long latency, cortically generated, and electrically evoked responses.

This chapter begins with an overview of how electrically evoked auditory responses are recorded and the kind of information that can be gained by doing so. The chapter focuses primarily on clinical applications with pediatric populations. Our goal is to have the reader come away with a better understanding of how this technology can be used to inform clinical practice today.

Recording Electrically Evoked Responses

There are a number of different auditory evoked neural potentials that can be recorded from CI users. These include, but are not limited to, EABR, ECAP, and electrically evoked middle and long latency responses (EMLR and ELLR). An illustration of each of these neural potentials is shown in Figure 7–1. In each case, the stimulus is a series of biphasic current pulses presented via a single intracochlear electrode. Note that both the time and amplitude scales are different on each plot and that these responses are quite different in terms of both latency and amplitude. Each of the electrically evoked responses share many features with their acoustically evoked counterpart (ECoG, ABR, and LLR). The acoustic electric cognates are presumed to reflect neural activity recorded from the same neural generators and typically respond to changes in stimulation and/or recording parameters in much the same way. The ECAP is particularly large in amplitude because it is recorded from an intracochlear electrode located very close to the auditory nerve, whereas surface electrodes positioned on the scalp are used to record the EABR and ELLR.

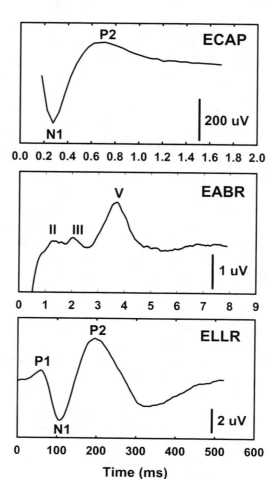

Figure 7–1. Electrically evoked auditory potentials recorded from a Nucleus CI24M cochlear implant user.

In order to record the EABR, the speech processor of the CI is typically bypassed, and the software provided by the manufacturer is used to directly control the implanted electronics. Although direct stimulation also can be used to evoke the ELLR (also referred to as the P1-N1-P2 complex), this long latency response is more frequently recorded in response to stimulation through the implant processor using brief tones or short speech tokens presented at supra-threshold levels in the sound field.

When using direct stimulation, measurement of neural potentials requires coordination of two different computer systems. One computer, equipped with a programming interface, is used for stimulation. A second computer, often a commercial evoked potential unit capable of being externally triggered, is used to record and average the associated neural response. Regardless of which recording system is used or how stimulation is accomplished, directly or through the sound field, the biggest challenge associated with measuring electrically evoked responses is finding a way to minimize contamination of the recorded responses by stimulus artifact. The stimulus artifact associated with electrical stimulation is often so large that it saturates the recording amplifier and distorts the recordings. To avoid this scenario, we typically increase the bandwidth of filters and decrease the amount of gain that is generally used for recording of acoustic responses.

The choice of stimulus characteristics also can impact the quality of the recordings. For example, stimulus artifact can be significantly reduced by shortening the duration of the stimulus pulses and by alternating the polarity of the stimulus in the average. Bipolar stimulation also results in significantly less stimulus artifact than monopolar stimulation.

Finally, the recording electrode montage that is used also can have a significant impact on the recordings obtained in response to electrical stimulation. Some evoked potential systems allow for simultaneous input from multiple electrode sites located around the head. These systems are frequently used when the evoked potential of interest is the cortically generated P1-N1-P2 complex. Typically, results of these studies have shown that the electrodes closest to

the implant receiver/stimulator are dominated by stimulus artifact and, as a result, are generally not used for data analysis. Although multiple electrode sites can help define the electrical field that results from activation of the CI and are critical if the intent is to define neural generators of the specific evoked potentials, they are not always practical in clinical settings that focus primarily on pediatric populations. For EABR recordings, we routinely use a contralateral or vertical electrode montage because Wave V of the EABR is not strongly affected by the location of the reference electrode. We have found that increasing the physical distance between the recording electrodes and receiver/stimulator of the CI is the best way to reduce the amount of stimulus artifact contamination in the recording.

Although finding ways to minimize stimulus artifact contamination is the key to obtaining quality electrically evoked auditory responses, there are instances where it can be helpful to focus on the artifact itself. Averaged electrode voltages (AEVs) are recordings of the stimulus artifact associated with activation of the CI. AEVs are typically recorded using an ipsilateral electrode montage. With blanking turned off, the recording epoch and stimulation parameters are chosen to allow good resolution of the response in the recorded time window and, perhaps most importantly, the gain of the differential amplifier typically is set very low so as to avoid saturation of the recording amplifier by the stimulus artifact. When a normally functioning device is tested, the recordings are expected to be biphasic and to change in a regular fashion as stimulation parameters are changed. It is possible to use these recordings to ensure that biphasic current pulses can be output from each electrode in the intracochlear array and to verify that changes in stimulation rate, level and/or pulse duration are, in fact, resulting in appropriate changes in the output of the CI.

Figure 7–2 shows a series of AEVs recorded from an individual with a normally functioning Nucleus CI24M cochlear implant. The recordings shown in this figure were obtained using an evoked potential unit, "The Crystal System," designed specifically for this purpose by Cochlear Corporation. The top two tracings show AEVs recorded using a low level current pulse that was presented either in common ground (CG) and monopolar stimulation modes on each of the 22 intracochlear electrodes. When the CG stimulation mode is used, the responses are largest when electrodes near the base of the cochlea are stimulated, they decrease in amplitude and often become difficult to resolve as the stimulating electrode is moved across the middle of the electrode array, they then reverse polarity and increase in amplitude as the stimulating electrode is moved further toward the apex. With monopolar stimulation, the responses recorded as the stimulating electrode is changed are similar in amplitude and polarity. The lower two traces show AEVs recorded as stimulation level and phase duration are systematically manipulated. A properly functioning implant will demonstrate changes in both amplitude and pulse duration as stimulus characteristics are varied as shown.

Recording AEVs does not require active participation by the subject. Additionally, recording AEVs is relatively quick because very few averages are needed. As a result, these responses can be recorded, even without sedation or sleep, from very young children. Average electrode voltages have been used to supplement the information about electrode impedance provided by the CI software to help diagnose electrode and/or device malfunctions (Franck & Shah, 2004; Heller, Sinopoli, Fowler-Brehm, & Shallop, 1991; Hughes, Brown, & Abbas, 2004; Kileny,

Meiteles, Zwolan, & Tellian, 1995; Mens, Brokx, & van den Broek, 1995; Mens, Oostendorp, & van den Broek, 1994). Although convenient, the Crystal System is not necessary for recording these responses. They can be recorded equally well with any commercial evoked potential unit. Some of the larger CI centers routinely record AEVs and use them to help diagnose potential problems with the implanted components of the CI. Other centers rely on personnel from the CI companies who can (and will) travel to the individual centers and bring the instrumentation appropriate for assessing device function in vivo.

Finally, all of the current CI systems have technology that makes it possible to use one of the intracochlear electrodes to record the response of the auditory nerve to electrical stimulation. Although the neural telemetry systems developed by these three CI manufacturers have different names and acronyms, they all measure the same evoked response: the ECAP. With all three systems, specialized software is used to control both stimulation and recording parameters. A stimulus pulse or series of pulses is applied to a specific intracochlear electrode and voltage on a nearby electrode is sampled, transmitted via a reverse telemetry system to an external coil and processed and displayed by the same computer used for stimulation. The close proximity of the recording electrode to the auditory nerve means that the recorded responses are relatively large in amplitude—often several hundred millivolts. Again, the challenge associated with recording the ECAP is to find a way effectively to minimize contamination by stimulus artifact. This is particularly problematic for this application because the stimulating and recording electrodes are located so close to each other (often only millimeters way) and the neural response has such a short latency (under 0.5 ms).

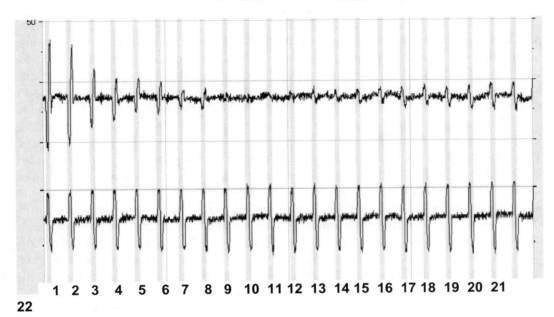

1 2 3 4 5 6 7 8 9 10 11 12 13 14 15 16 17 18 19 20 21
22

ELECTRODE

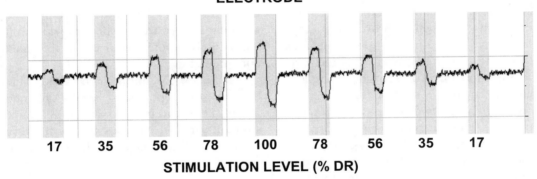

17   35   56   78   100   78   56   35   17

STIMULATION LEVEL (% DR)

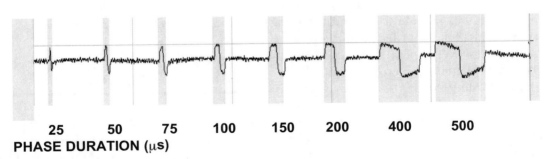

25   50   75   100   150   200   400   500

PHASE DURATION (μs)

Figure 7–2. Average Electrode Voltages (AEVs) recorded using the Crystal System from a single Nucleus CI24 cochlear implant user with a normally functioning device. The top panel shows AEVs recorded using common ground (*upper trace*) and monopolar (*lower trace*) modes. The middle and lower panels show the effect of systematic changes in stimulus level and duration for single electrode, monopolar stimulation.

As a result, much attention has been given to finding ways to minimize stimulus artifact in the ECAP recordings. The three major CI companies differ in how they approach this challenge.

Cochlear Corporation was the first to introduce software for measuring the ECAP. Typically that software, currently called Custom Sound EP, has been separate from the programming software but runs on the same platform. It is flexible and allows the user to record these responses manually or to run a fully automated version of the ECAP recording system that is designed to record ECAP thresholds on all 22 intracochlear electrodes in rapid succession (AutoNRT). Both the manual, clinician controlled software as well as the automated software use a forward masking technique originally described by Brown et al. (1990) to extract the neural response, the ECAP, from the stimulus artifact. This technique requires making one recording using a single current pulse, or probe, and a second recording using two pulses, a masker and a probe, presented with a very short interpulse interval (IPI). If the IPI is short enough, the auditory nerve will be refractory at the time the second pulse in the two-pulse sequence is presented. As a result, this recording will include a measure of the stimulus artifact associated with the probe without an overlapping neural potential. The ECAP is then extracted by subtracting the recording made in the two pulse sequence from the recording made using a single current pulse. This subtraction technique has been described in detail elsewhere (Abbas et al., 1999; Brown et al., 1990) and has been proven to be an effective method of eliminating artifact from the neural recordings.

Advanced Bionics and MED-EL corporations approached the task of reducing stimulus artifact in the intracochlear recordings a bit differently. The neural response recording system used by most clinicians who work with Advanced Bionics patients is part of the Soundwave programming software. With this system, artifact contamination is minimized by alternating the stimulus polarity in the average. MED-EL Corporation uses a template subtraction procedure to minimize contamination of the neural response by stimulus artifact. This approach requires making a recording of artifact by presenting the current pulse at a subthreshold level. They refer to this recording, which presumably consists of stimulus artifact without any neural response, as the template. Recordings are then obtained for pulses presented at suprathreshold levels. The template is scaled up to match the artifact in the suprathreshold recordings and subtracted from that response. The result is a neural response with minimal artifact contamination.

Miller, Abbas, and Brown (2000) published a study comparing results obtained using these three approaches. All have strengths and weaknesses and all three of the major CI manufacturers have reported success measuring the ECAP using their systems. The applications of these measures in clinical practice are similar, regardless of implant type or recording methodology.

Clinical Applications

When pediatric audiologists are asked to assess hearing in an infant or a very young child, a great deal of reliance is initially placed on the results of objective test procedures such as auditory brainstem response (ABR), auditory steady-state response (ASSR), otoacoustic emissions (OAE), and immittance. That information is supplemented by parent report, observation of the child's responses to auditory stimulation and the results of any age-appropriate behavioral testing procedures that may be possible. Typically, in the first few visits results from behavioral testing are limited. As the child grows, the emphasis shifts from one where greater reliance is placed on electrophysiologic or nonbehavioral measures of hearing to one where most decisions are based almost entirely on the results of behavioral testing. That said, however, no good audiologist would ignore the results of either form of assessment. What is important in a pediatric practice is to learn the limitations inherent in each type of assessment procedure and weigh the results accordingly. This is true regardless of whether or not the child is a CI user.

For CI users, regardless of their age and/or device type, optimal performance will depend on the speech processor being well fit. Achieving this goal with very young CI recipients can be time consuming. One area where objective measures of the auditory system response to electrical stimulation can be helpful is in programming the implant speech processor.

Additionally, CIs can fail. Some failures are obvious and easily detected, but much of the time, when a CI is failing the symptoms can be more subtle. Postlingually deafened adults can provide a great deal of information about the quality of the sound they hear and play an active role in trouble shooting malfunctions. The same is not true for congenitally deaf children who typically have limited communication skills, little or no auditory experience, and short attention spans. Diagnosing device malfunctions is another general area where electrically evoked auditory potentials can be useful.

Finally, there can be considerable variation in performance with a CI. Finding an evoked potential that correlates with performance would be important because

it could help us determine who might be a good candidate for cochlear implantation, drive ear selection and/or help explain why a given subject is not progressing with his/her device. The following sections focus specifically on clinical applications for electrically evoked auditory potentials in pediatric CI populations.

Determining Candidacy and/or Ear Selection

There are a number of reasons why one might want to record electrically evoked auditory potentials either prior to implantation or during the surgical procedure itself. For example, we know that postoperative performance with a CI varies widely. This is true, regardless of the type of CI. All of the major CI centers have had individuals with devices that appear to be functioning appropriately but who exhibit little or no measurable benefit. When this happens, particularly when it happens with a pediatric CI recipient, it can be devastating for all involved. Moreover, establishing that the child is truly not able to benefit from electrical stimulation in a meaningful way can take a great deal of time and effort on the part of the entire CI team. Historically, in order to avoid this scenario, some CI teams, both in the United States and abroad, have advocated the use of electrically evoked auditory potentials recorded prior to insertion of the CI as a method of establishing candidacy or to select the best ear to implant. Years ago it was common for a surgeon to place an electrode on the round window niche or the promontory of the middle ear and electrically stimulate the cochlea prior to insertion of the CI. The purpose of doing this was to allow the EABR to be recorded from surface electrodes. The idea was that patients (or ears) with particularly poor neural survival might be identified on the basis of either an absent EABR or significantly elevated EABR threshold (Kileny, Zimmerman-Phillips, Kemink, & Schmaltz, 1991; Mason, O'Donoghue, Gibbin, Garnham, & Jowett, 1997). The inherent assumption was that the EABR threshold, or more frequently the amplitude of wave V of the EABR, could be used to predict postoperative performance levels. In an effort to evaluate the validity of that assumption, Nikolopoulos and colleagues compared EABRs recorded using promontory stimulation with performance using a CI several months later (Nikolopoulos, Mason, Gibbin, & O'Donoghue, 2000; Nikolopoulos, Mason, O'Donoghue, & Gibbin, 1999). Although they did find that EABRs recorded from children who were deaf due to meningitis had less distinct morphologic characteristics and smaller amplitudes than similar measures made from children who were congenitally deaf, they did not find a significant correlation between the presence of a poor EABR measured preoperatively and performance outcomes. Similar results also were reported by Makhdoum, Groenen, Snik, and van den Broek (1998), Kubo et al. (2001), and Firszt, Chambers, and Kraus (2002). None of these studies found amplitude, latency, and/or growth of the EABR to be significantly correlated with performance. In particular, care should be taken not to conclude that an ear is not stimulable based on the absence of a promontory EABR. We have observed a number of instances when no response was obtained when the electrical stimulus was applied to the promontory of the middle ear, but clear electrically evoked auditory potentials could be recorded once the electrode array was inserted into the scala tympani. Many of these patients went on to become reasonably good CI users.

Today, few CI programs continue to include promontory stimulation as part of their routine preoperative assessment battery. There are, however, some fairly unusual cases where one may consider doing so. For example, there are times when there may be a reason to question the presence of an auditory nerve. Nikolopoulos et al. (2000) correctly noted that although lack of an EABR elicited from a stimulating electrode placed in the middle ear has little prognostic value, the presence of such a response in cases where there is cause for concern about the status of the auditory nerve (e.g., small internal auditory canal, auditory neuropathy) can be significant. A well-formed EABR suggests that the nerve is intact and the patient is likely to respond to stimulation.

Finally, this apparent lack of correlation between preoperative measures of EABR amplitude, latency or threshold and postoperative measures of word recognition, although somewhat disappointing, should come as no surprise. Acoustically evoked ABRs are not correlated with speech perception skills in less severely hearing-impaired populations.

Verifying Device Function

Although CIs are designed to last for the life of the recipient, the internal components of the CI can and do fail. Out of box failures, although rare, do occur. As a result, many surgeons require verification of device function even before the patient leaves the operating room. Unfortunately, malfunction of the internal components of the CI can occur months or even years following the surgery. Such failures result in percepts that can range from complete lack of stimulation, to intermittent overstimulation and/or a subtle change in the level or quality of stimulation provided by the implant. Although adult CI users can describe what they experience to the clinician, pediatric CI users are not always able to do so. Consequently, there is a need for objective tools that can be used to monitor the implanted components of the device for the life span of the individual user and most CI centers include measures of how the device is working at every postoperative visit.

There are two different ways that the function of the implanted components of the CI can be assessed. The most common approach is to use the software provided by the manufacturers for this purpose. All of the major CI manufacturers have included telemetry systems in the design of their implant and in the fitting software. These telemetry systems work by allowing the user to record voltages on individual electrodes during stimulation with a constant, low level current pulse. Based on these measures, the impedance of the individual electrodes in the CI can be computed. Performing this test is fast, does not require any participation by the CI user, nor does it require recording electrodes or use of an evoked potential system. Unfortunately, CIs manufactured prior to 1997 did not have reverse telemetry capabilities. Many of these devices are still in use today. For these patients, there is no way to assess electrode impedance directly.

The second approach to assessing device function is to measure Average Electrode Voltage(s). AEVs, such as those illustrated in Figure 7–2, can be recorded from any CI recipient regardless of the type or age of the CI they use. In order to record AEVs, a set of surface electrodes are applied including an active electrode positioned on the mastoid adjacent to the CI and a reference electrode on the contralateral mastoid. In a properly functioning CI, the AEV will be large in amplitude and biphasic. Changes in pulse duration, level, or rate are evident. Additionally, comparison of re-

sponse waveforms generated as the stimulating electrode is systematically changed can allow for abnormally functioning electrodes to be identified.

AEVs can be particularly useful for diagnosing problems with older CIs, such as the Nucleus 22 device, that does not have the reverse telemetry capabilities required for measuring electrode impedance. Several investigators have published reports demonstrating how these responses can be used to diagnose abnormal device function (Hughes et al., 2004; Kileny et al., 1995; Mahoney & Rotz Proctor, 1994, Mens et al., 1994). Even with current generation CIs, there may be advantages to recording AEVs in clinical practice. Both Hughes et al. (2004) and Franck and Shah (2004) have reported cases where abnormally functioning electrodes were not accurately identified on the basis of the clinical impedance measures, but could be diagnosed on the basis of abnormal AEVs. That said, the point should be made that the form of the AEV reflects more than simply the impedance of the stimulated electrode. It also is affected by factors such as the mode of stimulation, the spatial orientation of the stimulating and recording electrodes, and the current path within the ear itself. There is not a gold standard by which to calculate the relative sensitivity and specificity of the technique so care should be used in interpreting the results. We have encountered a number of cases where an adult or older child who is a good reporter of what they are hearing will have clearly abnormal AEVs but still report normal sensations when that electrode is stimulated. This is particularly true for older devices and for patients with unusual cochlear anatomy. Our goal for all CI users is to obtain baseline AEV measures during the first few months after surgery and then biannually thereafter. This information can prove invaluable if the child experiences a sudden decline in performance. When we find an abnormal AEV, we notify the programming audiologist. For adults or older children who are good reporters of what they hear, we leave the decision about whether or not to include that electrode in the program, or MAP, used by the speech processor to control stimulation levels up to the programming audiologist. Some of our adult CI users and families of older children will elect to continue using a MAP that includes the electrode with the abnormal AEV. Others will report that speech and environmental sounds are clearer if a MAP is created without that electrode. For very young CI users, who are not able to report abnormal percepts or distortions of the signal, we will err on the side of "programming out" the suspect electrode(s). CIs sometimes fail because they begin to have more and more individual electrodes that fail over time. Regardless of the decision about whether or not to continue using a specific electrode in the MAP, AEVs provide an objective and repeatable method of documenting device function (or malfunction). That information, particularly when interpreted in conjunction with electrode impedance and/or performance data, can be valuable in determining whether or not reimplantation should be considered.

Monitoring Changes in Response to Electrical Stimulation Over Time

Electrically evoked auditory potentials also can be used to assess changes in responsiveness to electrical stimulation over time. In theory, it is possible that long-term use of electrical stimulation could have deleterious effects. If that occurs, one might expect to see elevation of behavioral and/or electro-physiologic thresholds over time. In some cases, children who have been successful CI users for several years begin to resist wearing their device as they mature. Rejection of the device may happen for several reasons. In some cases, it is possible that the device may be failing. In other cases, where device malfunction has been ruled out, rejection of the CI or a decrease in performance with the CI may reflect a true change in the response of the auditory system. It is also possible that a child may begin to resist wearing the speech processor of the CI because of changes in his/her attitude and/or social environment. Electrophysiologic measures can be particularly helpful in determining which of those scenarios is more likely.

Prior to introduction of CIs with neural response measurement capabilities, it was fairly uncommon to see a patient for electrophysiologic testing multiple times. That was true regardless of whether acoustic or electrical stimuli were being used. ABR thresholds were obtained once, or perhaps twice, during the lifetime of most hearing-impaired children and the duration of these test sessions were limited. With the introduction of neural response telemetry circuits, it became possible to measure the ECAP efficiently, without sedation, and at each visit. As a result, for the first time it was possible to use an electrophysiologic measure of auditory sensitivity to assess changes over time in pediatric populations.

Research has shown that after the first few weeks or months of CI use, ECAP thresholds are very stable (Hughes et al., 2001; Lai, Aksit, Akdas, & Dillier, 2004). This is true even in the early postimplant period when the MAP can be changing dramatically, suggesting that changes such as those that are observed in uncomfortable loudness level over time are not based on changes in peripheral stimulation. Figure 7–3 is a box

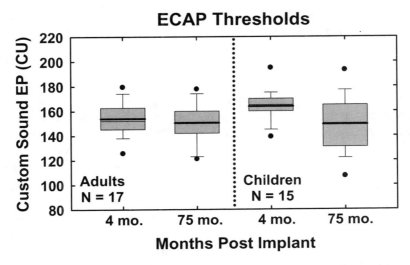

Figure 7–3. Box plots showing the distribution of ECAP thresholds recorded at two postoperative visits spaced approximately 6 years apart. The thick line indicates the mean. The upper and lower bounds of the box show the 25th and 75th percentile of the distribution. The whiskers show the 5th and 95th percentile and the dots show the full range of the data.

plot that shows the distribution of ECAP thresholds measured at two points in time for a group of 17 adults and 15 children. All of these patients used the Nucleus CI system. Paired comparison between thresholds recorded at 4 months postimplant and then again more than 6 years later are not statistically different for either age group. These results are reassuring and can be interpreted as evidence that the electrical stimulation provided by a CI is not, in and of itself, causing deleterious consequences over the long term. Based on such data, we suggest that ECAP thresholds, on a subset of electrodes spaced across the intracochlear electrode array, should be collected during the first few months of CI use and repeated periodically thereafter. These threshold measures can then serve as a point of comparison for years to come. Such information can prove invaluable when try-

ing to rule out a potential device failure or to determine why a child might be failing to progress with his/her implant. For example, we have worked with CI recipients who, based on behavioral testing, seem to require increasingly higher current levels in order to reach threshold or a maximum comfort level. A finding that the ECAP thresholds are also increasing over this time period can help corroborate those behavioral observations. On the other hand, stable ECAP thresholds may cause the clinician to question their behavioral results and explore other programming options with the child.

Many clinics will measure ECAP thresholds at the time of surgery. There are numerous reasons why these measures may not correlate well with similar measures made weeks to months later. Most changes in ECAP amplitude and threshold occur during the first months after implantation (Hughes et al., 2001). These changes could be due to a number of factors such as changes in electrode impedance or tissue growth in the cochlea that could impact both stimulation and recording. Obtaining baseline ECAP measures during one of the early postoperative visits, rather than in the operating room, ensures that the stimulus levels used will be tolerable for the subject and appropriate for repeated testing even years later.

Programming the Speech Processor

Of all the potential applications for electrophysiologic measures in clinical practice, perhaps the most significant application might be as a tool for estimating the stimulation levels needed to program the speech processor of the CI for an individual user. Young children with limited auditory experience and/or communication skills can be difficult or impossible to test using behavioral techniques. In some cases, although it is possible to use behavioral measures to estimate threshold, it may not be as easy to identify the stimulation levels where the electrical impulses are "most comfortable" or at a "maximum comfortable listening level." For many children, behavioral measures may be unreliable and/or may be relatively time consuming to obtain. Electrophysiologic measures such as the acoustically evoked ABR and ASSR are used routinely to estimate hearing thresholds and to determine how much gain a specific child requires from their hearing aid. Electrically evoked auditory potentials can, in some cases, serve a similar function. Several different groups of investigators began to explore the accuracy with which the levels needed to program the speech processor of the CI could be estimated for CI users of all ages.

Early studies showed that the EABR could be used to help guide the process of fitting the speech processor (Brown et al., 1994; Brown, Hughes, Lopez, & Abbas, 1999; Mason et al., 1993b; Shallop et al., 1991). Although promising, the reality was that for a variety of practical reasons few clinics actually used this approach to drive programming. The introduction of neural response telemetry, however, shifted focus almost overnight, from the EABR to the ECAP. The hope was that this technology would lead to the development of a prescriptive procedure that could be used reliably to program the speech processor of the CI. Toward that end, numerous investigators began to explore the relationship between ECAP thresholds and/or growth functions and the levels used to program the CI speech processor.

The first large scale studies that addressed this issue were studies published by Brown et al. (2000) and Hughes et al. (2000). Brown et al. (2000) reported results obtained from adult CI users. Hughes et al. (2000) reported similar data recorded from pediatric CI recipients. Both studies used a stimulation rate of 80 pulses per second (pps) to measure the ECAP and compared the physiologic thresholds with behavioral detection thresholds for a 500-msec burst of biphasic current pulses presented at a rate of 250 pps. This was the stimulus used to fit the SPEAK programming strategy. Brown et al. (2000) reported that mean ECAP thresholds were recorded at approximately 80% of the dynamic range for postlingually deafened adults. Hughes et al. (2000) reported finding mean ECAP thresholds for congenitally deaf children at approximately 60% of the dynamic range. The correlation between ECAP thresholds and the higher rate behavioral levels used to program the speech processor, although statistically significant, were only moderately strong and substantially lower than similar correlations obtained when the same low rate stimulus was used for both electrophysiologic and behavioral testing (Brown, et al. 2000). Examination of results from individual subjects revealed that, in some cases, the ECAP threshold versus stimulating electrode function was not parallel either to behaviorally determined threshold (T-level) versus electrode contours, or to the functions describing the relationship between maximum acceptable (C-level) or most comfortable (M-level) loudness and stimulating electrode position. These findings were corroborated later by a number of other investigators (Chen et al., 2002; Cullington, 2000; Di Nardo, Ippolito, Quaranta, Cadoni, & Galli, 2003; Gordon et al., 2002; McKay, Fewster, & Dawson, 2005; Thai-Van et al., 2001).

Since these first studies were published, the speech processing programs have changed significantly and now the gap between the stimulation rate used to record the ECAP (or EABR) and the stimulation rate used for programming the speech processors is even larger. Most of the early studies focused on the Nucleus CI users. Now it is possible to record the ECAP with other implant systems. Additionally, there is new software available that allows for automated recording of ECAP thresholds. Figures 7–4 through 7–6 illustrate the relationship we have found between ECAP thresholds recorded using a low stimulation rate and the levels needed to program the speech processors of individuals who use both the Nucleus and Advanced Bionics devices. Examination of Figures 7–4 through 7–6 shows that although speech processing technology has changed, the general relationship between the ECAP thresholds and

the levels needed to program the MAP of the speech processor has not.

Figure 7–4 shows ECAP thresholds plotted as a function of stimulating electrode for six different CI users. The three plots on the left in Figure 7–4 were recorded from Nucleus CI users. The three plots on the right were recorded from individuals who used the Advanced Bionics device. In all cases, the solid line shows variations in ECAP threshold as a function of stimulating electrode. For the Nucleus CI users (panels A through C), ECAP thresholds are contrasted with behavioral measures of threshold (T-level) and maximum comfort level (C-level). These behavioral measures of electrical dynamic range were obtained using stimulation rates ranging from 900 to 1200 pps. For the three Advanced Bionics CI users (panels D through F), ECAP thresholds are plotted relative to their estimates of most comfortable level (M-level) obtained using the HiRes-S and HiRes-P programming strategies. The stimulation rate used with the HiRes-P strategy is twice that used with HiRes-S and, as a result, M-levels are lower for the speech coding strategy with the faster rate. T-levels are not used to program the speech processor of the Advanced Bionics device and so are not shown. These results illustrate some common themes. All six subjects show variation in terms of how ECAP thresholds compare with the levels used for programming the speech processor. In some cases, ECAP thresholds exceed C-levels (Figure 7–4, panel B) or M-levels (Figure 7–4, panels E and F). For some CI users, the contour of the ECAP versus electrode function varies more across electrodes than do the behavioral measures of T-level, M-level or C-level (e.g., Figure 7–4, panel C or E). For all six subjects, ECAP thresholds indicate a stimulation level where the programming stimulus should be audible for the listener.

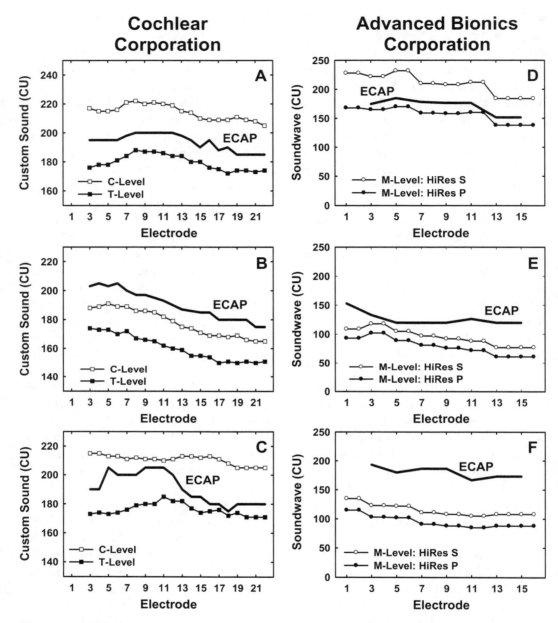

Figure 7–4. ECAP thresholds and stimulation levels used to program the speech processor are plotted as a function of the stimulating electrode for three Nucleus CI users (panels A–C) and three Advanced Bionics CI users (panels D–F).

Figure 7–5 shows group trends for both Nucleus and Advanced Bionics CI users. The upper panel shows data recorded from a group of 15 adults who used the Nucleus CI24RE system. They all used speech processors programmed using ACE and

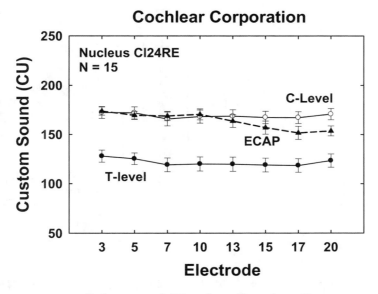

Cochlear Corporation

Advanced Bionics Corporation

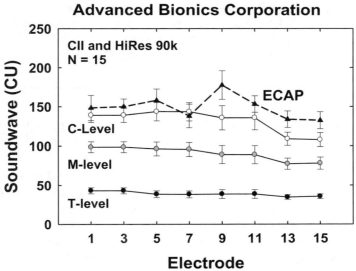

Figure 7–5. Comparisons between mean ECAP thresholds and MAP levels are shown for 15 Nucleus CI24RE cochlear implant users and 15 Advanced Bionics cochlear implant users. ECAP thresholds are shown with the dashed line and triangles. Programming levels are labeled and are shown with solid lines and circles. The error bar indicates one SE around the mean. The Nucleus CI users were all programmed in ACE and used stimulation rates between 900 and 1800 pps. The Advanced Bionics CI users all used the HiRes programming strategy.

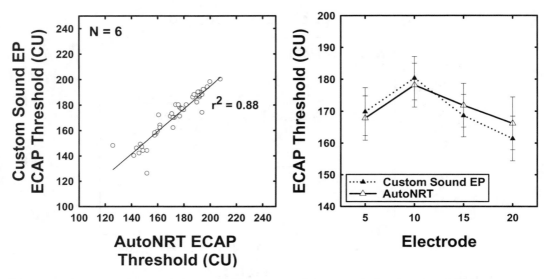

Figure 7–6. The left panel shows ECAP thresholds recorded using AutoNRT compared with similar measures obtained from the same subjects using the traditional recording software (Custom Sound EP). Data recorded from four different electrodes for each subject are shown. The right panel compares mean ECAP thresholds (±1 SD) recorded using AutoNRT and similar measures obtained using Custom Sound EP from the four electrodes assessed.

stimulation rates of 900 to 1800 pps. The lower panel of Figure 7–5 shows similar measures obtained from a set of 15 adult Advanced Bionics CI users. These subjects all used the HiRes-P or HiRes-M speech processing strategy. Although T- and C-levels are not used to program the speech processor of the Advanced Bionics CI, they were recorded to facilitate comparison to the results obtained from Nucleus CI users as shown in the upper panel of Figure 7–5. Regardless of implant type, mean ECAP thresholds are obtained at levels where the programming stimulus is near the upper boundary of the subject's dynamic range and more closely approximate C-level than M-level. The finding that on average ECAP thresholds approximate C-levels in this data set is different from similar measures reported earlier comparing ECAP thresholds with behavioral T- and C-levels for stimuli

presented at 250 pps (Brown et al., 2000). In that study, ECAP thresholds were recorded on average at 80% of the dynamic range for adult CI users. The difference between the data shown here and those reported previously likely is due to the fact that the behavioral T and C levels shown in Figure 7–5 were obtained using a stimulation rate that was significantly faster (900–1800 pps versus 250 pps) than the rate used in the Brown et al. (2000) study.

Recently Cochlear Corporation introduced a new automated method of recording ECAP thresholds. They refer to this as AutoNRT. This software automatically sweeps across the electrode array and estimates ECAP thresholds. Figure 7–6 shows data recorded from a set of six Nucleus CI24RE CI users. They were tested both using the traditional recording procedures that typically use a stimulation rate of 80 pps and with the AutoNRT software. For this admittedly small subject pool, the correlation between the two procedures is very strong (r^2 = 0.88), suggesting that the threshold estimates obtained using this streamlined, automated recording system are likely accurate.

A question that has received a fair amount of attention in the scientific literature is how can one account for the variation across subjects and improve the accuracy of ECAP-based MAP estimates? One reason ECAP thresholds do not more accurately predict the levels used to program the speech processor of the CI may be due to the fact that the physiologic threshold measures are peripherally generated and exhibit effects of adaptation (reduced amplitudes and elevated thresholds) with increasing stimulation rate, whereas behaviorally determined MAP levels are influenced by neural processing that occurs at higher levels within the auditory system and likely reflect the ability of the brain to integrate neural information over time. McKay et al. (2005) have shown that behavioral thresholds and maximum loudness levels tend to decrease as stimulation rate is increased even while ECAP amplitudes decrease and thresholds increase.

As early as 2000, methods were proposed by which the correlation between ECAP thresholds and speech processor programming levels could be improved (Brown et al., 2000; Hughes et al., 2000). This was accomplished by combining the ECAP threshold versus electrode information that could be obtained without behavioral participation in the recording process with a single measure of T- and/or C-level. The technique at least partially corrected for cross-user variance in temporal integration and should, in theory, work regardless of the stimulation rate used for programming the processor. The assumption that was inherent in this approach, however, was that

temporal integration is constant across the electrodes in the cochlea—an assumption which may not always be valid. Alternative methods for combining electrophysiologic estimates of detection for an electrical stimulus with behavioral measures of dyanamic range have been proposed and tested by other research groups (e.g., Franck & Norton, 2001; Smoorenburg, Willeboer, & van Dijk, 2002; Zimmerling & Hochmair, 2002). None of these methods has been completely satisfactory and all show evidence of worse performance as the difference between the stimulation rate used to record the physiologic measures and the rates used to program the speech processor of the CI increases.

So where does that leave us? It is not uncommon today for children under 1 year of age to receive a CI. Nor is it uncommon for children with multiple developmental delays to be considered for implantation. For these patients, there may be little choice but to rely on the ECAP (or other evoked potential) thresholds to drive the fitting process. If that is the case, the approach should be conservative—particularly if the speech processor to be programmed uses a rapid stimulation rate. With the exception of instances where a child may have cortical pathology, ECAP thresholds still can be interpreted as indicating a level where the programming stimulus will be audible. However, because this level may well be equal to or even exceed C-level, the stimulus used for programming the speech processor should be increased slowly and the child closely observed for any signs of discomfort. The current level where ECAP threshold is obtained, if tolerated by the child, may provide a good place to start the behavioral conditioning process.

An alternative approach is to use the ECAP versus electrode contour to set MAP thresholds, go into a live voice mode, and then shift this threshold versus electrode profile up until the child appears to detect sound in his or her environment. Then continue stimulating using this profile until the child begins to give some indication that the stimulation is beginning to become uncomfortable.

With time, as the speech processor programs are refined, the comparison between ECAP thresholds and behavioral measures of T- and/or C-level can reveal errors in the behavioral estimates of the MAP. For example, in our experience, the observation that the behavioral estimate of T-level for a given electrode is lower than ECAP threshold typically indicates that the behavioral response is set too high. Clearly, neural telemetry testing does not replace the behavioral fitting procedures, but can result in more rapid approximation of a final program or MAP. For developmentally delayed patients who never may be able to provide accurate behavioral responses, we typically create a set of programs with MAP levels that become progressively louder, but are based primarily on the ECAP threshold versus electrode contour. In some cases, we may opt to program the speech processor using a slower stimulation rate than is typical today (e.g., SPEAK) in order to further reduce the chance that we will be creating a MAP that is too loud. The loudest MAP will be created with C-levels set slightly above ECAP thresholds and T-levels set 20 to 30 clinical units lower.

Finally, it is important to note that much of the research to date has used behaviorally determined programming levels as a "gold standard" to which electrophysiologically based paradigms are compared. Several studies have compared performance with "electrophysiologically based MAPs" compared to clinically determined MAPs (Seyle & Brown, 2002; Smoorenburg et al., 2002). In both cases performance was similar, suggesting that programming the speech processor using ECAP threshold versus electrode data may not be unreasonable, and although not always optimal, may be sufficient to allow for some degree of speech understanding at a time when there may be few alternatives.

Future Directions

It is difficult to speculate about what the future holds in an area that changes as rapidly as the CI field does. It seems clear that whatever those changes are, there will always be a need for nonbehavioral methods of assessing hearing. Future CI designs will likely include innovations in the neural telemetry systems. These changes undoubtedly will make it possible to record the ECAP with even greater ease and accuracy. For instance, improvements in the recording system included in the Nucleus CI24RE system resulted in a significantly lower noise floor and consequently allowed for more reliable measures of small amplitude responses. This development, in turn, leads to improved automated approaches to recording ECAP thresholds. Future research may identify new or different ways in which these electrophysiologic measures can be used to predict the current levels needed to program the speech processor of the CI. Additionally, there is a great deal of research in both human and animal models that is currently underway and could expand our understanding of how the auditory nerve codes the kind of electrical impulses provided by the CI. Such information in turn could lead to the development of novel speech coding strategies or new ways to tailor a MAP for an individual user so as to optimize performance.

There is also interest in finding ways to use a future version of neural response telemetry systems, perhaps coupled with a novel and permanently implanted recording electrode array, to measure a wider range of electrically evoked responses. One example of such a response would be the cortically generated P1-N1-P2 response. These longer latency evoked potentials can be elicited using a passive listening paradigm and using a considerably wider range of stimuli than are typically used to record peripheral neural responses, such as the ECAP or the EABR. Such stimuli might include short speech tokens and/or long duration pulse trains. Electrically evoked cortical potentials:

1. have been shown to correlate with perceptual measures of loudness (Hoppe, Rosanowski, Iro, & Eysholdt, 2001);
2. may be more strongly correlated with performance than are peripherally generated, electrically evoked potentials (Beynon, Snik, & van den Broek, 2002);
3. can be used to assess an individual CI user's ability to detect change in an ongoing stimulus (Brown et al., 2008; Martin, 2007; Tremblay, Friesen, & Martin, 2003); and
4. appear to be influenced by factors known to affect performance with a CI, such as age at implant (Sharma, Dorman, & Spahr, 2002).

These findings are important because they suggest that these longer latency evoked potentials reflect the impact of higher level processing and, as such, may provide better estimates of factors, such as MAP and/or performance levels than are possible to obtain using peripherally generated, auditory evoked potentials. Although these measures can be recorded from CI users today, doing so requires additional recording equipment, often a fairly extensive recording electrode array, and a quiet but awake listener. If future research leads to the development of more pediatric friendly procedures for recording these evoked responses, it seems possible that such measures could revolutionize the way electrophysiologic potentials are used in clinical practice with CI users.

Acknowledgments. We acknowledge Grant DC00242 from the National Institutes of Health/NIDCD; and Grant RR59 from the General Clinical Research Centers Program, Division of Research Resources, NIH.

References

Abbas, P. J., & Brown, C. J. (1988). Electrically evoked brainstem potentials in cochlear implant patients with multi-electrode stimulation. *Hearing Research, 36,* 153-162.

Abbas, P. J., & Brown, C. J. (1991). Electrically evoked auditory brainstem response: Growth of response with current level. *Hearing Research, 51,* 123-138.

Abbas, P. J., Brown, C. J., Shallop, J. K., Firszt, J. B., Hughes, M. L., Hong, S. H., et al. (1999). Summary of results using the Nucleus CI24M implant to record electrically evoked compound action potential. *Ear and Hearing, 20,* 45-49.

Beynon, A. J., Snik, A. F., & van den Broek, P. (2002). Evaluation of cochlear implant benefit with auditory cortical evoked potentials. *International Journal of Audiology, 41,* 429-435.

Black, R. C., Clark, G. M., O'Leary, S. J., & Walters, C. (1983). Intracochlear electrical stimulation of normal and deaf cats investigated using brainstem response audiometry. *Acta Oto-Laryngologica Supplement, 399,* 5-17.

Brown, C. J., Abbas, P. J., Fryauf-Bertschy, H., Kelsey, D., & Gantz, B. J. (1994). Intraoperative and postoperative electrically evoked auditory brainstem responses in Nucleus cochlear implant users: Implications for the fitting process. *Ear and Hearing, 15,* 168-176.

Brown, C. J., Abbas, P. J., & Gantz, B. J. (1990). Electrically evoked whole-nerve action potentials: Data from human cochlear implant users. *Journal of the Acoustical Society of America, 88*, 1385-1391.

Brown, C. J., Etler, C., He, S., O'Brien, S., Erenberg, S., Kim, J. R., et al. (2008). The electrically evoked auditory change complex: Preliminary results from Nucleus cochlear implant users. *Ear and Hearing, 29*, 704-717.

Brown, C. J., Hughes, M. L., Lopez, S. M., & Abbas, P. J. (1999). The relationship between EABR thresholds and levels used to program the Clarion Speech Processor. *Annals of Otology, Rhinology, and Laryngology, 108* (Suppl. 177), 50-57.

Brown, C. J., Hughes, M. L., Luk, B., Abbas, P. J., Wolaver, A., & Gervais, J. (2000). The Relationship between EAP and EABR thresholds and levels used to program the Nucleus CI24M speech processor: Data from adults. *Ear and Hearing, 21*, 151-163.

Chen, X., Han, D., Zhao, X., Wang, S., Kong, Y., Liu, S., et al. (2002). Comparison of neural response telemetry thresholds with behavioral T/C levels. *Zhonghua Er Bi Yan Hou Ke Za Zhi—Chinese Journal of Otorhinolaryngology, 37*, 435-439.

Cullington, H. E. (2000). Preliminary neural response telemetry results. *British Journal of Audiology, 34*, 131-140.

Di Nardo, W., Ippolito, S., Quaranta, N., Cadoni, G., & Galli, J. (2003). Correlation between NRT measurement and behavioral levels in patients with the Nucleus 24 cochlear implant. *Acta Otorhinolaryngologica Italica, 23*, 352-355.

Dobie, R. A., & Kimm, J. (1980). Brainstem responses to electrical stimulation of cochlea. *Archives of Otolaryngology, 106*, 573-577.

Firszt, J. B., Chambers, R. D., & Kraus, N. (2002). Neurophysiology of cochlear implant users II: Comparison among speech perception, dynamic range, and physiological measures. *Ear and Hearing, 23*, 516-531.

Franck, K. H., & Norton, S. J. (2001). Estimation of psychophysical levels using the electrically evoked compound action potential measured with the neural response telemetry capabilities of Cochlear Corporation's CI24M device. *Ear and Hearing, 22*, 289-299.

Franck, K. H., & Shah, U. K. (2004). Averaged electrode voltage testing to diagnose an unusual cochlear implant internal device failure. *Journal of the American Academy of Audiology, 15*, 643-648.

Game, C., Gibson, W., & Pauka, C. (1987). Electrically evoked brainstem auditory potentials. *Annals of Otology, Rhinology, and Laryngology, 96*(Suppl. 128), 94-95.

Gordon, K. A., Ebinger, K. A., Gilden, J. E., & Shapiro, W. H. (2002). Neural response telemetry in 12- to 24-month old children. *Annals of Otology, Rhinology, and Laryngology, 111*(Suppl. 189), 42-48.

Heller, J. W., Sinopoli, T., Fowler-Brehm, N., & Shallop, J. K. (1991). Characterization of averaged electrode voltages from the Nucleus cochlear implant. *Proceedings of the Annual International Conference of the IEEE Engineering in Medicine and Biology Society, 13*, 1907-1908.

Hoppe, U., Rosanowski, F., Iro, H., & Eysholdt, U. (2001). Loudness perception and late auditory evoked potentials in adult cochlear implant users. *Scandinavian Audiology, 30*, 119-125.

Hughes, M. L., Brown, C. J., & Abbas, P. J. (2004). Sensitivity and specificity of averaged electrode voltage (AEV) measures in cochlear implant recipients. *Ear and Hearing, 25*, 431-446.

Hughes, M. L., Brown, C. J., Abbas, P. J., Wolaver, A. A., & Gervais, J. P. (2000). Comparison of EAP and EABR thresholds with map levels in the Nucleus CI24M speech processor: Data from children. *Ear and Hearing, 21*, 164-174.

Hughes, M. L., Vander Werff, K. R., Brown, C. J., Abbas, P. J., Kelsay, D. M. R., Teagle, H. F. B., & Lowder, M. W. (2001). A longitudinal study of electrode impedance, the electrically evoked compound action potential, and behavioral measures in Nucleus 24 cochlear implant users. *Ear and Hearing, 22*, 471-486.

Jewett, D. L., Romano, M. N., & Williston, J. S. (1970). Human auditory evoked potentials: Possible brain stem components detected on the scalp. *Science, 167*, 1517-1518.

Kileny, P. R., Meiteles, L. Z., Zwolan, T. A., & Tellian, S. A. (1995). Cochlear implant device failure: Diagnosis and management. *American Journal of Otology, 16*, 164-171.

Kileny, P. R., Zimmerman-Phillips, S., Kemink, J. L., & Schmaltz, S. P. (1991). Effects of preoperative electrical stimulability and historical factors on performance with multichannel cochlear implants. *Annals of Otology, Rhinology, and Laryngology, 100,* 563-568.

Kubo, T., Yamamoto, K., Iwaki, T., Matsukawa, M., Doi, K., & Tamura, M. (2001). Significance of auditory evoked responses (EABR and P300) in cochlear implant subjects. *Acta Otolaryngologica, 121,* 257-261.

Lai, W. K., Aksit, M., Akdas, F., & Dillier, N. (2004). Longitudinal behaviour of neural response telemetry (NRT) data and clinical implications. *International Journal of Audiology, 43,* 252-263.

Mahoney, M. J., & Rotz Proctor, L. A. (1994). The use of averaged electrode voltages to assess the function of Nucleus internal cochlear implant devices in children. *Ear and Hearing, 15,* 177-183.

Makhdoum, M. J., Groenen, P. A., Snik, A. F., & van den Broek P. (1998). Intra- and inter-individual correlations between auditory evoked potentials and speech perception in cochlear implant users. *Scandinavian Audiology, 27,* 13-20.

Martin, B. A. (2007). Can the acoustic change complex be recorded in an individual with a cochlear implant? Separating neural responses from cochlear implant artifact. *Journal of the American Academy of Audiology, 18,* 126-140.

Mason, S. M., Cope, Y., Garnham, J., O'Donoghue, G. M., & Gibbin, K. P. (2001). Intra-operative recordings of electrically evoked auditory nerve action potentials in young children by use of neural response telemetry with the Nucleus CI24M cochlear implant. *British Journal of Audiology, 35,* 225-235.

Mason, S. M., O'Donoghue, G. M., Gibbin, K. P., Garnham, C. W., & Jowett, C.A. (1997). Perioperative electrical auditory brain stem response in candidates for pediatric cochlear implantation. *American Journal of Otology, 18,* 466-471.

Mason, S. M., Sheppard, S., Garnham, C. W., Lutman, M. E., O'Donoghue, G. M., & Gibbin, K. P. (1993a). Application of intraoperative recordings of electrically evoked ABRs in a paediatric cochlear implant programme. Nottingham Paediatric Cochlear Implant Group. *Advances in Oto-Rhino-Laryngology, 48,* 136-141.

Mason, S. M., Sheppard, S., Garnham, C. W., Lutman, M. E., O'Donoghue, G. M., & Gibbin, K. P. (1993b). Improving the relationship of intraoperative EABR thresholds to T-level in young children receiving the Nucleus cochlear implant. In I. J. Hochmair-Desoyer & E. S. Hochmair (Eds.), *Advances in cochlear implants* (pp. 44-49). Vienna: Manz.

McKay, C. M., Fewster, L., & Dawson, P. (2005). A different approach to using neural response telemetry for automated cochlear impant processor programming. *Ear and Hearing, 26*(Suppl.), 38S-44S.

Mens, L. H., Brokx, J. P., & van den Broek, P. (1995). Averaged electrode voltages: Management of electrode failures in children, fluctuating threshold and comfort levels, and otosclerosis. *Annals of Otology, Rhinology, and Laryngology, 104*(Suppl. 166), 169-172.

Mens, L. H. M., Oostendorp, T., & van den Broek, P. (1994). Identifying electrode failures with cochlear implant generated surface potentials. *Ear and Hearing, 15,* 330-338.

Miller, C. A., Abbas, P. J., & Brown, C. J. (2000) An improved method of reducing stimulus artifact in the electrically evoked whole nerve potential. *Ear and Hearing, 21,* 280-290.

Miyamoto, R. T., & Brown, D. D. (1987). Electrically evoked brainstem responses in cochlear implant recipients. *Otolaryngology-Head and Neck Surgery, 96,* 34-38.

Nikolopoulos, T. P., Mason, S. M., Gibbin, K. P., & O'Donoghue, G. M. (2000). The prognostic value of promontory electric auditory brain stem response in pediatric cochlear implantation. *Ear and Hearing, 21,* 236-241.

Nikolopoulos, T. P., Mason, S. M., O'Donoghue, G. M., & Gibbin, K. P. (1999). Integrity of the auditory pathway in young children with congenital and postmeningitic deafness. *Annals of Otology, Rhinology, and Laryngology, 108,* 327-330.

Seyle, K., & Brown, C. J. (2002). Speech perception using maps based on neural response telemetry measures. *Ear and Hearing, 23*(Suppl.), 72S-79S.

Shallop, J. K., Beiter, A. L., Goin, D. W., & Mischke, R. E. (1990). Electrically evoked auditory brainstem responses (EABR) and middle latency responses (EMLR) obtained from patients with the Nucleus multichannel cochlear implant. *Ear and Hearing, 11,* 5–15.

Shallop, J. K., VanDyke, L., Goin, D. W., & Mischke, R. E. (1991). Prediction of behavioral threshold and comfort values for Nucleus 22-channel implant patients from electrical auditory brain stem response test results. *Annals of Otology, Rhinology, and Laryngology, 100,* 896–898.

Sharma, A., Dorman, M. F., & Spahr, A. J. (2002). A sensitive period for the development of the central auditory system in children with cochlear implants: Implications of age of implantation. *Ear and Hearing, 23,* 532–539.

Smith, L., & Simmons, F. B. (1983). Estimating eighth nerve survival by electrical stimulation. *Annals of Otology, Rhinology, and Laryngology, 92,* 12–23.

Smoorenburg, G. F., Willeboer, C., & van Dijk, J. E. (2002). Speech perception in Nucleus CI24M cochlear implant users with processor settings based on electrically evoked compound action potential thresholds. *Audiology and Neuro-Otology, 7,* 335–347.

Sohmer, H., & Feinmesser, M. (1967). Cochlear action potential recorded from the external ear in man. *Annals of Otololgy, Rhinology, and Laryngology, 76,* 427–436.

Thai-Van, H., Chanal, J. M., Coudert, C., Veuillet, E., Truy, E., & Collet, L. (2001). Relationship between NRT measurements and behavioral levels in children with the Nucleus 24 cochlear implant may change over time: Preliminary report. *International Journal of Pediatric Otorhinolaryngology, 58,* 153–162.

Tremblay, K. L., Friesen, L., Martin, B. A., & Wright, R. (2003). Test-retest reliability of cortical evoked potentials using naturally produced speech sounds. *Ear and Hearing, 24,* 225–232.

van den Honert, C., & Stypulkowski, P. H. (1986). Characterization of the electrically evoked auditory brainstem response in cats and humans. *Hearing Research, 21,* 109–126.

Wilson, B. S., Finley, C. C., Lawson, D. T., & Zerbi, M. (1997). Temporal representations with cochlear implants. *American Journal of Otology, 18*(Suppl.), S30–S34.

Yoshie, N., Ohashi, T., & Suzuki, T. (1967). Nonsurgical recording of auditory nerve action potentials in man. *Laryngoscope, 77,* 76–85.

Zimmerling, M. J., & Hochmaier, E. S. (2002). EAP recordings in Ineraid patients: Correlations with psychophysical measures and possible implications for patient fitting. *Ear and Hearing, 23,* 81–91.

CHAPTER 8

Vestibular Assessment

SHARON L. CUSHING
BLAKE C. PAPSIN

Introduction

In many centers, vestibular end-organ function testing has long been a part of the evaluation of adults preparing for cochlear implantation in order to predict the potential for vestibular complications and in some instances has guided surgical decisions (i.e., side of implantation). In contrast, preoperative vestibular evaluation has not been consistently utilized in the pediatric population. This is likely because vestibular function testing can be challenging in infants and children and this group often does not exhibit obvious signs of vestibular dysfunction post-operatively. In the last five years, however, evaluation of vestibular end-organ function in the setting of profound sensorineural hearing loss (SNHL) has garnered increased attention because of its relevance to the safety of bilateral cochlear implantation and the potential risk of bilateral vestibular injury that this intervention carries. This concern has led to the evaluation of vestibular function in even very young children and has led us to a better under-

standing of the vestibular correlates of severe to profound SNHL in this population. With this in mind, the current chapter discusses the relevance and feasibility of vestibular testing in the pediatric population as well as provide details regarding the tools currently available. There is much that remains to be learned about the developing vestibular system and vestibular assessment in children. In this continually evolving field, this chapter should be viewed as a summary of the current state of knowledge as opposed to well-defined recommendations for testing in cochlear implant candidates.

In the context of the pediatric patient undergoing evaluation for cochlear implantation we discuss the following:

1. Relationship between the auditory and vestibular systems
2. Evaluation of vestibular end-organ function
3. Evaluation of static and dynamic balance function
4. Effects of etiology of sensorineural hearing loss on vestibular and balance function

5. Importance of evaluating vestibular and balance function
6. Proposed mechanisms for compensation following vestibular injury
7. Potential pediatric test battery.

The Auditory and Vestibular Systems Are Closely Related

The cochlea shares an anatomic proximity as well as histologic and physiologic similarity to the neighboring vestibular end organs. In both systems, the sensory epithelium is composed of hair cells which are mechanoreceptors whose stereocilia are embedded in an overlying layer of inertial mass. Movement of the inertial mass in both the vestibular and auditory systems translates into small deflections of the stereocilia and leads to changes in the activity of the primary afferents. Distinguishing features between the systems are limited to the nature of the overlying layer (i.e., basilar membrane versus otoconia, etc.), the organization of the hair cells within the sensory epithelium (organ of Corti versus macula versus cupula, etc.) and the mechanical stimulus that leads to excitation.

Because the cochlea and vestibular end organs are so closely related, it is reasonable to theorize that, in some instances, lesions or insults that lead to auditory dysfunction also may lead to dysfunction of the vestibular end organs. In turn, dysfunction of the vestibular end organs may cause disruption in the ability to maintain static and dynamic balance. Reports of vestibular dysfunction in children with hearing impairment indicate that somewhere between 20 and 70% of children with hearing loss demonstrate some form of vestibular end-organ dysfunction (Arnvig, 1955). The prevalence of vestibular dysfunction also appears to correlate with the severity of the cochlear loss although this is true more consistently on a group rather than an individual level (Goldstein, Landau, & Kleffner, 1958; Sandberg & Terkildsen, 1965). The variability in vestibular responsiveness across different etiologies of SNHL is readily apparent in the limited available literature (Huygen, van Rijn, Cremers, & Theunissen, 1993; Rapin, 1974). More recently our ability to identify the etiology of deafness has improved with the advent of more sophisticated imaging and molecular genetic techniques. This likely represents the first step in improving our ability to identify the vestibular phenotype of various congenital, hereditary, and acquired causes of SNHL.

Evaluation of Vestibular End-Organ Function

Ideally in our quest to characterize the vestibular system, we would employ a single test that would probe the overall function of the peripheral vestibular system, isolate individual end-organ function, test the integrity of the peripheral pathways, and predict functional balance outcomes. In reality, the available tests assess only single vestibular end-organ function. The majority of clinical tests of the peripheral vestibular system reflect the function of the horizontal semicircular canal solely. More recently, the measurement of saccular function also has been undertaken. As a result, we do not have a comprehensive way to assess vestibular function or dysfunction. The following sections provide a description of available measures of vestibular end-organ function and a summary of their use in the pediatric implant population, followed by a general discussion of compliance and reliability related issues.

Horizontal Canal Function

The horizontal canal is the best understood of the vestibular end organs, likely because it is the end organ that can be most effectively tested. Responsive to head rotation about its axis, input from the horizontal canal sets up the vestibuloocular reflex (VOR) which serves to maintain a stable retinal image during head/body motion. This is a primitive and vital function of mammalian survival. The integrity of the horizontal canal function is typically determined using either a caloric or a rotational stimulus and a discussion of the advantages and disadvantages of each follows below.

Caloric Testing

The horizontal canal is most commonly assessed by caloric stimulation using either air or water irrigation (hot, cold ± ice water). Indeed, caloric stimulation has long been considered 'the gold standard' of vestibular function measurement. An advantage of caloric stimulation is that each ear can be tested individually and the responses can be compared. There are, however, some important requirements for obtaining reliable caloric results particularly in children. In addition to age, a multitude of factors predispose children to incorrect (usually false negative) results on this and other tests of vestibular function; malposition of irrigation tubing, presence of cerumen, crying, agitation, and inadequate mental tasking (Rapin, 1974). In addition, inattention and frequent random eye movement are more common in children and create difficulties in analyzing electronystagmography(ENG) traces obtained during caloric or rotational stimuli to the point of requiring an individual trace by trace analysis (Snashall, 1983). Vestibular testing in hearing impaired children is further complicated by the ability of

this group to suppress nystagmic responses. In these children with hearing loss, normal nystagmic responses that are present during mental alerting are rapidly eliminated when this mental alerting (tasking) is stopped. Therefore, inadequate tasking carries with it the risk of inappropriately labeling a child with reduced or absent vestibular responses (Brookhouser, Cyr, & Beauchaine, 1982). In normal-hearing children, verbal alerting typically is used whereas in children with SNHL, tactile alerting may be necessary. Despite these challenges, clinicians have succeeded in performing vestibular function tests in even the most challenging pediatric patients and the importance of repeated testing should be underscored. Clearly, the testing becomes more straightforward as the children age. In the adult implant literature, reported rates of horizontal canal dysfunction as measured by caloric stimulation vary widely from 25 to 100% with this range narrowing slightly from 23% to 76% when only studies with larger numbers (n >15) are included (Buchman, Joy, Hodges, Telischi, & Balkany, 2004; Enticott, Tari, Koh, Dowell, & O'Leary, 2006; Fina et al., 2003; Huygen et al., 1995; Kiyomizu, Tono, Komune, Ushisako, & Morimitsu, 2000; Vibert, Hausler, Kompis, & Vischer, 2001). In our cohort of children with unilateral cochlear implants, the incidence of horizontal canal dysfunction in response to a caloric stimulus was 50% (16/32), with a large proportion of these (6/16, 38%) reflecting mild (n = 5) to moderate (n = 1) unilateral abnormalities. Nine children (28%) demonstrated complete horizontal canal dysfunction (areflexia) bilaterally and one child had complete unilateral canal dysfunction (areflexia) (Cushing, Papsin, Rutka, James, & Gordon, 2008b). In comparison, in a second series of children (n = 22), a larger percentage (68%) demonstrated absent or low intensity responses to caloric irrigation preoperatively (Buchman et al., 2004). In summary, the reported rate of horizontal canal dysfunction in the pediatric population also is variable with anywhere from one-third to two-thirds of implant candidates demonstrating dysfunction (Buchman et al., 2004; Cushing et al., 2008b).

Rotational Testing

The integrity of horizontal canal function also can be assessed by measuring the VOR in response to rotation. A rotational stimulus can be administered through several means but the most standardized is the rotational chair. The chair provides sinusoidal harmonic rotation which allows the horizontal VOR to be measured. One limitation of rotational testing, however, is that it may miss a unilateral decrease or loss of horizontal canal function given that the VOR is subject to physiologic compensation. For example, a patient with a unilateral loss of horizontal canal function may yield any of the following results: (1) decreased VOR gain (the measure of VOR strength) as the head is rotated toward the lesioned side, (2) bilateral decreased VOR gain, or (3) bilaterally normal VOR gain, depending on the degree of dysfunction and subsequent compensation that has occurred.

Just as the auditory system operates over a wide range of sound frequencies, the vestibular system also operates over a range of motion frequencies. For example the semicircular canals are sensitive to a frequency range of angular accelerations between 0.10 Hz to 10 Hz with low-frequency performance extended to 0.01 Hz through central mechanisms (Carey & Della Santina, 2005; Newlands & Wall, 2006). One of the current deficiencies of using a caloric stimulus to assess horizontal canal function is that it routinely measures only the very lowest frequencies within the functional range of the horizontal canal (0.002 to 0.004 Hz)

and, as such, does not reflect the "real world" operating range of the system (0.5 to 7 Hz) (Hamid, 2000; Hess, Baloh, Honrubia, & Yee, 1985; Shepard & Telian, 1996). This might be akin to using an audiogram which measured thresholds from 250 to 500 Hz only (a frequency range much narrower than the operating range of functional speech which is from 500 to 4000 Hz). The use of a high-frequency rotational stimulus improves on caloric stimulation in that it allows access to responses to higher frequencies of motion, including those that fall within this "real world" range. Measuring the responsiveness of the system to high-frequency motion is important given that abnormalities in symptomatic patients might only be revealed using high-frequency rotational testing (Prepageran, Kisilevsky, Tomlinson, Ranalli, & Rutka, 2005). In summary, using high-frequency rotational chair testing not only allows us access to a spectrum of higher frequency function, it also may allow us to distinguish those with losses that lead to functional balance problems versus those that do not. Also, we understand that isolated high-frequency losses occur and can be symptomatic, carrying with them functional consequences for balance (Prepageran et al., 2005). These abnormalities can be missed when we assess horizontal canal function using calorics or low-frequency rotational testing alone. In a subgroup of our pediatric cochlear implant population we demonstrated that 38% (14/37) demonstrated abnormalities in horizontal canal function in response to rotation; the majority (10/14, 71%) demonstrated a loss that spanned all frequencies (0.25 to 5 Hz) whereas 4 children displayed bilateral losses detectable only at high frequencies of rotation (>1 Hz in 2 children and >3 Hz in 2 children) (Cushing et al., 2008b). In comparison, studies which include mostly adult cochlear implant candidates and employ low-frequency rotational chair testing estimate the incidence of unilateral vestibular deficits to be approximately 14% and bilateral deficits to be 28% (Chiong, Nedzelski, McIlmoyl, & Shipp, 1994; Vibert et al., 2001). Those studies using velocity step tests report an incidence of approximately 3% of unilateral and 63% bilateral vestibular dysfunction in the same population (Huygen et al., 1995).

Saccular Function

Vestibular Evoked Myogenic Potential (VEMP) Testing

Although much of the adjunctive vestibular end-organ testing focuses on the horizontal canal, assessment of saccular function, the sacculocollic pathway and the integrity of the inferior vestibular nerve is possible using the vestibular evoked myogenic potential (VEMP). The saccule is the vestibular end-organ that is most closely associated with the cochlea. During early development the otic vesicle divides into several chambers including a utricular chamber, which gives rise to the utricle and the semicircular canals, and a saccular chamber which gives rise to the saccule and the cochlea (O'Rahilly, 1963). In some nonmammalian species, the saccule functions as a hearing organ (Furukawa & Ishii, 1967). The original function of the inner ear is presumed to be a vestibular proprioceptor and throughout evolution transformations have occurred allowing for the detection of sound. Based on this notion of specialization, the inner ear often is viewed to consist of two separate divisions; the superior division, consisting of the three semicircular canals and the utricle, and the inferior division which includes the saccule and the cochlea (Lowenstein, 1936). Given the anatomic compartmentalization of the saccule and the cochlea, one might predict that saccular function is more likely to be affected than utricular or semicircular canal function in the presence of an inner ear injury leading to SNHL. Saccular function can be examined by eliciting a VEMP response which is a transient, biphasic, short latency muscle relaxation potential generated by the synchronous discharges of motor units within the sternocleidomastoid (SCM) muscle in response to a loud sound, most often a click. This myogenic potential is felt to reflect a disynaptic vestibulocollic reflex originating in the saccule and transmitted via the ipsilateral medial vestibulospinal tract to SCM motoneurons (Kushiro, Zakir, Ogawa, Sato, & Uchino, 1999). It is presumed that the VEMP arises from the saccule given that this is the vestibular end-organ most sensitive to auditory stimulation (Didier & Cazals, 1989; Young, Fernandez, & Goldberg, 1977). Further evidence is that click sensitive neurons in the vestibular nerve respond to tilts of the head and generally are located in the saccular macula (Murofushi & Curthoys, 1997; Murofushi, Curthoys, Topple, Colebath, & Halmagyi, 1995).

Measurement of saccular responses using vestibular evoked myogenic potentials has been successful in young children 3 to 11 years of age. Normative data have been established and describes high compliance with testing (Kelsch, Schaefer, & Esquivel, 2006). The latencies of the VEMP amplitude peaks (the P1 and N1 waves) increase significantly with age (particularly for the negative peak (N1) and, thus, age needs to be considered when determining the appropriate time window to record and detect these responses (Figure 8–1) (Kelsch et al., 2006). In contrast to the high compliance described in the literature, we found that children had difficulty maintaining head elevation throughout the test and that most children could only tolerate the testing for

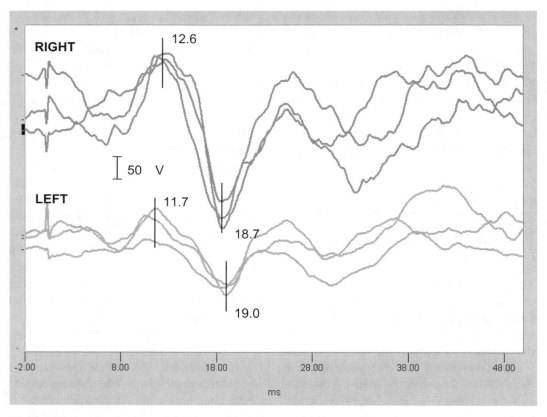

Figure 8–1. Vestibular evoked myogenic potential obtained using parameters outlined above. Note the mean latency of the P1 (12.15 msec) and N1 (18.85 msec).

short periods. As a result, proper assessment of the VEMP was questionable in a number of young patients. Specifically, the absence of a myogenic response in many children could have been related to an inability to produce sufficient and consistent tonic activation of the SCM to allow for reliable and replicable averaged evoked potential measures. This meant that VEMP data was excluded in many cases thus lowering our diagnostic yield for VEMP testing. The ability to obtain reliable VEMPs may be improved by incorporating a video feedback system that promotes and monitors ongoing tonic contraction of the SCM. VEMP data

obtained in children who were able to elevate their head during testing frequently indicated an overall disruption of saccular function as measured by the absence of a VEMP response. This was common in our pediatric cohort with 10 of 26 (38%) demonstrating an abnormality; VEMP was absent bilaterally in 5 of 26 (19%) and unilaterally in 5 of 26 (19%) (Cushing et al., 2008b). These findings are consistent with a smaller study by Jin, Nakamura, Shinjo, and Kaga (2006) who reported that 6/12 children with profound SNHL had abnormalities of saccular function and VEMP responses before surgery for a cochlear implant.

Clinical Neuro-Otologic Testing

Clinical examination is central to the evaluation of vestibular function in any child with SNHL. There are several clinical tests which make up the battery of neuro-otologic testing and these are listed in Table 8–1. Of these tests, the high-frequency head thrust test (Halmagyi) and a test of dynamic visual acuity (DVA) have the highest yield in identifying children with vestibular and balance dysfunction. For literate children, a Sloan letters chart is used, whereas a LEA symbols chart is used for younger children to test dynamic visual acuity. Dynamic visual acuity (DVA) is tested using passive head rotation at roughly 2 Hz at an amplitude of approximately 20°. We would expect oscillopsia on DVA in those children with bilateral vestibular losses due to their inability to use the VOR to stabilize the retinal image during rapid self-motion. Abnormalities of the high-frequency head-thrust test are predicted to occur in children with significant unilateral or bilateral losses resulting in an inability of their VOR to generate accurate production of equal, but opposite conjugate movements of the eyes relative to the head. We therefore were surprised in our recent study to find that some children with significant vestibular losses demonstrated subjectively normal clinical tests. When the caloric test result was used as the gold standard for horizontal canal function, we found the sensitivity of the head thrust maneuver was 29% (4/14) and its specificity was 100% (15/15). Similarly, the sensitivity and specificity of DVA testing was 73% (8/11) and 93% (14/15), respectively, based on a gold standard of rotational chair testing in light. This finding corroborates a previous study which demonstrated that the clinical Halmagyi was not a strong predictor of test results on the Halmagyi when using a scleral coil (Kessler et al., 2008).

TABLE 8–1. Standard Battery of Clinical Neuro-Otologic Tests and Function Tested

Neuro-Otologic Test	Function Tested
Vestibulo-ocular function	
VOR Suppression	Visual suppression of horizontal VOR
High Acceleration Head Thrust Test (Halmagyi)	Unilateral horizontal canal function
Dynamic Visual Acuity	Bilateral horizontal VOR dysfunction leading to retinal slip
Head-shaking nystagmus	Symmetry of the horizontal VOR
Vestibulo-spinal function	
Romberg ± vision	Postural stability with/without vision
Tandem Gait	Postural stability
Other	
Unterberger's step test	Labyrinthine asymmetry
Dix-Hallpike	Paroxysmal positional vertigo of posterior canal

It is clear that although clinical examination is a very important part of evaluating the child with SNHL, significant vestibular disturbance can be missed. Coupling the clinical exam with adjunctive tests or adding to it an objective component (i.e., head thrust with DC-ENG or sclera coil monitoring) therefore may dramatically increase the yield and accuracy of the diagnosis. The same is true for subjective tests of static balance function. For example, one might assume that the Romberg test is an accurate means of assessing static balance in children, but in our experience even children with the most profound losses perform a standard Romberg without difficulty. This observation has been reported in the literature where a comparison between responses to caloric stimulation and performance in a standard and modified Romberg demonstrated that the standard Romberg, even with eyes closed, was of little benefit in the identification of bilateral or unilateral caloric weaknesses (Brookhouser et al., 1982; Horak, Shumway-Cook, Crowe, & Black, 1988). A tandem Romberg using the Jendrassik maneuver (hands are hooked together by flexed fingers while attempting to pull them apart) which increased the difficulty of the test, was more consistent with caloric test abnormalities in a significant number of subjects (Brookhouser et al., 1982).

Compliance and Reliability of Vestibular End-Organ Testing in Children

In our experience, children 3 years of age and older are able to comply with vestibular testing in most cases. However, this high degree of compliance somewhat underestimates the challenges involved in testing this population and the time commitment for testing and retesting that is necessary to achieve reliable results. Yet, despite modifications in technique, caloric or rotational chair testing of young children often yields only qualitative results. Qualitatively normal results can be quite helpful whereas qualitatively abnormal results may only signal the need for repeat testing at an older age (Rapin, 1974). In cases where quantifiable results are obtained, the level of accuracy is hard to determine. The accuracy of vestibular testing in the pediatric setting depends equally on the test-retest reliability and also requires an understanding of the potential risk of confounding due to normal developmental changes in vestibular function that may occur early on. Minimizing this risk requires a thorough understanding of the time course to maturation of the vestibular end organs and their measurable responses. Several studies have examined both of these issues. In a study of caloric function in neonates, repeat caloric tests within 24 hours produced identical results (Donat, Donat, & Lay, 1980). Similarly, in children over the age of 5 years, the test-retest reliability was found to be excellent (Kenyon, 1988). These two studies, however, did not include children aged 12 to 36 months which undoubtedly represents the most challenging age group for testing. When this group was included, the disagreement between caloric ENG testing was as high as 24%, where an initial absent response was followed by a positive response in all cases (Rapin, 1974). Age and patient compliance were most certainly an issue in these false negative responses with two of the children in the above study being 18 months of age. Assessment of horizontal canal function by sinusoidal, harmonic acceleration, rotational chair testing may be less affected by age. This is an accurate and nonaversive tool to assess vestibular function in infants and children as young as 2 days of age as all subjects older than 9 months have been shown to generate consistent nystagmic responses over a range of frequencies (Staller, Goin, & Hildebrandt, 1986). This finding supports a short maturational time course of the VOR. The gain, phase, and symmetry in children (3 months to 6 years) are similar to the currently established adult normative values during harmonic sinusoidal rotation at 0.08 Hz. No significant differences were detected in the gain, phase, and symmetry of the responses of full-term versus premature infants (Cyr, Brookhouser, Valente, & Grossman, 1985).

Evaluation of Static and Dynamic Balance Function

Clinically, the importance of vestibular function testing is that it provides an indication of a child's ability to achieve and maintain adequate static and dynamic balance to participate in daily activities. However, the functional outcomes of vestibular end-organ dysfunction are much less commonly measured and reported in the literature. This is particularly true of children receiving cochlear implants. The maintenance of posture and the control of gait are complex functions that rely on the appropriate acquisition of motor control patterns with feedback modulation resulting from inputs to and from the vestibular, visual, and somatosensory systems. The labyrinths are known to play a role in postural responses (Mergner & Rosemeier, 1998) and, therefore, it is natural to think that their hypofunction would lead to delays in the acquisition of gross motor milestones. Although the failure to acquire language alerts us to hearing disorders, failure to achieve motor milestones should alert us to potential vestibular dysfunction. Identifying a periph-

eral vestibular loss based on measures of functional balance in a child, however, can be difficult. There is considerable variation in the interval during which children acquire these skills and parents often only notice significant differences when they compare motor function between their children. The motor clues that lead us to suspect vestibular dysfunction may be subtle and include delay of gross motor development such as sitting and walking, head tilt, "floppy" or weak neck, "wobbly" head, and crawling with head hanging. These children might be labeled as uncoordinated, awkward, or clumsy. Although even children with the most profound losses routinely achieve adequate gait, they may fail to develop the skills necessary for more complex motor functions such as skating or riding a bicycle.

In children with SNHL, the relationship between specific deficits of the peripheral vestibular system and deficiencies in motor coordination can be difficult to establish given the variability of etiology and degree of the hearing loss. As a group, children with profound SNHL do tend to perform more poorly on tests of gross motor or balance activities compared to their normal hearing peers (Cushing, Chia, James, Papsin, & Gordon, 2008a; Potter & Silverman, 1984; Rapin, 1974); however, on an individual level there is immense variability. For example, a group of children with SNHL (various etiologies) who had decreased or absent responses to caloric stimuli showed a wide range of ages at which developmental milestones were reached (Rapin, 1974). The age at which children first began to sit ranged from 6 to 24 months ($\mu = 10.6$ months) and first steps occurred at age ranges of 10 to 48 months ($\mu = 20$ months). Nearly half of the group began walking at 18 months or later (Rapin, 1974) which meant that many children, including some children with absent responses bilaterally (confirmed by repeated testing), walked at ages expected in normally developing children. Therefore, we cannot assume that the emergence of walking at a normal age negates the presence of a significant vestibular disturbance (Rapin, 1974).

The assessment of static and dynamic balance in children with or without hearing loss is not straightforward and requires that testing be sufficiently challenging to detect deficits although sufficiently easy so that the testing can be completed by young children. Gross motor skills such as bilateral coordination, strength, running speed, skipping, and hopping are often unaffected by peripheral vestibular dysfunction whether complete or partial, symmetric or asymmetric and thus are not useful in differentiating children with isolated vestibular losses from children with normal function (Fisher, Mixon, & Herman, 1986; Horak et al., 1988). Additional tests used commonly to assess static balance include rail walking and one-foot standing with eyes open and eyes closed (Lindsey & O'Neal, 1976; McCarron & Ludlow, 1981; Myklebust, 1964; Potter & Silverman, 1984; Scanlon & Goetzinger, 1969). However, no clear relationship has been established between reaction to caloric stimuli and the rail walking test (Davey, 1954).

When children with SNHL are challenged by sufficiently difficult balance tasks that appropriately emphasize the contribution of the peripheral vestibular system, deficiencies in balance function surface (Cushing et al., 2008a; Shumway-Cook & Woollacott, 1985). Computerized dynamic posturography (CDP) provides one means of producing these challenging environments to test the vestibular system. CDP is a technique that allows for the assessment of postural stability during controlled alterations of the sensory environment. Both the platform and the visual surround can be moved and a foam spacer can be placed between the subject's feet and the platform to alter proprioception. The ability to remove and alter sensory inputs such as vision and proprioception allows an evaluation of the relative contributions of different sensory information to the maintenance of balance in a given patient. Unfortunately, children with normal vestibular function who are under the age of 5 to 7 years, typically fall in conditions when vision and surface inputs are eliminated and/or inaccurate. Therefore, to date, posturography has limited sensitivity in younger children (Shumway-Cook & Woollacott, 1985).

In our center we have adapted an inexpensive but standardized means of testing static and dynamic balance in children as young as 4 years of age. The balance subset of the Bruininks Oseretsky Test of Motor Proficiency II (BOT 2) (Bruininks & Bruininks, 2005) has met the need of providing a spectrum of sufficiently difficult tasks that remain appropriate in younger children and it has become our routine measure of static and dynamic balance in children with SNHL (Cushing et al., 2008a). The BOT 2 is one of the most commonly used, age-standardized tests of developmental motor function in the realm of physical and occupational therapy. It contains a number of subtests designed to assess gross and fine motor skills in children over 4 years of age. A number of the subtests are relevant to the study of peripheral vestibular function, in particular the balance subset which contains nine balance related tasks, four of which are performed alternately with eyes open and eyes closed (Table 8–2). One clear advantage of this test is that it has been standardized and population norms by age are provided. The raw score, typically the timed duration during which the child maintains position up to a maximum of 10 seconds, is converted into a point score, and the point scores for

TABLE 8–2. Bruininks-Oseretsky Test of Motor Proficiency 2 (BOT 2) Balance Subtest Items and Grading Scheme

Balance Subtest Items		Maximum Score
Standing with feet apart on a line	Eyes Open	10 sec
	Eyes Closed	10 sec
Walking forward on a line		6 steps
Standing on one leg on a line	Eyes Open	10 sec
	Eyes Closed	10 sec
Walking forward heel to toe on a line		6 steps
Standing on one leg on a balance beam	Eyes Open	10 sec
	Eyes Closed	10 sec
Standing heel-to-toe on a balance beam		10 sec

each of the 9 items are summed to produce a total point score (range 0 to 37 points). The total point score and the subject's age at the time of testing are then used to obtain an age-matched scale score based on population norms provided by the test.

The published age-adjusted mean ($n = 1520$) for the BOT 2 Balance Subset is 15 ± 5 (SD) (scale range 1 to 35). We obtained statistically similar results for a separate control group ($n = 19$, $\mu = 17 \pm 5$ (SD) units). However when we tested children with SNHL who were using unilateral cochlear implants, performance was significantly poorer ($\mu = 12.9 \pm 5.2$(SD) than both the population norms and our own control group ($t_{(37.3)} = 2.98$, $p = 0.005$; $t_{(29)} = 2.72$, $p = 0.01$, respectively) (Cushing et al., 2008a). Importantly, these children had not been otherwise subjectively identified by their families as having motoric or balance difficulties. It appears that motor skills develop in children with peripheral vestibular dysfunction; although at times development proceeds on a protracted timeline. Even children who show no evidence of peripheral vestibular func-

tion learn to walk, run, and jump eventually (Rapin, 1974). As a result, clinically significant vestibular dysfunction can be easily overlooked in children with congenital or early onset severe to profound hearing impairment. This is especially true given that hearing and vestibular impairments are not reflected in scores on tests of fine motor coordination and visual motor coordination (Brunt & Broadhead, 1982; Geddes, 1978; Holderbaum, Ritz, Hassaneim, & Goetzinger, 1979) but rather surface only on tasks that discretely isolate reliance on sensory vestibular input (Horak et al., 1988).

The balance subset of the BOT 2 (see Table 8–2) appears to be particularly well suited to identify vestibular dysfunction in children with SNHL in comparison to a number of other clinical tests (Crowe & Horak, 1988). The variety of tasks that make up the balance subset of the BOT 2 provide this necessary gradation in level of difficulty and place emphasis on peripheral vestibular function. It is, therefore, deemed to be an appropriate tool that will adequately uncover functional deficits in children with SNHL over a wide range of ages (4 to 22 years) (Horak et al., 1988). In particular, those items that involve standing across a narrow balance beam limiting ankle torque and disabling the ability of children with peripheral vestibular dysfunction to adjust their body center of mass using hip movements, provide the difficulty level required to uncover vestibular deficits in this group (Supance & Bluestone, 1983). More importantly on an individual level, use of the BOT 2 has allowed us to identify accurately which children with profound SNHL have concurrent abnormalities of balance. Although some children with deafness performed at or above the normative mean on the BOT 2, the performance of 70% falls below it. It is only those with the poorest scores that demonstrate concurrent deficits on vestibular end-organ testing. An additional advantage of the BOT 2 is that because the overall score is standardized by age, the test can be repeatedly administered and scores compared over time in a single child. This is particularly useful in determining the impact of sequential interventions.

Unfortunately, like computerized dynamic posturography, the BOT 2 cannot be administered to very young children (<4 years) which excludes the majority of children being considered for cochlear implantation. Alternatively, the Peabody Developmental Motor Scales 2 (PDMS 2) (Folio & Fewell, 2000) is a well-standardized test of motor function in children that can be applied to children of all ages starting at birth. As such, it may represent an appropriate tool for the evaluation of the youngest children being considered for cochlear implantation. The PDMS 2 is composed of a number of subtests including the Stationary Skill Subtests which measure a child's ability to sustain control of his or her body within its center of gravity and maintain

equilibrium. The Locomotion Subtest also may be appropriate as it assesses a child's ability to move from one place to another and measures actions such as crawling, walking, running, hopping, and jumping forward. These items can be combined with other subtests such as reflexes and object manipulation to calculate a gross motor quotient. The test is scored in much the same fashion as the BOT 2 with age-standardized scores available for comparison (Folio & Fewell, 2000).

Effects of Etiology of SNHL on Vestibular and Balance Function

Given that there is still much to learn about vestibular function in children with SNHL, one could argue that vestibular end-organ testing should be performed in all children undergoing evaluation for cochlear implantation. This approach, however, is not always feasible and targeted assessment more effectively uses test resources and may provide more reliable results. As shown in Figure 8–2, we found that children with SNHL secondary to meningitis or abnormal cochleovestibular anatomy were most likely to demonstrate abnormalities of vestibular end-organ function. Based on these data, perhaps these two groups should be targeted to undergo formal end-organ evaluation. On the other hand, some children with SNHL due to connexin 26 mutations or of unknown etiology also demonstrated dysfunction in our studies. How then do we identify all of the children who should progress to more formal testing? One method would be to target those children who regardless of etiology perform poorly on a

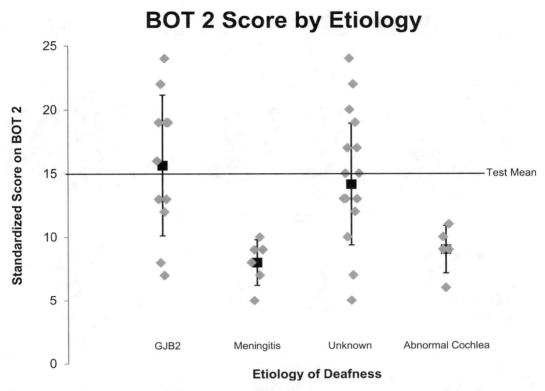

Figure 8–2. Age standardized score on balance subset of BOT-2 plotted by etiology. (■ Mean ± 1 standard deviation).

test of static or dynamic balance such as the BOT 2 or the PDMS 2 described in the previous section. As shown in Figure 8–3, there was a wide spread of performance on the BOT 2 across and within all etiologies of SNHL. In the following section we describe what is currently known about the vestibular phenotype in typical etiologic groups that make up our implant population.

Meningitis

It is estimated that 5 to 35% of patients who survive meningitis experience partial to pro-

found SNHL (Baldwin, Sweitzer, & Freind, 1985; Berlow, Caldarelli, Matz, Meyer, & Harsch, 1980; Dodge et al., 1984; Keane, Potsic, Rowe, & Konkle, 1979; Nadol, 1978). Although not as well studied, the incidence of vestibular loss in the same population appears to be lower and in the range of 3 to 12% (Kaplan, Goddard, Van Kleeck, Catlin, & Feigin, 1981; Lindberg, Rosenhall, Nylen, & Ringner, 1977). It is well known that bacterial meningitis can lead to precipitous ossification of the inner ear (Figure 8-4). The pathophysiology of the hearing and/or vestibular loss that occurs in the setting of bacterial meningitis results from injury occurring early on in the disease course.

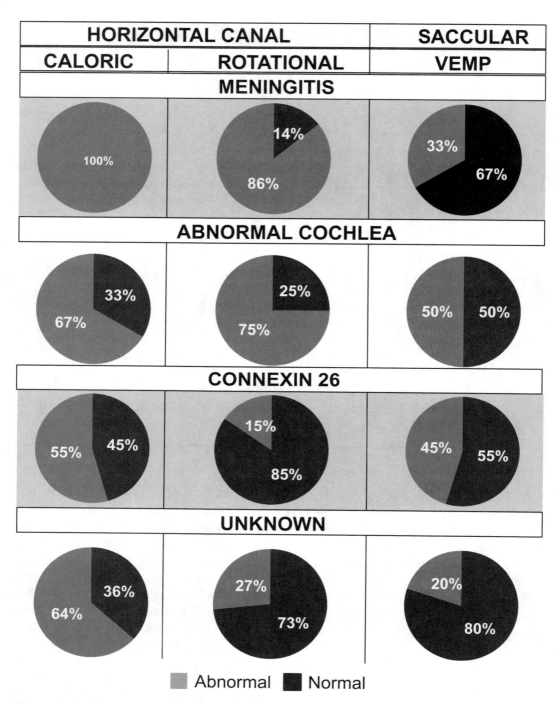

Figure 8–3. Graphical representation of vestibular end-organ (dys)function as measured by caloric, rotational, and VEMP testing. Results are categorized by etiology of SNHL.

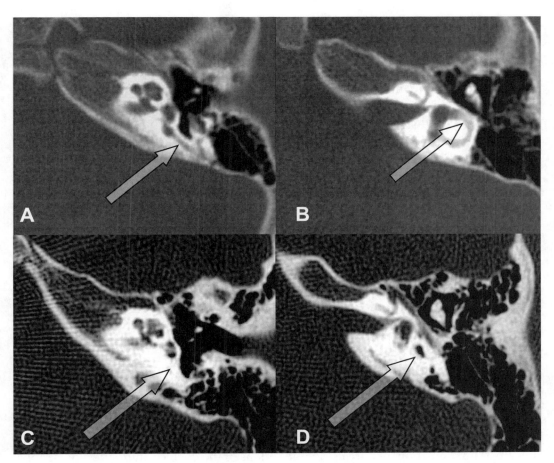

Figure 8–4. High-resolution nonenhanced computed tomography (NECT) of left temporal bone in a child with acquired meningitis. Axial section through posterior semicircular canal with arrow denoting left anterior portion of the horizontal canal (**A, C**). Axial section through horizontal semicircular canal with arrow denoting superior portion of the posterior canals (**C, D**) Images in A and B obtained several weeks following acute bacterial meningitis. Follow-up images (**C** and **D**) were obtained at 10 years and demonstrate bony obliteration of both the horizontal (**C**) and posterior (**D**) canals. Images courtesy of Dr. S. Blaser.

Many studies have demonstrated that ataxia felt to be labyrinthine in origin can be either a presenting or early sign of bacterial meningitis (Bergstrand, Fahlen, & Thilen, 1957; Kaplan et al, 1981; Landthaler & Andrieu-Guitrancourt, 1975; Liebman, Lovrinic, Ronis, & Katinsky, 1969; Lindberg et al., 1977; Roeser, Campbell & Daly, 1975; Schwartz, 1972; Sproles, Azerrad, Williamson, & Merrill, 1969). Although the details of the inner ear damage secondary to bacterial meningitis is not fully understood, spread of infection to the inner ear appears to occur primarily via the cochlear aqueduct and occasionally via the cochlear modiolus (Merchant & Gopen, 1996). Histopathologic studies of temporal bones following meningitis have suggested that SNHL results from suppurative labyrinthitis which occurs in the acute phase of the disease (Merchant & Gopen, 1996).

Despite the inflammatory response seen in these specimens, the sensory and neural elements of the auditory and vestibular systems generally were intact in these bones. A minority of specimens, however, demonstrated variable losses of the organ of Corti and spiral ganglion cells and of the sensory cells of the cristae and maculae. Leukocytic infiltration of the cochlear and vestibular nerves also was seen. Neurosensory structures generally also are intact in animal models even in cases with confirmed profound hearing loss (Bhatt et al., 1991). This suggests perhaps that the SNHL or vestibular impairment resulting from meningitis results from biochemical alteration of the inner ear milieu or by ultrastructural changes not seen by light microscopy. With respect to the distribution of the inner ear injury, temporal bone studies suggest that the scala tympani was the most likely to be affected by suppurative labyrinthitis with the most inflammation occurring in the basal turn. The scala vestibuli was affected in 50% of the temporal bones and the horizontal semicircular canal was commonly involved. Inflammation did not involve the saccule or utricle in any cases (Merchant & Gopen, 1996). The distribution of inflammation reported in these temporal bone studies parallels the pattern of ossification that we have observed in serial CT imaging in our cohort of children with meningitis (see Figure 8–4). This finding is also consistent with the fact that horizontal canal function was almost universally affected in our population, whereas saccular function was well preserved in the majority of the children studied, as shown in Figure 8–2 (Cushing et al., 2008b). The resistance of the saccule to injury in the face of a suppura-

tive labyrinthitis that so dramatically affects the surrounding cochlea and semicircular canals is difficult to explain. If utrical function likewise was preserved in these children, this may support the theory that the more primitive otolithic organs are more resistant to injury from meningitis although it would still remain difficult to determine the pathophysiologic basis of this apparent resistance. In spite of the preservation of saccular function, static and dynamic balance function as measured by the BOT 2 was poorest in those children with acquired hearing loss due to meningitis. Despite these poor scores, however, these children participated in a wide variety of activities that would be considered balance intensive such as horseback riding, dancing, and bicycle riding.

Abnormal Cochleovestibular Anatomy

We have found that static and dynamic balance ability in five children with malformations of the cochlea and/or vestibular apparatus was poor and only marginally better than that of children with acquired hearing loss due to meningitis (see Figure 8–2). Balance dysfunction was accompanied by loss of horizontal canal function in 2 of 3 (67%) children using caloric stimuli and in 3 of 4 (75%) based on rotational stimuli. Of the 5 children with temporal bone anomalies, more than half (3) demonstrated abnormalities of the vestibule and semicircular canal on CT imaging (Figure 8–5) and ranged from mild dysplasia to significant posterior labyrinthine dysplasia. Only a single child demonstrated abnormal horizontal canal function without an apparent abnormality of the semicircular canals. It is possible then that vestibular dysfunction in the setting of cochleovestibular anomalies is the

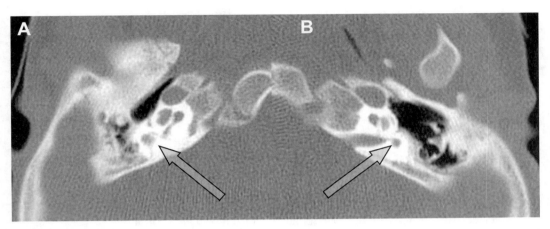

Figure 8–5. High-resolution NECT of the temporal bone of a child with features of CHARGE association (**A, B**). Arrows denotes severe left sided vestibular hypoplasia with rudimentary anlage in the usual location of the horizontal semicircular canals at the level of the cochlea (**A**) and the IAC (**B**). Images courtesy of Dr. S. Blaser.

result of gross abnormalities in the formation of the vestibular end-organs. A second possibility may be that malformation of the cochlea and or vestibular end organs are an indicator of ultrastructural abnormalities within the inner ear and not themselves directly responsible for the dysfunction.

GJB2-Related Deafness

Mutations in the GJB2 gene that encodes the connexin 26 protein lead to altered gap junction coupling in the inner ear. The SNHL is believed to result from changes in potassium homeostasis causing impairment of the endocochlear potential (Forge et al., 2003). Similarly, it has been shown that the vestibular receptors of the otolithic organs and the semicircular canals are coupled by a network of gap junctions (Kikuchi, Adams, Paul, & Kimura, 1994). This network is responsible for creating a depolarization-dependent increase of potassium around the vestibular hair cell synapses (Furukawa,

1985) as is the case for the outer hair cells of the cochlea (Johnstone, Patuzzi, Syka, & Sykova, 1989). Based on these commonalities one might predict that vestibular end-organ function may also be affected by mutations in the GJB2 gene. However, as shown in Figure 8–2, the balance performance as measured by the BOT 2 was significantly better in children with GJB2-related SNHL compared to children with hearing loss due to meningitis or cochleovestibular anomalies. There was, however, much more variability within the GJB2 group and performance spanned the spectrum from above average to well-below average. The incidence of vestibular end-organ dysfunction in GJB2-related SNHL measured by caloric, rotational and VEMP testing was also lower (see Figure 8–3) compared with other etiologies. The majority of children with SNHL due to GJB2 had relatively normal horizontal canal function with a small number demonstrating mild unilateral dysfunction on the implanted side. All the children with mild unilateral losses demonstrated normal

VOR during rotation, highlighting the mild and/or compensated nature of these losses. Saccular function was absent bilaterally in a minority of children with GJB2 related deafness (1/9) and several demonstrated absent VEMPs on only the implanted side (4/9). Two of the 9 children with GJB2 deafness, however, demonstrated very different results; both showed complete horizontal canal dysfunction in response to caloric and rotational stimuli. We have begun to test the hypothesis that these phenotypic differences reflect differences in the particular GJB2 mutations expressed in these children. However, presently it is unclear whether these GJB2 mutations are disease causing or simply polymorphisms.

Overall, there are limited reports on the evaluation of vestibular function in the setting of GJB2-related deafness to date. A second study that included 7 adult patients with variable degrees of SNHL and different GJB2 mutations demonstrated normal horizontal canal function in all but one patient and absent saccular function in the majority (5/7) (Todt, Hennies, Basta, & Ernst, 2005). Although our results for horizontal canal function are similar with the exception of our 2 patients with complete dysfunction, saccular function was preserved in the majority of our patients (Cushing et al., 2008b). Absence of saccular function in the setting of GJB2 related deafness has also been demonstrated in two other single patient reports (Jun et al., 2000; Tsuzuku, Kaga, Kanematsu, Shibata, & Ohde, 1992). Again, we question how the type of GJB2 mutation as well as its expression in one or both alleles affects the vestibular and cochlear systems. Although we tend to group together all subjects with GJB2 related deafness, already over 100 mutations have been described in the GJB2 gene (Ballana, Ventayol, Rabionet, Gaspaarini, & Estivill, 2007)

and certainly support for phenotypic differences exists (Cohn et al., 1999; Snoeckx et al., 2005). If there is a variable impact of specific GJB2 mutations on auditory and vestibular end-organ function, we also would expect to find differences in other areas of the two systems such as in the efferent inputs or in the composition and response properties of ionic channels. Clearly, further study is warranted.

Unknown Etiology

Our ability to identify the etiology of deafness has increased with improved imaging and molecular genetic diagnostics; however, the etiology still is not identified in a significant proportion of our implant population. Balance ability in the setting of SNHL of unknown etiology was on average relatively normal; however, individual performance did again span a large spectrum with some children demonstrating very poor abilities (see Figure 8–2). Forty-two percent of children with SNHL of unknown etiology demonstrated horizontal canal dysfunction based on caloric testing (see Figure 8–3). The degree of dysfunction ranged from mild unilateral losses in the implanted ear to bilateral areflexia. Twenty-six percent demonstrated dysfunction of the horizontal canal based on an abnormal VOR on rotational chair testing. Given the likely heterogeneity of the underlying causes of SNHL in this group it becomes difficult to discuss the association between SNHL and vestibular end-organ and balance dysfunction. This highlights the importance of thoroughly investigating the etiology of the SNHL as well as continuing to identify additional genetic causes of deafness that likely comprise the majority of the currently unknown etiologies within this group. Alternatively, identifying dysfunction of the vestibular end organs in a child with SNHL also can help direct the search for an underlying genetic cause known to be associated with severe vestibular dysfunction such as Usher's syndrome Type I.

Time Course of Hearing Loss: Progressive Versus Nonprogressive

Although many different etiologies of SNHL exist and influence the likelihood of concurrent vestibular dysfunction, likewise the time course of the SNHL is also variable and can range from congenital to acquired, sudden versus progressive. Certainly such differences also may reflect differences in the time course of an accompanying vestibular loss and this is considered in the following section. Just as children with progressive auditory losses are able to develop speech and language given even minimal access to sound, there may be a parallel mechanism which occurs within the vestibular system in relation to developing adequate balance in the presence of a progressive vestibular loss. We found that differences in balance ability as estimated by BOT 2 performance were both observed and demonstrated statistically when comparing the results of children with progressive versus nonprogressive SNHL (Figure 8–6). Although we

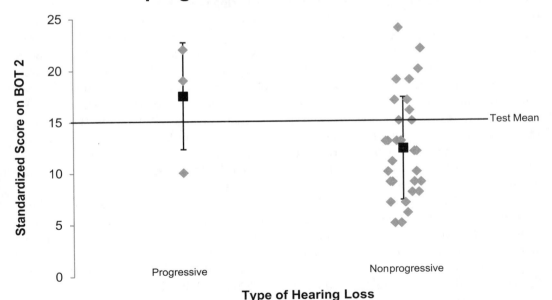

Figure 8–6. Age standardized score on balance subset of BOT-2 plotted by type of hearing loss (progressive vs. nonprogressive). (■ Mean ± 1 standard deviation).

examined only a small number of children with progressive losses ($n = 4$), as a group these children demonstrated better performance on the BOT 2 irrespective of horizontal canal function. Presumably, a slow progressive loss of vestibular function would allow access to at least weak vestibular signals over a period of time and that may be sufficient to generate appropriate motor responses. Depending on the time course of the loss of function, perhaps even a gradual substitution or shift of the importance of other sensory inputs (visual, proprioceptive and possibly even vestibulospinal) in the maintenance of balance may have occurred.

Compensatory Mechanisms for Vestibular Dysfunction

The maintenance of balance and stability results from a complex interplay between the peripheral vestibular, visual, and somatosensory system. Fortunately, considerable overlap in the handling of sensory information between these systems exists. This redundancy promotes and facilitates adequate function in the presence of perceptual and physical disturbances, as well as when the function of any one of these systems is lost, compromised, or distorted. The time course of an insult is also important given that differences in the compensatory strategies employed likely exist and change over time. The relative importance and contribution of each of the sensory and motor systems that work together to maintain balance is not static but rather fluctuates according to the characteristics of the sensory information at any one point in time. How children with combined cochleovestibular loss compensate in order to maintain their balance cannot be answered without understanding the characteristics of the sensory environment in which these children find themselves.

Attempts have been made to identify the compensatory strategies for maintaining postural control employed by subjects with congenital or early acquired bilateral vestibular loss. Theoretically, models of postural orientation suggest that when somatosensory and vestibular information interpret the surface as stable, one can rely on somatosensory information alone to control and maintain posture. However, the maintenance of postural control when a surface is interpreted as unstable, results from a decreased reliance on surface somatosensory information and an increased reliance on vestibular information (Mergner & Rosemeier, 1998). More specifically, some studies have aimed to determine the relative weighting of different sensory receptor systems in the congenital or early acquired absence of peripheral vestibular input by examining postural control using posturography under a number of sensory conditions which target the three sensory systems important for balance (visual, vestibular, proprioceptive) (Enbom, Magnusson, & Pyykko, 1991). Visual manipulations are typically eyes open versus eyes shut or light versus dark. Proprioception can be manipulated by changing the platform the subject stands on from a solid surface to foam rubber or by applying vibration to the calves. Under these settings challenges are presented to the vestibular system through perturbations of the platform. It has been shown that children with normal cochleovestibular function and those with bilateral vestibular loss are indistinguishable based on postural sway when only one of the three sensory systems distorted (Enbom et al., 1991). However, when two sensory distortions were applied simultaneously, children with bilateral vestibular loss were easily distinguished from controls. The degree to which these sensory perturbations disrupt postural control however was variable. For example, the increase in body sway elicited by eye closure was similar in the two groups, regardless of the presence of foam surface or calf vibration.

Similarly, the application of muscle vibration while standing on a solid surface increased sway velocity to a similar degree in children with normal versus abnormal cochleovestibular function. However, when either the eyes were closed and/or in the presence of muscle vibration, the simultaneous distortion of pressor reception caused by standing on foam rubber, led to a proportionally larger increase in sway in children with bilateral vestibular loss. This suggests that, in the presence of bilateral vestibular dysfunction, the strategy for postural control is unevenly redistributed to the visual, proprioceptive, and exteroceptive receptors with increasing importance placed on pressor reception and proprioception whereas the relative importance of vision on postural control remains unchanged. This is in sharp contrast to the findings in a number of adult studies that used similar tasks. In those studies, adults with acquired vestibular loss were found to depend much more heavily on visual cues and eye closure resulted in proportionally worse postural instability compared to control subjects (Bles & de Jong, 1986; Buchanan & Horak, 2001). It has been suggested also that the ability to control the head independent of the trunk is important for postural compensation following vestibular loss. Individuals who suffer vestibular loss in infancy retain their ability to separate head and trunk motion and thus control their head in a manner more similar to age-matched controls than do adults with later onset vestibular loss and thus perform better on tasks of static and dynamic balance (Buchanan & Horak, 2001; Shupert & Horak, 1996).

Other studies in children have corroborated the relative importance of somatosensory information in the setting of a bilateral vestibular loss. These studies demonstrate near-normal postural sway in sensory conditions when either accurate surface or visual information is available whereas sway significantly increases when the surface is sway referenced, suggesting again that compensation is highly dependent on pressor and proprioceptive inputs even when eyes are open (Black & Nashner, 1984; Black, Wall, & Nashner, 1983; Horak, 1987; Shumway-Cook & Horak, 1986). Using the BOT 2 we have demonstrated that the relative importance of vision on the maintenance of balance is unchanged in the presence of a bilateral vestibular loss. This was reflected in the finding that all children, normal hearing, deaf, with and without concurrent vestibular dysfunction, suffered a proportionally identical decrement in performance on certain items on the BOT 2 when the eyes were closed (Cushing et al., 2008a).

In summary, in the presence of bilateral vestibular dysfunction, the strategy for postural control in children likely is unevenly redistributed to the visual, proprioceptive, and exteroceptive receptors with increasing importance placed on pressor reception and proprioception whereas the relative importance of vision on postural control remains unchanged. As a consequence of the efficacy of the compensatory mechanisms for sensorimotor control, tests of static and dynamic balance must be adequately sensitive; otherwise, even bilateral vestibular areflexia may be missed by employing simple tests such as the Romberg. In addition, the visual and somatosensory conditions should be manipulated systematically and incrementally in order to partition the use of alternative interacting sensory components of postural control.

Importance of Vestibular and Balance Evaluation

Implications for Implantation

Just as anomalies of the auditory system due to genetic defects, meningitis, or other causes may be associated with parallel injuries of the vestibular end organs, so too might cochlear implantation iatrogenically cause injury to the vestibular system. More recently, evaluation of vestibular end-organ function in the setting of profound SNHL has garnered increased attention because of its relevance to the topic of bilateral cochlear implantation and the potential risk of bilateral vestibular injury. There are a number of potential mechanisms by which the act of cochlear implantation may disturb vestibular function. Specifically, surgically induced injuries to the labyrinth may occur secondary to (1) the induction of a serous labyrinthitis due to opening of the membranous labyrinth, (2) the introduction of blood into the inner ear, (3) mechanical injury due to the insertion of the electrode array, and (4) high-speed drilling within the temporal bone (Molony & Marais, 1996; Spector, 1973). Although the electrode array itself and its insertion appears quite delicate, cochlear implantation has been shown to lead to mechanical disruption of inner ear structures including rupture of the basilar membrane, fracture of the osseous spiral lamina, transection of the scala media, and fracture of the modiolus (Eshraghi, Yang, & Balkany, 2003; Gstoettner et al., 1997; Kennedy, 1987; Richter et al., 2001; Richter, Jaekel, Aschendorff, Marangos, & Laszig, 2001; Rossi & Bisetti, 1998; Welling, Hinojosa, Ganta, & Lee, 1993). More specifically, with respect to the histopathology of the vestibular end organs following implantation, fibrosis, hydrops with saccular membrane distortion, osteoneogenesis, and reactive neuromas are described in the vestibule and semicircular canals (Tien & Linthicum, 2002). These observed histologic injuries did not always translate into physiologic dysfunction, however (Tien & Linth-icum, 2002). Histopathologic analysis of temporal bones and the vestibular apparatus following cochlear implantation has demonstrated injury in more than half of patients. Histologic abnormalities following implantation have included fibrosis of the vestibular apparatus, saccular membrane distortion, osteoneogenesis, and reactive neuromas. In addition, involvement of the scala vestibuli as a result of damage to the osseous spiral lamina or basilar membrane in the cochlear basal turn, correlated strongly with vestibular end-organ damage (Tien & Linthicum, 2002).

In addition to structural injuries of the labyrinth following cochlear implantation, measurable damage to vestibular function following cochlear implantation has been described (Black, 1977). Subjective complaints of dizziness following cochlear implantation occur in 2 to 49% of patients and are more likely to occur with increasing age in adulthood (Black, Lilly, Peterka, Fowler, & Simmons, 1987; Cohen, Hoffman, & Stroschein, 1988; Enticott et al., 2006; Huygen, van den Broek, Spies, Mens, & Admiraal, 1994; Ito, 1998; Kempf, Johann, & Lenarz, 1999; Kubo, Yamamoto, Iwaki, Doi, & Tamura, 2001; Ribari, Kustel, Szmirmai, & Repassy, 1999; Webb et al., 1991). Adults undergoing cochlear implantation more often experience transient vestibular systems postoperatively in comparison to their pediatric counterparts. In our program, approximately 1% of children (8/758) have experienced transient symptoms of vestibular dysfunction with the only identifiable risk factors being, cochleovestibular anomaly (± CSF gusher at the time of surgery), symptomatic episodic vertigo prior to implantation and, in the case of reimplantation, dizziness at the time of their first surgery as well as reimplantation itself. In these 8 children, some combination of observed or reported direction fixed horizontal nystagmus, disequilibrium, and vomiting leading to delayed discharge, repeat visit, or telephone notification was seen.

The reported and estimated risk of losing or significantly diminishing horizontal canal function based on caloric testing postimplantation ranges between 0 and 77% (Black et al., 1987; Brey et al., 1995; Buchman et al., 2004; Chiong et al., 1994; Chouard, Chouard, Fugain, Meyer, & Gegu, 1984; Eisenberg, Nelson, & House, 1982; Higgins, Chen, Nedzelski, Shipp, & McIllmoyl, 2002; Huygen et al., 1995; Ito, 1998; Kiyomizu et al., 2000; Ribari et al., 1999; Rossi, Solero, Rolando, & Spadola Bisetti, 1998; van den Broek, Huygen, Mens, Admiraal, & Spies, 1993; Vibert et al., 2001). However, these results vary with increasing duration between implantation and postoperative testing; this interval is important to consider as some individuals may exhibit a transient loss or decrease in function followed by recovery (Vibert et al., 2001). Longitudinal measures of horizontal canal function by caloric stimulus postcochlear implantation suggest that by 4 months postimplantation caloric function has stabilized and few improvements in function occur subsequent to that (Buchman et al., 2004). In adults and children, postimplant vestibular function was reduced in 29% of those "at risk" for vestibular effects after cochlear implantion (i.e., those with normal or reduced but not absent horizontal canal function preimplant in response to a caloric stimulus). In this setting, significant reduction of vestibular function was defined as a reduction of the total caloric response of 21° per second or greater. Changes in horizontal canal function as measured by a loss of caloric function often were paralleled by changes in VOR phase and gain in response to rotation (Buchman et al., 2004).

In one of the most thorough evaluations of the horizontal and vertical semicircular canal function using head impulse testing, Migliaccio and colleagues demonstrated preoperative hypofunction of the horizontal canal in 36% and decreased gain in one or more of the vertical canals in 50%. Postoperatively, only a single patient (9%) experienced a significant decrease in function of all three semicircular canals on the implanted side accompanied by transient vertigo and oscillopsia (Migliaccio, Della Santina, Carey, Niparko, & Minor, 2005). The current subject population allows for a limited evaluation of the impact of cochlear implantation on balance and vestibular end organ function given that at the time of testing they already had a unilateral implant. However, of those children with mild to moderate unilateral hypofunction ($n = 6$) of the horizontal canal, all but one (83%) occurred on the side of implantation. This difference, however, did not reach statistical significance and the study was not powered primarily to detect such differences. We also examined the difference in VOR gain in response to a rotational stimulus on the implanted versus nonimplanted side. In our analysis, no significant asymmetry was found suggesting little effect of implantation on VOR gain measured by rotational chair testing (Cushing et al., 2008b).

Most studies to date have focused on the effect of cochlear implantation on horizontal canal function; thus, little is known about the impact of cochlear implantation on the otolithic organs. However, the saccule may be more susceptible to damage than the utricle or semicircular canals because of its proximity to the insertion path of the implant's electrode array (Tien & Linthicum, 2002). We demonstrated a trend for unilateral saccular dysfunction to occur more commonly on the implanted side (Cushing et al., 2008b). In a separate study, 50% of 12 children demonstrated bilaterally normal saccular function as measured by VEMP prior to surgery (Jin et al., 2006), which was subsequently obliterated given the disappearance of VEMP responses after cochlear implantation. There was one exception: a VEMP measured postoperatively in one child but the response was smaller in amplitude than that seen preoperatively (Jin et al., 2006). In comparison, utricular function measured using off-vertical axis rotation was not found to be impaired following cochlear implantation (Vibert et al., 2001).

Although age (>70 years) and a partial loss prior to surgery may increase the risk of a postoperative diminution in vestibular function, no consistent and reliable means have yet been established for determining the likelihood of experiencing a vestibular disturbance after cochlear implantation (Enticott et al., 2006).

Given the high degree of non- and hypofunctioning vestibular systems prior to implantation, some authors suggest that the risk of a significant vestibular lesion secondary to implantation is quite low (Buchman et al., 2004). In contrast, we have shown that the majority of children demonstrate sufficient peripheral vestibular function to be considered "at risk" of sustaining an injury due to implantation. In our cohort, only one third of patients would be considered to be "at low risk" for further vestibular injury from cochlear implantation due to sufficiently little or absent vestibular end-organ function. It is of great interest that despite the severity of the vestibular losses in this "low risk" group, all children whose hearing loss was caused by meningitis, ambulated without difficulty and many of those with even the most profound losses were involved in many activities that challenge balance (e.g., skating, dancing, horseback riding). The overall function of these children in the face of their severe losses of vestibular function is likely a reflection of compensation secondary to a reliance on other inputs (i.e., visual and somatosensory) that contribute to the maintenance of stability. It is this ability to compensate for such profound deficits in vestibular end-organ function that has reassured us with regard to the safety of bilateral implantation.

Clinical Relevance of Identifying Vestibular and Balance Dysfunction

Over the last decade increasing emphasis has been placed on the need for early identification of children with SNHL with the target of having such children aided by 6 months of age, a goal that now is routinely achieved. In the setting of hearing rehabilitation, there is a clear relationship between early intervention and outcome. Although difficult to estimate because of the impact of etiology and residual thresholds, for all children with severe to profound SNHL the incidence of a simultaneous vestibular lesion likely is around 30%. Despite this incidence we have not taken the same aggressive approach to identifying and rehabilitating concurrent vestibular impairment. There are a number of reasons why we should strive to do so. First, identifying peripheral vestibular dysfunction prevents the false labeling of children as having global delay, central lesions, or multiple handicaps. Second, different therapeutic approaches can be used for the rehabilitation of children with either loss of vestibular sensitivity or deficits of sensory organization. For example, children with SNHL and reduced or absent vestibular dysfunction may benefit from balance strategies in various environmental contexts in an effort to prime their visual and somatic senses facilitating compensation. More specifically, interventions as simple as a 10-day exercise program focused on activities of static balance activities led to significant improvement in standing balance duration in children with SNHL compared to untreated hearing-impaired controls (Effgen, 1981).

At a minimum, bilateral vestibular loss carries with it a number of clinical safety concerns that should certainly be relayed to patients. These include the potential for loss of spatial orientation when swimming under water as well as in the dark, and reports of drowning have occurred in patients where loss of bilateral loss of vestibular function was suspected (Verhagen, Huygen, & Horstink, 1987). Although such limitations are obvious to clinicians, they often are not to patients and their parents. Excellent, although incomplete, compensation appears to occur in many children with bilateral vestibular deficits; therefore, eliciting abnormalities on functional testing may be quite difficult. Also, given the absence of normal vestibular input since infancy, these individuals and/or their parents may not recognize the child's difficulties when riding a bicycle, walking on a balance beam, or orienting in the dark. In order to be sensitive indicators of peripheral vestibular loss, tests of balance must place individuals in an environment without redundant visual and surface sensory inputs or require movement patterns in which vestibular input is critical.

Potential Pediatric Test Battery

Just as it may not be practical to test all children who are implant candidates, it also may not be practical to perform an extended battery of vestibular tests in any one child. Of the tests of vestibular end-organ function employed in our study, performance on high-frequency rotational chair testing displayed the strongest and most robust

correlation with static and dynamic balance ability as measured by the BOT 2 (Cushing et al., 2008b). Horizontal canal dysfunction based on caloric areflexia also was correlated with balance ability; however, horizontal canal function based on rotational chair testing allowed us to identify an additional population of children with isolated high frequency loss. This loss was deemed clinically significant based on the children's poor performance on the BOT 2. It is important to note that this population would have been missed by caloric testing alone. Another advantage of rotational chair testing is that it is better tolerated by children than caloric testing, particularly given that confirmation of bilateral areflexia requires the use of ice water caloric irrigation. In summary, our results suggest that caloric testing may identify horizontal canal dysfunction that is not clinically significant likely as a result of physiologic compensation and also may miss clinically significant high-frequency losses of function identified by rotational chair testing. For these reasons, we feel that the true incidence of vestibular dysfunction in our study population likely is best predicted by abnormalities of the VOR response to high-frequency rotation. Although it is still our preference to perform an extended battery of vestibular and balance tests on children undergoing assessment for cochlear implantation, high-frequency rotational testing combined with a measure of static and dynamic balance such as the BOT 2 or PDMS 2 comprises a reasonable evaluation.

Summary

"The testing of children rarely fulfills all the conditions for an ideal vestibular study" (Rapin, 1974, p. 934). This quote certainly reflects the sentiment that surrounds testing of any kind in a pediatric clinical setting. Identifying a peripheral vestibular loss or balance dysfunction in a child can be difficult for a number of reasons. The primary challenge lies in ensuring compliance with testing protocols. In the setting of SNHL these compliance issues become even more difficult given the added communication barriers. The ability to effectively convey verbal reinforcement is a hallmark in the success of pediatric testing and this is compromised in children who have delayed oral speech-language development resulting from hearing loss. Identifying a pure and isolated peripheral vestibular dysfunction may be more elusive (Rapin, 1974). The identification of vestibular losses, particularly in children, requires not only tests of balance function that attempt to isolate the contribution of the vestibular end organs by removing or distorting other sensory inputs, but also that the tasks be sufficiently difficult. Current mainstream tests of peripheral vestibular function provide a useful but limited assessment of a subset of the vestibular end organs, in particular, the horizontal canal and the saccule. Finally, before we can even begin to understand the implications of unilateral and/or bilateral cochlear implantation on vestibular end-organ and balance function, we need to be certain that our baseline measures are accurate and adequately reflect functional outcome. An understanding of baseline vestibular function also may allow us to experiment with the properties of cochlear implants in an effort to increase the quality of the sensory information provided to children with concurrent lesions of the cochlea and the labyrinth. As we are identifying an ever increasing number of genes responsible for SNHL, the vestibular phenotype of these children has already begun to narrow and dictate the search for the genetic etiology of their hearing loss (i.e., any child with bilateral areflexia is tested for the gene responsible for Usher's Type I) and most certainly will continue to do so in the future.

Future Directions

Limited evaluation of the impact of implantation on static and dynamic balance has been performed to date. There has been some indication, however, that cochlear implantation actually may positively influence balance function; small improvements in performance have been documented on CDP in some individuals following implantation when their implants are activated (Buchman et al., 2004; Eisenberg et al., 1982). We also have demonstrated that children with SNHL and unilateral implants perform slightly, although significantly, better on the BOT 2 balance subset with their implants on versus their implants off, although this certainly requires additional study with proper control of the directional information contained in the auditory signals presented to the implant (Cushing et al., 2008a).

Although a beneficial effect of implantation on vestibular and balance function may exist, at this point we can only speculate as to the underlying mechanism that could account for this. With this in mind, such benefits may relate to the fact that the poorer performance of children with profound SNHL without an identifiable injury of the vestibular end organs may be attributed to a lack or poor quality of spatial cues that occur in the setting of deafness and exist even after rehabilitation with a unilateral implant. Although we are quick to recognize the importance of visual, somatosensory, and vestibular cues in the maintenance of balance, the contribution of hearing is rarely considered and may explain the overall poor balance performance seen preimplantation in this study. A second theoretical possibility is that the improvement somehow is related to extracochlear spread of current. Spread of current to the facial nerve leads to demonstrable EMG activity in the facial musculature of nearly 50% of children with cochlear implants with translation into clinically evident facial movement in a much smaller proportion (Cushing, Papsin, & Gordon, 2006). The vestibular end organs are within even closer proximity to the implant electrode than the facial nerve and are also housed within the same fluid-filled environment. As such, it is certainly possible that electrophysiologic changes may occur at the level of the vestibular end organs and afferents in response to activation of a cochlear implant. Certainly further study is required to determine if this indeed is the case and if so what the impact may or may not be on functional outcomes. Much can also be learned from the longitudinal study of vestibular and balance function in our pediatric implant patients as changes in their ability to compensate for a vestibular loss may occur over time as visual acuity and proprioceptive sensitivity decrease with age and concurrent illness.

Irrespective of whether the observed improvements in balance are occurring secondary to increased access to auditory cuing and spatial information in sound or as a result of the delivery of low level electrical stimulation via the implant to the vestibular end organs and primary afferents, the thought that we could positively affect functional balance using a cochlear implant is an exciting proposition. Further study most certainly is required to elucidate these potential benefits and this may be particularly relevant to those children who demonstrate severe bilateral peripheral vestibular dysfunction. As a final note, it is without question, however, that the study of vestib-

ular and balance function in children with SNHL and cochlear implant(s) has a bright and exciting future.

Acknowledgments. Special thanks to Dr. Karen Gordon for her thorough review and input to this chapter. Thanks also to Dr. Adrian James, Dr. Susan Blaser, Dr. John Rutka, and Dr. Neil Bailie for their contributions to this work and to Heather, Al, Julie, Wanda, Eileen, Barb, Melissa, and Georgette for their role in the vestibular and balance testing.

References

Arnvig, J. (1955). Vestibular function in deafness and severe hardness of hearing. *Acta Oto-Laryngologica, 45*, 283–288.

Baldwin, R. L., Sweitzer, R. S., & Freind, D. B. (1985). Meningitis and sensorineural hearing loss. *Laryngoscope, 95*, 802–805.

Ballana, E., Ventayol, M., Rabionet, R., Gasparini, P., & Estivill, X. (2007). *Connexins and deafness*. Retrieved March 09, 2008, from: http://www.crg.es/deafness .

Bergstrand, C. G., Fahlen, T., & Thilen, A. (1957). A follow-up study of children treated for acute purulent meningitis. *Acta Paediatrica, 46*, 10–17.

Berlow, S. J., Caldarelli, D. D., Matz, G. J., Meyer, D. H., & Harsch, G. G. (1980). Bacterial meningitis and sensorineural hearing loss: A prospective investigation. *Laryngoscope, 90*, 1445–1452.

Bhatt, S., Halpin, C., Hsu, W., Thedinger, B. A., Levine, R. A., Tuomanen, E., et al. (1991). Hearing loss and pneumococcal meningitis: An animal model. *Laryngoscope, 101*, 1285–1292.

Black, F. O. (1977). Present vestibular status of subjects implanted with auditory prostheses. *Annals of Otology, Rhinology, and Laryngology, 86*(Suppl. 34), 49–56.

Black, F. O., Lilly, D. J., Peterka, R. J., Fowler, L. P., & Simmons, F. B. (1987). Vestibulo-ocular and vestibulospinal function before and after cochlear implant surgery. *Annals of Otology, Rhinology, and Laryngology, 96*(Suppl. 128), 106–108.

Black, F. O., & Nashner, L. M. (1984). Vestibulospinal control differs in patients with reduced versus distorted vestibular function. *Acta Oto-Laryngologica, Supplement 406*, 110–114.

Black, F. O., Wall, C. III, & Nashner, L. M. (1983). Effects of visual and support surface orientation references upon postural control in vestibular deficient subjects. *Acta Oto-Laryngologica, 95*, 199–201.

Bles, W., & de Jong, J. (1986). Uni- and bilateral loss of vestibular function. In W. Bles & T. Brandt (Eds.), *Disorders of posture and gait* (pp. 127–141). Amsterdam: Elsevier Science.

Brey, R. H., Facer, G. W., Trine, M. B., Lynn, S. G., Peterson, A. M., & Suman, V. J. (1995). Vestibular effects associated with implantation of a multiple channel cochlear prosthesis. *American Journal of Otology, 16*, 424–430.

Brookhouser, P. E., Cyr, D. G., & Beauchaine, K. A. (1982). Vestibular findings in the deaf and hard of hearing. *Otolaryngology-Head and Neck Surgery, 90*, 773–777.

Bruininks, R., & B. Bruininks. (2005). *BOT-2 Bruininks-Oseretsky Test of Motor Proficiency* (2nd ed., p. 263). Circle Pines, MN: AGS.

Brunt, D., & Broadhead, G. D. (1982). Motor proficiency traits of deaf children. *Research Quarterly for Exercise and Sport, 53*, 236–238.

Buchanan, J. J., & Horak, F. B. (2001). Vestibular loss disrupts control of head and trunk on a sinusoidally moving platform. *Journal of Vestibular Research, 11*, 371–389.

Buchman, C. A., Joy, J., Hodges, A., Telischi, F. F., & Balkany, T. J. (2004). Vestibular effects of cochlear implantation. *Laryngoscope, 114*, 1–22.

Carey, J. P., & Della Santina, C. C. (2005). Principles of applied vestibular physiology. In C. W. Cummings, P. W. Flint, L. A. Harker, B. H. Haughey, M. A. Richardson, K. T. Robbins, et al. (Eds.), *Otolaryngology head and neck surgery* (4th ed., pp. 3115–3159). Philadelphia: Elsevier Mosby.

Chiong, C. M., Nedzelski, J. M., McIlmoyl, L. D., & Shipp, D. B. (1994). Electro-oculographic findings pre- and post-cochlear implantation. *Journal of Otolaryngology, 23*, 447–449.

Chouard, C. H., Fugain, C., Meyer, B., & Gegu, D. (1984). Prognostic evaluation of the multichannel cochlear implant. *Acta Oto-Laryngologica, Supplement 411*, 161–164.

Cohen, N. L., Hoffman, R. A., & Stroschein, M. (1988). Medical or surgical complications related to the Nucleus multichannel cochlear implant. *Annals of Otology, Rhinology, and Laryngology, Supplement 135*, 8–13.

Cohn, E. S., Kelley, P. M., Fowler, T. W., Gorga, M. P., Lefkowitz, D. M., Kuehn, H. J., et al. (1999). Clinical studies of families with hearing loss attributable to mutations in the connexin 26 gene (GJB2/DFNB1). *Pediatrics, 103*, 546–550.

Crowe, T. K., & Horak, F. B. (1988). Motor proficiency associated with vestibular deficits in children with hearing impairments. *Physical Therapy, 68*, 1493–1499.

Cushing S. L., Chia, R., James, A. L., Papsin, B. C., & Gordon, K. A. (2008a). The Vestibular Olympics: A test of static and dynamic balance function in children with cochlear implants. *Archives of Otorhinolaryngology-Head and Neck Surgery, 134*, 34–38.

Cushing, S. L., Papsin, B. C., & Gordon, K. A. (2006). Incidence and characteristics of facial nerve stimulation in children with cochlear implants. *Laryngoscope, 116*, 1787–1791.

Cushing, S. L., Papsin, B. C., Rutka, J. A., James, A. L., & Gordon, K. A. (2008b). Evidence of vestibular and balance dysfunction in children with profound sensorineural hearing loss using cochlear implants. *Laryngoscope, 118*, 1814–1823.

Cyr, D. G., Brookhouser, P. E., Valente, M., & Grossman, A. (1985). Vestibular evaluation of infants and preschool children. *Otolaryngology-Head and Neck Surgery, 93*, 463–468.

Davey, P. R. (1954). Observations on equilibrium in deaf children. *Journal of Laryngology and Otology, 68*, 329–331.

Didier, A., & Cazals, Y. (1989). Acoustic responses recorded from the saccular bundle on the eighth nerve of the guinea pig. *Hearing Research, 37*, 123–127.

Dodge, P. R., Davis, H., Feigin, R. D., Holmes, S. J., Kaplan, S. L., Jubelirer, D. P., et al. (1984). Prospective evaluation of hearing impairment as a sequela of acute bacterial meningitis. *New England Journal of Medicine, 311,* 869-874.

Donat, J. F., Donat, J. R., & Lay, K. S. (1980). Changing response to caloric stimulation with gestational age in infants. *Neurology, 30,* 776-778.

Effgen, S. K. (1981). Effect of an exercise program on the static balance of deaf children. *Physical Therapy, 61,* 873-877.

Eisenberg, L. S., Nelson, J. R., & House, W. F. (1982). Effects of the single-electrode cochlear implant on the vestibular system of the profoundly deaf adult. *Annals of Otology, Rhinology, and Laryngology, 91*(Suppl. 91), 47-54.

Enbom, H., Magnusson, M., & Pyykko, I. (1991). Postural compensation in children with congenital or early acquired bilateral vestibular loss. *Annals of Otology, Rhinology, and Laryngology, 100,* 472-478.

Enticott, J. C., Tari, S., Koh, S. M., Dowell, R. C., & O'Leary, S. J. (2006). Cochlear implant and vestibular function. *Otology and Neurotology, 27,* 824-830.

Eshraghi, A. A., Yang, N. W., & Balkany, T. J. (2003). Comparative study of cochlear damage with three perimodiolar electrode designs. *Laryngoscope, 113,* 415-419.

Fina, M., Skinner, M., Goebel, J. A., Piccirillo, J. F., Neely, J. G., & Black, O. (2003). Vestibular dysfunction after cochlear implantation. *Otology and Neurotology, 24,* 234-242; discussion 242.

Fisher, A., Mixon, J., & Herman, R. (1986). The validity of the clinical diagnosis of vestibular dysfunction. *Occupational Therapy Journal of Research, 6,* 3-20.

Folio, M. R., & Fewell, R. R, (2000). *PDMS-2: Peabody Developmental Motor Scales* (2nd ed.). Austin, TX: Pro-Ed.

Forge, A., Becker, D., Casalotti, S., Edwards, J., Marziano, N., & Nevill, G. (2003). Gap junctions in the inner ear: Comparison of distribution patterns in different vertebrates and assessment of connexin composition in mammals. *Journal of Comparative Neurology, 467,* 207-231.

Furukawa, T. (1985). Slow depolarizing response from supporting cells in the goldfish saccule. *Journal of Physiology, 366,* 107-117.

Furukawa, T., & Ishii, Y. (1967). Neurophysiological studies on hearing in goldfish. *Journal of Neurophysiology, 30,* 1377-1403.

Geddes, D. (1978). Motor development profiles of preschool deaf and hard-of-hearing children. *Perceptual and Motor Skills, 46,* 291-294.

Goldstein, R., Landau, W. M., & Kleffner, F. R. (1958). Neurological assessment of some deaf and aphasic children. *Annals of Otology, Rhinology, and Laryngology, 67,* 468-479.

Gstoettner, W., Plenk, H., Jr., Franz, P., Hamzavi, J., Baumgartner, W., Czerny, C., & Ehrenberger, K. (1997). Cochlear implant deep electrode insertion: Extent of insertional trauma. *Acta Oto-Laryngologica, 117,* 274-277.

Hamid, M. A. (2000) Contemporary neurovestibular physiologic assessment. *Current Opinion in Otolaryngology and Head and Neck Surgery, 8,* 391-397.

Hess, K., Baloh, R. W., Honrubia, V., & Yee, R. D. (1985). Rotational testing in patients with bilateral peripheral vestibular disease. *Laryngoscope, 95,* 85-88.

Higgins, K. M., Chen, J. M., Nedzelski, J. M., Shipp, D. B., & McIlmoyl, L. D. (2002). A matched-pair comparison of two cochlear implant systems. *Journal of Otolaryngology, 31,* 97-105.

Holderbaum, F. M., Ritz, S., Hassaneim, K. M., & Goetzinger, C. P. (1979). A study of otoneurologic and balance tests with deaf children. *American Annals of the Deaf, 124,* 753-759.

Horak, F. B. (1987). Clinical measurement of postural control in adults. *Physical Therapy, 67,* 1881-1885.

Horak, F. B., Shumway-Cook, A., Crowe, T. K., & Black, F. O. (1988). Vestibular function and motor proficiency of children with impaired hearing, or with learning disability and motor impairments. *Developmental Medicine and Child Neurology, 30,* 64-79.

Huygen, P. L., Hinderink, J. B., van den Broek, P., van den Borne, S., Brokx, J. P., Mens, L. H, & Admiraal, R. J. (1995). The risk of vestibular function loss after intracochlear implantation. *Acta Oto-Laryngologica, Supplement 520,* 270-272.

Huygen, P. L., van den Broek, P., Spies, T. H., Mens, L. H., & Admiraal, R. J. (1994). Does intracochlear implantation jeopardize vestibular function? *Annals of Otology, Rhinology, and Laryngology, 103,* 609–614.

Huygen, P. L., van Rijn, P. M., Cremers, C. W., & Theunissen, E. J. (1993). The vestibulo-ocular reflex in pupils at a Dutch school for the hearing impaired: Findings related to acquired causes. *International Journal of Pediatric Otorhinolaryngology, 25,* 39–47.

Ito, J. (1998). Influence of the multichannel cochlear implant on vestibular function. *Otolaryngology-Head and Neck Surgery, 118,* 900–902.

Jin, Y., Nakamura, M., Shinjo, Y., & Kaga, K. (2006). Vestibular-evoked myogenic potentials in cochlear implant children. *Acta Oto-Laryngologica, 126,* 164–169.

Johnstone, B. M., Patuzzi, R., Syka, J., & Sykova, E. (1989). Stimulus-related potassium changes in the organ of Corti of guinea-pig. *Journal of Physiology, 408,* 77–92.

Jun, A. I., McGuirt, W. T., Hinojosa, R., Green, G. E., Fischel-Ghodsian, N., & Smith, R. J. (2000). Temporal bone histopathology in connexin 26-related hearing loss. *Laryngoscope, 110,* 269–275.

Kaplan, S. L., Goddard, J., Van Kleeck, M., Catlin, F. I., & Feigin, R. D. (1981). Ataxia and deafness in children due to bacterial meningitis. *Pediatrics, 68,* 8–13.

Keane, W. M., Potsic, W. P., Rowe, L. D., & Konkle, D. F. (1979). Meningitis and hearing loss in children. *Archives of Otolaryngology, 105,* 39–44.

Kelsch, T. A., Schaefer, L. A., & Esquivel, C. R. (2006). Vestibular evoked myogenic potentials in young children: Test parameters and normative data. *Laryngoscope, 116,* 895–900.

Kempf, H. G., Johann, K., & Lenarz, T. (1999). Complications in pediatric cochlear implant surgery. *European Archives of Oto-Rhino-Laryngology, 256,* 128–132.

Kennedy, D. W. (1987). Multichannel intracochlear electrodes: Mechanism of insertion trauma. *Laryngoscope, 97,* 42–49.

Kenyon, G. S. (1988). Neuro-otological findings in normal children. *Journal of the Royal Society of Medicine, 81,* 644–648.

Kessler, P., Zarandy, M. M., Hajioff, D., Tomlinson, D., Ranalli, P., & Rutka, J. (2008). The clinical utility of search coil horizontal vestibulo-ocular reflex testing. *Acta Oto-Laryngologica, 128,* 29–37.

Kikuchi, T., Adams, J. C., Paul, D. L., & Kimura, R. S. (1994). Gap junction systems in the rat vestibular labyrinth: Immunohistochemical and ultrastructural analysis. *Acta Oto-Laryngologica, 114,* 520–528.

Kiyomizu, K., Tono, T., Komune, S., Ushisako, Y., & Morimitsu, T. (2000). Dizziness and vertigo after cochlear implantation. *Advances in Otorhinolaryngology, 57,* 173–175.

Kubo, T., Yamamoto, K., Iwaki, T., Doi, K., & Tamura, M. (2001). Different forms of dizziness occurring after cochlear implant. *European Archives of Oto-Rhino-Laryngology, 258,* 9–12.

Kushiro, K., Zakir, M., Ogawa, Y., Sato, H., & Uchino, Y. (1999). Saccular and utricular inputs to sternocleidomastoid motoneurons of decerebrate cats. *Experimental Brain Research, 126,* 410–416.

Landthaler, G., & Andrieu-Guitrancourt, J. (1975) Ataxia and deafness secondary to meningitis in children: The role of labyrinth diseases. *Archives Françaises de Pédiatrie, 32,* 319–335.

Liebman, E. P., Lovrinic, J. H., Ronis, M. L., & Katinsky, S. E. (1969). Hearing improvement following meningitis deafness. *Archives of Otolaryngology, 90,* 470–473.

Lindberg, J., Rosenhall, U., Nylen, O., & Ringner, A. (1977). Long-term outcome of Hemophilus influenzae meningitis related to antiobiotic treatment. *Pediatrics, 60,* 1–6.

Lindsey, D., & O'Neal, J. (1976). Static and dynamic balance skills of eight year old deaf and hearing children. *American Annals of the Deaf, 121,* 49–55.

Lowenstein, O. (1936). The equilibrium function of the vertebrate labyrinth. *Biological Reviews, 11,* 113–145.

McCarron, L., & Ludlow, G. (1981). Sensorineural deafness and neuromuscular dysfunctions: Considerations for vocational evaluation and job placement. *Journal of Rehabilitation, 47,* 59–79.

Merchant, S. N., & Gopen, Q. (1996). A human temporal bone study of acute bacterial meningogenic labyrinthitis. *American Journal of Otology, 17,* 375–385.

Mergner, T., & Rosemeier, T. (1998). Interaction of vestibular, somatosensory and visual signals for postural control and motion perception under terrestrial and microgravity conditions —a conceptual model. *Brain Research. Brain Research Reviews, 28*, 118-135.

Migliaccio, A. A., Della Santina, C. C., Carey, J. P., Niparko, J. K., & Minor, L. B. (2005). The vestibulo-ocular reflex response to head impulses rarely decreases after cochlear implantation. *Otology and Neurotology, 26*, 655-660.

Molony, N. C., & Marais, J. (1996). Balance after stapedectomy: The measurement of spontaneous sway by posturography. *Clinical Otolaryngology and Allied Sciences, 21*, 353-356.

Murofushi, T., & Curthoys, I. S. (1997). Physiological and anatomical study of click-sensitive primary vestibular afferents in the guinea pig. *Acta Oto-Laryngologica, 117*, 66-72.

Murofushi, T., Curthoys, I. S., Topple, A. N., Colebatch, J. G., & Halmagyi, G. M. (1995). Responses of guinea pig primary vestibular neurons to clicks. *Experimental Brain Research, 103*, 174-178.

Myklebust, H. (1964). *The psychology of deafness: Sensory deprivation, learning and adjustment* (2nd ed.), New York: Grune & Stratton.

Nadol, J. B., Jr. (1978). Hearing loss as a sequela of meningitis. *Laryngoscope, 88*, 739-755.

Newlands, S., & Wall, C., III. (2006). Vestibular function and anatomy. In B. Bailey, J. Johnson, & S. Newlands, (Eds.), *Head and neck surgery-Otolaryngology* (pp. 1905-1915). Philadelphia: Lippincott Williams & Wilkins.

O'Rahilly, R. (1963). The early development of the otic vesicle in staged human embryos. *Journal of Embryology and Experimental Morphology, 11*, 741-755.

Potter, C. N., & Silverman, L. N. (1984). Characteristics of vestibular function and static balance skills in deaf children. *Physical Therapy, 64*, 1071-1075.

Prepageran, N., Kisilevsky, V., Tomlinson, D., Ranalli, P., & Rutka, J. (2005). Symptomatic high frequency/acceleration vestibular loss: Consideration of a new clinical syndrome of vestibular dysfunction. *Acta Oto-Laryngologica, 125*, 48-54.

Rapin, I. (1974). Hypoactive labyrinths and motor development. *Clinical Pediatrics, 13*, 922-923, 926-929, 934-937.

Ribari, O., Kustel, M., Szirmai, A., & Repassy, G. (1999). Cochlear implantation influences contralateral hearing and vestibular responsiveness. *Acta Oto-Laryngologica, 119*, 225-228.

Richter, B., Aschendorff, A., Lohnstein, P., Husstedt, H., Nagursky, H., & Laszig, R. (2001). The nucleus contour electrode array: A radiological and histological study. *Laryngoscope, 111*, 508-514.

Richter, B., Jaekel, K., Aschendorff, A., Marangos, N., & Laszig, R. (2001). Cochlear structures after implantation of a perimodiolar electrode array. *Laryngoscope, 111*, 837-843.

Roeser, R. J., Campbell, J. C., & Daly, D. D. (1975). Recovery of auditory function following meningitic deafness. *Journal of Speech and Hearing Disorders, 40*, 405-411.

Rossi, G., & Bisetti, M. S. (1998). Cochlear implant and traumatic lesions secondary to electrode insertion. *Revue de Laryngologie-Otologie-Rhinologie, 119*, 317-322.

Rossi, G., Solero, P., Rolando, M., & Spadola Bisetti, M. (1998). Vestibular function and cochlear implant. *ORL: Journal for Oto-Rhino-Laryngology and Its Related Specialties, 60*, 85-87.

Sandberg, L. E., & Terkildsen, K. (1965). Caloric tests in deaf children. *Archives of Otorhinolaryngology, 81*, 350-354.

Scanlon, S. L., & Goetzinger, C. P. (1969). The health rails and Fukuda vestibular tests with deaf and hearing subjects. *Eye, Ear, Nose, and Throat Monthly, 48*, 8-15.

Schwartz, J. F. (1972). Ataxia in bacterial meningitis. *Neurology, 22*, 1071-1074.

Shephard, N. T., & Telian, S. (Eds.) (1996). Rotational chair testing in practical management of the balance disorder patient. *Practical management of the balance disordered patient* (pp. 109-128). San Diego, CA: Singular.

Shumway-Cook, A., & Horak, F. B. (1986). Assessing the influence of sensory interaction of balance. Suggestion from the field. *Physical Therapy, 66*, 1548-1550.

Shumway-Cook, A., & Woollacott, M. H. (1985). The growth of stability: Postural control from a development perspective. *Journal of Motor Behavior, 17,* 131–147.

Shupert, C. L., & Horak, F. B. (1996). Effects of vestibular loss on head stabilization in response to head and body perturbations. *Journal of Vestibular Research, 6,* 423–437.

Snashall, S. E. (1983). Vestibular function tests in children. *Journal of the Royal Society of Medicine, 76,* 555–559.

Snoeckx, R. L., Huygen, P. L., Feldmann, D., Marlin, S., Denoyelle, F., Waligora, J., et al. (2005). GJB2 mutations and degree of hearing loss: A multicenter study. *American Journal of Human Genetics, 77,* 945–957.

Spector, M. (1973). Electronstagmography after stapedectomy. *Annals of Otology, Rhinology, and Laryngology, 82,* 374–377.

Sproles, E. T. III, Azerrad, J., Williamson, C., & Merrill, R. E. (1969). Meningitis due to Hemophilus influenzae: Long-term sequelae. *Journal of Pediatrics, 75,* 782–788.

Staller, S. J., Goin, D. W., & Hildebrandt, M. (1986). Pediatric vestibular evaluation with harmonic acceleration. *Otolaryngology-Head and Neck Surgery, 95,* 471–476.

Supance, J. S., & Bluestone, C. D. (1983). Perilymph fistulas in infants and children. *Otolaryngology-Head and Neck Surgery, 91,* 663–671.

Tien, H. C., & Linthicum, F. H., Jr. (2002). Histopathologic changes in the vestibule after cochlear implantation. *Otolaryngology-Head and Neck Surgery, 127,* 260–264.

Todt, I., Hennies, H. C., Basta, D., & Ernst, A. (2005). Vestibular dysfunction of patients with mutations of Connexin 26. *Neuroreport, 16,* 1179–1181.

Tsuzuku, T., Kaga, K., Kanematsu, S., Shibata, A., & Ohde, S. (1992). Temporal bone findings in keratitis, ichthyosis, and deafness syndrome. Case report. *Annals of Otology, Rhinology, and Laryngology, 101,* 413–416.

van den Broek, P., Huygen, P. L., Mens, L. H., Admiraal, R. J., & Spies, T. (1993). Vestibular function in cochlear implant patients. *Acta Oto-Laryngologica, 113,* 263–265.

Verhagen, W. I., Huygen, P. L., & Horstink, M. W. (1987). Familial congenital vestibular areflexia. *Journal of Neurology, Neurosurgery, and Psychiatry, 50,* 933–935.

Vibert, D., Hausler, R., Kompis, M., & Vischer, M. (2001). Vestibular function in patients with cochlear implantation. *Acta Oto-Laryngologica, Supplement 545,* 29–34.

Webb, R. L., Lehnhardt, E., Clark, G. M., Laszig, R., Pyman, B. C., & Franz, B. K. (1991). Surgical complications with the cochlear multiple-channel intracochlear implant: Experience at Hannover and Melbourne. *Annals of Otology, Rhinology, and Laryngology, 100,* 131–136.

Welling, D. B., Hinojosa, R., Gantz, B. J., & Lee, J. T. (1993). Insertional trauma of multichannel cochlear implants. *Laryngoscope, 103,* 995–1001.

Young, E. D., Fernandez, C., & Goldberg, J. M. (1977). Responses of squirrel monkey vestibular neurons to audio-frequency sound and head vibration. *Acta Oto-Laryngologic, 84,* 352–360.

CHAPTER 9

Assessment of Auditory Speech-Perception Capacity

ARTHUR BOOTHROYD

Definition

For present purposes, auditory capacity is defined as the ability of the peripheral auditory system to generate useful sensory evidence about sound patterns. In this context, "useful" implies the sensitivity, resolution, and consistency needed by central systems for detection, discrimination, and recognition. We begin with four basic assumptions:

1. *Auditory capacity* is a combination of sensitivity (i.e., threshold), spectrotemporal resolution (i.e., detail), and consistency. Consistency requires that invariant features of sound patterns are represented by invariant features of neural excitation.
2. *Unaided* auditory capacity depends on the properties of cochlear and peripheral neural systems.

3. *Aided* auditory capacity depends on the properties of the hearing aid, the properties of cochlear and peripheral neural systems, and the relationships among them.
4. *Implanted* auditory capacity depends on the properties of the implant, the properties of the peripheral neural system, and the relationship between them.

These assumptions are encapsulated in Figure 9–1, in which the clamps indicate the fixed nature of cochlear and peripheral neural systems and the diagonal arrows indicate the adjustable nature of aid and implant properties. Note, also, that auditory capacity with the cochlear implant is assumed to be independent of the integrity of the cochlea and, therefore, of preimplant threshold (Boothroyd, Geers, & Moog, 1991).

Valid and reliable methods for measuring sensitivity in young children are well

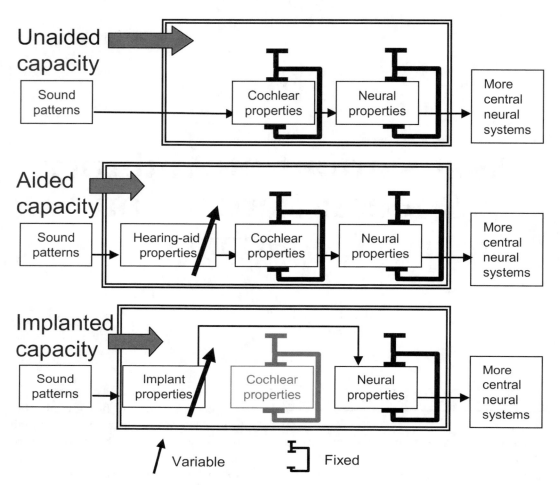

Figure 9–1. Fixed and variable factors contributing to auditory capacity, as defined in this chapter.

established. This chapter focuses on the assessment of suprathreshold resolution and consistency.

Role of Auditory Capacity

The assumptions just outlined are incorporated into the model of auditory perception illustrated in Figure 9-2. In this model, the role of auditory capacity is to provide the listener's central auditory system with sensory evidence about sound patterns and their sources. Perceptual decisions are based on this evidence together with evidence from the physical, social, and linguistic context (Boothroyd, 1991, 1997a, 1997b, 1998, 2002; Boothroyd & Nittrouer, 1988; Nittrouer & Boothroyd, 1990). The ability to make these perceptual decisions accurately and speedily depends on the listener's knowledge and skill. Experience is assumed to enhance

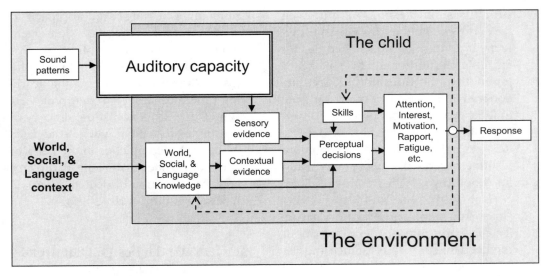

Figure 9–2. Auditory performance involves perceptual decisions based on four factors: sensory evidence, contextual evidence, listener knowledge, and listener skill. Perceptual decisions provide experience that may advance knowledge, skill, or both (*the broken lines*). The presence of perceptual and behavioral responses depends on multiple nonauditory factors.

knowledge and skill, but not auditory capacity—at least, as it is defined here.

In both natural and clinical situations, we seek evidence of perceptual decisions from a child's behavioral responses. Unfortunately, the presence of these responses depends not only on auditory capacity and perceptual abilities but also on several nonauditory factors. These include attention, comfort, interest, motivation, rapport with others present, motor skills (including speech skills), emotional state, and fatigue. These factors create a major challenge when developing or applying pediatric tests of auditory perception.

To summarize, auditory perception depends on four factors: sensory evidence, contextual evidence, knowledge, and skill. The role of auditory capacity is to provide the sensory evidence.

Why Measure Auditory Capacity?

There are several reasons for measuring both threshold and suprathreshold resolution in young children with hearing loss. For example:

1. Threshold alone is of limited value as the sole predictor of suprathreshold resolution, or as a criterion for the choice of sensory assistance (Cone-Wesson, 2003). Aided and implanted thresholds can confirm adequate audibility of conversational-level speech signals but otherwise are of no value in predicting suprathreshold resolution. It is true that, in children using hearing aids, unaided thresholds can be used to predict

suprathreshold resolution but even here, the predictions are far from perfect. In a study of aided children, for example, the author and his colleagues found that individual differences accounted for around 40% of the variance in a measure of phonetic contrast perception after the variables of hearing loss, sensation level, age, and random test-retest variability were accounted for (Boothroyd, 1995; Boothroyd, Eran, & Hanin, 1996).

2. Unassisted measures of auditory capacity can contribute to decisions about the need for sensory assistance and the choice between cochlear implants and hearing aids.

3. Postfitting measures can indicate how well one has met the immediate, or short-term, goal of sensory assistance—namely, the optimization of sensory evidence. Moreover, such measures may do so early enough to guide device adjustment and to inform decisions about habilitative intervention. Of course, the ultimate goals of hearing aids and implants in children is to facilitate spoken language acquisition and psychosocial development (NIDCD, 1995). But spoken language acquisition takes time and depends on interactions between auditory capacity and habilitative intervention (Boothroyd & Boothroyd-Turner, 2002; Boothroyd et al., 1996). Evidence of success or failure in meeting this long-term goal may come too late to ensure optimum sensory or habilitative management.

4. Knowledge of aided or implanted auditory capacity can help determine the need for, and type of, habilitative intervention. Convincing evidence of negligible auditory capacity, for example, can throw into question the advisability of pursuing a hearing-based approach to spoken language acquisition. Conversely, detailed evidence of specific capacities may help set hearing-related goals and justify the allocation of valuable learning time to hearing-based approaches.

5. Cumulative evidence of the efficacy of sensory management will help advance evidence-based practice in the fields of audiology, speech-language pathology, and the education of deaf and hard-of-hearing children (Cox, 2005).

Behavioral Approaches to Assessing Auditory Capacity

Because the primary long-term goal of sensory assistance is spoken language acquisition, behavioral techniques for assessing auditory capacity have used speech, or speechlike, stimuli. More simple stimuli such as pure-tones and broadband noise have been used in psychoacoustic research with young hearing children (Werner & Rubel, 1992), and these techniques can work well in group studies. They have not, however, been adapted for clinical use with individuals. Moreover, our ability to predict speech perception capacity from basic psychoacoustic data is extremely limited (Kuhl, 1992)—hence, the focus on speech stimuli.

One problem with the use of speech stimuli is the potential contribution of spoken language knowledge and skills, as illustrated in Figure 9–2. To minimize these effects, one needs to use basic tasks, such as the detection of phonemic contrasts, previously referred to by the author as Speech-Pattern Contrasts (SPAC) (Boothroyd, 1984, 1985a, 1995). The ability to perceive phonemic contrasts is necessary (though insufficient) for the eventual development of speech perception skills at the word and sentence levels. By embedding the contrasts in nonword stimuli we minimize lexical, syntactic, and semantic effects. This precaution does not, however, eliminate the potential effects of phonological development. Nevertheless, the child who has yet to develop a phonology may still hear, and respond to, the acoustic changes responsible for phonemic contrasts (Kuhl, Williams, Lacerda, Stevens, & Lindblom, 1992).

Criteria for an Effective Pediatric Test

In clinical testing we seek three characteristics: validity, reliability, and efficiency (Boothroyd, 1995). In other words, the test should measure what it claims to measure, variability of scores on repeated testing should be small, and the test time should be short. We achieve validity by careful choice of perceptual and response tasks. We improve reliability by increasing the number of test items, increasing the information collected on each trial, and/or reducing the effects of fluctuations in extraneous variables. Efficiency requires that adequate reliability can be attained in a short time. These three requirements interact and are often in conflict. The task of the test designer then becomes one of finding an appropriate compromise.

The foregoing comments suggest several criteria for an ideal clinical test of auditory speech-perception capacity:

1. In the interests of validity, the results should reflect the ability to detect phonologically significant contrasts among the sound patterns of speech without confounding from maturational level, cognitive status, language knowledge, language competence, reading ability, or motor speech skills.
2. Nevertheless, the results should be predictive of the potential for development of spoken language competence.
3. Phonemic contrasts should be presented in a varying phonetic context to ensure that the child is responding to invariant cues rather than to context-specific cues.
4. The procedure should be interesting enough to maintain motivation and compliance for the length of time needed for testing.
5. It should be possible to obtain a reasonably small standard deviation of repeated scores (say, under 10 percentage points) in a time that is commensurate with the limitations of attention, interest, and compliance.

What follows is an account of the author's search for appropriate ways to satisfy these criteria.

The Spac (Speech-Pattern Contrast) Test

The original Spac test was developed for studies of auditory speech-perception capacity in orally trained deaf children. Stimuli were real words produced at the end of a carrier phrase—for example, "Underline the word 'pan.'" The response was selection from four printed alternatives. To optimize efficiency each response was scored twice, once for each of two binary contrasts. Consider, for example, a stimulus of Pan and possible responses of Pan, Ban, Fan, and Van. Responses of Pan or Fan would be scored correct for initial consonant voicing whereas responses of Pan or Ban would be scored correct for initial consonant continuance.

The Spac test was administered from recordings, under headphones, at the highest comfortable level, to 120 prelingually hearing-impaired listeners between the ages of 11 and 18 years (Boothroyd, 1984). Three-frequency average hearing loss ranged from 55 dB to 123 dB HL. All listeners were students in an oral school for the deaf. As in previous studies of this type (Erber, 1972, 1979; Hack & Erber, 1982; Pickett et al., 1972; Risberg, 1976), some contrasts were found to be more resistant to the effects of hearing loss than others. Suprasegmental contrasts were perceived better than segmental contrasts and vowel contrasts were perceived better than consonant contrasts. Among vowels, height contrasts were perceived better than place (front/back) contrasts. Among consonants, voicing and continuance contrasts were perceived better than place-of-articulation contrasts. Mean performance on all contrasts fell with increasing hearing loss. The 3-frequency average pure-tone threshold accounted for 61% of the variance in composite contrast score.

The obvious drawback to the original Spac test was the need for reading skills. In the study just described, this was not a serious problem because the curriculum of the students' school placed a strong emphasis on the early development of reading in parallel with spoken language. But the need for reading prevents application to children younger than 7 or 8 years, or even to older children if they have poor reading skills.

Other researchers have developed forced-choice tests of speech perception performance involving picture identification (Ross, Kessler, Philips, & Lerman, 1972; Tyler, 1993). These tests avoid the issue of reading and are applicable to children younger then 7 years. They do, however, retain potential effects of vocabulary knowledge.

Three-Interval Forced-Choice Test of Speech-Pattern Contrast Perception (ThriftSpac)

Reading and vocabulary effects were eliminated in ThriftSpac. In this test, the stimulus consisted of three nonword syllables of which two were the same and one differed along a single phonetic dimension. The response task was to indicate the position of the odd man out (Boothroyd, 1995). The oddity approach already had been used successfully in psychoacoustic studies with normally hearing 3-year-olds by Allen and colleagues (Allen, Wightman, Kistler, & Dolan, 1989) and also by Most (1985) in a study of intonation perception in hearing and hearing-impaired 3-year-olds.

Application of a computer-assisted version of ThriftSpac to hearing adults listening to low-pass filtered speech showed a strong association between composite contrast scores and sentence-level performance (Boothroyd, 1991). Studies of children with normal hearing (Hnath-Chisolm, Laippley, & Boothroyd, 1998) and aided and implanted children with hearing loss (Boothroyd, 1995) confirmed the usability and reliability of ThriftSpac, but only for children above 7 years of age. Even after age 7 there was evidence that performance continued to improve with age. Although ThriftSpac is suitable for research in adults and older children, it is boring, cognitively demanding, and not very efficient. It remains to be seen whether these problems could be overcome in a more appealing video-game format.

Imitative Test of the Perception of Speech-Pattern Contrasts (ImSpac)

The issue of age was addressed in ImSpac (Boothroyd, 1997a, 1998; Boothroyd et al., 1996). Children were presented with non-word utterances, and asked to repeat them. Responses were recorded for subsequent evaluation. Testing was carried out in two phases: the first by hearing plus vision (plus text and/or finger spelling, if appropriate) and the second by hearing alone. Performance on the first phase was intended to provide an estimate of the child's best production. Performance on the second phase was intended to provide an estimate of auditory perception capacity—at least up to any limits imposed by production skills.

The child's recorded utterances were extracted, digitized, and prepared for evaluation in which teams of four auditors selected, from four alternatives, the one they thought the child was trying to imitate. The forced-choice approach to evaluating production minimizes the effect of listener experience in evaluating the speech of children with hearing loss (Boothroyd, 1985b). As with the original Spac test, each response provided information on the perception of two binary contrasts, thereby increasing efficiency.

ImSpac proved appropriate for children down to around 3 years of age and was used effectively in studies of the relative efficacy of hearing aids and cochlear implants in children with hearing loss (Boothroyd, 1997a, 1998; Boothroyd et al., 1996). In a group of 97 hearing-aid users between the ages of 3 and 15 years, age accounted for only an insignificant 1.5% of the variance in auditory-only composite ImSpac score, and

mode of communication (oral versus total communication) accounted for none (Boothroyd et al., 1996). This finding suggested that we were moving closer to a test of auditory capacity that was unaffected by knowledge, skill, maturation and other nonauditory factors. The auditory-visual ImSpac score, however, improved significantly with age and oral training. And in six children who were followed longitudinally after receiving multichannel cochlear implants, both auditory-only and auditory-visual ImSpac performance improved for one or two years after surgery (Boothroyd, 1998; Boothroyd et al., 1996). The last two findings imply that the ImSpac score is by no means a pure measure of capacity.

Although the effectiveness of ImSpac as a research tool was demonstrated in the work just cited, there were two obvious limitations to its application as a clinical tool. The first was the time, personnel, and cost involved in editing and auditing the child's recorded utterances. Kosky, however, demonstrated that the technique could be used online by a single tester/listener who is visually and auditorily blinded to the stimuli presented to the child (Kosky & Boothroyd, 2003). Further work led to the development of an on-line version (OlimSpac), described below.

The second problem with an imitative approach is the need for speech production skills on the part of the child. This problem limits the application of the test to children who are postlingually deafened or, if prelingually deafened, have had the opportunity to acquire speech production skills through appropriate management—including optimal use of hearing. In most of the studies conducted with ImSpac using children with hearing loss, auditory-visual performance has exceeded auditory-only performance by between 10 and 20 percentage points

(Boothroyd & Boothroyd-Turner, 2002; Boothroyd et al., 1996). This finding implies that production skills have not placed a limit on the ability to imitate auditorily presented stimuli, at least in the populations tested. Indeed, it is more likely that, for children trained in an auditory-oral program, auditory speech-perception capacity is the determinant of speech production skill rather than the reverse. Note, also, that the forced-choice approach requires only that the child produces detectable and consistent differences. The child does not need to produce each phoneme accurately. The fact remains, however, that the test is unsuitable for children who have not developed reasonable production skills. It also is unsuitable for children younger than 3 years of age.

On-Line Imitative Test of Speech-Pattern Contrast Perception (OlimSpac)

The on-line version of ImSpac is one of a battery of tests developed by the author and his colleagues at the House Ear Institute for ongoing research into the early development and assessment of hearing, speech, and language skills in aided and implanted children (Eisenberg, Martinez, & Boothroyd, 2003, 2007). The concept behind the test battery is that the perceptual task and test stimuli should remain constant across all tests but that the response tasks should differ according to the maturation and interest level of the child. The goal is to allow within-child, within-group, and across-group comparisons of scores obtained with different tests.

The computer-assisted version of Olim-Spac is designed to be used with a single computer, supplemented with a slave monitor. The basic test arrangement is shown in Figure 9–3, taken from the software manual. Visual stimuli are shown on the left side of the screens and the tester's controls and response options are shown on the right. The child is prevented from seeing the controls by a simple cardboard mask. The tester is blinded to the visual component of a stimulus by a second cardboard mask, and to the auditory component by a broad-band masking noise. The masking noise lasts only as long as the auditory stimulus, so that the tester can hear and respond to the child's imitation. There are eight response alternatives, allowing the simultaneous collection of information on three binary contrasts (Figure 9–4). A single test presentation consists of eight trials using one set of response alternatives and another eight trials using a second set—giving information on six contrasts. The contrasts are:

1. Vowel Height (VH) as in /oo/ versus /ah/
2. Vowel Place (VP) as in /oo/ versus /ee/
3. Consonant Voicing (CV) as in /d/ versus /t/
4. Consonant Continuance (CC) as in /t/ versus /s/
5. Consonant Place front (CPf) as in /d/ versus /b/
6. Consonant Place rear[1] (CPr) as in /s/ versus /sh/

A combination of data for the first two contrasts provides information on vowel-contrast perception. A combination of data for the last four contrasts provides information on consonant-contrast perception.

---

[1]In this context, "front" and "rear" mean pre- and postalveolar, respectively. Prealveolar consonant contrasts are typically more visible.

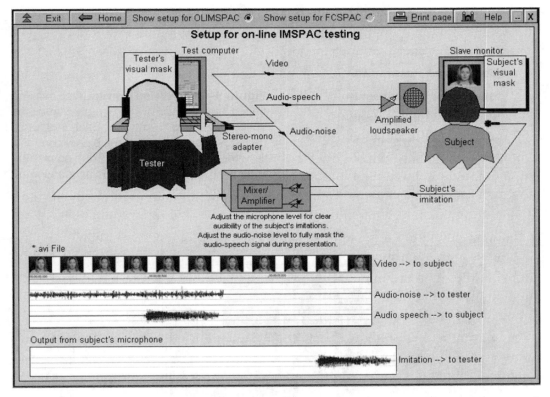

Figure 9–3. The test setup for the On-Line Imitative test of Speech-Pattern Contrast perception (OlimSpac). The tester is prevented from seeing or hearing the stimulus presented to the child. The child is prevented from seeing the tester's controls.

A combination of data for all six contrasts provides weighted information on phoneme-contrast perception.[2]

Two things should be noted about this contrast set. First, it involves only segmental contrasts. Unlike the earlier Spac tests, there is no attempt to evaluate suprasegmentals. Second, this contrast set is used, not only for OlimSpac, but also for the four tests still to be described. These five tests form the House Ear Institute's Battery of Auditory speech-perception Tests for Infants and Toddlers (BATIT) (Eisenberg et al., 2007).

A complete OlimSpac administration consists of 16 auditory-visual trials and 16 auditory-only trials.[3] The software generates a profile of performance on each contrast plus an average (composite) score together with confidence limits for scores based on random guessing. As an example, Figure 9–5 shows the contrast profile for a 5-year-old cochlear implant user, several

---

[2]The contribution of consonant contrasts to the composite score is twice that of vowel contrasts. Among the consonant contrasts, the contribution of place is twice that of either voicing or continuance. The goal is to reflect, albeit crudely, the relative contributions of the segmental contrasts to word- and sentence-level speech perception.
[3]The option is also provided for visual-only presentation, if required.

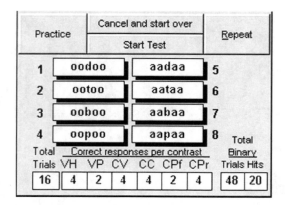

Figure 9–4. When testing via OlimSpac, the tester must decide which of eight stimuli the child was trying to imitate. Each response provides information on three binary contrasts —in this case, vowel height (VH), consonant voicing (CV), and prealveolar consonant place (CPf).

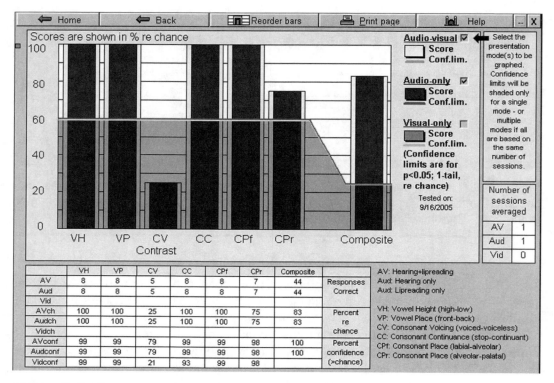

Figure 9–5. The contrast-perception profile of a 5-year-old user of a multichannel cochlear implant, obtained with audio-only and audio-visual presentation of OlimSpac. This child passed five of the six contrasts at a confidence level of 98%. The exception was consonant voicing (CV).

years postimplant. These data were collected by the author during formative evaluation of the test. Note the apparent difficulty with the consonant voicing contrast (CV).

Figure 9–6 shows the composite auditory-visual and auditory-only scores (corrected for guessing) as a function of age for five small groups of children with normal

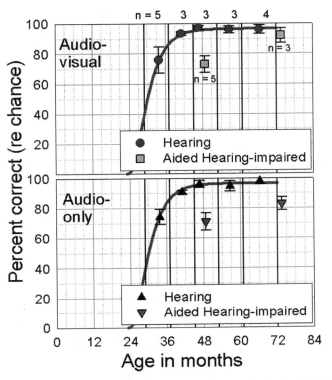

Figure 9–6. Composite audiovisual and audio-only OlimSpac scores, as functions of mean age, for five small groups of children with normal hearing and two small groups of aided children with hearing loss.

hearing and two small groups of aided children with hearing loss. These data were collected during formative evaluation and norming of the test by Laurie Eisenberg and Amy Martinez of the House Ear Institute. Means are fit by cubed exponential growth functions (Boothroyd, 2008). The data support the conclusion that one should expect scores of 90% or higher for hearing children who have passed their third birthday. Further analysis showed that the reduced scores for younger children were attributable to contrasts of consonant voicing, continuance, and postalveolar place. There was little evidence from these normally hearing data that auditory-visual performance was better than audio-only. The 6-year-old hearing-impaired children, however, did provide weak evidence of the expected audio-visual advantage.

Video-Game Test of Speech-Pattern Contrast Perception (VidSpac)

VidSpac is one of a series of tests in which the listener is rewarded for a response to a temporary phonemic change (deviant utterances) in a continuous string of nonword standard utterances. This approach was originally developed for research into auditory development in children with normal hearing

(Eilers, Wilson, & Moore, 1977; Kuhl, 1979, 1991; Kuhl et al., 1992; Marean, Werner, & Kuhl, 1991; Nittrouer, 1996) and has been adapted for clinical evaluation of children with hearing loss (Boothroyd, 2005; Daemers et al., 2006; Dawson, Nott, Clark, & Cowan, 1998; Eisenberg et al., 2007; Govaerts et al., 2006; Martinez, Eisenberg, Boothroyd, & Visser-Dumont, 2008). The approach has similarities to the change-no change test which was developed in the early days of pediatric cochlear implant research. In this test, the child is presented with strings of eight syllables and is asked to respond verbally, by button push, or by some play activity, to the strings in which the last four syllables are different from the first four (Carney et al., 1993; Osberger et al., 1991; Sussman, 1993).

The game format in VidSpac is intended to enhance motivation, prolong participation, and, if appropriate, allow self-testing. Once the program is started, the child effectively tests herself (Figure 9–7). A software-selectable cartoon playmate produces the utterances while holding a box (Figure 9–8). Hits are positively reinforced by adding the box to a collection on the screen. False positives are negatively reinforced by discarding the box. After a run of four trials for a given contrast, the saved boxes vanish to reveal hidden characters and the listener chooses one to watch in a short cartoon

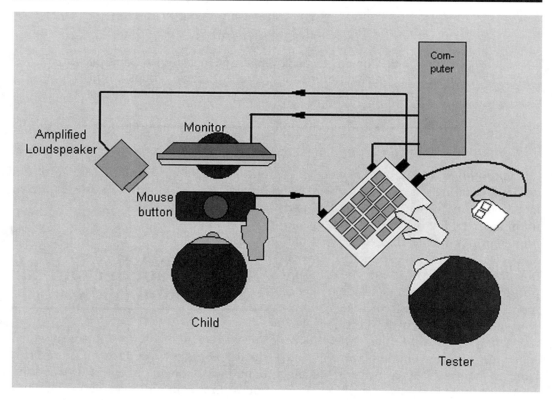

Figure 9–7. A simple setup for sound-field testing with the video-game test of Speech-Pattern Contrast Perception (VidSpac).

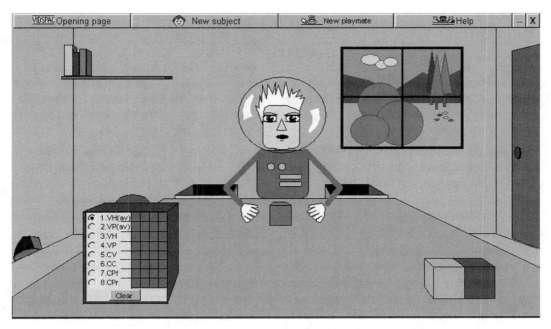

Figure 9–8. In VidSpac, a cartoon "playmate" retrieves a colored box and begins to produce a string of standard utterances. The child's task is to press a button when a deviant utterance is produced. Hits are rewarded by collecting boxes at the front of the table. False positives are "punished" by discarding the box. After four deviant trials, the boxes open to reveal cartoon characters and the child selects one to watch in a short animated cartoon before returning to the listening task.

before returning to testing. The test uses the same recorded stimuli and the same contrasts as in OlimSpac. For training purposes, the two vowel contrasts are shown with changing mouth shapes.

Results are automatically logged and displayed as a profile, with confidence limits based on the measured false-positive rate. Figure 9–9 illustrates the contrast profile generated by the same listener shown in Figure 9–5. Note the persistence of problems with consonant voicing.

VidSpac was used in a study of the effects of spectral degradation on speech perception by hearing children as young as five (Eisenberg, Shannon, Martinez, Wygon-

ski, & Boothroyd, 2000). Further experience has shown it suitable for children down to about four years of age.

Visual-Response and Interactive-Play Tests of Speech-Pattern Contrast Perception (V.I.P.Spac)

A variation on the change detection approach is V.I.P.Spac. Like VidSpac, this test also measures responses to a temporary phonemic change in an otherwise unchanging string of nonword utterance.

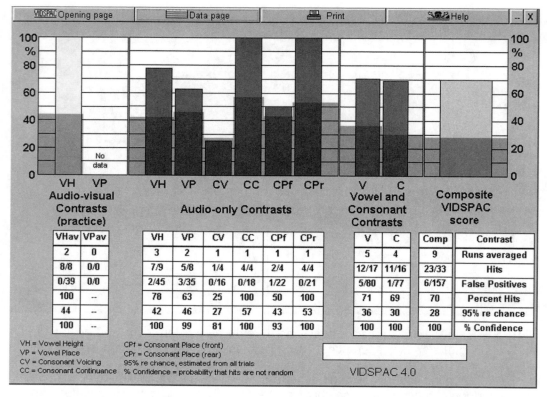

Figure 9–9. A contrast-perception profile generated by VidSpac. The shaded areas show the 95% confidence limits for scores based on random responses—estimated from false-positive responses. This profile is for the same child whose OlimSpac data were shown in Figure 9–5. Note the persistence of problems with consonant voicing (CV).

One of the problems with pediatric tests of contrast perception is that each is only applicable over a limited age range, making it difficult to track changes within a subject, or to compare subject groups of different ages. To address this problem, V.I.P.Spac incorporates three tests using different response modes appropriate to children of different age (Eisenberg et al., 2007; Martinez et al., 2008). The three tests are:

1. VRASpac, which requires a conditioned head turn response, rewarded by animated toy, cartoon, or video-clip (Figure 9-10). This test is suitable for children between about 6 and 18 months of age.[4]
2. PlaySpac, which requires a play response such as placing a block on a tower or dropping it into a bucket (Figure 9-11). The reward is intrinsic, enhanced by social approval. PlaySpac is suitable for children over 3 years of age.

---

[4]A similar test (VRSID) is commercially available, at the time of writing, from Intelligent Hearing Systems (www.ihsys.com).

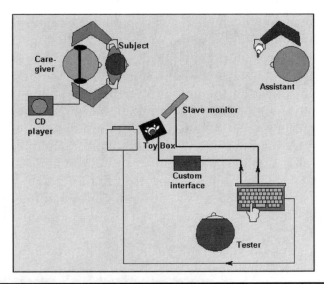

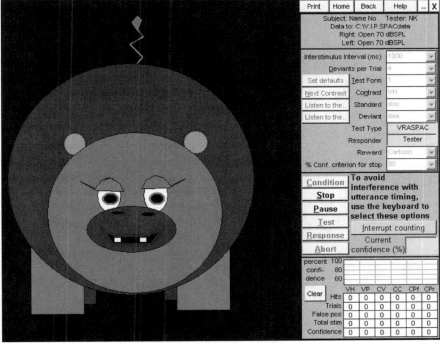

Figure 9–10. The upper panel shows the basic setup for contrast-perception testing via VraSpac. The lower panel shows the tester's controls on the right and an example of an animated cartoon reinforcer on the left. A simple cardboard mask hides the tester's controls from the child.

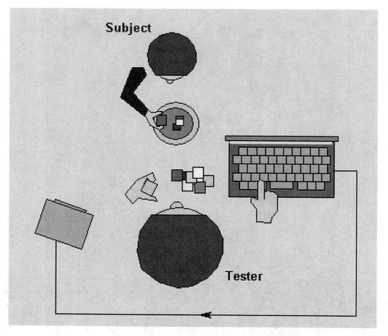

Figure 9–11. A simple setup for sound-field testing via PlaySpac.

3. ButtonSpac, which requires a button or keyboard press, rewarded by advancing an on-screen jigsaw puzzle (Figure 9–12). This test is suitable for children over about 4 years of age.

The reader will recognize that these variations are adapted from pediatric threshold audiometry. The difference is that the stimulus is a change from standard to deviant utterance rather than a change from silence to sound.

In all three of the V.I.P.Spac tests, the onset interval of the repeated utterances is selectable from 500 to 1200 msec. The number of deviant utterances that will be played before returning to the standard is selectable from one to seven. The standard utterance is selectable as either "ootoo" or "oodoo," giving two forms of the test. It is also possible for users to substitute other stimuli (Uhler, 2008). All responses are logged in the computer and are automatically classified as hits or false positives. The "hit" window begins with the second deviant utterance and lasts for 1.5 times the duration of the deviant utterances. The software computes a running estimate of the probability that the child is not responding at random and testing stops either when this estimate reaches a criterion (selectable between 75 and 95%) or after a fixed number of "change" trials. The purpose of the stopping rules is to take as much advantage as possible of the limited testing time that is available when working with young children. Although scores can be reported as percent correct, they are usually based on very few trials. It makes more sense, therefore, to record performance in terms of

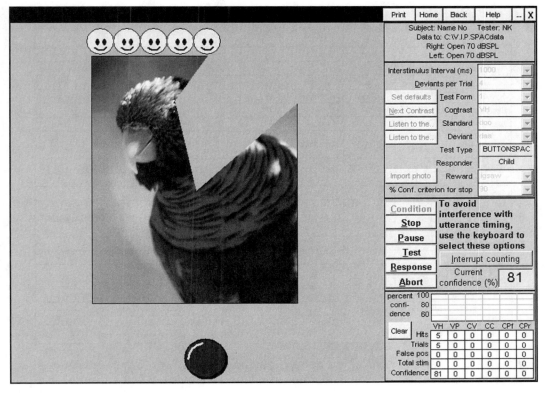

Figure 9–12. In ButtonSpac, a response to change is rewarded by adding a piece to an on-screen jigsaw.

Pass/Fail, at a given level of confidence, for each contrast tested. Testing time for six contrasts depends on the false-positive rate, the time taken for conditioning or training, and the stopping criterion. It can average around 20 minutes for VRASpac and around 12 minutes for the other two tests.

Summary of the Speech-Pattern Contrast Tests

For reference, Figure 9–13 provides a summary of the eight tests just described.

When examining this figure, please note the following.

Computer Assistance

Most of the tests are designed for computer-based application, that is, a computer is used for presentation of stimuli, logging of responses, and computation of scores and/or confidence levels. Exceptions were the original Spac test which was a pencil and paper test, and the original ImSpac test in which only the task of the auditors was computerized.

	Original Spac	Thrift-Spac	ImSpac	OlimSpac	VidSpac	VRASpac	PlaySpac	Button-Spac
			Speech Pattern Contrast Tests					
Computerized	No	Yes	Partial	Yes	Yes	Yes	Yes	Yes
Stimuli	Words	non-words	non-words	non-words	non-words	non-words	non-words	non-words
Auditory	Yes	Yes	Yes	Yes	Yes	Yes	Yes	Yes
Visual	No	Yes	Yes	Yes	No	No	No	No
Contrasts/trial	2	1	2	3	1	1	1	1
Game format	No	Could be	No	No	Yes	No	Yes	Yes
Response	Word-choice	Odd man out	Imitation	Imitation	Button press	Head turn	Play action	Button press
Needs reading	Yes	No	No	No	No	No	No	No
Needs speech	No	No	Yes	Yes	No	No	No	No
Stopping rule	No	No	No	No	No	Yes	Yes	Yes
Score	%	%	%	%	%	Pass/Fail plus confidence	Pass/Fail plus confidence	Pass/Fail plus confidence
Est. time (min)	5	10	10	5	20	20	12	12
Age-range (y)	7+	7+	3+	3+	4+	0.5 to 1.5	3+	4+
Availability at time of writing	No	No	No	Yes*	Yes**	Yes*	Yes*	Yes*
* contact: leisenberg@hei.org				<----------	---------------	Same stimulus set --	---------->	
** contact: aboothroyd@cox.net						<----------	V.I.P.Spac	---------->
				<----------	HEI Battery of Auditory Tests		---------->	
					for Infants and Toddlers (BATIT)			

Figure 9–13. Characteristics of the Speech-Pattern Contrast tests described in this chapter. See the text for more detailed information on the criteria listed in the first column.

Stimuli

All but one of the tests uses non-word stimuli to avoid lexical and semantic influences. The exception is the original Spac test, which used meaningful words. The five tests of the BATIT battery have used both consonant-vowel and vowel-consonant-vowel utterances. The latter were introduced to provide the listener with both pre- and postvocalic coarticulation cues to consonant contrasts.

Modality

All tests obviously provide information on auditory contrast perception. ThriftSpac and the two imitative tests can also provide information on visual and auditory-visual perception.

Contrasts Per Trial

In the interests of efficiency, the original Spac test was designed to provide information on two contrasts at each trial. This feature was extended to three contrasts per trial in OlimSpac. Unfortunately, the "change" tests cannot take advantage of this feature.

Response Task and Game Format

The forced-choice word identification response task of the original Spac test and the three-interval forced-choice response task of ThriftSpac render them unsuitable for children below 7 or 8 years of age. Imitation, however, is a natural behavior for young children, making it suitable as a response task down to around 3 years. Moreover, if the child has a hearing loss, there is a good chance that he will have become very familiar with imitative activities during habilitative intervention. Similarly the head turn, to locate and identify interesting events, is natural for very young children and can be conditioned down to around 6 months of age. Depending on the skills and affect of the tester, children who have reached 3 years of age usually are prepared to interact in a game whose rules are determined by an adult. Simple button pushing is by no means an ideal response but can be effective if the consequences of a correct response are interesting enough.

Reading and Speech

The original Spac test is the only one that requires reading skills. The two imitation tests require motor speech skills and therefore cannot be used with children who have not had an opportunity to develop the phonology and motor speech skills required for spoken language.

Stopping Rule

In Spac, ThriftSpac, ImSpac, OlimSpac, and VidSpac there is no stopping rule. As a result, the time of administration depends on the intrinsic structure of the test, time taken for explanation or training, and the response time of the subject. In the original ImSpac test, there was, of course, additional time involved in editing and auditing the child's imitations but this did not impact clinical testing time. In the three tests of V.I.P.Spac, testing stops either when the results provide reasonable confidence in the conclusion that the child is not responding at random, or when a certain number of changes have been presented. Consequently, the time taken for these three tests depends on the preset confidence criterion, the false-positive rate, and the frequency with which the tester initiates the change to a different utterance. Interestingly, a prolonged period of no change, without false positives, steadily increases confidence in the conclusion that prior hits were not the result of random responses. In the case of VRASpac, total test time must, unfortunately, include the time needed to condition (and sometimes recondition) the child.

Type of Score

Whereas the early Spac tests sought a percent correct score, more recent efforts in V.I.P.Spac have focused on estimating confidence that the child is not responding at random, the aim being to minimize valuable testing time. Performance on a single contrast therefore, is reported as pass/fail with an associated confidence level. A composite score can be expressed as the number of contrasts (out of six) meeting the criterion for a pass, but this is not equivalent to the percent correct composite scores of the other tests.

Esimated Test Times

The estimated times are based on the assumption that a complete test will evaluate performance on six contrasts. The original Spac, ThriftSpac, and ImSpac tests actually used more contrasts, but the more recent tests focus on just six segmental contrasts. In terms of time taken, OlimSpac clearly has an advantage because each trial provides simultaneous information on three contrasts. This advantage, however, is offset by the need for production skills and, to a certain extent, by the increased complexity of the test setup, as illustrated in Figure 9–3.

Age Range

VraSpac is the only test that is suitable for children below 3 years of age. Unfortunately, its suitability diminishes rapidly after around 18 months of age.[5] This leaves a gap of around two years during which, at the time of writing, we have no appropriate behavioral test of phonemic contrast perception.

Discussion

Validity

Do the tests just described actually measure auditory speech-perception capacity? For reasons explained earlier, tests of the ability to detect phonologically significant changes in a varying phonetic context have face validity as an *indicator* of capacity. It is important to remember, however, that behavioral tests are measures of performance. They are not direct measures of capacity. The best we can hope for is that we have minimized the influence of other factors so that the primary determinant of performance, in fact, is the underlying capacity.

With the exception of the original Spac, the tests described here clearly eliminate the effects of lexical, syntactic, and semantic development. But their very nature implies that they can be sensitive to phonological development. In the case of the imi-

tative tests, motor speech skills also are involved. And for the other tests, we make the untested assumption that a child whose phonological development is incomplete can deal with the task at an acoustic level rather than a phonetic level. Then there is the basic issue of perceptual development —that is, the development of the knowledge and skills needed to take full advantage of sensory and contextual evidence when making auditory perceptual decisions. A relevant anecdote in this connection comes from the implanted child whose performance data are illustrated in Figure 9–5 and Figure 9–9. After the difficulties with consonant voicing were brought to the attention of the speech pathologist, she spent some time focusing on the voice/voiceless distinction. Very soon the child was able to perform perfectly on this contrast.

Added to learning issues are those of attention, comfort, motivation, interest, boredom, fatigue, and compliance. In short, only if a child scores 100% on these tests, can we infer that the underlying capacity is present. If the score is less than 100% we can only conclude that the capacity is at least as good as indicated but it may be better. But we cannot, with confidence, attribute departures from 100% to a loss of capacity rather than to other factors. There is, in fact, plenty of evidence of learning effects for children newly fitted with cochlear implants. The assumption that we can immediately determine auditory speech-perception capacity in newly implanted children, using tests of phonemic contrasts perception, is clearly false.

Associated with issues of validity and learning is that of neural plasticity. The separation between peripheral and central mechanisms implied in the introduction is

---

[5]The conditioned head turn can be used for threshold assessment up to the age of three (Madell, 2008), but interest and motivation fall rapidly after 18 months of age—seriously limiting available testing time when the task is used for contrast-perception assessment.

open to question. One can argue that the ability of peripheral mechanisms to deliver useful information is, in part, dependent on the adaptation of central mechanisms to deal with that information. Moreover, communication between peripheral and central mechanisms is a two-way street. We know that efferent fibers in the auditory nerve carry signals that can modify the properties of the cochlea. It is difficult to see how such fibers can have any effect on the properties of a cochlear implant, but it is likely that such two-way communication also operates at every level in the brainstem, the cortex, and association areas. In other words, changes in neural organization may well increase the ability of more central systems to take advantage of any detail being generated at the periphery. We certainly have clear evidence from animal research of cortical reorganization in response to auditory stimulation (Stanton & Harrison, 1996). And there is evidence from human research of experience-mediated changes in cortical electrophysiological responses to speech (Tremblay, Kraus, & McGee, 1998).

If, in fact, inexperienced perceptual systems are unable to take full advantage of auditory capacity, as defined in this chapter, then the search for a behavioral measure of that capacity in children who are either very young, or are only recently provided with sensory assistance, may well be futile.

From the analysis just presented, we must conclude that a single administration of any of these tests is not necessarily a valid indicator of capacity unless the child performs perfectly. This does not mean, however, that the tests have no clinical value. One of the benefits of tests of contrast detection is that they can be administered to children as young as six months. Moreover any learning is likely to be completed in a much shorter time than that required for tasks involving higher levels of knowledge and skill, both perceptual and

linguistic (Uhler, 2008). To address learning effects, it becomes imperative that tests are repeated over time. The resulting longitudinal performance data offer two benefits. First, one can discard low outliers as attributable to non-auditory factors such as motivation, fatigue, irritability, and so on. Second, the scores that are not discarded most likely will show an exponential growth pattern, the asymptote of which may be taken as a valid indicator of capacity. One of the theoretical benefits of the BATIT test battery is that longitudinal data can be collected as the child passes through several maturational stages, using different response tasks.

Reliability

It will not have escaped the reader's notice that Figure 9–13 contains no data on reliability. There are several reasons for this omission. First, reliability depends, in part, on the number of trials on which a single score is based. Second, reliability for an individual child may well depend on the consistency of the many nonauditory factors that influence performance. In other words, inherently good reliability of a test procedure can well be undermined by poor reliability of the child.

Of the tests described here, only Thrift-Spac has been used in empirical measures of reliability (Boothroyd, 1995). Test-retest data were collected from older children with hearing loss, using six trials for each of nine contrasts. Composite scores therefore were based on 54 trials. The measured standard deviation of repeated scores (after correction for guessing) was 9 percentage points. This value compared favorably with the worst case of 10 percentage points predicted from the application of binomial theory (Boothroyd, 1968; Thornton & Raffin, 1978), supporting the conclusion that we were measuring the inherent reliability of the procedure and that the subjects themselves were performing consistently.

Among the current BATIT tests, only OlimSpac and VidSpac lend themselves to application of binomial theory. In OlimSpac there are eight trials for each of six contrasts, giving 48 trials for the composite score. The predicted worst case gives a standard deviation of repeated scores of 14.4 percentage points—after correction for guessing (which, unfortunately, is 50% for all contrasts). The virtue of OlimSpac is that three contrasts are tested simultaneously, thus reducing testing time. For VidSpac, there are four trials for each of six contrasts giving only 24 trials for the composite score. The worst case prediction for the standard deviation of repeated scores is 10.2 percentage points. This value assumes there is no correction for guessing—an assumption that becomes invalid if there is a high false-positive rate. These numbers seem quite high but they apply to the worst case, when the probability of a correct response is close to 50%. The predicted standard deviation falls as scores move closer to 100%. Remember, also, that the worst case standard deviation predicted by binomial theory for a word recognition score based on a 50-word list is not much better—at around 7.1 percentage points.

The foregoing discussion deals only with composite scores—averaged across several contrasts. For single contrasts, test-retest variability is very high and it makes more sense to think in terms of pass/fail. A pass requires that the score is significantly higher, at some level of confidence, from that predicted from random guessing. For OlimSpac a score of seven correct out of the eight trials is needed for a pass, with 95% confidence, on a single contrast.

As indicated earlier, the pass/fail approach is used for the three "change" tests of V.I.P.Spac but the expected performance from random responses has to be measured as the test progresses. We cannot, therefore, apply binomial theory to obtain an a priori estimate of inherent reliability.

In summary, we can only estimate inherent reliability for some of the tests described here. When we do this, reliability is only fair. It could be improved by increasing the number of trials per contrast but, unfortunately, one would then encounter a law of diminishing returns. By extending testing time, we increase the likelihood that inattention, boredom, or some other non-auditory variable will undermine not only reliability but also validity. These considerations provide yet one more reason for the collection of longitudinal data.

Prediction of Sentence Level Performance from Contrast Perception Data

One criterion for validity, mentioned earlier, is that the results should be predictive of eventual sentence-level performance. The author has developed formulae for such predictions, based on probability theory. The formulae make use of two factors. The j-factor deals with the perception of wholes as predicted from the perception of the constituent parts. The k-factor deals with the perception of parts in context as predicted from the perception of the same parts in isolation (Boothroyd, 1978, 1985b, 2002; Boothroyd & Nittrouer, 1988; Nittrouer & Boothroyd, 1990). The equation relating contrast perception to the perception of words in sentences is as follows:

$$p_{ws} = 1-(1-(1-(1-p_c^{jp})^{kw})^{jw})^{ks} \quad (1)$$

Where:

p_{ws} = the probability of recognizing words in sentences.

p_c = the probability of detecting binary phonemic contrasts.

jp = the effective number of independent binary contrasts required for recognition of a phoneme.

kw = the effect of CVC word context on phoneme recognition.

jw = the effective number of independent phonemes in a CVC word.

ks = the effect of sentence context on word recognition.

Figure 9–14 illustrates this relationship for competent listeners under the following assumptions, based partly on empirical data (Boothroyd, 1991; Boothroyd & Nittrouer, 1988; Nittrouer & Boothroyd, 1990):

1. An average of 4 independent binary contrasts are needed to define a phoneme (jp = 4).
2. CVC word context multiplies the effective number of channels of independent information in a phoneme by a factor of 1.3 (kp = 1.3).
3. There are effectively 2.5 independent phonemes in a CVC word (jw =2.5).
4. The effect of sentence context is to multiply the effective number of channels of independent information in a word by between 2 (difficult sentences) and 10 (easy sentences) (ks).

Also shown in Figure 9–14 are group mean data for 8 children using multichannel cochlear implants. Average age at testing was 11 years. Average age at implantation was 6 years. Average duration of implant use was 5 years. Average composite score on ImSpac was 85% (= 70% after correction for guessing). Word recognition in preschool-level sentences was 62%. Word recognition in Grade-5-level sentences was 83%. The average k-factors for preschool- and grade-5-level sentences were 7 and 3, respectively. All data are for hearing alone (Boothroyd & Boothroyd-Turner, 2002).

Findings such as these suggest that information about phonemic contrast perception can be used to make realistic predictions about the probable development of sentence-level perception in children with hearing loss.

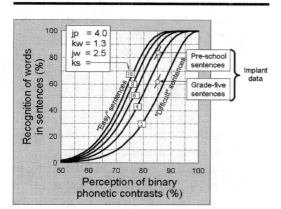

Figure 9–14. Predicted relationships between phoneme-level contrast perception and sentence-level word recognition, based on equation (1). The two data points are means for a group of cochlear implant users listening to, and repeating, both preschool-level sentences and grade-five-level sentences.

Electrophysiologic Approaches

It is possible that developmental and non-auditory barriers to the behavioral assessment of peripheral capacity can be overcome by the use of electrophysiology. Certainly, electrophysiology has solved many of the problems associated with threshold measurement in infants.

At the time of writing, several researchers are exploring the possibility of assessing suprathreshold auditory resolution by means of electrophysiology. To this end, the author and his colleagues have focused on the Acoustic Change Complex (ACC). The ACC is an N1P2 cortical response to a change in the middle of an ongoing stimulus. We first observed this complex in response to the transition from consonant to vowel in a consonant-vowel syllable (Ostroff, Martin, & Boothroyd, 1999). We subsequently showed that the complex could be evoked by changes of amplitude, spectrum, and periodicity in speechlike sounds (Martin & Boothroyd, 1999, 2000). We also showed that the threshold for detection of the ACC in response to a second formant shift during a synthetic 3-formant vowel could be detected in hearing adults at levels that are close to those found behaviorally (Ostroff, 1999). Since that initial work, Martin has demonstrated the possibility of removing the electrical artifact from the ACC when testing individuals with cochlear implants (Martin, 2007).

MisMatch Negativity (MMN) also has received attention as a possible electrophysiologic index of contrast perception. MMN is a difference between responses to standard and deviant stimuli in a paradigm that resembles the "change" tests of V.I.P.Spac (Henkin, Kileny, Hildesheimer, & Kishon-Rabin, 2008; Kraus, 1996; Kraus, McGee, Carrell, et al., 1993; Kraus, McGee, Micco, et al., 1993; Kraus, McGee, Sharma, Carrell, & Nicol, 1992; Kraus, Micco, et al., 1993; Ponton & Don, 1995; Sandridge & Boothroyd, 1996; Sharma, Kraus, McGee, Carrell, & Nicol, 1993).

Work on speech-evoked electrophysiologic responses has been ongoing for several years and has generated potentially valuable research data. At the time of writing, however, it still remains to be seen whether these techniques can provide a valid and reliable clinical tool for the assessment of auditory speech-perception capacity in individual subjects who are very young, hearing-impaired, or both.

Conclusions

The work described above leads to several conclusions:

1. The search for a valid behavioral test of auditory speech perception capacity, as defined here, is probably futile. Behavioral tests measure performance, not capacity. They can, however, be used to make inferences about capacity if scores are very high, or if they approach an asymptote after an appropriate period of training and/or experience.

2. Moreover, performance on tests of phonemic contrast perception can (or could) make a valuable contribution to clinical practice as an early indicator of progress on the building blocks required for the development of more advanced speech perception skills. They can (or could) also indicate directions for effective habilitative intervention.

3. The evidence of learning effects points to the need for the accumulation of longitudinal data. In addition to measuring progress, such data would help identify scores that are unusually low because of nonauditory factors.

4. We still need to explore behavioral measures of phonemic contrast perception in children between the ages of 1.5 and 3.5 years. One possibility is the use of partially scripted play interactions between child and caregiver.

5. Further research is needed to determine the most appropriate utterance form, contrast set, and test parameters for optimization of validity, reliability, and efficiency of behavioral tests.

6. It is possible that electrophysiologic indicators, such as the acoustic change complex, will provide valid and reliable objective measures of peripheral audi-

tory capacity, but this has yet to be determined.

Acknowledgments. This chapter provides a narrative of research and discovery by a single researcher and is, therefore, noticeably egocentric. The work described, however, would not have been possible without the previous and parallel efforts of numerous distinguished researchers, many of whom are referenced here. Nor would it have been possible without the efforts of many talented colleagues. These include, at the City University of New York, Teresa Hnath-Chisolm, Laurie Hanin, Larry Medwetsky, Liat Kishon-Rabin, Orna Eran, Christine Kosky, Eddy Yeung, Charlie Chen, Gary Chant, Jodi Ostroff, and Bethany Mulhearn, and, at the House Ear Institute, Laurie Eisenberg and Amy Martinez.

Funding for much of the research on which this chapter is based came from federal grants including: DC00178, DC004433, and DC006238 from NIH and G008302511 and H1343E9800 from NIDRR. Preparation of this chapter was supported by NIH grant DC006238.

References

Allen, P., Wightman, F., Kistler, D., & Dolan, T. (1989). Frequency resolution in children. *Journal of Speech and Hearing Research*, *32*, 317-322.

Boothroyd, A. (1968). Developments in speech audiometry. *British Journal of Audiology (formerly Sound)*, *2*, 3-10.

Boothroyd, A. (1978). Speech Perception and Sensorineural Hearing Loss. In M. Ross & T. G. Giolas (Eds.), *Auditory management of hearing impaired children* (pp. 117-144). Baltimore: University Park Press.

Boothroyd, A. (1984). Auditory perception of speech contrasts by subjects with sensorineural hearing loss. *Journal of Speech and Hearing Research*, *27*, 134-144.

Boothroyd, A. (1985a). Auditory capacity and the generalization of speech skills. In J. L. Lauter (Ed.), *Speech planning and production in normal and hearing-impaired children. ASHA Reports #15* (pp. 8-14). Rockville, MD: American Speech-Language-Hearing Association.

Boothroyd, A. (1985b). Evaluation of speech production in the hearing-impaired: Some benefits of forced-choice testing. *Journal of Speech and Hearing Research*, *28*, 185-196.

Boothroyd, A. (1991). Speech perception measures and their role in the evaluation of hearing aid performance in a pediatric population. In J. A. Feigin & P. G. Stelmachowicz (Eds.), *Pediatric amplification* (pp. 77-91). Omaha, NE: Boys Town National Research Hospital.

Boothroyd, A. (1995). Speech perception tests and hearing-impaired children. In G. Plant & K. E. Spens (Eds.), *Profound deafness and speech communication* (pp. 345-371). London: Whurr.

Boothroyd, A. (1997a). Auditory capacity of hearing-impaired children using hearing aids and cochlear implants: Issues of efficacy and assessment. *Scandinavian Audiology Supplementum*, *46*, 17-25.

Boothroyd, A. (1997b). Auditory development of the hearing child. *Scandinavian Audiology Supplementum*, *46*, 9-16.

Boothroyd, A. (1998). Evaluating the efficacy of hearing aids and cochlear implants in children who are hearing-impaired. In F. H. Bess (Ed.), *Children with hearing impairment: Contemporary trends* (pp. 249-260). Nashville, TN: Bill Wilkerson Center Press.

Boothroyd, A. (2002). *Influencia del Contexto en la Percepción del Lengaje Hablado*. Paper presented at the Congreso Internacional de Foniatría, Audiología, Logopedia y Psicología del lenguaje, Salamanca, Spain.

Boothroyd, A. (2005). Measuring auditory speech-perception capacity in young children. In R. C. Seewald & J. M. Bamford (Eds.), *A sound foundation through early amplification: Proceedings of the 3rd International Conference* (pp. 129-140). Zurich: Phonak AG.

Boothroyd, A. (2008). The Performance/Intensity function: an underused resource. *Ear and Hearing, 29,* 479-491.

Boothroyd, A., & Boothroyd-Turner, D. (2002). Post-implantation audition and educational attainment in children with prelingually-acquired profound deafness. *Annals of Otology, Rhinology, and Laryngology, 111* (Suppl. 189), 79-84.

Boothroyd, A., Eran, O., & Hanin, L. (1996). Speech perception and production in children with hearing impairment. In F. H. Bess, J. S. Gravel, & A. M. Tharpe (Eds.), *Amplification for children with auditory deficits* (pp. 55-74). Nashville, TN: Bill Wilkerson Center Press.

Boothroyd, A., Geers, A. E., & Moog, J. S. (1991). Practical implications of cochlear implants in children. *Ear and Hearing, 12*(Suppl.), 81S-89S.

Boothroyd, A., & Nittrouer, S. (1988). Mathematical treatment of context effects in phoneme and word recognition. *Journal of the Acoustical Society of America, 84,* 101-114.

Carney, A. E., Osberger, M. J., Carney, E., Robbins, A. M., Renshaw, J., & Miyamoto, R. T. (1993). A comparison of speech discrimination with cochlear implants and tactile aids. *Journal of the Acoustical Society of America, 94,* 2036-2049.

Cone-Wesson, B. (2003). Pediatric audiology: A review of assessment methods for infants. *Audiological Medicine, 1,* 175-184.

Cox, R. M. (Ed.). (2005). Evidence-based practice in audiology. *Journal of the American Academy of Audiology, 16,* 408-409.

Daemers, K., Yperman, M., De Beukelaer, C., De Saegher, G., De Ceulaer, G., & Govaerts, P. J. (2006). Normative data of the A§E® discrimination and identification tests in preverbal children. *Cochlear Implants International, 7,* 107-116.

Dawson, P. W., Nott, P. E., Clark, G. M., & Cowan, R. S. (1998). A modification of play audiometry to assess speech discrimination ability in severe-profoundly deaf 2- to 4-year-old children. *Ear and Hearing, 19,* 371-384.

Eilers, R. E., Wilson, W. R., & Moore, J. M. (1977). Developmental changes in speech discrimination in infants. *Journal of Speech and Hearing Research, 20,* 766-780.

Eisenberg, L. S., Martinez, A. S., & Boothroyd, A. (2003). Auditory-visual and auditory-only perception of phonetic contrasts in children. *Volta Review, 102,* 327-346.

Eisenberg, L. S., Martinez, A. S., & Boothroyd, A. (2007). Assessing auditory capabilities in young children. *International Journal of Pediatric Otorhinolaryngology, 71,* 1339-1350.

Eisenberg, L. S., Shannon, R. V., Martinez, A. S., Wygonski, J., & Boothroyd, A. (2000). Speech recognition with reduced spectral cues as a function of age. *Journal of the Acoustical Society of America, 107,* 2704-2710.

Erber, N. P. (1972). Auditory, visual, and auditory-visual recognition of consonants by children with normal and impaired hearing. *Journal of Speech and Hearing Research, 15,* 413-422.

Erber, N. P. (1979). Speech perception by profoundly hearing-impaired children. *Journal of Speech and Hearing Disorders, 44,* 255-270.

Govaerts, P., Daemers, K., Yperman, M., De Beukelaer, C., De Saegher, G., & De Ceulaer, G. (2006). Auditory speech sounds evaluation (A§E®): A new test to assess detection, discrimination and identification in hearing impairment. *Cochlear Implants International, 7,* 92-106.

Hack, Z. C., & Erber, N. P. (1982). Auditory, visual, and auditory-visual perception of vowels by hearing-impaired children. *Journal of Speech and Hearing Research, 25,* 100-107.

Henkin, Y., Kileny, P. R., Hildesheimer, M., & Kishon-Rabin, L. (2008). Phonetic processing in children with cochlear implants: An auditory event-related potentials study. *Ear and Hearing, 29,* 239-249.

Hnath-Chisolm, T. E., Laippley, E., & Boothroyd, A. (1998). Age-related changes on a children's test of sensory-level speech perception capacity. *Journal of Speech and Hearing Research, 41,* 94-106.

Kosky, C., & Boothroyd, A. (2003). Validation of an on-line implementation of the Imitative Test of Speech Pattern Contrast Perception (IMSPAC). *Journal of the American Academy of Audiology, 14,* 72-83.

Kraus, N. (1996). The discriminating brain: MMN and acoustic change. *Hearing Journal, 49,* 10.

Kraus, N., McGee, T., Carrell, T., Sharma, A., Micco, A., & Nicol, T. (1993a). Speech-evoked cortical potentials in children. *Journal of the American Academy of Audiology, 4,* 238–248.

Kraus, N., McGee, T., Micco, A., Sharma, A., Carrell, T., & Nicol, T. (1993b). Mismatch negativity in school-age children to speech stimuli that are just perceptibly different. *Electroencephalography and Clinical Neurophysiology, 88,* 123–130.

Kraus, N., McGee, T., Sharma, A., Carrell, T., & Nicol, T. (1992). Mismatch negativity event-related potential elicited by speech stimuli. *Ear and Hearing, 13,* 158–164.

Kraus, N., Micco, A. G., Koch, D. B., McGee, T., Carrell, T., Sharma, A., Wiet, R. J., & Weingarten, C. Z. (1993c). The mismatch negativity cortical evoked potential elicited by speech in cochlear-implant users. *Hearing Research, 65,* 118–124.

Kuhl, P. K. (1979). Speech perception in early infancy: Perceptual constancy for spectrally dissimilar vowel categories. *Journal of the Acoustical Society of America, 66,* 1668–1679.

Kuhl, P. K. (1991). Human adults and human infants show a "perceptual magnet effect" for the prototypes of speech categories, monkeys do not. *Perception and Psychophysics, 50,* 93–107.

Kuhl, P. K. (1992). Psychoacoustics and speech perception: Internal standards, perceptual anchors, and prototypes. In L. A. Werner & E. W. Rubel (Eds.), *Developmental psychoacoustics* (pp. 293–332). Washington, DC: American Psychological Association.

Kuhl, P. K., Williams, K. A., Lacerda, F., Stevens, K. N., & Lindblom, B. (1992). Linguistic experience alters phonetic perception in infants by 6 months of age. *Science, 255,* 606–608.

Madell, J. R. (2008). Using visual reinforcement audiometry to evaluate hearing in infants from 5 to 36 months. In J. R. Madell & C. Flexer (Eds.), *Pediatric audiology: Diagnosis, technology, and management* (pp. 65–75). New York: Thieme Medical.

Marean, G. C., Werner, L. A., & Kuhl, P. K. (1992). Vowel categorization by very young infants. *Developmental Psychology, 28,* 396–405.

Martin, B. A. (2007). Can the acoustic change complex be recorded in an individual with a cochlear implant? Separating neural responses from the cochlear implant artifact. *Journal of the American Academy of Audiology, 18,* 126–140.

Martin, B. A., & Boothroyd, A. (1999). Cortical, auditory, evoked potentials in response to periodic and aperiodic stimuli with the same spectral envelope. *Ear and Hearing, 20,* 33–44.

Martin, B. A., & Boothroyd, A. (2000). Cortical, auditory, evoked potentials in response to changes of spectrum and amplitude. *Journal of the Acoustical Society of America, 107,* 2155–2161.

Martinez, A., Eisenberg, L., Boothroyd, A., & Visser-Dumont, L. (2008). Assessing speech pattern contrast perception in infants: Early results on VRASPAC. *Otology and Neurotology, 29,* 183–188.

Most, T. (1985). *Assessment of the perception of intonation by severely and profoundly hearing-impaired children.* Doctoral dissertation, City University of New York.

National Institute on Deafness and Other Communication Disorders. (1995). Cochlear Implants in Adults and Children. *NIH Consensus Statement, 13*(2), 1–30.

Nittrouer, S. (1996). Discriminability and perceptual weighting of some acoustic cues to speech perception by 3-year-olds. *Journal of Speech and Hearing Research, 39,* 278–297.

Nittrouer, S., & Boothroyd, A. (1990). Context effects in phoneme and word recognition by young children and older adults. *Journal of the Acoustical Society of America, 87,* 2705–2715.

Osberger, M. J., Miyamoto, R. T., Zimmerman-Phillips, S., Kemink, J. L., Stroer, B. S., Firszt, J. B., & Novak, M. A. (1991). Independent evaluation of the speech perception abilities of children with the Nucleus 22-channel cochlear implant system. *Ear and Hearing, 12*(Suppl. 4), 66–80.

Ostroff, J. (1999). *Parametric study of the acoustic change complex elicited by second formant change in synthetic vowel stimuli.* Doctoral dissertation, City University of New York.

Ostroff, J. M., Martin, B. A., & Boothroyd, A. (1998). Cortical evoked response to acoustic change within a syllable. *Ear and Hearing, 19*, 290–297.

Pickett, J. M., Martin, E. S., Johnson, D., Brandsmith, S., Daniel, Z., Willis, D., & Otis, W. (1972). On patterns of speech feature perception by deaf listeners. In G. Fant (Ed.), *International symposium on speech communication ability and profound deafness* (pp. 119–134). Washington, DC: Alexander Graham Bell Association for the Deaf.

Ponton, C. W., & Don, M. (1995). The mismatch negativity in cochlear implant users. *Ear and Hearing, 16*, 131–146.

Risberg, A. (1976). *Diagnostic rhyme test for speech audiometry with severely hard of hearing and profoundly deaf children* (Quarterly Progress and Status Report, 2–3, 40–55). Stockholm: Karolinska Technical Institute, Speech Transmission Laboratory.

Ross, M., Kessler, M., Phillips, M., & Lerman, J. (1972). Visual, auditory, and combined mode presentation of the WIPI test to hearing impaired children. *Volta Review, 74*, 90–96.

Sandridge, S. A., & Boothroyd, A. (1996). Using naturally produced speech to elicit mismatch negativity. *Journal of the American Academy of Audiology, 7*, 105–112.

Sharma, A., Kraus, N., McGee, T., Carrell, T., & Nicol, T. (1993). Acoustic versus phonetic representation of speech as reflected by the mismatch negativity event-related potential. *Electroencephalography and Clinical Neurophysiology, 88*, 64–71.

Stanton, S. G., & Harrison, R. V. (1996). Abnormal cochleotopic organization in the auditory cortex of cats reared in a frequency augmented environment. *Auditory Neuroscience, 2*, 97–107.

Sussman, J. E. (1993). Auditory processing in children's speech perception: Results of selective adaptation and discrimination tasks. *Journal of Speech and Hearing Research, 36*, 380–395.

Thornton, A. R., & Raffin, M. J. (1978). Speech discrimination scores modeled as a binomial variable. *Journal of Speech and Hearing Research, 21*, 507–518.

Tremblay, K., Kraus, N., & McGee, T. (1998). The time course of auditory perceptual learning: neurophysiological changes during speech-sound training. *Neuroreport, 9*, 3557–3560.

Tyler, R. S. (Ed.). (1993). Speech perception by children. *Cochlear implants: Audiological foundations* (pp. 191–256). San Diego, CA: Singular.

Uhler, K. (2008). *Longitudinal study of infant speech perception in young cochlear implant candidates: Three case studies*. Doctoral dissertation, University of Colorado.

Werner, L. A., & Rubel, E. W. (Eds.). (1992). *Developmental psychoacoustics*. Washington DC: American Psychological Association.

CHAPTER 10

Assessing Spoken Word Recognition in Children with Cochlear Implants

KAREN ILER KIRK
BRIAN F. FRENCH
SANGSOOK CHOI

Introduction

Cochlear implantation has been used in the medical management of children with profound deafness for more than two decades. Over time, the field has seen advances in the design of cochlear implant systems, evolving pediatric candidacy criteria, and the implementation of new sensory aid configurations for cochlear implant recipients. The earliest cochlear implant recipients were adults with postlingual, profound, bilateral hearing loss. However, candidacy quickly evolved to include persons with prelingual, profound hearing loss, most commonly children. The vast majority of these children were monaurally implanted and used no other sensory aid. Today cochlear implants are approved for children as young as 12 months of age with profound hearing loss,

and for children aged 2 years or older with severe-to-profound hearing loss. Bilateral implantation has increased markedly in the last few years in an effort to improve speech understanding in noise and sound localization abilities, thereby enhancing incidental learning and promoting language development in children. For similar reasons, monaural cochlear implantation has been combined with hearing aid use on the ipsilateral and/or contralateral ear in children with good residual hearing. The variety of cochlear implant options, with their associated candidacy criteria and expected outcomes, presents new challenges for clinicians who determine cochlear implant candidacy and postimplant benefits. Tests of spoken word recognition provide the most direct evidence of sensory aid benefit. Thus, they should be included in testing protocols used to evaluate cochlear implant candidates and recipients whenever possible. But which tests to use?

In this chapter, we review factors that influence spoken word recognition in listeners with normal hearing and those with hearing loss, and consider factors that impact the development and selection of spoken word recognition tests for children. We also review currently available tests for children and present alternative strategies for selecting and administering tests within a protocol. Finally, we describe our current efforts to develop a new theoretically motivated, norm-referenced test of audiovisual speech recognition for children.

Factors Influencing Spoken Word Recognition

Traditionally, spoken word recognition was thought to involve several underlying perceptual processes in which the speech signal is converted into an acoustic-phonetic representation, normalized for talker differences and then identified by matching these transformed internal representations to those stored in long-term lexical memory (Studdert-Kennedy, 1974). Processing at these higher levels influences spoken word recognition and lexical access. A more recent, alternative view of the speech perception process is compatible with a large and growing body of literature in cognitive science dealing with "exemplar" or "episodic" models of categorization and "multiple-trace" models of memory (Hintzman, 1986; Kruschke, 1992; Nosofsky, 1986). This approach assumes that highly detailed stimulus information in the speech signal is processed and encoded by the listener (Goldinger, 1996, 1997, 1998). Pisoni and his colleagues have demonstrated that indexical information about a talker's

voice and face and detailed information about other episodic properties of speech are encoded into memory representations, becoming part of the long-term representational knowledge a listener has about the words of his or her language (Pisoni, 1997). Thus, the human perceptual system encodes and retains very fine episodic details of the perceptual event.

Auditory-Visual Integration

Sumby and Pollack (1954) were the first researchers to document that the addition of visual speech cues to the auditory speech signal yielded substantial improvements in speech perception for listeners with normal hearing, especially in adverse listening conditions such as noise. Similar results have been obtained by other investigators for listeners with normal hearing (Demorest, Bernstein, & DeHaven, 1996; Massaro & Cohen, 1995; Sommers, Tye-Murray, & Spehar, 2005; Summerfield, 1987), and for listeners with hearing loss (Erber, 1972; Moody-Antonio et al., 2005; Walden, Prosek, & Worthington, 1975). The cognitive processes by which individuals combine and integrate auditory and visual speech information with lexical and syntactic knowledge have become an important area of research in the field of speech perception. Visual cues provide segmental and suprasegmental information that is complementary to the acoustic speech cues. Spoken word recognition, therefore, appears to be more than the simple addition of auditory and visual information (Bernstein, Demorest, & Tucker, 2000). However, substantial individual variability is noted in the ability to integrate the two types of speech cues (Demorest & Bernstein, 1992). One factor that appears to influence auditory-visual, or multimodal integration is degree of hearing loss. Individuals with lesser degrees of hearing loss obtain better auditory-only (A-only) and auditory-visual (AV) performance than individuals with greater degrees of hearing loss (Erber, 1972).

The nature of a listener's early linguistic experience also influences multimodal speech perception. Individuals with an earlier onset of deafness demonstrate better visual-only (V-only) spoken word recognition than listeners with a late onset of deafness (Bergeson & Pisoni, 2004). Grant and Seitz (1998) proposed that variability in multimodal spoken word recognition depends not only on how lexical access is influenced by an individual's access to auditory and visual speech cues, but also on the processes by which the two types of cues are integrated, and by the impact of top-down contextual constraints and memory processes.

Stimulus Variability

Listeners with normal hearing reliably extract abstract phonological and semantic information from speech, despite enormous variability in the acoustic signal introduced by different talkers using different speaking rates or dialects (Pisoni, 1993, 1996). The processes by which listeners recognize words and recover meaning from widely divergent acoustic signals are often referred to as perceptual constancy or perceptual normalization. Creelman (1957) conducted one of the first studies to examine the effects of talker variability on spoken word recognition. He found that listeners with normal hearing were poorer at recognizing words in lists containing words produced by two or more talkers compared with lists produced by only one talker. Subsequent studies demonstrated that as stimulus vari-

ability increases, either by increasing the number of talkers or by varying the speaking rate, word identification accuracy decreases and response latency increases (Mullennix & Pisoni, 1990; Mullennix, Pisoni, & Martin, 1989; Nygaard & Pisoni, 1998; Nygaard, Sommers, & Pisoni, 1992; Sommers, Nygaard, & Pisoni, 1994). Presumably this occurs because perceptual normalization consumes common processing resources. Similar results have been demonstrated for listeners with hearing impairment using A-only stimuli (Kirk, Pisoni, Sommers, Young, & Evanson, 1994; Sommers, Kirk, & Pisoni, 1997) and AV presentation of isolated words (Kaiser, Kirk, Lachs, & Pisoni, 2003).

Although stimulus variability in the form of multiple talkers results in short-term deficits in word recognition, it appears to have long-term benefits. The perceptual normalization process appears to encode episodic information about talker characteristics that is preserved in memory to facilitate recall of words (Goldinger, 1991; Mullennix, Pisoni, & Martin, 1989). Talker characteristics are not irrelevant sources of "noise"; they are considered an important source of information in the speech signal that listeners make use of in recognizing spoken words (Bradlow, Akahane-Yamada, Pisoni, & Tohkura, 1999; Bradlow & Pisoni, 1999; Pisoni, 1993).

Lexical Characteristics of the Stimuli

The lexical properties of words also have been shown to influence spoken word recognition. Word frequency (i.e., the frequency of occurrence of words in the language) and lexical density (i.e., the number of phonemically similar words to the target) have been shown to affect the accuracy and speed of spoken word recognition performance (Elliott, Clifton, & Servi, 1983; Luce, Pisoni, & Goldinger, 1990; Treisman, 1978a, 1978b). One measure of lexical similarity is the number of "lexical neighbors" or words that differ by one phoneme from a target word (Greenburg & Jenkins, 1964; Landauer & Streeter, 1973). For example, the words *bat, cap, cut, scat,* and *at* are all lexical neighbors of the target word *cat.* Words with many lexical neighbors come from "dense" lexical neighborhoods, whereas those with few lexical neighbors come from "sparse" neighborhoods. The neighborhood activation model (NAM) (Luce & Pisoni, 1998) offers a two-stage account of how the sound pattern of words in memory contribute to the perception of spoken words. According to NAM, a stimulus input activates a set of similar acoustic-phonetic patterns in memory in a multidimensional acoustic-phonetic space, with activation levels proportional to the degree of similarity to the target word. This initial activation stage is followed by "lexical selection" among a large number of potential candidates that are consistent with the acoustic-phonetic input. Word frequency is assumed to act as a biasing factor in this model by multiplicatively adjusting the activation levels of the acoustic-phonetic patterns. In lexical selection, the activation levels are then summed and the probability of choosing each pattern is computed based on the overall activation level. Word recognition occurs when a given acoustic-phonetic representation is chosen based on the computed probabilities.

Figure 10-1 illustrates two lexical neighborhoods. The wide bars in Figure 10-1 represent the target word to be identified and the narrow bars represent the lexical neighbors competing for lexical selection. Word frequency is represented by the height of the bars. Luce and his colleagues (Cluff & Luce, 1990; Luce, Pisoni, & Goldinger, 1990) showed that word frequency, neighborhood density (i.e., the number of lexical neighbors for the target word), and the neighborhood frequency (i.e., the average word frequency of the words in the lexical neighborhood) all influence A-only spoken word recognition. Lexically "easy" words (high-frequency words from sparse neighborhoods) were recognized with greater accuracy and speed than lexically "hard" words (low-frequency words from dense neighborhoods). These results demonstrate that the structure and organization of sound patterns in memory affect spoken word recognition performance by listeners with normal hearing.

A number of studies have been carried out over the last decade to investigate lexical effects on spoken word recognition by adults and children with hearing loss. Like individuals with normal hearing, adults and children with hearing loss identify lexically easy words better than lexically hard words. These results have been demonstrated for isolated words (Dirks, Takayanagi, Moshfegh, Noffsinger, & Fausti, 2001; Frisch, Meyer, Pisoni, Svirsky, & Kirk, 2000; Kirk, Hay-McCutcheon, Sehgal, & Miyamoto, 1998; Kirk, Pisoni, & Miyamoto, 2000; Kirk, Pisoni, & Osberger, 1995) and for sentences containing lexically controlled key words in an A-only format (Bell & Wilson, 2001; Eisenberg, Martinez, Holowecky, & Pogorelsky, 2002; Wilson, Bell, & Koslowski, 2003). Lexical effects also have been shown to influence AV presentation of isolated words (Kaiser, et al., 2003). Although individuals with hearing loss may receive a degraded auditory input from their sensory aid and thus their word recognition performance is reduced, they appear to organize and access words from lexical memory in a similar fashion to listeners with normal hearing.

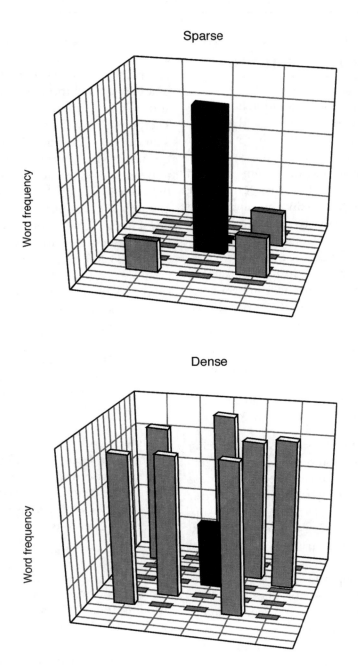

Figure 10–1. Two hypothetical lexical neighborhoods showing target words that are easy or hard to identify. The dark bars represent the target word to be identified and the remaining bars are lexical neighbors (i.e., they differ by one phoneme from the target word). Word frequency is represented by bar height. Words that are easy to identify occur often and come from sparse neighborhoods whereas words that are hard to identify have the opposite lexical characteristics.

Clinical Tests of Spoken Word Recognition

Tests of spoken word recognition have been used clinically in the diagnosis and management of individuals with hearing loss for the last 60 years. They are used to assess the effects of hearing loss on communication abilities (Hudgins, Hawkins, Karling, & Stevens, 1947), to classify the degree and type of hearing loss, to determine candidacy for cochlear implantation (Kirk, 2000), to measure objectively the benefit provided by a cochlear implant or hearing aid, and to provide information that will inform aural (re)habilitation programs (Mackersie, 2002). The usual goal of such testing is to:

> . . . provide a measure of how well listeners understand speech in a controlled environment as a reflection of how they may do in everyday listening situations. (Mendel & Danhauer, 1997a, p. 3)

In research settings, listeners with hearing loss may be administered spoken word recognition tests to evaluate the effectiveness of signal processing strategies, to better understand perceptual processes that support spoken word recognition, or to identify factors that contribute to individual variability. Obviously, no one test can achieve all of the clinical and research aims. However, clinical test protocols should include measures designed to assess speech perception skills ranging from speech sound detection and discrimination through open-set word recognition.

Considerations in the Development of Spoken Word Recognition Tests

According to Bilger (1984), tests of spoken word recognition are analogous to tradi-

tional psychological tests of mental ability in their development and standardization. The principles of psychometric theory and practice should apply to the development and standardization of these instruments. The preliminary stages of test development include: (a) specifying the construct (i.e., the underlying abstract ability) purported to be measured by the test, (b) determining the domain of possible test items and procedures for sampling that domain (i.e., developing the test blueprint), and (c) specifying the response format and scoring procedures. Later stages include developing multiple test forms and assessing test score validity and reliability using participants drawn from the population for whom the test is intended. Following these procedures will allow an instrument to be in accord with standard test development practice as specified in Standards for Educational and Psychological Testing (1999). Furthermore, gathering the necessary score reliability and validity data will assist in gaining support for the instrument and overcoming legal and technical challenges that may arise from the research community and the general public (Brennan, 2004) with such tests that are used for clinical or placement decisions.

Test Construct

The test construct shapes the selection of stimulus items and response format. Boothroyd (1991) has proposed that successful spoken word recognition requires the listener to utilize two types of evidence: sensory information produced by the sense organs in response to physical signals, and contextual information contained in the linguistic, physical and social context of the language pattern. If the test construct is to measure sensory or auditory capacity, then linguistic or contextual cues should be minimized. Speech perception tests intended for this purpose typically require the listener to identify nonsense syllables or to discriminate between minimally contrastive word pairs (Kirk, Diefendorf, Pisoni, & Robbins, 1997). A closed-set response format (e.g., wherein the listener selects a response from a limited set of alternatives) is used routinely to minimize learning effects (Mackersie, 2002) and responses are scored to reflect how well consonant features (i.e., manner, place, or voicing) or vowel features (e.g., vowel height or vowel place) are perceived. Boothroyd and colleagues have developed a family of tests designed to assess speech feature perception in adults (Boothroyd, 1984) and in children of varying ages (Boothroyd, 1991; Eisenberg, Martinez, & Boothroyd, 2003, 2004; Hnath-Chisolm, Laippley, & Boothroyd, 1998). At the opposite end of the spectrum are "perceptually robust tests" of speech perception and spoken word recognition (Pisoni, 1990, 1996, 2000) that are designed to measure a listener's ability to recognize or comprehend spoken language under robust listening conditions. These tests use isolated words (Egan, 1948; Hirsch et al., 1954; Peterson & Lehiste, 1962; Tillman & Carhart, 1966), sentences (Bilger, 1984; Boothroyd, Hanin, & Hnath, 1985; Dirks et al., 2001; Kalikow, Stevens, & Elliott, 1977; Takayanagi, Dirks, & Moshfegh, 2002; Wilson et al., 2003), or passages of connected speech (Cox, Alexander, & Gilmore, 1987; Cox, Alexander, Gilmore, & Pusakulich, 1988) to assess spoken word recognition. Listeners typically repeat or write their response using an open-set format (i.e., wherein no response alternatives are provided). Responses are scored as the percent of words correctly identified at a given presentation level, or as the signal-to-noise level needed to reach a certain performance criterion such as 50% words correct (McArdle, Wilson, & Burks, 2005; Nilsson, Soli, & Sullivan, 1994). Performance on such open-set

tests reflects phonological and/or lexical discrimination processes as well as higher level cognitive and linguistic processes such as vocabulary knowledge, lexical access, and working memory (Paatsch, Blamey, Sarant, Martin, & Bow, 2004; Pisoni, 2000).

Test Score Validation

Test score validation involves gathering multiple forms of evidence to demonstrate that the desired ability or trait is being measured. That is, multiple sources contribute to a body of evidence to support the construct validity, or intended interpretation of test scores for the intended purpose. Sources of evidence include, but are not limited to, mapping of skills to test items and expert reviews of items, the relationship between scores from established tests and the test under development, and the relationship between test scores and performance on a criterion (Messick, 1989). The interested reader is directed to a discussion of validity issues in *Educational Researcher* (2007) for recent trends in score validity.

There are three main types of validity evidence to consider when developing a test instrument. Please note these are not the only sources of validity evidence that should be considered. Additionally, traditional validity language has been used here because these are terms most often used and what readers likely will see in past and recent writings. Note that this language is changing slowly (e.g., Cizek, 2008) to reflect current validity theory. Construct validity refers to how well the test measures the underlying ability; according to Messick (1989), this is the most important form of validity and is the overarching idea which all validity evidence is to support. Speech perception is an abstract construct that is difficult to define; it cannot be measured directly, but only inferred from a listener's responses (Robbins & Kirk, 1996). Furthermore, as noted above, both sensory and higher level cognitive abilities contribute to speech perception. Thus, most tests of spoken word recognition focus on concrete measures, such as phoneme, word, or sentence recognition (Mendel & Danhauer, 1997b). These manifestations of the construct can be used to assess the fit of the data to the theoretical model through confirmatory factor analysis, as one assessment of construct validity.

Criterion-related validity (i.e., concurrent and predictive), refers to the ability of a given test score to estimate performance at present or in the future, as measured by another instrument (i.e., the criterion) under realistic listening situations. The predictive validity of spoken word recognition tests is not well known (Walden, 1984). Content validity refers to the extent to which the test items reflect the construct, as judged by a panel of content experts. Content validity guides item selection, such as phonetic balancing or equivalence across lists. However, because construct and criterion validity evidence can be difficult to determine, most test developers of spoken word recognition assessment instruments have focused on assessing content validity. This lack of focus on the other forms of validity for spoken word recognition assessments is problematic; it cannot be determined how well these tests are measuring the construct or whether the scores have the intended meaning to make clinical decisions. Without this evidence, scores and decisions may be meaningless and even harmful to the consumer.

Test Reliability

Score reliability is the extent to which variance in scores of a given test is reflective of variance in the trait measured by the test (Anastasi & Urbina, 1997). Scores cannot be valid if reliability evidence is not first established. One generally looks for consistency between: (a) test items (i.e., internal consistency reliability), (b) test-taking sessions (i.e., test-retest reliability), and (c) test forms (i.e., parallel forms reliability) (Anastasi & Urbina, 1997). As with validity evidence, it is important to gather several forms of score reliability as scores may be unreliable due to a variety of extraneous sources of error. For example, examinees should maintain their position in the score distribution upon retesting with the same instrument after a given time interval. A high correlation between time 1 and 2 scores indicates consistency across time and minimal influences of errors associated with time. A high correlation also is sought between scores obtained from two forms of the same test. The idea is that the examinees's score should not depend on the form completed. Both test-retest and parallel forms reliability require the completion of two tests by the same group of examinees. In contrast, internal consistency reliability (e.g., Cronbach's coefficient alpha) requires only one test administration and assesses the extraneous effects due to a lack of content homogeneity. At the minimum, this should be reported for tests. For more information on score reliability, the interested reader is directed to Traub and Rowley (1991).

Selecting Appropriate Outcome Measures

As noted above, the individual variability among cochlear implant recipients, both in terms of their demographic characteristics (e.g., age, residual hearing, etc.) and their speech perception, production and language skills, presents challenges to researchers in the selection of appropriate outcome measures. The primary benefit of cochlear implant use for adults with profound, post-lingual deafness is improved speech perception and spoken word recognition. In contrast cochlear implantation in children may have a profound impact on all aspects of communication, and the assessment battery employed for children should be broad enough to reflect these changes. Finally, individuals with bilateral auditory input, either from two cochlear implants or from the simultaneous use of a cochlear implant and hearing aid(s), may also experience improved directional hearing (Buss et al., 2008; Ching, van Wanrooy, Hill, & Incerti, 2006; Litovsky et al., 2004) and clinical tests have been developed to assess these skills in both adults and children (Garadat & Litovsky, 2007; Tyler, Noble, Dunn, & Witt, 2006). Thus, clinical researchers must have available a wide array of age-appropriate outcome measures that allows them to target different aspects of auditory performance and communication development.

Considerations in the Use of Speech Perception Tests

A comprehensive speech perception test battery should permit the evaluation of a hierarchy of skills, ranging from discrimination of vowel and consonant speech features through the comprehension of connected speech. Several methodological factors are likely to affect results. These include internal factors inherent in the tests themselves, such as whether they are objective or subjective, the type of response format they employ, or the number and equivalence of test lists. External factors concerning the way in which the tests are administered also influence outcomes. External factors include the use of recorded versus live voice tests, the stimulus presentation level, the use of competing noise during presentation, and the sensory modality in which the speech signal is presented.

Objective Versus Subjective Measures. Objective measures of speech perception and spoken word recognition present various stimuli (syllables, words, phrases, connected speech) to the listener and require the listener to respond. In contrast, subjective measures ask the listener or someone else to report on listening behaviors that are demonstrated in various environments. Subjective measures often are employed when assessing speech perception or communicative performance in very young children with limited reporting capabilities; they also may be used with individuals who cannot participate in objective testing. A number of such questionnaires have been developed specifically for use with pediatric cochlear implant recipients (Archbold, Lutman, & Marshall, 1995; Archbold, Lutman, & Nikolopoulos, 1998; Cox, Alexander, & Gilmore, 1991; Lin et al., 2007; Purdy, Farrington, Moran, Chard, & Hodgson, 2002; Zimmerman-Phillips, Robbins, & Osberger, 2000). Subjective measures also can be used to estimate performance outside of the clinic or lab environment (Cox, Alexander, & Gilmore, 1991; Purdy, Farrington, Moran, Chard, & Hodgson, 2002). The questionnaires may be completed by the patient, a family member, a teacher or a clinician. One must be cautious in interpreting subjective data because they are prone to informer bias. It is best if subjective measures can be supplemented with at least some objective data. If that is not possible, comparing responses from more than one informant may be helpful.

Open- Versus Closed-Set Test Formats. Most cochlear implant test batteries utilize both open- and closed-set objective test measures of speech understanding in auditory-only conditions. Open-set tests are those in which the listener theoretically has an unlimited number of response possibilities. On hearing the test item, no response alternatives are provided and the listener typically repeats what is heard. Closed-set tests are those that restrict the listener to one of a fixed number of possible responses.

Open-set tests are advantageous in that the demands simulate those encountered in natural listening situations. Performance on open-set tests of spoken word recognition is influenced by cognitive processing, just as is real-world speech comprehension. Cognitive processing is facilitated by an individual's general knowledge including vocabulary and linguistic knowledge, and by expectations based on the context of the speech act.

Sometimes researchers wish to evaluate an individual's sensory capabilities without the influence of cognitive factors (Boothroyd, 1985, 1995; Eisenberg et al., 2003, 2004; Mackersie, 2002). For example, researchers may wish to determine which speech features are well conveyed by a particular cochlear implant system. Closed-set tests of word or nonsense syllable recognition often are used for this purpose. The target speech signal is embedded among foils that are acoustically or phonetically similar. Such closed-set tests of speech feature perception also are useful in assessing implant performance in those with minimal open-set speech understanding through audition alone. These listeners may have fairly good speech understanding when certain speech features that are well conveyed by the cochlear implant (such as manner of consonant articulation) are combined with lipreading cues.

List Number and Equivalency. Open-set tests of spoken word recognition vary in the number of lists that are provided; those that do have multiple lists do not always report interlist equivalency. If repeated testing is necessary, as in a longitudinal study or when testing a patient in multiple sensory aid configurations this becomes a particularly important consideration. Learning effects are to be expected if the same list is administered repeatedly in a short period of time. However, if multiple lists of a test are not equivalent, spurious data will be obtained.

Recorded Versus Live-Voice Stimulus Presentation. The use of recordings as opposed to live-voice administration of speech perception tests has been debated widely. Proponents of recorded materials point out that speakers differ and, therefore, results obtained with live voice presentation are not comparable across clinics or research centers unless speaker equivalence can be demonstrated. Subtle changes in presentation may improve performance over the testing interval. Indeed, several clinicians and researchers have argued that consistency in presentation between listeners or over time can be maintained only through the use of recorded test stimuli (Carhart, 1965; Mendel & Danhauer, 1997c). However, there may be as much difference between recordings as between two different talkers administering live-voice tests (Hood & Poole, 1980). Live-voice testing provides greater flexibility for the examiner. It often takes less time than using recorded versions. In general, the use of recorded tests is preferred for assessing performance in adults and older children so that results can be compared across centers and testing intervals. Very young children frequently require flexible testing situations. The need to customize the length and pace of testing often necessitates live-voice testing.

Presentation Level. Historically, cochlear implant speech perception outcomes were evaluated using speech materials presented at 70 dB SPL (Gantz et al., 1988; Owens, Kessler, Raggio, & Schubert, 1985; Tyler et al., 1984; Tyler, Lowder, Parkinson, Woodworth, & Gantz, 1995). More recent investigators have suggested that speech perception testing should be carried out at lower presentation levels that are more representative of conversational speech such as 50 or 60 dB SPL. Skinner and colleagues measured speech perception performance in 10 adult cochlear implant recipients using word and sentence stimuli presented at 50, 60 and 70 dB SPL (Skinner, Holden, Holden, Demorest, & Fourakis, 1997). Performance was highest when the stimuli were presented at 70 dB SPL; speech perception scores dropped with each reduction in presentation level. A follow-up study carried out with 78 adult participants yielded similar results (Firszt et al., 2004). Participants in this later study demonstrated substantial speech recognition abilities at all three presentation levels. However, significant level effects were noted. Firszt et al. found that performance was similar when stimuli were presented at 60 or 70 dB SPL; when the presentation level was reduced to 50 dB SPL, speech perception performance dropped significantly. These authors recommended developing new candidacy criteria based on performance at 50 or 60 dB SPL because these levels are more reflective of conversational speech.

The Use of Competing Noise. Tests of speech perception and spoken word recognition in quiet yield estimates of speech understanding under optimum listening situations. However, they may not accurately estimate performance in daily living where there are many sources of competing noise. Also, test administration in quiet may produce "ceiling" effects for cochlear implant recipients with excellent spoken word recognition. Conversely, testing only in noise can produce floor effects for individuals with poor speech recognition skills. Ceiling and floor effects can interfere with a clinician's decision regarding the best device settings. These effects also can reduce the accuracy with which researchers identify and weight factors that influence outcomes. Whenever possible, it is best to evaluate word recognition in both quiet and noise.

One approach to testing in noise is to present the stimuli at a fixed signal-to-noise ratio (SNR) and to measure the percent of words or sentences correctly identified (Firszt et al., 2004; Holt, Kirk, Eisenberg, Martinez, & Campbell, 2005). This approach has been followed in most FDA clinical trials that include testing in the presence of competing noise. The difficulty with this approach lies in finding an SNR that avoids floor and ceiling effects across all participants. An alternative approach employs a procedure in which the signal is held constant and the noise is adaptively varied to converge on a particular percent-correct value, such as 50% (Holt et al., 2005; Nilsson et al., 1994). The dependent measure is the SNR that yields the target value. This adaptive approach avoids floor and ceiling effects. It is used routinely in research settings, but can be difficult to implement clinically.

Stimulus Presentation Format. Speech is a multimodal signal. It has an auditory component, the acoustic waveform, and a visual component, the visible articulatory gestures generated during speech production (e.g., lip rounding). Under natural conditions, listeners use both auditory and visual speech cues to extract meaning from speech signals containing many sources of variability introduced by different talkers, dialects, speaking rates, and background noise. The addition of visual cues to the acoustic signal yields substantial gains in spoken word recognition, especially in adverse listening conditions (Erber, 1972; MacLeod & Summerfield, 1987; Massaro & Cohen, 1995; Sumby & Pollack, 1954). Visual cues are particularly important because they help to specify place of articulation, a speech feature that is fragile acoustically and often not accessible to many individuals with significant hearing loss (Erber, 1972; Grant & Walden, 1996; Walden, Grant, & Cord, 2001). However, in most clinical settings, speech perception and spoken word recognition performance have been assessed routinely using A-only presentation of monosyllabic word lists produced by a single talker using carefully articulated speech (Martin, Champlin, & Chambers, 1998). Such measures currently serve as the gold standard for determining candidacy for and/or benefit from cochlear implants. A-only tests may not adequately characterize the performance of listeners with hearing loss. For example, although some adults and children with cochlear implants demonstrate substantial A-only word recognition, others obtain high levels of speech understanding only when auditory *and* visual speech cues are available (Bergeson, Pisoni, & Davis, 2003, 2005; Hay-McCutcheon, Pisoni, & Kirk, 2005; Kaiser et al., 2003). Furthermore, the ability to combine and integrate auditory and visual speech information has been found to be an important predictor of speech perception benefit with a sensory aid (Bergeson & Pisoni, 2004; Bergeson, Pisoni, & Davis, 2003, 2005; Lachs, Pisoni, & Kirk, 2001) and thus has important implications for understanding the underlying representation and processing of speech in listeners who use these devices. Whenever possible, performance should be assessed in all three presentation modalities: A-only, V-only and AV. When combined, results from independent and multimodality testing provide information, not only about how well speech is conveyed through an implant alone, but also about speech perception enhancement that is obtained when auditory and visual cues are provided.

Outcome Measures for Children

Historically, two approaches have been used in the development of a speech perception battery for children with profound deafness that use cochlear implants or other sensory aids. One approach, previously followed by Geers and her colleagues at the Central Institute for the Deaf (CID) (Geers & Moog, 1989), assumes that children acquire speech perception abilities in a hierarchical fashion starting from simple detection through spoken word comprehension (Erber, 1982). Test administration follows this hierarchy and children are required to reach criterion scores at each level before being administered more difficult measures. The outcome of this testing is used to categorize the children's speech perception abilities and determine auditory training goals. Table 10–1 gives an example of the speech perception categories used by the CID researchers.

An advantage of the hierarchical approach is that less time is required to complete testing. This may be especially important for assessing young children with limited attention spans. However, there are potential disadvantages of hierarchical testing and categorization of performance. First, some skills may develop in parallel rather than hierarchically, and administering only part of a test battery might not reveal the development of more sophisticated listening skills. Secondly, categorizing children's responses often obscures individual differences in performance and may make it more difficult to identify factors that influence spoken word recognition (Tyler, 1993).

TABLE 10–1. Speech Perception Categories in the CID Test Battery

Category	Speech Perception Skills
0	No detection of speech (e.g., aided speech detection threshold >65 dB HL)
1	Speech detection
2	Pattern perception (discrimination based on temporal or stress cues; e.g., airplane vs. baby)
3	Beginning word identification (closed-set word identification based on phoneme information; e.g., airplane vs. lunchbox)
4	Word identification via vowel recognition (closed-set word identification based on vowel information; e.g., boat vs. bat)
5	Word identification via consonant recognition (closed-set word identification based on consonant information; e.g., pear vs. chair)
6	Open-set word recognition (word recognition without contextual cues through listening alone)

Source: Information adapted from Geers (1994).

An alternative approach makes no a priori assumptions concerning the sequence of auditory skill development. Instead, children are administered a battery of tests that evaluates a range of speech perception abilities and are then assigned scores for each test in the battery. This approach has been followed at the Indiana University School of Medicine (IUSM) (Kirk, 2000), and in more recent investigations by Geers and her colleagues (Geers, Brenner, & Davidson, 2003). A strength of this approach is that it allows the clinician or researcher to describe all aspects of a child's communication abilities. However, this approach has disadvantages as well. It requires greater time to administer and score a large number of tests. Also, because the speech perception tasks and materials must be appropriate for the age, developmental and linguistic levels of the children being tested, it is difficult to find tests that are suitable for children of varying ages and abilities. To address these considerations, researchers at the IUSM compiled two different batteries, one for preschool-aged children and one for school-aged children.

As part of a multicenter, longitudinal cohort study titled Childhood Development after Cochlear Implantation (CDaCI), Eisenberg and her colleagues used a hybrid approach to compile a test battery for assessing speech perception in young children (Eisenberg et al., 2006). The hierarchical approach was adopted from the CID battery and the age-based approach was adopted from the IUSM protocol. For each measure in the CDaCI hierarchy, a criterion level of performance must be reached before children move on to more difficult tests. Testing on a specific measure is discontinued once a ceiling is reached at two consecutive test intervals spaced six months apart. Like the previous two batteries, the CDaCI hierarchy utilizes both closed- and open-set test formats. Closed-set tests are used to assess pattern perception, word and sentence recognition. Open-set tests assess word and sentence recognition. At the more difficult levels, testing can be conducted in quiet or in background noise. For children who are too young to participate in objective testing, parent questionnaires are employed to obtain subjective information about auditory performance.

Subjective Measures of Performance

The Meaningful Auditory Integration Scale (MAIS) (Robbins, Renshaw, & Berry, 1991) uses a structured parent interview format. Parents are asked 10 questions about the auditory behaviors their child demonstrates in daily activities. The questions probe a hierarchy of behaviors; initial questions probe the child's attachment to the sensory aid and simple auditory detection. Later questions examine the recognition and comprehension of speech. Each probe receives a score of 0 to 4 depending on how frequently the child demonstrates the behavior. In the CDaCI battery, this measure is used with parents whose children are 4 years of age or older. The Infant-Toddler Meaningful Auditory Integration Scale (IT-MAIS) (Zimmerman-Phillips et al., 2000) was later developed for use with very young children. This measure shares many of the same questions with the MAIS. It differs in questions that specifically explore an infant's vocal behavior. The CDaCI battery uses this measure with parents of children who are between the ages of 1 to 3 years.

Closed-Set Tests of Speech Perception/Spoken Word Recognition

Table 10-2 lists tests that frequently have been used to assess closed-set speech perception in children with cochlear implants. The CID Early Speech Perception Test (ESP) (Moog & Geers, 1990) requires children to select a word from a number of different alternatives presented. Subtests assess the children's pattern perception (i.e., differen-tiating stimuli on the basis of syllable number), spondee recognition, and monosyllabic word recognition. In the monosyllabic subtest, the target and foils have similar consonants but different vowels. In the standard version, children are presented with 12-picture plates from which to select their response. The CDaCI battery includes this test for children who are at least 3 years of age. The low-verbal version may be used for children with limited vocabularies. This version uses a smaller response set and presents the children with real objects from which to make a selection. The CDaCI battery includes this test for children aged 2 years or older.

The Word Intelligibility by Picture Identification Test (WIPI) (Ross & Lehrman, 1971) uses a picture-pointing response. One stimulus word is presented per six-picture plate. The target and six foils have similar vowels but different consonants. As pointed out by Geers, Brenner, and Davidson, 2003, the WIPI is more difficult than the ESP because both the auditory task (recognizing words using consonant cues) and the vocabulary demands are greater in the WIPI.

The Grammatical Analysis of Elicited Language—Pre-Sentence Level (Moog, Kozak, & Geers, 1983) has been adapted for use as a closed-set speech perception test. It assesses recognition of 30 isolated words representing familiar vocabulary. Children are first familiarized with the 30 objects in the auditory-plus-visual modality. During test administration, the 30 objects are presented in sets of 4 and the child must identify the target through listening alone. The four-item set changes after every trial. The item presentation has been reordered from that suggested by Moog et al. so that the 11 multisyllabic words are presented first followed by the 19 monosyllabic words. This eliminates syllable number as a cue to word recognition.

TABLE 10–2. Closed-Set Tests of Spoken Word Recognition for Children

Test	Stimuli	Presentation Mode	Test Condition	Presentation Format	Response Format	Test Age
ESP— Low verbal[a]	1-, 2-, or 3-syllable words, Spondees	Monitored-live-voice (MLV) or Recorded	Quiet	A only	Object selection (Sets of 4 alternatives)	2 years +
ESP— Standard[a]	1-, 2-, or 3-syllable words, Spondees	MLV or Recorded	Quiet	A only	Picture selection (12-picture plates)	3 years +
WIPI[b]	Monosyllabic words	MLV or Recorded	Quiet	A only	Picture selection (6-picture plates)	4 years +
GAEL-P[c]	1-, 2-, or 3-syllable words	MLV	Quiet	A only	Object selection (Sets of 4 alternatives)	2 years +
PSI[d]	Monosyllabic words, sentences	Recorded	Quiet and com-petition	A-only	Picture selection (5-picture or 6-picture* plates)	3 years +
CRISP[e]	Spondees	Recorded	Adaptive testing in quiet or in noise	A only	Picture selection (≤25 pictures**)	4 years +
CRISP-Jr[e]	1- or 2-syllable words	Recorded	Adaptive testing in quiet or in noise	A only	4-alternative-pictures**	2.5–3 years

[a](Moog & Geers, 1990); [b](Ross & Lehrman, 1971); [c](Moog, Kozak, & Geers, 1983); [d](Jerger, Jerger, & Lewis, 1981); [e](Garadat & Litovsky, 2007).

*The IUSM protocol presents children with six-picture plates to minimize their ability to use a "process of elimination" (Kirk & Choi, in press).

**Test words are familiarized before testing. The words that are not easily identified by a child are eliminated from the closed-set alternatives (Garadat & Litovsky, 2007).

The Pediatric Speech Intelligibility Test (Jerger, Jerger, & Lewis, 1981; Jerger, Lewis, Hawkins, & Jerger, 1980) evaluates word and sentence recognition using five-picture plates. The IUSM protocol presents children with six-picture plates to minimize their ability to use a "process of elimination" in target selection. The CDaCI battery uses a recorded version (Eisenberg & Dirks, 1995) and presents the stimuli in quiet and in the presence of single-talker competition at message-to-competition ratios ranging from +10 to −10 dB. The message is presented via a loudspeaker at 0 degrees azimuth and the competition is presented from a loudspeaker located at 90 degrees on the side of the nonimplanted ear. The CDaCI battery introduces this test when children are at least 3 years of age. More details on test administration may be found in Eisenberg et al. (2006).

The Children's Realistic Intelligibility and Speech Perception (CRISP) test (Garadat & Litovsky, 2007) was developed by Litovsky and colleagues to measure the speech reception threshold (i.e., 50% correct) in very young children. Two different versions are available. The CRISP is suitable for children aged 4 years and older. It contains 25 spondee words selected from the Children's Spondee list (CID W-1) that have been recorded by a male talker. The CRISP-Jr. utilizes 16 words, 12 monosyllabic and 4 bisyllabic, recorded by a male talker. The target words in the CRISP-Jr. are inspired by the Mr. Potato Head toy, and represent vocabulary that is appropriate for children aged 2.5 to 3 years of age, such as the names of objects and body parts. Both the CRISP and CRISP-Jr present words at fixed presentation levels in quiet and in the presence of different types of noise. Adaptive testing also can be performed wherein a speech reception threshold is obtained (i.e., the SNR that yields 50% words cor-

rect). Prior to testing, children are familiarized with the vocabulary through the use of pictures. During testing, children respond by pointing to pictures representing the target word. The CRISP recently has been used to assess directional hearing and release from masking in children with bilateral cochlear implants or children who use a cochlear implant and a hearing aid on the nonimplanted ear (Litovsky et al., 2004).

Open-Set Tests of Spoken Word Recognition

Table 10–3 lists tests that are used to assess open-set word or sentence recognition in children with cochlear implants. In open-set testing, children are presented with the target word or sentence and asked to repeat what they hear. The responses typically are scored as the percent of words correctly identified.

Traditional Clinical Tests

The Mr. Potato Head task was developed as a modified open-set task (Robbins, 1994). Children are asked to carry out commands in assembling a Mr. Potato Head toy through listening alone. Two percent-correct scores are generated: a sentence score for the percent of commands correctly carried out, and a word score for the percent of key words correctly identified, even if the command was not followed correctly. This test is considered to be a modified open-set test because the number of items that can be used is large (20 or more), but not unlimited. Because children could touch an object representing a key word by chance, 5% was set as chance performance for key words. No chance score is assigned for sentence recognition as children cannot complete this task through guessing alone.

TABLE 10–3. Open-Set Speech Perception Tests for Children

Test	Stimulus Format	Presentation Mode	Test Condition	Presentation Format	Lists	Test Age
Mr. Potato Head[a]	Words, sentences	Monitored Live Voice (MLV)	Quiet	A only	2 lists of 10 sentences	3 years +
MLNT[b]	2- or 3-syllable words	Recorded (single- or multitalker versions)	Quiet	A only	2 lists of 24 words	3 years +
LNT[b]	Monosyllabic words	Recorded (single- or multitalker versions)	Quiet	A only	2 lists of 50 words	4 years +
PB-K[c]	Monosyllabic words	MLV or Recorded	Quiet	A only	4 lists of 50 words*	5 years +
CAVET[d]	1-, 2-, or 3- syllable words	Recorded (CD-ROM, VHS)	Quiet	A only V only A + V	2 list of 20 words	7–9 years + for children with profound prelingual hearing loss
BKB[e]	Sentences	MLV or Recorded	Quiet	A only	21 lists of 16 sentences	6 years +
HINT–C[f]	Sentences	Recorded	Quiet or Noise (Adaptive)	A only	13 lists of 10 sentences	5 years +
AV-LNST[g]	Sentences	Recorded (Quick Time movie files)	Quiet	A only V only A + V	6 lists of 8 sentences	4 years +

[a](A. M. Robbins, 1994); [b](K. I. Kirk, Pisoni, & Osberger, 1995); [c](Haskins, 1949); [d](Tye-Murray & Geers, 2001); [e](Bench, Kowal, & Bamford, 1979); [f](Gelnett, Sumida, Nilsson, & Soli, 1995); [g](R. F. Holt, Kirk, & Howell, 2007).

*Although there are 4 lists developed by Haskins (1949), only lists 1, 3, and 4 are similar in difficulty.

**An American English version of BKB sentences was adapted by Kenworthy et al. (Kenworthy, Klee, & Tharpe, 1990).

The Phonetically Balanced Kindergarten Word List (PBK) (Haskins, 1949) is one of the oldest and most widely used tests of spoken word recognition in children. It consists of four lists of 50 words. As noted in Table 10–3, only three of the lists were found to be equivalent in Haskins' original study. Within each list the 50 words are phonetically balanced. The test is scored as the percent of words or phonemes correctly recognized. In the CDaCI battery, this test is used for children aged 5 years and above.

The Bamford-Kowal-Bench Sentences (BKB) (Bamford & Wilson, 1979) consists of lists of 16 simple sentences that include 50 key words. They were developed to be suitable for hearing-impaired children aged 8 to 15 years. Children are asked to imitate the sentence. The child's entire response is noted, but the responses are scored only as the percent of key words correctly identified.

The Hearing-in-Noise Test for Children (HINT-C) (Gelnett, Sumida, Nilsson, & Soli, 1995) is composed of 130 sentences derived from the original 250 sentences of the HINT (Nilsson et al., 1994). The sentences are arranged into 13 lists of 10 sentences. Vocabulary was selected to be familiar to young children. A recorded version of the test is used to test children in quiet or in the presence of speech-spectrum-shaped noise. The HINT-C has been administered in two ways. As the test was designed, the speech reception threshold for sentences is determined adaptively with the speech presented in speech-spectrum-shaped noise. In an alternative method often used in clinics, the tests are administered in quiet or at a fixed SNR. This test is administered to children age 5 years and above in the CDaCI battery.

Theoretically Motivated Tests

Development of the Lexical Neighborhood Tests

Traditional open-set tests yield descriptive information regarding spoken word recognition abilities but reveal little about the underlying perceptual processes that support spoken word recognition. To address this problem, in the early 1990s the senior author and colleagues developed new measures designed to assess spoken word recognition in children with cochlear implants. Stimuli were selected according to two criteria. First, the test words had to be familiar to young children with relatively limited vocabularies. Thus, stimuli were drawn from the Child Language Data Exchange System database (MacWhinney & Snow, 1985) which contains transcripts of young children's verbal exchanges with a caregiver or another child. All tokens were drawn from productions by typically developing children between the ages of 3 to 5 years and thus represent early-acquired vocabulary. The second criterion was that the new measures should be based on what currently is known about spoken word recognition and lexical access using a model of spoken word recognition. The tests thus were theoretically motivated by the assumptions underlying the Neighborhood Activation Model (Luce & Pisoni, 1998). Based on computational analyses, word lists were constructed to allow systematic examination of the effects of word frequency, lexical density, and word length. The resulting Lexical Neighborhood Test (Kirk et al., 1995) consists of 2 lists of 50 monosyllabic words, whereas the Multisyllabic Lexical Neighborhood Test (MLNT) consists of 2 lists of 24 two- to three-syllable words. On each list, half of the words are lexically easy (i.e., occur often and have few phonemically similar neighbors with which to compete for lexical selection) and half are lexically hard (i.e., occur infrequently and come from dense lexical neighborhoods).

In the first of a series of studies, Kirk et al. (1995) used these new measures to examine the effect of lexical characteristics on spoken word recognition performance by children with cochlear implants and to compare their performance on the LNT and MLNT with their performance on a traditional pediatric test, the PBK. Participants were 27 children with profound deafness who had used a cochlear implant for at least one year. Test stimuli were presented in an auditory-only format via live voice at approximately 70 dB SPL; children responded by repeating the word they heard using spoken and/or signed English. The percentage of words correctly identified was significantly higher for lexically easy words than for hard words. Furthermore, performance was consistently higher on the lexically controlled lists than on the PBK. These early results demonstrated that pediatric cochlear implant users are sensitive to the acoustic-phonetic similarity among words, that they organize words into similarity neighborhoods in long-term memory, and that they use this structural information in recognizing isolated words in an open-set response format. The results also suggested that the PBK underestimated the participants' spoken word recognition abilities, perhaps because of the vocabulary constraints inherent in creating phonetically balanced word lists.

In an effort to determine the minimum participant age at which these tests should be attempted, we tested spoken word recognition in 3- and 4-year-old children with normal hearing using the PBK, LNT

and MLNT (Kluck, Pisoni, & Kirk, 1997). Stimulus presentation and response collection procedures were the same as described above. Both the 3- and 4-year-old groups of children completed the tasks with scores that were close to ceiling. High scores and lack of variability in this population precluded establishing test-retest reliability for children with normal hearing. However, performance by these children provided a "benchmark" for assessing the spoken word recognition abilities of children with hearing loss; children with normal hearing ≥3 years of age can complete these tasks. In the CDaCI battery, both the MLNT and LNT may be introduced when children are at least 3 years of age. The IUSM protocol suggests using the MLNT when the child is 3 years of age and the LNT when the child is 4 or 5 years of age; this is determined, in part, by their vocabulary knowledge.

Kirk, Sehgal, and Hay-McCutcheon (2000) compared pediatric cochlear implant recipients' familiarity with words on the PBK, LNT and MLNT using parent ratings on a seven-point scale. Results showed a significant difference in familiarity between words on the three lists; words on the LNT were rated as most familiar followed by the MLNT and the PBK, respectively. Poor performance on the PBK may result, in part, because children with profound deafness are unfamiliar with the test items. There were no significant differences in familiarity between the lexically easy and hard words on the LNT and MLNT. Additionally, word familiarity was significantly related to chronological age for the MLNT and PBK, but not the LNT. These results provide further support for the appropriateness of the LNT as a spoken word recognition test for children of widely varying ages.

Studies have shown that performance on the LNT and MLNT is strongly correlated with other traditional measures of spoken word recognition and spoken language processing in children with cochlear implants (Geers, Brenner, & Davidson, 2003; Pisoni, Svirsky, Kirk, & Miyamoto, 1997). We examined the relationship among measures of spoken language processing in pediatric cochlear users with exceptionally good speech perception abilities (Pisoni et al., 1997). The results revealed that performance on the LNT was strongly correlated with open-set sentence recognition, receptive vocabulary, receptive and expressive language abilities, speech intelligibility, nonword repetition, and working memory span. The pattern of results suggests that the LNT and MLNT are measuring the same underlying construct. That is, they are measuring phonological coding processes that are used to encode, store, retrieve, and manipulate spoken language.

Development of Audio-Recorded Versions of the LNT and MLNT

Kirk (1999) subsequently developed audio-recorded versions of both the LNT and MLNT using three male and three female talkers. In a pilot study, the intelligibility of the target words was determined by a group of 60 college students with normal hearing (10 listeners per talker). They heard the tokens from each talker presented in quiet under headphones at 70 dB SPL and wrote down the word they heard. The mean intelligibility of the six talkers ranged from 92–100% words correct. These intelligibility results were used to create equivalent recorded LNT and MLNT lists in single-talker and multiple-talker conditions. Tokens from one male were used for the single-talker version because his intelligibility score was closest to mean for the six talkers. The multiple-talker version contained tokens

produced by the remaining two males and three females.

Kirk and colleagues (Kirk, Eisenberg, Martinez, & Hay-McCutcheon, 1999) examined the test-retest reliability and interlist equivalency of the audio-recorded versions of the LNT and MLNT in 16 children with profound, prelingual hearing loss who used a cochlear implant. Stimuli were presented at approximately 70 dB SPL via loudspeaker at 0 degrees azimuth. Children responded by repeating the word they heard in spoken and/or signed English. Each child was tested twice, with the time between sessions ranging from 3 hours to 15 days, depending on availability. The LNT and MLNT had high test-retest reliability and good interlist equivalency. Spoken word recognition scores were higher for lexically easy words than for lexically hard words, replicating the earlier findings obtained with live voice stimuli (Kirk et al., 1995).

We later used the recorded versions of the LNT and MLNT to examine the effects of lexical competition, talker variability, and word length on auditory-only spoken word recognition in 20 children with cochlear implants (Kirk, Hay-McCutcheon, Sehgal, & Miyamoto, 1998). Each participant was administered one LNT and one MLNT word list in the single-talker condition and the remaining LNT list and MLNT list in the multiple-talker condition. Lexically easy words were recognized more accurately than lexically hard words regardless of talker condition or word length. Multisyllabic words were identified better than monosyllabic words, presumably because longer words contain more linguistic redundancy and have few lexical neighbors with which to compete for selection. The children in this study also were sensitive to talker characteristics, with differences in performance noted between the single-talker and multiple-talker lists.

Utility of the LNT and MLNT

The results summarized above demonstrate that the LNT and MLNT provide reliable measures of auditory-only spoken word recognition abilities of children with profound hearing loss who use a cochlear implant. These tests are commercially available in a single-talker format (one male voice) and a multi-talker format (two males and three females) from Auditec of St. Louis. Since their introduction in the 1990s, the LNT and MLNT have been used to help determine CI candidacy and postimplant benefit in the majority of FDA pediatric clinical trials of new CI systems. These tests also have been used by a number of different researchers to examine factors that influence cochlear implant outcomes (Geers, Brenner, & Davidson, 2003; Kirk, Pisoni, & Miyamoto, 2000; Wang et al., 2008).

Development of an Audio-Recorded Lexical Sentence Test for Children

Eisenberg et al. (2002) created lexically controlled sentences from the subset of words used to develop the LNT and MLNT. Sentence lists were generated using the definitions and procedures of Kirk et al. (1995) in accordance with the Neighborhood Activation Model. Three key words were used in constructing each of the five- to seven-word sentences. These sentences were combined into two lists, each with 5 practice and 20 test sentences that were syntactically correct but semantically neutral. One list contained sentences with lexically easy key words; the other list contained key words that were lexically hard. Eisenberg et al. (2002) then used these sentences to investigate the effects of word frequency and lexical density on the children's recognition of isolated words and the same words pro-

duced in a sentence context. The lexically controlled sentences and the isolated key words comprising the sentences were audio-recorded separately as two different tests and used in three experiments. In Experiment 1, 48 children with normal hearing between the ages of 5 to 12 years repeated the isolated words and sentences at one of six different levels to generate performance-intensity functions. In Experiment 2, 12 normal-hearing children aged 5 to 14 years repeated the words and sentences under spectrally degraded conditions intended to simulate cochlear implant speech processing. In Experiment 3, 12 children with cochlear implants aged 5 to 14 years repeated the unprocessed stimuli. Children also completed a test of vocabulary recognition. In all three experiments, sentences containing lexically easy key words were recognized more accurately than sentences containing lexically hard key words. Sentence scores were significantly higher than word scores for the children with normal hearing and nine high-performing children with cochlear implants. Three low-performing children with cochlear implants showed the opposite pattern for isolated word and sentence stimuli. A statistically significant relationship was observed between chronologic age and sentence scores for children with normal hearing who heard degraded speech. For children with cochlear implants, the relationship between language abilities and spoken word recognition was strong and significant. This result demonstrates the influence of linguistic knowledge on phonological processing of words.

Auditory-Visual Tests of Spoken Word Recognition for Children

The Children's Audio-Visual Enhancement Test (CAVET) (Tye-Murray & Geers, 2001) was designed to estimate auditory-visual enhancement (i.e., the improvement noted in speech understanding when auditory information is added to lipreading). The CAVET consists of 3 different stimulus lists, each containing 20 words. Vocabulary for the stimuli was judged to be familiar to young deaf children. In order to avoid floor and ceiling effects, half of each list consists of low-visibility items in a vision-only condition; the remaining items are high visibility. One list is presented in an AV format and another list is presented in a V-only format. Children repeat the target words. Visual enhancement (VE) is calculated as: VE = (AV−A)(1−A).

Theoretically Motivated Tests

The Audiovisual-Lexical Neighborhood Sentence Test (AV-LNST) (Holt, Kirk, Pisoni, Burckhartzmeyer, & Lin, 2005) is an audiovisually recorded test derived from the Lexical Sentence Test described above. The 50 sentences created by Eisenberg et al. (2002) were audiovisually recorded using a professional Caucasian female announcer who spoke a General American dialect of English in a conversational speaking style. The resulting AV-LNST contains six lists of eight sentences that can be administered in three different presentation formats: V-only, A-only, and AV. The sentence lists are equally difficult within each presentation format. Children respond by repeating the sentences. The test is scored as the percent of lexically easy and hard key words identified correctly. The remaining words in each sentence are lexically neutral and are not scored.

New Directions: Perceptually Robust Tests of Auditory-Visual Sentence Recognition

As noted above, traditional clinical tests of spoken word recognition routinely employ isolated words or sentences produced by a single talker in an auditory-only presentation format. The more central cognitive processes used during multimodal integration, perceptual normalization and lexical discrimination that may contribute to individual variations in spoken word recognition performance are not assessed in conventional tests of this kind. We believe that there is a need for perceptually robust pediatric tests (i.e., incorporating stimulus variability) that can be administered in an auditory-visual format. Data also are needed about how children with differing degrees of hearing and different sensory aids perform on multimodal tests as a function of presentation format (A-only, V-only, and AV). Such standardization data are needed to guide decisions about sensory aid use and intervention strategies.

In collaboration with Dr. Laurie Eisenberg at the House Ear Institute in Los Angeles and Dr. Nancy Young at Children's Memorial Hospital in Chicago, we are developing new auditory-visual, multitalker sentence tests for adults and children. This work is supported by the National Institute on Deafness and Other Communication Disorders. Test development builds on basic research concerning spoken language processing by listeners with normal hearing or with hearing loss. Like our earlier tests, the new Multimodal Lexical Sentence Test for Children (MLST-C) is theoretically motivated by the Neighborhood Activation Model and contains lexically controlled stimulus items. It expands on our earlier tests in that the lexical characteristics of word frequency and lexical density are independently manipulated. Furthermore, it incorporates a wider range of stimulus variability by including sentences produced by 10 different talkers. This 5-year project, which was initiated in 2007, encompasses the following development milestones as described below. These milestones are presented to illustrate the concrete steps involved in test development.

It is noted that this work is ongoing and, at the time of this writing, only Milestone 1 has been completed and Milestone 2 is in the process of being completed.

Milestone 1: Construct sentence lists containing key words with equivalent lexical characteristics

The MLST-C utilizes the 50 Eisenberg et al. (2002) sentences and an additional, 50 new sentences created to allow for the independent manipulation of word frequency and lexical density. Words with many lexical neighbors come from sparse lexical neighborhoods, whereas words with few lexical neighbors come from dense lexical neighborhoods. Within the sentence sets, key words represent four different lexical categories: (1) High Frequency-Sparse, (2) High-Frequency-Dense, (3) Low-Frequency-Sparse, and (4) Low-Frequency-Dense. Category 1 contains key words that are easy to identify in a spoken word recognition task, whereas Category 4 contains key words that are hard to identify. We have used words from these two lexical categories in our previous tests of spoken word and sentence recognition. Categories 2 and 3 contain key words that are presumed to represent an intermediate level of difficulty.

Milestone 2: Create audiovisually recorded, multitalker versions of the sentence

Talker Selection. Twenty-five adults with normal hearing were recruited from the Purdue University community as potential talkers. All had normal hearing and were native speakers of a General American dialect of English. Each participant completed a brief survey to allow us to obtain demographic information and to verify that there was no history of speech, language or hearing disorders. Vision and hearing were screened and speech samples were obtained while participants were seated inside a sound-treated booth. Participants were asked to produce the sustained vowels, /a/ and /i/, twice for 5 seconds each at a comfortable pitch and intensity. Subjects also read the first paragraph of the Rainbow Passage using a conversational speaking style. The samples were digitally audio-recorded and acoustic analyses of each speech sample were carried out to aid in the selection of 10 participants to serve as talkers. Fundamental frequency (F_0) was measured during the steady state portion of each vowel and at selected points throughout the Rainbow Passage. F_0 was extracted using an autocorrelation pitch extraction algorithm as described in Boersma (Boersma, 1993). Table 10–4 presents the mean and range of F_0 values as a function of participant gender.

The senior author and two research assistants next made perceptual judgments concerning voice quality, speech intelligibility, and dialect region of the participants while listening to the Rainbow Passage. Participants who were perceived to have an unusual voice quality or a regional dialect were excluded from further consideration. Ten talkers (5 males and 5 females)

TABLE 10–4. Mean and Range of F_0 (In Hz) as a Function of Participant Gender

Participant Gender	/a/		/i/		Rainbow Passage	
	Mean	Range	Mean	Range	Mean	Range
Females (N = 13)	210	144–244	221	147–274	185	79–480
Males (N = 12)	115	92–141	118	94–145	116	80–309

representing diverse racial and/or ethnic groups were selected to maximize the range of F_0 within each gender. Table 10–5 presents demographic information as well as the mean and range of F_0 for each selected talker.

Talker Recording. Talker recording took place inside an Industrial Acoustics Company (IAC) sound-attenuated booth to eliminate extraneous noise. Each talker was digitally audiovisually recorded in High-Definition Digital Format (HD) to be sure that our materials will be compatible with future television technology. Fixed distances were maintained between each talker and the camera, microphone, lighting and background. Lighting was controlled to eliminate unwanted shadows on the talkers' faces. Sentences and isolated key words were produced at a normal conversational rate with the talker looking directly at the camera/teleprompter and assuming a neutral expression in between words and sentences. Words or sentences that were mispronounced were re-recorded immediately during the session. All talkers wore a black t-shirt and the video shot composition was adjusted to accommodate each talker's physiologic characteristics.

Editing of AV Stimuli. Editing of the digital files was carried out at Purdue University and the House Ear Institute. Individual QuickTime (Apple Computer, 2004) movie files were created for the sentences. The auditory waveform was used to remove the silence from the beginning and end of each sentence. The visual signal then was examined to ensure that the talker's face and articulators were in a steady-state position at the beginning and end of each movie file;

TABLE 10–5. Talker Characteristics

Talker	Gender	Age (Yrs)	Race	Primary Residence	/a/	/i/	Rainbow Passage Mean	Rainbow Passage Range
1	F	25	Asian	Indiana	244	274	207	(77–366)
2	F	23	White	Arizona	231	232	201	(78–308)
3	F	21	White	Midwest	222	227	183	(104–322)
4	F	24	Black	New Jersey	172	179	172	(78–452)
5	F	36	White	Illinois	144	147	145	(84–334)
6	M	27	Black/White	Indiana	131	135	137	(80–295)
7	M	20	White	Midwest/East Coast	119	118	124	(90–181)
8	M	27	White	Utah	119	121	116	(81–191)
9	M	28	White	California	134	145	113	(103–175)
10	M	28	Black/White	Indiana	104	106	113	(76–271)

The F_0 (Hz) column spans /a/, /i/, and Rainbow Passage (Mean, Range).

adjustments were made as necessary. Once editing was completed, two research assistants compared the two recordings of each sentence for each talker and selected the best one. When the research assistants did not agree, the senior author selected the token to be used.

Equating Intensity Across Sentences. The auditory and visual speech signals were separated using custom software. We then measured the root mean square (RMS) amplitude of the auditory signal for each sentence using Audition software. The average RMS amplitude was calculated across all sentences and talkers and the amplitude of the individual sentences was adjusted to match this level. The auditory and visual portions of the signals were merged in Final Cut Pro, taking care not to alter the temporal aspects of the two types of signals.

Generating Equivalent Multitalker Lists. The 100 sentences produced by the talkers will be used to generate 12 lists of eight sentences (24 key words per sentence); each MLST-C list will contain two sentences per lexical category. Adults with normal hearing will participate in speech perception testing to determine the intelligibility of each sentence produced by the talkers. The participants will be divided randomly into 30 groups of 10 listeners. Each group of 10 listeners will be presented with all of the sentences produced by one talker in one presentation format. To avoid ceiling effects, the speech signal in the auditory only and auditory-plus-visual presentation formats will be presented in the presence of noise shaped to match the long-term average spectrum of the sentence stimuli. To date, we have completed a pilot project with 25 adults to adaptively determine the signal-to-noise ratio that yields performance near 75% key words correct. When testing of normal hearing listeners is completed, we will use the intelli-gibility scores to generate multitalker lists that have equivalent talker difficulty within (but not across) each presentation format.

Milestone 3: Measure reliability and establish validity of the sentence sets in listeners with hearing loss

Once Milestones 1 and 2 are achieved, we will have multitalker sentence lists that are equivalent to listeners with normal hearing. However, it has been found that lists which are equivalent to listeners with normal hearing may not be equivalent to listeners with hearing loss (Cox, Alexander, Gilmore, & Pusakulich, 1988). Therefore, we will carry out our studies to verify that the lists are similar, reliable and valid when used with the target clinical population (i.e., children with hearing loss).

Milestone 4: Collect normative data from children

We will administer the MLST-C to children with normal hearing and with hearing loss to collect data concerning performance in the A-only, V-only and AV presentation formats. These normative data can be used for future test interpretation. Normative data from children with normal hearing will serve as a benchmark for comparing results obtained from clinical populations. Pyschometric analyses carried out under Milestone 3 will be replicated with the standardization sample and reported in the technical manual to be developed.

Milestone 5: Dissemination of the new test materials

The end product of this 5-year project will be a psychometric analysis kit comprising a DVD containing the MLST-C, an instruction booklet for delivering the test, data gathering forms, and a manual for data interpretation. The proposed test materials will be broadly disseminated and can be utilized for sensitive and objective testing in clinical decision matrices.

Summary

We believe that these new norm-referenced, multimodal sentence tests should provide important insights into the spoken word recognition differences and enormous variability noted among individuals with hearing loss and lead to better diagnosis, evaluation, and assessment paradigms. Information obtained from these new measures should prove useful in selecting sensory aids and in developing intervention programs that are targeted to an individual's specific needs. Finally, these tests should better reflect real-world listening abilities than traditional speech discrimination tests employing highly constrained auditory stimulus materials.

Acknowledgments. This work was supported in part by Grant Numbers R01DC 00064 and R01DC008875 from the National Institute on Deafness and Other Communication Disorders. The content is solely the responsibility of the authors and does not necessarily represent the official views of the National Institute on Deafness and Other Communication Disorders. We would like to thank Lindsay Prusick and Jennifer Karpicke for their assistance in manuscript preparation.

References

American Educational Research Association, American Psychological Association, and National Council on Measurement in Education. (1999). *Standards for educational and psychological testing.* Washington, DC: American Educational Research Association.

Anastasi, A., & Urbina, S. (1997). *Psychological testing* (7th ed.). Upper Saddle River, NJ: Prentice Hall.

Archbold, S., Lutman, M. E., & Marshall, D. H. (1995). Categories of auditory performance. *Annals Otology, Rhinology, and Laryngology 104*(Suppl. 166), 312–314.

Archbold, S., Lutman, M. E., & Nikolopoulos, T. (1998). Categories of auditory performance: Inter-user reliability. *British Journal of Audiology, 32,* 7–12.

Bamford, J., & Wilson, I. (1979). Methodological considerations and practical aspects of the BKB sentence lists. In J. Bench & J. Bamford (Eds.), *Speech-hearing tests and the spoken language of hearing-impaired children* (pp. 147–187). London: Academic Press.

Bell, T. S., & Wilson, R. H. (2001). Sentence recognition materials based on frequency of word use and lexical confusability. *Journal of the American Academy of Audiology, 12,* 514–522.

Bench, J., Kowal, A., & Bamford, J. (1979). The BKB (Bamford-Kowal-Bench) sentence lists for partially-hearing children. *British Journal of Audiology, 13,* 108–112.

Bergeson, T. R., & Pisoni, D. B. (2004). Audiovisual speech perception in deaf adults and children following cochlear implantation. In G. A. Calvert, C. Spence, & B. E. Stein (Eds.), *The handbook of multisensory perception* (pp. 749–772). Cambridge, MA: MIT Press.

Bergeson, T. R., Pisoni, D. B., & Davis, R. A. (2003). A longitudinal study of audiovisual speech perception by children with hearing loss who have cochlear implants. *Volta Review, 103,* 347–370.

Bergeson, T. R., Pisoni, D. B., & Davis, R. A. O. (2005). Development of audiovisual comprehension skills in prelingually deaf children with cochlear implants. *Ear and Hearing, 26,* 149–164.

Bernstein, L. E., Demorest, M. E., & Tucker, P. E. (2000). Speech perception without hearing. *Perception and Psychophysics, 62,* 233–252.

Bilger, R. C. (1984). *Speech recognition test development (No. 14).* Rockville, MD: ASHA Reports.

Boersma, P. (1993). Accurate short-term analysis of the fundamental frequency and the harmonics-to-noise ratio of a sampled sound. *Proceedings of the Institute of Phonetic Sciences, 17,* 97-110.

Boothroyd, A. (1984). Auditory perception of speech contrasts by subjects with sensorineural hearing loss. *Journal of Speech and Hearing Research, 27,* 134-144.

Boothroyd, A. (1985). Evaluation of speech production of the hearing impaired: Some benefits of forced-choice testing. *Journal of Speech and Hearing Research, 28,* 185-196.

Boothroyd, A. (1991). Assessment of speech perception capacity in profoundly deaf children. *American Journal of Otology, 12*(Suppl.), 67-72.

Boothroyd, A. (1995). Speech perception tests and hearing impaired children. In G. Plant & K. E. Spens (Eds.), *Profound deafness and speech communication* (pp. 345-371). London: Whurr.

Boothroyd, A., Hanin, L., & Hnath, T. (1985). A sentence test of speech perception: Reliability, set equivalence and short term learning. *City University of New York Internal Report No. RCI 10.* New York: City University of New York.

Bradlow, A. R., Akahane-Yamada, R., Pisoni, D. B., & Tohkura, Y. (1999). Training Japanese listeners to identify English /r/ and /l/: Long-term retention of learning in perception and production. *Perception and Psychophysics, 61,* 977-985.

Bradlow, A. R., & Pisoni, D. B. (1999). Recognition of spoken words by native and non-native listeners: talker-, listener-, and item-related factors. *Journal of the Acoustical Society of America, 106,* 2074-2085.

Brennan, R. L. (2004). *Revolutions and evolutions in current educational testing (CASMA Research Report No. 6).* Iowa City: University of Iowa, Center for Advanced Studies in Measurement and Assessment.

Buss, E., Pillsbury, H. C., Buchman, C. A., Pillsbury, C. H., Clark, M. S., Haynes, D. S., et al. (2008). Multicenter U. S. bilateral MED-EL cochlear implantation study: Speech perception over the first year of use. *Ear and Hearing, 29,* 20-32.

Carhart, R. (1965). Problems in the measurement of speech discrimination. *Archives of Otolaryngology, 82,* 253-260.

Ching, T. Y., van Wanrooy, E., Hill, M., & Incerti, P. (2006). Performance in children with hearing aids or cochlear implants: Bilateral stimulation and binaural hearing. *International Journal of Audiology, 45*(Suppl. 1), 108-112.

Cizek, G. J., Rosenberg, S. L., & Koons, H. H. (2008). Sources of validity evidence for educational and psychological tests. *Educational and Psychological Measurement, 68,* 397-412.

Cluff, M. S., & Luce, P. A. (1990). Similarity neighborhoods of spoken two-syllable words: Retroactive effects on mulitple activation. *Journal of Experimental Psychology: Human Perception and Performance, 16,* 551-563.

Cox, R. M., Alexander, G. C., & Gilmore, C. (1987). Development of the Connected Speech Test. *Ear and Hearing, 8*(Suppl. 5), 119-126.

Cox, R. M., Alexander, G. C., & Gilmore, C. (1991). Objective and self-report measures of hearing aid benefit. In G. A. Studebaker, F. H. Bess, & L. B. Beck (Eds.), *The Vanderbilt hearing aid report, II* (pp. 201-213). Parkton, MD: York Press.

Cox, R. M., Alexander, G. C., Gilmore, C., & Pusakulich, K. M. (1988). Use of the connected speech test (CST) with hearing-impaired listeners. *Ear and Hearing, 9,* 198-207.

Creelman, C. D. (1957). Case of the unknown talker. *Journal of the Acoustical Society of America, 29,* 655.

Demorest, M. E., & Bernstein, L. E. (1992). Sources of variability in speechreading sentences: A generalizability analysis. *Journal of Speech and Hearing Research, 35,* 876-891.

Demorest, M. E., Bernstein, L. E., & DeHaven, G. P. (1996). Generalizability of speechreading performance on nonsense syllables, words, and sentences: Subjects with normal hearing. *Journal of Speech and Hearing Research, 39,* 697-713.

Dirks, D. D., Takayanagi, S., Moshfegh, A., Noffsinger, P. D., & Fausti, S. A. (2001). Examination of the Neighborhood Activation Theory in normal and hearing-impaired listeners. *Ear and Hearing, 22,* 1-13.

Educational Researcher. (2007). *Special issue on validity, 36*(8).

Egan, J. P. (1948). Articulation testing methods. *Laryngoscope, 58*, 955–991.

Eisenberg, L. S., & Dirks, D. D. (1995). Reliability and sensitivity of paired comparisons and category rating in children. *Journal of Speech, Language, and Hearing Research, 38*, 1157–1167.

Eisenberg, L. S., Johnson, K. J., Martinez, A. S., Cokely, C. G., Tobey, E. A., Quittner, A. L., Fink, N. E., Wang, N-Y., Niparko, J. K., & the CDaCI Investigative Team. (2006). Speech recognition at 1-year follow-up in the Childhood Development after Cochlear Implantation Study: Methods and preliminary findings. *Audiology and Neurotology, 11*, 259–268.

Eisenberg, L. S., Martinez, A. S., & Boothroyd, A. (2003). Auditory-visual and auditory-only perception of phonetic contrasts in children. *Volta Review, 103*, 327–346.

Eisenberg, L. S., Martinez, A. S., & Boothroyd, A. (2004). Perception of phonetic contrasts in infants: Development of the VRASPAC. In R. Miyamoto (Ed.), Proceedings of the 8th International Cochlear Implant Conference. *International Congress Series, 1273* (pp. 364–367). Netherlands: Elsevier.

Eisenberg, L. S., Martinez, A. S., Holowecky, S. R., & Pogorelsky, S. (2002). Recognition of lexically controlled words and sentences by children with normal hearing and children with cochlear implants. *Ear and Hearing, 23*, 450–462.

Elliott, L. L., Clifton, L. A., & Servi, D. G. (1983). Word frequency effects for a closed-set word identification task. *Audiology, 22*, 229–240.

Erber, N. P. (1972). Auditory, visual, and auditory-visual recognition of consonants by children with normal and impaired hearing. *Journal of Speech and Hearing Disorders, 15*, 413–422.

Erber, N. P. (1982). *Auditory training*. Washington, DC: Alexander Graham Bell Association for the Deaf.

Firszt, J. B., Holden, L. D., Skinner, M. W., Tobey, E. A., Peterson, A., Gaggl, W., Runge-Samuelson, C. L., & Wackym, P. A. (2004). Recognition of speech presented at soft to loud levels by adult cochlear implant recipients of three cochlear implant systems. *Ear and Hearing, 25*, 375–387.

Frisch, S., Meyer, T. A., Pisoni, D. B., Svirsky, M. A., & Kirk, K. I. (2000). Using behavioral data to model open-set word recognition and lexical organization by pediatric cochlear implant users. *Annals of Otology, Rhinology, and Laryngology, 109*(Suppl. 185), 60–62.

Gantz, B. J., Tyler, R. S., Knutson, J. F., Woodworth, G., Abbas, P., McCabe, B. F., Hinrichs, J., Tye-Murray, N., Lansing, C., & Kuk, F. (1988). Evaluation of five different cochlear implant designs: Audiologic assessment and predictors of performance. *Laryngoscope, 98*, 1100–1106.

Garadat, S. N., & Litovsky, R. Y. (2007). Speech intelligibility in free field: Spatial unmasking in preschool children. *Journal of the Acoustical Society of America, 121*, 1047–1055.

Geers, A. E. (1994). Techniques for assessing auditory speech perception and lip-reading enhancement in young deaf children. *Volta Review, 96*, 85–96.

Geers, A., Brenner, C., & Davidson, L. (2003). Factors associated with development of speech perception skills in children implanted by age five. *Ear and Hearing, 24*(Suppl. 1), 24S–35S.

Geers, A. E., & Moog, J. S. (1989). Evaluating speech perception skills: Tools for measuring benefits of cochlear implants, tactile aids, and hearing aids. In E. Owens & D. Kessler (Eds.), *Cochlear implant in young deaf children* (pp. 227–256). Boston: College-Hill Press.

Gelnett, D., Sumida, A., Nilsson, M., & Soli, S. D. (1995, March). *Development of the Hearing-in-Noise Test for Children (HINT-C)*. Paper presented at the annual meeting of the American Academy of Audiology, Dallas, TX.

Goldinger, S. D. (1996). Words and voices: Episodic traces in spoken word identification and recognition memory. *Journal of Experimental Psychology: Learning, Memory, and Cognition, 22*, 1166–1183.

Goldinger, S. D. (1997). Speech perception and production in an episodic lexicon. In K. Johnson & J. W. Mullennix (Eds.), *Talker variability in speech processing* (pp. 33–66). New York: Academic Press.

Goldinger, S. D. (1998). Echoes of echoes? An episodic theory of lexical access. *Psychological Review, 105*, 251–279.

Goldinger, S. D., Pisoni, D. B., & Logan J. S. (1991). On the nature of talker variability effects on the recall of spoken word lists. *Journal of Experimental Psychology: Learning, Memory, and Cognition, 17*, 152–162.

Grant, K. W., & Seitz, P. F. (1998). Measures of auditory-visual integration in nonsense syllables and sentences. *Journal of the Acoustical Society of America, 104*, 2438–2450.

Grant, K. W., & Walden, B. E. (1996). Evaluating the articulation index for auditory-visual consonant recognition. *Journal of the Acoustical Society of America, 100*, 2415–2424.

Greenburg, J. H., & Jenkins, J. J. (1964). Studies in the psychological correlates of the sound system of American English. *Word, 20*, 157–177.

Haskins, H. (1949). *A phonetically balanced test of speech discrimination for children.* Master's thesis, Northwestern University, Evanston, IL.

Hay-McCutcheon, M. J., Pisoni, D. B., & Kirk, K. I. (2005). Audiovisual speech perception in elderly cochlear implant recipients. *Laryngoscope, 115*, 1887–1894.

Hintzman, D. L. (1986). "Schema abstraction" in a multiple-trace memory model. *Psychological Review, 93*, 411–428.

Hirsch, I. J., Davis, H., Silverman, S. R., Reynolds, E. G., Eldert, E., & Benson, R. W. (1952). Development of materials for speech audiometry. *Journal of Speech and Hearing Disorders, 17*, 321–337.

Hnath-Chisolm, T. E., Laippley, E., & Boothroyd, A. (1998). Age-related changes on a children's test of sensory-level speech perception. *Journal of Speech, Language, and Hearing Research, 41*, 94–106.

Holt, R. F., Kirk, K. I., Eisenberg, L. S., Martinez, A. S., & Campbell, W. (2005). Spoken word recognition development in children with residual hearing using cochlear implants and hearing aids in opposite ears. *Ear and Hearing, 26*(Suppl. 4), 82S–91S.

Holt, R. F., Kirk, K. I., & Howell, S. (2007, April). *The Audiovisual Lexical Neighborhood Sentence Test: Test development and preliminary results from pediatric cochlear implant recipients.* Presented at the 11th International Conference on Cochlear Implants in Children, Charlotte, NC.

Holt, R. F., Kirk, K. I., Pisoni, D. B., Burckhartzmeyer, L., & Lin, A. (2005). Lexical and context effects in children's audiovisual speech recognition. Presented at the 150th Meeting of the Acoustical Society of America, Minneapolis, MN. *Journal of the Acoustical Society of America, 118*, 162.

Hood, J. D., & Poole, J. P. (1980). Influence of the speaker and other factors affecting speech intelligibility. *Audiology, 19*, 434–455.

Hudgins, C. V., Hawkins, J. E., Karling, J. E., & Stevens, S. S. (1947). The development of recorded auditory tests for measuring hearing loss of speech. *Laryngoscope, 57*, 57–89.

Jerger, S., Jerger, J., & Lewis, S. (1981). Pediatric speech intelligibility test. II. Effect of receptive language age and chronological age. *International Journal of Pediatric Otorhinolaryngology, 3*, 101–118.

Jerger, S., Lewis, S., Hawkins, J., & Jerger, J. (1980). Pediatric speech intelligibility test. I. Generation of test materials. *International Journal of Pediatric Otorhinolaryngology, 2*, 217–230.

Kaiser, A. R., Kirk, K. I., Lachs, L., & Pisoni, D. B. (2003). Talker and lexical effects on audiovisual word recognition by adults with cochlear implants. *Journal of Speech, Language, and Hearing Research, 46*, 390–404.

Kalikow, D. N., Stevens, K. N., & Elliott, L. L. (1977). Development of a test of speech intelligibility in noise using sentence materials with controlled word predictability. *Journal of the Acoustical Society of America, 61*, 1337–1351.

Kenworthy, O. T., Klee, T., & Tharpe, A. M. (1990). Speech recognition ability of children with unilateral sensorineural hearing loss as a function of amplification, speech stimuli and listening condition. *Ear and Hearing, 11*, 264–270.

Kirk, K. I. (1999). Assessing speech perception in listeners with cochlear implants: The development of the Lexical Neighborhood Tests. *Volta Review, 100*, 63–85.

Kirk, K. I. (2000). Challenges in the clinical investigation of cochlear implant outcomes. In J. K. Niparko, K. I. Kirk, N. K. Mellon, A. McConkey Robbins, D. L. Tucci, & B. S. Wilson (Eds.), *Cochlear implants: Principles and practices* (pp. 225–259). Philadelphia: Lippincott Williams & Williams.

Kirk, K. I., & Choi, S. (in press). Results and outcomes of cochlear implantation. In J. K. Niparko (Ed.), *Cochlear implants: Principles and practice* (2nd ed.). Philadelphia: Lipincott, Williams & Wilkins.

Kirk, K. I., Diefendorf, A. O., Pisoni, D. B., & Robbins, A. M. (1997). Assessing speech perception in children. In L. L. Mendel & J. L. Danhauer (Eds.), *Audiologic evaluation and management and speech perception assessment* (pp. 101–132). San Diego, CA: Singular.

Kirk, K. I., Eisenberg, L. S., Martinez, A. S., & Hay-McCutcheon, M. (1999). Lexical neighborhood test: Test-retest reliability and interlist equivalency. *Journal of the American Academy of Audiology, 10,* 113–123.

Kirk, K. I., Hay-McCutcheon, M., Sehgal, S. T., & Miyamoto, R. T. (2000a). Speech perception in children with cochlear implants: Effects of lexical difficulty, talker variability, and word length. *Annals of Otology, Rhinology, and Laryngology, 109*(Suppl. 185), 79–81.

Kirk, K. I., Pisoni, D. B., & Miyamoto, R. T. (2000b). Lexical discrimination by children with cochlear implants: Effects of age at implantation and communication mode. In S. B. Waltzman & N. L. Cohen (Eds.), *Cochlear implants* (pp. 252–256). New York: Thieme.

Kirk, K. I., Pisoni, D. B., & Osberger, M. J. (1995). Lexical effects on spoken word recognition by pediatric cochlear implant users. *Ear and Hearing, 16,* 470–481.

Kirk, K. I., Pisoni, D. B., Sommers, M. S., Young, M., & Evanson, C. (1995). New directions for assessing speech perception in persons with sensory aids. *Annals of Otology, Rhinology, and Laryngology, 104*(Suppl. 166), 300–303.

Kirk, K. I., Sehgal, S. T., & Hay-McCutcheon, M. (2000c). Comparison of children's familiarity with tokens on the PBK, LNT, and MLNT. *Annals of Otology, Rhinology, and Laryngology, 109*(Suppl. 185), 63–64.

Kluck, M., Pisoni, D. B., & Kirk, K. I. (1997). Performance of normal-hearing children on open-set speech perception tests. *Research in Spoken Language Processing* (Progress Report No. 21, pp. 349–366). Bloomington: Indiana University, Speech Research Laboratory.

Kruschke, J. K. (1992). ALCOVE: An exemplar-based connectionist model of category learning. *Psychological Review, 99,* 22–44.

Lachs, L., Pisoni, D. B., & Kirk, K. I. (2001). Use of audiovisual information in speech perception by prelingually deaf children with cochlear implants: A first report. *Ear and Hearing, 22,* 236–251.

Landauer, T. K., & Streeter, L. A. (1973). Structural differences between common and rare words: Failure of equivalence assumptions for theories of word recognition. *Journal of Verbal Learning and Verbal Behavior, 12,* 119–131.

Lin, F. R., Ceh, K., Bervinchak, D., Riley, A., Miech, R., & Niparko, J. K. (2007). Development of a communicative performance scale for pediatric cochlear implantation. *Ear and Hearing, 28,* 703–712.

Litovsky, R. Y., Parkinson, A., Arcaroli, J., Peters, R., Lake, J., Johnstone, P., & Yu, G. (2004). Bilateral cochlear implants in adults and children. *Archives of Otolaryngology-Head and Neck Surgery, 130,* 648–655.

Luce, P. A., & Pisoni, D. B. (1998). Recognizing spoken words: The Neighborhood Activation Model. *Ear and Hearing, 19,* 1–36.

Luce, P. A., Pisoni, D. B., & Goldinger, S. D. (1990). Similarity neighborhoods of spoken words. In G. T. M. Altmann (Ed.), *Cognitive models of speech processing: Psycholinguistic and computational perspectives* (pp. 122–147). Cambridge, MA: MIT Press.

Mackersie, C. L. (2002). Tests of speech perception abilities. *Current Opinions in Otolaryngology-Head and Neck Surgery, 10,* 392–397.

MacLeod, A., & Summerfield, A. Q. (1987). Quantifying the contribution of vision to speech perception in noise. *British Journal of Audiology, 21,* 131–141.

MacWhinney, B., & Snow, C. (1985). The child language data exchange system. *Journal of Child Language, 12,* 271–295.

Martin, F. N., Champlin, C. A., & Chambers, J. A. (1998). Seventh survey of audiometric practices in the United States. *Journal of the American Academy of Audiology, 9,* 95–104.

Massaro, D. W., & Cohen, M. M. (1995). Perceiving talking faces. *Current Directions in Psychological Science, 4,* 104–109.

McArdle, R. A., Wilson, R. H., & Burks, C. A. (2005). Speech recognition in multitalker babble using digits, words, and sentences. *Journal of the American Academy of Audiology, 16,* 726–739.

Mendel, L. L., & Danhauer, J. L. (Eds.) (1997a). Historical review of speech perception assessment. In *Audiologic evaluation and management and speech perception assessment* (pp. 1–5). San Diego, CA: Singular.

Mendel, L. L., & Danhauer, J. L. (Eds.) (1997b). Test development and standardization. In *Audiologic evaluation and management and speech perception assessment* (pp. 7–13). San Diego, CA: Singular.

Mendel, L. L., & Danhauer, J. L. (Eds.). (1997c). Test administration and interpretation. In *Audiologic evaluation and management and speech perception assessment* (pp. 15–57). San Diego, CA: Singular.

Messick, S. (1989). Meaning and values in test validation: The science and ethics of assessment. *Educational Researcher, 18,* 5–11.

Moody-Antonio, S., Takayanagi, S., Masuda, A., Auer, E. T., Fisher, L., & Bernstein, L. E. (2005). Improved speech perception in adult congenitally deafened cochlear implant recipients. *Otology and Neurotology, 26,* 649–654.

Moog, J. S., & Geers, A. (1990). *Early Speech Perception Test for profoundly hearing-impaired children.* St. Louis, MO: Central Institute for the Deaf.

Moog, J. S., Kozak, V. J., & Geers, A. E. (1983). *Grammatical analysis of elicitied language —Pre-Sentence Level.* St. Louis, MO: Central Institute for the Deaf.

Mullennix, J. W., & Pisoni, D. B. (1990). Stimulus variability and processing dependencies in speech perception. *Perception and Psychophysics, 47,* 379–390.

Mullennix, J. W., Pisoni, D. B., & Martin, C. S. (1989). Some effects of talker variability on spoken word recognition. *Journal of the Acoustical Society of America, 85,* 365–378.

Nilsson, M., Soli, S. D., & Sullivan, J. A. (1994). Development of the Hearing-in-Noise Test for the measurement of speech reception thresholds in quiet and in noise. *Journal of the Acoustical Society of America, 95,* 1085–1099.

Nosofsky, R. M. (1986). Attention, similarity, and the identification-categorization relationship. *Journal of Experimental Psychology: General, 115,* 39–61.

Nygaard, L. C., & Pisoni, D. B. (1998). Talker-specific learning in speech perception. *Perception and Psychophysics, 60,* 355–376.

Nygaard, L. C., Sommers, M. S., & Pisoni, D. B. (1992). The effects of speaking rate and amplitude variability on perceptual identification. *Journal of the Acoustical Society of America, 91,* 2430.

Owens, E., Kessler, D. K., Raggio, M. W., & Schubert, E. D. (1985). Analysis and revision of the minimal auditory capabilities (MAC) battery. *Ear and Hearing, 6,* 280–290.

Paatsch, L. E., Blamey, P. J., Sarant, J. Z., Martin, L. F., & Bow, C. P. (2004). Separating contributions of hearing, lexical knowledge, and speech production to speech-perception scores in children with hearing impairments. *Journal of Speech, Language, and Hearing Research, 47,* 738–750.

Peterson, G. E., & Lehiste, I. (1962). Revised CNC lists for auditory tests. *Journal of Speech and Hearing Disorders, 27,* 62–70.

Pisoni, D. B. (1990, November). *Effects of talker variability on speech perception: Implications for current research and theory.* Paper presented at the first International Conference on Spoken Language Processing, Kobe, Japan.

Pisoni, D. B. (1993). Long-term memory in speech perception: Some new findings on talker variability, speaking rate and perceptual learning. *Speech Communication, 13,* 109–125.

Pisoni, D. B. (1997). Some thoughts on "normalization" in speech perception. In K. Johnson & J. W. Mullennix (Eds.), *Talker variability in speech processing* (pp. 9–32). San Diego, CA: Academic Press.

Pisoni, D. B. (2000). Cognitive factors and cochlear implants: Some thoughts on perception, learning, and memory in speech perception. *Ear and Hearing, 21*, 70-78.

Pisoni, D., Svirsky, M., Kirk, K., & Miyamoto, R. (1997). Looking at the "Stars": A first report on intercorrelations among measures of speech perception, intelligibility, and language in pediatric cochlear implant users. *Research on spoken language processing* (Progress Report No. 21 , pp. 51-92). Bloomington: Indiana University, Speech Research Laboratory.

Purdy, S. C., Farrington, D. R., Moran, C. A., Chard, L. L., & Hodgson, S. A. (2002). A parental questionnaire to evaluate children's Auditory Behavior in Everyday Life (ABEL). *American Journal of Audiology, 11*, 72-82.

Robbins, A. M. (1994). *Mr. Potato Head task.* Indianapolis: Indiana University School of Medicine.

Robbins, A. M., & Kirk, K. I. (1996). Speech perception assessment and performance in pediatric cochlear implant users. *Seminars in Hearing, 17*, 353-369.

Robbins, A. M., Renshaw, J. J., & Berry, S. W. (1991). Evaluating meaningful auditory intergration in profoundly hearing-impaired children. *American Journal of Otology, 12*(Suppl.), 144-150.

Ross, M., & Lehrman, J. (1971). *Word Intelligibility by Picture Identification.* Pittsburgh, PA: Stanwix House.

Skinner, M. W., Holden, L. K., Holden, T. A., Demorest, M. E., & Fourakis, M. S. (1997). Speech recognition at simulated soft, conversational and raised-to-loud vocal efforts by adults with cochlear implants. *Journal of the Acoustical Society of America, 101*, 3766-3782.

Sommers, M. S., Kirk, K. I., & Pisoni, D. B. (1997). Some considerations in evaluating spoken word recognition by normal-hearing, noise-masked normal-hearing, and cochlear implant listeners. I: The effects of response format. *Ear and Hearing, 18*, 89-99.

Sommers, M. S., Nygaard, L. C., & Pisoni, D. B. (1994). Stimulus variability and the perception of spoken words: Effects of variations in speaking rate and overall amplitude. *Journal of the Acoustical Society of America, 96*, 1314-1324.

Sommers, M. S., Tye-Murray, N., & Spehar, B. (2005). Auditory-visual speech perception and auditory-visual enhancement in normal-hearing younger and older adults. *Ear and Hearing, 26*, 263-275.

Studdert-Kennedy, M. (1974). The perception of speech. In T. A. Sebeok (Ed.), *Current Trends in Linguistics* (Vol. 2, pp. 1-62). The Hague: Mouton.

Sumby, W. H., & Pollack, I. (1954). Visual contribution of speech intelligibility in noise. *Journal of the Acoustical Society of America, 26*, 212-215.

Summerfield, Q. (1987). Some preliminaries to a comprehensive account of audio-visual speech perception. In B. Dodd & R. Campbell (Eds.), *Hearing by eye: The psychology of lipreading* (pp. 3-51). Hillsdale, NJ: Lawrence Erlbaum Associates.

Takayanagi, S., Dirks, D. D., & Moshfegh, A. (2002). Lexical and talker effects on word recognition among native and non-native listeners with normal and impaired hearing. *Journal of Speech, Language, and Hearing Research, 45*, 585-597.

Tillman, T. W., & Carhart, R. (1966). An expanded test for speech discrimination utilizing CNC monosyllabic words. Northwestern University Auditory Test No. 6. *USAF School of Aerospace Medicine Technical Report.*

Traub, R. E., & Rowley, G. L. (1991). Understanding reliability. *Educational Measurement, Issues and Practice, 10*, 37-45.

Treisman, M. (1978a). Space or lexicon? The word frequency effect and the error response frequency effect. *Journal of Verbal Learning and Verbal Behavior, 17*, 35-59.

Treisman, M. (1978b). A theory of identification of complex stimuli with an application to word recognition. *Psychological Review, 85*, 525-570.

Tye-Murray, N., & Geers, A. (2001). *Children's Audio-Visual Enhancement Test.* St. Louis, MO: Central Institute for the Deaf.

Tyler, R. S. (Ed.). (1993). Speech perception by children. In *Cochlear implants: Audiological foundations* (pp. 191-256). San Diego, CA: Singular.

Tyler, R. S., Lowder, M. W., Otto, S. R., Preece, J. P., Gantz, B. J., & McCabe, B. F. (1984). Initial Iowa results with the multichannel cochlear implant from Melbourne. *Journal of Speech and Hearing Research, 27,* 596-604.

Tyler, R. S., Lowder, M. W., Parkinson, A. J., Woodworth, G. G., & Gantz, B. J. (1995). Performance of adult Ineraid and Nucleus cochlear implant patients after 3.5 years of use. *Audiology, 34,* 135-144.

Tyler, R. S., Noble, W., Dunn, C., & Witt, S. (2006). Some benefits and limitations of binaural cochlear implants and our ability to measure them. *International Journal of Audiology, 45*(Suppl. 1), 113-119.

Walden, B. E. (1984). *Validity issues in speech recognition testing.* Rockville, MD: ASHA Reports.

Walden, B. E., Grant, K. W., & Cord, M. T. (2001). Effects of amplification and speechreading on consonant recognition by persons with impaired hearing. *Ear and Hearing, 22,* 333-341.

Walden, B. E., Prosek, R. A., & Worthington, D. W. (1975). Auditory and audiovisual feature transmission in hearing-impaired adults. *Journal of Speech and Hearing Research, 18,* 272-280.

Wang, N. Y., Eisenberg, L. S., Johnson, K. C., Fink, N. E., Tobey, E. A., Quittner, A. L., Niparko, J. K., & CDaCI Investigative Team. (2008). Tracking development of speech recognition: Longitudinal data from hierarchical assessments in the Childhood Development after Cochlear Implantation (CDaCI) study. *Otology and Neurotology, 29,* 240-245.

Wilson, R. H., Bell, T. S., & Koslowski, J. A. (2003). Learning effects associated with repeated word-recognition measures using sentence materials. *Journal of Rehabilitative Research and Development, 40,* 329-336.

Zimmerman-Phillips, S., Robbins, A. M., & Osberger, M. J. (2000). Assessing cochlear implant benefit in very young children. *Annals of Otology, Rhinology, and Laryngology, 109* (Suppl. 185), 42-43.

CHAPTER 11

The Speech-Language Specialist on the Pediatric Cochlear Implant Team

SOPHIE E. AMBROSE
DIANNE M. HAMMES-GANGULY
KATHLEEN M. LEHNERT

Introduction

The goals of this chapter are to outline the role of the speech-language specialist on a pediatric cochlear implant (CI) team and to explain, in detail, the various steps in carrying out the responsibilities associated with that role. An additional goal is to outline the different factors that are considered in the candidacy process; factors that the speech-language specialist will need to understand in order to serve as a member of the CI team. Fulfilling these goals is not a straightforward task, considering that not all CI teams even include a speech-language specialist as a team member. Instead, some CI teams run on a strictly medical model which includes primarily an otologist and audiologist. Other CI teams include speech-language specialists, psychologists, educational liaisons, social workers, and/or teachers of the deaf (TOD) in addition to otologists and audiologists. However, even on these more comprehensive teams, the responsibilities of the speech-language specialist will vary greatly from one team to another. For example, at some CI centers, the speech-language specialist's responsibilities begin when the child enters the CI candidacy process and end when the candidacy decision is made. Thus the speech-language specialist's responsibilities are fulfilled over a relatively short period of time. At other centers, the speech-language specialist may continue interacting with a child who receives a CI until the child transitions to adult services, thus allowing for a long-term relationship with the child and family. At different centers, the speech-language specialist's responsibilities may begin the day the child is identified with hearing loss and continue, regardless of whether the child is determined to be a CI candidate, until the child transitions to adult services.

In this chapter, the reader will find information about the responsibilities of the speech-language specialist from the moment the child enters the CI candidacy process through the point at which a pediatric CI recipient transitions to adult services. Additionally, the reader will find a few notes about the ways in which the speech-language specialist's responsibilities could differ if his or her involvement was to begin or end at earlier or later points in time. Specifically, the chapter begins with a description of who serves as the speech-language specialist and the responsibilities of that person. The subsequent section outlines the candidacy considerations of the CI team. Following this section, the chapter is broken into a segment on the CI candidacy speech and language evaluation and a segment on the post-CI speech and language evaluation. Finally, there is a brief discussion of aural habilitation.

The authors are speech-language pathologists by training who offer different perspectives that are colored by experiences at two CI centers. Currently, all three authors share the role of speech-language specialist at the House Ear Institute (HEI) Children's Auditory Research and Evaluation (CARE) Center in Los Angeles. Additionally, the second author spent 11 years working at the Carle Foundation Expanding Children's Hearing Opportunities (ECHO) CI Program in Urbana, Illinois. These two programs differ significantly in the way the speech-language specialist is utilized on the CI team. This chapter integrates experiences and knowledge gained from participating on these two differing teams.

The Speech-Language Specialist: Roles and Responsibilities

The position of the speech-language specialist has been filled by a variety of professionals in the numerous CI centers across the country. For example, there are audiologists and TOD who have received post-degree training in language development and thus have developed the skills necessary to fill this position on the CI team. These professionals have often been certified as auditory-verbal therapists following completion of a program involving study and mentorship on the auditory, speech, and language development of oral deaf children. Most commonly, a certified speech-language pathologist who is educated extensively on both normal and abnormal language development fills this role. This allows the speech-language pathologist not only to identify how the child's auditory experience has affected his or her language development, but also to identify the presence of speech and language disorders that are not secondary to hearing loss. For example, the speech-language pathologist's education makes him or her uniquely qualified to identify stuttering, voice disorders, and developmental phonological disorders. This education, when coupled with the appropriate training in auditory skill development, typically makes the speech-language pathologist ideally suited to fill the speech-language specialist position on a CI team. For this reason, and because having a speech-language pathologist fill this role is standard practice in the field of CIs, throughout the rest of the chapter the person who is responsible for evaluating speech and language development is referred to as a speech-language pathologist, or SLP.

Responsibilities of the SLP During the Candidacy Process

The responsibilities of the SLP can be divided into those during the CI candidacy process and those following the decision regarding implantation. During the CI candidacy process, the SLP serves collaboratively as a CI candidacy team member. The SLP provides information regarding the child's speech and language skills and describes how this information impacts the prognosis for developing or advancing spoken language skills following the receipt of a CI.

In fulfilling the responsibilities as a team member, the SLP spends the majority of time in two separate processes: collecting information regarding the child and evaluating the speech and language skills of the child. The process of collecting information involves reviewing medical records, talking with the professionals who work with the child (e.g., the child's SLP, TOD, and classroom teacher), and interviewing the child's family. Later in this chapter, detailed descriptions of the information to be attained from each of these sources can be found in the segment entitled "Speech and Language Evaluation for Cochlear Implant Candidacy" (or more specifically: "Step 1: Chart or Record Review," "Step 2: Speaking with Other Professionals," and "Step 4: Parental Interview," respectively).

In addition to collecting information, the SLP will directly evaluate the speech and language skills of the child. Two primary purposes of the evaluation are to gather information that will be critical in the decision-making process regarding CI candidacy and to establish a baseline for the child's speech and language abilities. This information will be necessary in documenting a child's speech and language progress if he or she becomes a CI recipient. A thorough description of the process of carrying out these evaluations can be found later in the chapter. The SLP is also responsible for helping to guide, educate, and counsel the family on topics such as the family's expectations for post-CI speech and language outcomes, the options for post-CI aural (re)habilitation, and techniques for facilitating language development.

Responsibilities of the SLP After the Candidacy Decision

If the child is determined not to be a CI candidate, the SLP on a CI team generally has two responsibilities after the candidacy decision is made: advising the family on options for communication modalities and educational placements, and connecting the family with appropriate professionals to help them make or follow through with their choices. If the child is determined to be a candidate for a CI and the family follows through with implantation, the general responsibilities of the SLP remain similar to those during the CI candidacy process. However, the process of carrying out those roles changes slightly as does the goal of each role. For example, the SLP continues to serve as a member of the child's CI team and provide the team with information about the child's speech and language skills. Such information will allow the team to discuss whether any changes should be recommended in the child's post-CI habilitation plan. For example, if the SLP provides information indicating that a child's speech and language growth is significantly poorer or better than expected after implantation, the team may recommend a change in the focus, intensity, or frequency of the child's aural habilitation services. More drastic recommendations may include recommending a change in communication modality or educational placement (e.g., from an oral deaf and hard of hearing, or DHH, classroom to a total communication DHH classroom, or from an oral DHH classroom to a mainstream classroom).

The SLP will spend the majority of his or her time collecting information about the child and directly evaluating the child's speech and language skills. In regard to collecting information, the SLP is no longer gathering information to make a prognosis about how the child's speech and language progress will be impacted by receipt of a CI. Instead, the SLP's goal is to determine whether the child is meeting speech and language milestones as expected with his or her CI. The SLP will ask the child's intervention or education team about how the child communicates with the CI, their perspectives on the child's progress, and how the child functions in his or her school setting (if applicable). The SLP also will talk with the child's parent(s) about the child's rate of language progress and functioning as a communicator in the home environment. In the process, the SLP asks questions to determine the presence or level of communication frustration the child or family may be experiencing.

The SLP will again directly evaluate the speech and language skills of the child. The goal at this point is to measure the child's rate of progress to determine whether the child is closing the gap between his or her speech and language abilities and those of his or her hearing peers or if that gap is widening (if such a gap was present). This information is used when discussing appropriate recommendations with the CI team and the child's parents.

As in the CI candidacy process, the SLP continues to guide, counsel, and educate the child's family. However, the topics shift toward the current aural habilitation services and educational placement. The SLP, with input from other team members, determines whether the services are appropriate and

what may be the most effective way to facilitate specific areas of speech or language that appear to be delayed. Additional topics will be family driven, as parents inevitably have questions about the speech and language development and abilities of their child.

Following the CI candidacy decision, the SLP also may become more involved with the child's education or intervention team. As an increasing number of children with CIs are mainstreamed, more professionals will need to be educated regarding CIs, auditory skill development, and aural habilitation techniques. Similarly, many professionals in the field of deaf education may have extensive experience working with children who are DHH, but not with oral children who utilize CIs. These professionals will need continuing education on the ways in which aural habilitation techniques differ for children with CIs. Although some CI teams have a person who is specifically responsible for educating the professionals working with children with CIs, such as an educational liaison, other teams rely on the SLP to fill this role.

Another new responsibility the SLP may undertake is providing aural habilitation. This, however, is a topic broad enough to fill an entire textbook. Nonetheless, a short description of the process of carrying out this responsibility can be found later in this chapter in the section entitled "Aural Habilitation."

General Candidacy Considerations of the Cochlear Implant Team

In addition to understanding the responsibilities of the SLP on the CI team and the processes involved in fulfilling those responsibilities, the SLP must be generally informed on all of the factors relevant to CI candidacy that will be discussed by the team. The following sections outline a number of factors that are typically considered regarding CI candidacy. The direct impact factors that the team collectively considers include pre-CI language abilities, implant age and timing factors, the presence of multiple disabilities, the intended mode of communication and educational placement post-CI, the child's support services, and the family's expectations and support. Other direct impact factors that are not discussed in the following section, because they fall strictly in the domain of the otologist or audiologist, include medical and audiologic candidacy criteria. A child may be deemed an inappropriate candidate for a CI due to the absence of an auditory nerve or due to malformations of the cochleae, depending on the severity. When a child presents with malformed cochleae such as a common cavity or with severe ossification, the otologist will make the decision about whether cochlear implantation is advisable from a medical standpoint. From an audiologic perspective, the child may be ruled out as a candidate if the child (1) has full aided access to the speech spectrum, (2) has not completed a hearing aid trial (except in extreme cases such as meningitis), or (3) has not consistently worn hearing aids, due to parents' inability to enforce hearing aid use or the child's unwillingness to wear the hearing aids (providing some evidence that the child is unlikely to wear his or her CI consistently).

In addition to these direct-impact factors that are, in conjunction with one another, often used to rule out children as being candidates for a CI, there are many factors with less direct impact on candidacy decisions that will be discussed by the team. These include the impact of residual hearing (in this case, hearing that allows the child some access to sound, but not enough for full access to the speech spec-

trum), nonverbal IQ (above the level at which a child would be diagnosed as having an intellectual disability), a difference in the home and intervention or school language, and additional family characteristics. Although these latter factors do not necessarily have a direct impact on the candidacy decision, they are important when counseling families on the prognosis for spoken language development following receipt of a CI and for developing a post-CI aural habilitation plan.

It is absolutely critical that everyone involved in the CI candidacy process understands the interconnectedness of the factors considered during the candidacy process and that none of the factors other than clear medical contraindications independently rule out a child as a CI candidate. In order to represent the interconnectedness of the many candidacy considerations, many CI centers utilize a candidacy profile, such as the Children's Implant Profile (ChIP) (Hellman et al., 1991) or adaptations of the ChIP including the Graded Profile Analysis (GPA) (Daya et al., 1999) and the Nottingham version of the ChIP (NChIP) (Nikolopoulos, Gibbin, & Dyar, 2004b). These scales include a variety of factors that can be considered when making a decision regarding a child's candidacy for a CI. The child is given a score for each of these factors. A negative score in one area is not enough to rule out a child as a candidate. Instead, a child must have a negative score in a number of areas. These areas are rarely mutually exclusive. For example, children with negative scores regarding implant age and other timing factors (e.g., duration of deafness) are more likely to have negative scores regarding pre-CI language abilities. Similarly, children with multiple disabilities also may be more likely to have negative scores regarding their pre-CI language abilities. A number of these factors are considered in the following sections.

Direct Impact Candidacy Factors

Pre-Cochlear Implant Language Abilities

As previously mentioned, the candidacy characteristic that falls strictly within the domain of the SLP is the child's pre-CI language abilities. The pre-CI language abilities of children presenting for CI candidacy are common considerations of CI teams when making decisions regarding candidacy and a common area of concern regarding the prognoses of children in the candidacy process (Nikolopoulos, Dyar, & Gibbin, 2004a). This is true whether the child is at the prelinguistic or linguistic stage of language development. The reason that CI teams consider pre-CI language ability stems from the hypothesis that children who have developed some language skill prior to receipt of a CI, whether through sign language or spoken language, will have a language base from which to build after receipt of the CI.

Evidence to support this hypothesis comes from three different areas of research. First, it is well established that prelinguistic skills are significantly correlated with later language outcomes for typically developing children who have normal hearing. For example, Watt, Wetherby, and Shumway (2006) found that joint attention, gesture ability, and language comprehension during the second year of life were highly correlated with receptive and expressive language outcomes in the third year of life. Second, it is clear that even for children with developmental disabilities, prelinguistic skills are significantly correlated with language outcomes (Calandrella & Wilcox, 2000). Finally, although the number of studies in the area is limited, there is evidence to suggest that pre-CI language abilities are correlated with

post-CI language outcomes. In one study, Kane, Schopmeyer, Mellon, Wang, and Niparko (2004) used the *Communication and Symbolic Behavior Scales* (Wetherby & Prizant, 1993), a measure of prelinguistic communication and early language, prior to cochlear implantation to predict performance on a later, more formalized measure of language development. Although high prelinguistic scores did not necessarily predict high scores on the formal language measure, low scores "tended strongly toward" low scores on the formalized measure (p. 622). In another study, Connor and Zwolan (2004) examined the effects of language pre- and post-CI in a very different way. They found that a measure of vocabulary that was utilized prior to implantation predicted vocabulary skill on the same measure an average of over four years post CI implantation. Edwards (2003) found that the degree of concern regarding speech and language abilities prior to implantation (as recorded on the ChIP) was significantly predictive of receptive language, speech perception, and speech intelligibility three years after implantation.

Despite the findings that pre- and post-CI language outcomes are related, many CI teams may not consider a child's language abilities to be part of the candidacy process. However, at the House Ear Institute CARE Center the child's language abilities are very important in deciding CI candidacy. For example, with all other factors being equal, at the CARE Center a 4-year-old child with at least some functional spoken language will more likely be approved for a CI than a 4-year-old child with no spoken language abilities. Furthermore, the CI team is more likely to implant a 4-year-old child with strong sign language abilities than a 4-year-old child with no language abilities. The children who sign have a language base from which to build; they have already succeeded in developing some language skills and understand key communication concepts (e.g., objects have labels, the actions of caregivers can be manipulated with the use of language). These abilities are important because by this age, children require an established language base to support academic skill and social skill development. In addition, these children have the skills and concepts needed to participate in the CI programming and subsequent aural habilitation that they would undergo following implantation. In contrast, when a child lacks language at 4 years of age, spoken language development even with a CI will be a slow process. Even with 18 to 24 months of experience with the CI, this child typically demonstrates extremely delayed language skills. Limited language development at this age poses a serious challenge for academic skill development and the child's ability to actively participate in programming. The primary goal at this point would be to establish the most efficient means for the child to develop language, which, depending on the full array of circumstances, may or may not include a CI.

Implant Age and Timing Factors

The most widely considered candidacy factors relate to age and timing factors. The three primary considerations are the age at which the child is implanted, the age at onset of deafness, and the duration of deafness prior to cochlear implantation. Notably, these three characteristics are interrelated. For example, if the age of onset of deafness and the age at which the child was implanted are known, the duration of deafness prior to cochlear implantation can be determined.

Age of Implantation. The most studied of these three factors is the age of implantation. The results of studies examining this factor vary greatly. Although the authors of most studies agree this factor is of the utmost importance, not all studies have yielded similar results. For example, Geers (2004) examined the speech perception, speech production, language, and reading skills of 181 8- to 9-year-old children who received CIs prior to the age of 5 years. She compared the performances of children implanted at 2, 3, and 4 years of age and did not find a statistically significant advantage of age at implantation for any of the outcome measures. In an attempt to explain this finding, Geers suggested that 2 years of age may not have been young enough to show the advantages of early input or that any advantage may have disappeared by 8 years of age.

Other studies have pointed directly toward age of implantation as a key factor for predicting communication outcomes. For example, Tomblin, Barker, Spencer, Zhang, and Gantz (2005) examined age of initial stimulation following cochlear implantation in 29 young children implanted between 11 and 40 months of age. The investigators found that age at initial stimulation accounted for 14.6% of the variance in expressive language growth rates. Manrique, Cervera-Paz, Huate, and Molina (2004) determined that children implanted before 2 years of age, unlike children implanted between 2 and 6 years of age, performed similarly to their hearing peers on the *Peabody Picture Vocabulary Test* (Dunn & Dunn, 1998) and the *Reynell Developmental Language Scales* (Reynell & Gruber, 1990) after 36 months of experience with their CI. Similarly, Svirsky, Teoh, and Neuburger (2004) found a large and statistically strong benefit for implantation prior to 2 years of age when they utilized developmental trajectory analysis. More recently, Holt and Svirsky (2008) examined the developmental trajectories of children implanted before the age of 4, including six children who were implanted under the age of 12 months. The authors found that earlier cochlear implantation typically led to better spoken language scores. However, the differences in spoken language scores between the group implanted from 13 to 24 months of age and the group implanted before 12 months of age were minimal. Although the U.S. Food and Drug Administration does not endorse CIs for children under 12 months of age in the United States (at the time of this writing), CI teams both within (e.g., Waltzman & Roland, 2005) and outside (e.g., Colletti et al., 2005; Dettman et al., 2007) the United States have been implanting children before their first birthday. For example, the pediatric CI research team in Melbourne, Australia recently reported outcomes for 19 infants who were implanted from 7 to 12 months of age and 87 toddlers who were implanted from 12 to 24 months of age (Dettman, Leigh, Dowell, Pinder, & Briggs, 2007). The team found that the infants were able to make one year of language progress for each year following implantation. However, the toddlers demonstrated significantly slower growth in both receptive and expressive language.

Although these studies do not definitively outline a critical time window for cochlear implantation, studies on the plasticity of the central auditory system (CAS) in children are beginning to outline a sensitive window for normal central auditory development. For example, Sharma, Dorman, and Spahr (2002) found that the CAS is maximally plastic during the first 3.5 years after a child is born with a congenital hearing loss or after a child loses his or her hearing. Additionally, Dorman, Sharma, Gilley, Martin, and Roland (2007) found that delays in synaptic transmission could be normalized within 3 to 6 months after initial stimulation of a CI if the child spent less than 3.5 years without access to auditory infor-

mation. However, synaptic transmission will remain delayed or may never normalize in children implanted after 3.5 years of age.

Clearly, the research dedicated to age at time of implantation is not sufficiently conclusive to determine that a CI is inadvisable beyond a particular age. However, it is compelling enough for most CI teams to assume that, all other factors being equal, the earlier a child is implanted, the more positive the prognosis for auditory and spoken language development.

Age at Onset of Deafness. Another age and timing consideration relates to the age at onset of deafness. Osberger, Todd, Berry, Robbins, and Miyamoto (1991) found an advantage in speech perception ability for the children whose age at onset of deafness was after 5 years of age. However, they did not find the same advantage for children who lost their hearing in the first 3 years of life. This result was attributed to the fact that the later deafened children had the advantage of a strong language base. More recently, Geers (2004) studied 39 implanted children who became deaf prior to 3 years of age, including 14 who became deaf prior to 1 year of age. She found that children who had even a brief period of hearing, coupled with a CI shortly after the onset of hearing loss, demonstrated better outcomes than implanted children who did not have any history of normal hearing.

Duration of Deafness. A third implant age and timing characteristic is duration of deafness. Geers (2004) found that for children with later onset of deafness, it was the interval between onset of deafness and age of implantation that was important. If the gap was less than 1 year, children had an 80% chance of developing speech and language within normal limits. In another study, Edwards (2003) found that age at implantation was not a significant predictor of understanding spoken language, but duration of deafness was.

Assuming that all other factors are equal, the House Ear Institute CARE Center CI team might not implant a 7-year-old child who has been deaf for 6 years, but would likely implant a 7-year-old who has been deaf for less than 1 year. Of course, all other factors are typically not equal in this case. The child with 6 years of hearing experience should have stronger pre-CI language abilities. However, even without looking at language ability, there still appears to be an advantage for a shorter duration of deafness when examining the role of duration of deafness on the development of the central auditory pathway.

In summary, it is expected that the three implant age and timing characteristics (i.e., earlier age at implantation, older age at onset of deafness, and shorter duration of deafness) lead to more positive prognoses following cochlear implantation. As a result, these factors impact candidacy decisions. However, as previously mentioned, all factors rarely are equal but, rather, are intertwined, affecting prognoses as they relate to pre-CI language ability.

Additional Disabilities

With regard to candidacy, children who have disabilities in addition to their hearing loss that might hinder their participation in audiologic assessment, CI programming, or aural habilitation, typically have not been considered CI candidates at the CARE Center. This cautionary stance has been taken because, as previously mentioned, at the CARE Center the primary consideration is the child's potential for the development of oral language. For children who have disabilities that may hinder audiologic management and aural habilitation, the CI team

must be extremely cautious about determining whether the development of spoken language is a realistic goal (Winter, Johnson, & Vranesic, 2004).

Despite this general policy, there are a number of children with intellectual and/or behavioral disabilities who utilize a CI and who receive services at the CARE Center. These children typically fit into one of two categories. The first group includes children who were implanted at such an early age that the presence of an additional disability was not readily apparent. The second group includes select children whose parents had realistic expectations, were committed to appropriate post-CI habilitation services, and who agreed to allow the research team to track their child's progress in a number of areas. This research examines whether these children receive any nontraditional benefits from the CI and explores the best way to identify and document these benefits.

In contrast to the policy of the CARE Center, the ECHO program is much less conservative in regard to implanting children with multiple disabilities. When a child presents with multiple disabilities at the ECHO program, the team focuses less on prognosis for oral language development but more on whether the child can receive other meaningful benefits from the receipt of a CI. These benefits may include allowing the family to feel more connected to the child and allowing the child to become more aware of his or her environment. Thus, for these children, the goal of evaluations during the CI candidacy stage is to determine whether the SLP feels the child will be able to make any meaningful use of sound information from the implant and whether the auditory information from hearing will benefit the child's overall development and enable a greater level of interaction with those around the child.

Communication Mode and Educational Placement

Communication mode and educational placement are important considerations during the CI pre-evaluation, particularly as they impact post-CI outcomes. Although the influence of mode of communication has been explored in multiple studies in the literature, the results are complicated by a number of factors. First, children may not utilize the same mode of communication at home as they do at school. Additionally, the mode of communication used at home or school may change multiple times in the first years of a child's life. Parents may spend the first year of their child's life using the auditory oral (AO) modality to attempt to communicate with their child. Then, when they learn that their child is deaf, they may switch to using sign language and may enroll their child in a total communication (TC) program that utilizes oral language and sign language. After their child receives a CI, the family may wish to switch back to use of the AO modality and re-enroll in an AO program. Finally, if the child makes insufficient progress with the development of oral language, the parents may switch the child back to using TC in the home and/or school setting. Thus, it can be difficult to draw conclusions from crossectional studies on the impact of mode of communication and educational placement on the language development of children with CIs.

Robbins, Bollard, and Green (1999) noted an additional complication related to studying mode of communication with children with CIs. Although they found no significant difference on a language measure when comparing performance between a TC and an AO group, they did see a trend toward faster language learning by the AO group. However, the authors noted that their findings were biased because the TC children had more profound hearing impairments than the AO children. They also noted that "this difference suggests that children with more limited auditory potential with hearing aids are placed in TC programs" (p. 118).

Another complicating factor is the range of education provided by TC classrooms. Although some TC classrooms emphasize sign and speech equally, many emphasize one skill almost to the exclusion of the other. Parents often have little say in the emphasis of their child's program as their child often must attend the only TC program in the area. Geers (2002) hypothesized that the difference in quality of TC education may have led to the differences in the findings of her study and a study by Connor, Hieber, Arts, and Zwolan (2000). Although Geers (2002) found that AO education (as opposed to TC) was more beneficial for auditory and spoken language development than any of the other factors she examined, Connor et al. (2000) did not see similar results. It was noted that the Connor et al., study was conducted in Michigan, a state known for quality TC programming. Geers, on the other hand, conducted her study with children from 33 different states and 5 Canadian provinces. Thus, the quality of TC education varied greatly amongst her participants. Similarly, it has been noted that children in AO programs often are provided with more individualized speech and language intervention than children in TC programs (Tobey et al., 2000).

Despite conflicting results from research, at the House Ear Institute CARE Center and Carle ECHO the CI teams generally are reluctant to implant children who will be placed in educational classrooms where the teacher doesn't use or encourage spoken language. That is, when all other factors are equal, if a child is placed in a classroom where he or she will not be exposed to consistent AO input (with or without the addition of sign language), the child may be deemed a poorer CI candidate than a child who will be receiving consistent AO input throughout the school day.

Support Services

Another important prognostic factor contributing to the development of spoken language is the child's participation in appropriate post-CI aural habilitation services. These services can be obtained from a variety of sources including early intervention programs for infants and toddlers through Part C of the Individuals with Disabilities Education Act (IDEA), a child's local school district or office of education, private oral deaf schools, private aural habilitation providers, and nonprofit organizations. In some instances, children can receive aural habilitation services directly from the CI center. Of course, not all services are equal in quality and parents must work with the CI team to ensure that the services their child will be receiving following implantation are appropriate. This can be difficult to ensure even in urban areas and may require the parents to advocate extensively for the needs of their child.

For children in rural settings, parents may have even more difficulty identifying appropriate support services for their child. It is still not uncommon for children in rural areas to be the first CI recipient in their county or school district. In these instances, there may not be anyone in the child's immediate geographic area with experience providing aural habilitation services to CI recipients. In these instances, families generally have three options. The first is driving a great distance to receive services from a qualified aural habilitation provider that may practice far away. Families may arrange these services on a weekly or biweekly basis with the understanding that the primary goal of aural habilitation is for the service provider to teach the parents how

to facilitate language and listening between appointments. In some states, if the child's Part C provider or school district is cognizant of the fact that they do not have a professional qualified to provide the family with aural habilitation services, they may reimburse the family for mileage. Another option is finding a professional in the family's area who is willing to learn about auditory skill development and CIs. The professional will need to travel to the CI center or to workshops in other areas to develop his or her skills in the area of aural habilitation. Families also may choose to move either permanently or temporarily to an area where appropriate services can be accessed. Again, in some areas, in addition to providing mileage for traveling between a temporary living placement and the family's permanent residence, a family may advocate for reimbursement of rent near an appropriate educational placement during the school year. Finally, some families take on the role of attending professional training programs that teach how to facilitate the language and listening development of their child. Although having parents serve as their child's only interventionist is not ideal, the parents can work with an SLP or TOD to combine their knowledge and skills in order to develop an aural habilitation program for their child. At the CARE Center and Carle ECHO, the CI teams will never rule out a child as a candidate for a CI simply because the child lives in a rural area with few services available. Instead, the CI team will help the family devise a plan for attaining appropriate services.

Family Expectations and Support

As is apparent in the previous section, families are often required to spend an extraordinary amount of time and effort advocating for and working with their child who receives a CI. In order to accomplish this, families generally must have realistic expectations, signifying that the family understands that the CI is not an instant fix and will require that they support their child's development by investing in and advocating for appropriate post-CI aural habilitation services. Nikolopoulos, Gibbin, and Dyar (2004b) found that of the 12 factors considered on the NChiP, family structure and support was one of the four most important predictors of the outcomes of children's speech perception abilities (in addition to children's learning style, short duration of deafness, and young age at implantation).

CI teams should be especially concerned about a family's ability and willingness to support their child if the family regularly does not show up for appointments, cancels multiple appointments for inappropriate reasons, repeatedly arrives late for appointments, or regularly arrives without their child's hearing aids. However, when families demonstrate this type of behavior, the child is not immediately ruled out as a CI candidate. Instead, the CI team may schedule a counseling appointment with the family to discuss the family's expectations and the expectations of the family. It is best when as many members of the CI team as possible attend this appointment. If the child is a candidate both medically and audiologically, the team members should explain that the child would be a candidate if the family establishes appropriate follow-up care, and that the child would not be a candidate if follow-up will not be consistent. The team can then work to help the parents outline a plan that will allow the CI team to be assured of the family's ability to follow through. This may include the family arriving on time for repeated hearing tests, or establishing intervention services through an outside source and regularly attending those appointments for a period of time. This may also include the family attending training with their CI center's SLP, who can teach the parents how to facilitate speech and language with their child. If parents are unable to follow-through with the plan, then the team may make the very difficult decision not to implant the child, despite the fact that the child would have otherwise been a candidate.

Factors with Less Direct Impact on Candidacy Decisions

The factors discussed thus far directly impact whether cochlear implantation is recommended. There are additional factors that may not directly impact the candidacy decision but do affect how the family is counseled regarding the child's prognosis for success with a CI and recommendations for developing appropriate post-CI habilitation services.

Residual Hearing

One factor with less direct impact on candidacy is whether the child has some usable residual hearing, despite not having full access to the speech-spectrum with hearing aids. Studies examining the relationship between pre-CI residual hearing and post-CI outcomes have pointed toward an advantage for children with more residual hearing prior to receipt of their CI. Nicholas and Geers (2006) studied a group of children who had unaided pure tone averages ranging from 77 to 120 dB HL and aided pure tone averages ranging from 32 to 110 dB HL. They found that children who received benefit from hearing aids prior to implantation were more likely to have higher language scores following implantation than their peers who had less residual hearing and thus received less benefit from their hearing aids. Similarly, in a study with German-speaking children, Szagon (2001) found pre-CI hearing to be a better predictor of later vocabulary and utterance length than age at implantation. That is, children with better pre-CI hearing were more likely to have better post-CI language skills than were their peers with more significant hearing losses.

Despite the relationship between pre-CI residual hearing and later speech perception and communication outcomes, children are not excluded from implantation based on lack of residual hearing. If, however, the children's residual hearing is adequate for the development of AO language, they are not considered typical CI candidates. Although the impact of a lack of pre-CI residual hearing on prognoses for success with a CI is not used when making candidacy decisions, this information is used in counseling parents regarding expectations following implantation. Research has demonstrated that children who gain some benefit from a hearing aid in their non-CI ear are more likely to have better speech perception scores (Francis, Yeagle, Bowditch, & Niparko, 2005). Similarly, children with a severe loss as opposed to a profound loss in their implanted ear may have more intact auditory pathways and better experience perceiving speech with their hearing aids. Again, this may lead to a better prognosis for development of speech perception skills and thus oral language development and therefore should be discussed in counseling sessions regarding appropriate parental expectations.

Nonverbal Intelligence Quotient (IQ)

Another characteristic that has the ability to impact a child's prognosis for post-CI language success is nonverbal IQ. When Geers (2002) examined six different child and family characteristics (age, age at onset, age at implant, performance IQ, family size, and parent's education), she found that performance IQ had the greatest effect on all five speech and language measures, including reading. Likewise, in a study examining predictors of language ability in 8- to 9-year-old children with implants, nonverbal IQ was found to be one of four significant predictors (Geers, Nicholas, & Sedey, 2003).

At the CARE Center, a licensed psychologist sees all children during the CI candidacy evaluation. It is very important that a psychologist who has experience with children who have hearing loss and is knowledgeable about the CI process complete this evaluation. A psychologist without experience in this area may over identify children as having developmental delays if he or she is unable to parse out which tasks the child is unable to do due to limited language ability and which tasks are true indicators of the child's intelligence. If the psychologist determines that the child has a cognitive delay significant enough to be considered an intellectual disability, then that finding is considered in the CI candidacy process. However, a child with a nonverbal IQ score in the low-average range will not be considered a poorer candidate for a CI than a child with a nonverbal IQ score in the high-average or even above-average range. Instead, considering the research in this area, nonverbal IQ may be considered when determining prognoses and talking with families about their child's potential for success.

Differences Between the Home and Intervention/School Language

Another topic that often arises when counseling parents during the candidacy process is the impact of multiple languages in the child's life. Daya, Ashley, Gysin, and Papsin (2000) note that originally they were concerned about the families under their care whose first language was not English. However, the investigators found that children from multilingual backgrounds were just as likely to end up in mainstream classrooms as their monolingual peers. Thomas, El-Kashlan, and Zwolan (2008) found no significant differences in language outcomes for 12 matched pairs of children with CIs who resided in either monolingual or bilingual homes. Similarly, McConkey Robbins, Green, and Waltzman (2004) found that, on average, the 12 children with CIs in their study who were being raised in bilingual homes developed oral English language skills within the average range. Although their second language abilities were not as high as their first, children did show evidence of growth between year one and year two in their second language.

The previous studies examined homes in which both the majority language (i.e., English) and minority language were being spoken. Stronger concerns exist when a child is exposed to a minority language at home and the majority language only during intervention or school. Thus, the child's first language is not English as in the McConkey Robbins et al. (2004) study, but rather the child's first language is a minority language and English is their second language. In a situation such as this, it is suggested that a program designed to teach parents how to facilitate language and listening in their native language will be beneficial for parents who are not fluent in the majority language. The parents should be encouraged to learn English so that they are able to more readily access resources in their area and have productive conversations with their child's intervention team (McConkey Robbins et al., 2004).

Considering the research regarding outcomes for children with CIs who are raised in bilingual homes, it is reasonable to council parents that speaking both languages to their child is advisable, assuming the parents are not providing incomplete input in either language. The lack of research regarding outcomes for children with CIs who are raised in monolingual homes where the language differs from the majority language makes recommendations for this group more difficult. When there are differences between the home and school or intervention language, it is strongly recommended that parents speak in their native language and not the school language if speaking in the school language will limit the amount of input (e.g., require the parent to speak in two-word sentences) or the quality of input (grammatically, semantically, or otherwise). As McConkey Robbins et al. (2004) suggested, these parents should be encouraged to enroll in programs that assist them in learning to facilitate language and listening skills via their native language. However, even though the parents are encouraged to use their native language at home, parents also are advised to put equal effort into learning English. This not only allows parents to reinforce what children are learning in intervention and at school, but also helps parents when advocating for their children. To encourage the learning of a second language, it is helpful if the CI center can share references with parents for audio-learning that can be accessed via the local library system.

Additional Family Characteristics

The literature on post-CI outcomes also points to a variety of other family characteristics that may impact post-CI prognoses. Geers et al. (2002) examined the role of parents' education on children's speech and language skills for 136 children across the United States and Canada. They found that family size and parents' education were significant predictors of a language variable that combined oral and sign language skill (with smaller family size and higher parental education resulting in higher language skills when speech and sign were considered together). However, these were not significant predictors of speech production, spoken language, or reading. In another publication, Geers et al. (2003) noted that family size and socioeconomic status (SES) were significant predictors of children's language abilities via spoken language and via the child's preferred language modality for 181 8- to 9-year-old children. Similarly, Connor and Zwolan (2004) found that children from low SES families (as determined by insurance status) achieved significantly lower reading comprehension scores on average than did children from middle SES families. In each of these studies, however, it is unclear why these factors had such an impact on these variables. It is possible that lower SES families or families with more children have less time to dedicate to supporting their child's post-CI listening and language development. In any case, the CI teams at the CARE Center and Carle ECHO never directly consider SES as part of the candidacy decision. However, they may discuss whether the family's other responsibilities, such as caring for multiple children in the home or working multiple jobs to pay for rent in a safe area, may make the child's aural habilitation less of a priority. If this may be the case, the CI team can devise a plan for helping the family to meet each of their responsibilities.

Speech and Language Evaluation for Cochlear Implant Candidacy

In this segment of the chapter, the goals of the preimplantation speech and language evaluation are described and the reader is provided with information about each age group of children that may present for a CI candidacy evaluation. The reader also is provided with explicit information about how to plan and prepare for candidacy evaluations as well as how to execute the candidacy evaluations. Finally, information is provided about how diagnostic therapy and contracts can be utilized when the candidacy decision is uncertain.

Goals of the Speech and Language Evaluation for Cochlear Implant Candidacy

There are generally two important goals in accomplishing the speech-language evaluation. The first goal is to gather the information necessary to determine whether the child is a good candidate for a CI from a speech and language perspective. The second goal is to establish a baseline marker of the child's speech and language abilities. In rare instances, only the latter of these two goals will be relevant during the evaluation. This may occur if a child has had meningitis and is clearly a medical and audiologic candidate. The decision to implant immediately due to concerns regarding impending ossification may be made before the speech and language candidacy evaluation occurs. This also may occur if a child has been receiving aural habilitation and audiologic services at the CI center for a period of several months. In these cases, necessary medical and audiometric data have been collected, much is already known about the child and his or her communication skills, and the child has demonstrated lack of or inadequate spoken language progress with hearing aids. In addition, the families have been enrolled in parent-infant therapy or an aural habilitation program for a minimum of 6 months and have learned about and made decisions regarding communication options.

Furthermore, the families have demonstrated an understanding of the impact hearing loss can have on their child's communication development, and have made a decision to have their child implanted. Despite the existence of these unique situations, for the purpose of simplicity, the expression "candidacy evaluation" will be used throughout the rest of this chapter to refer to the speech and language evaluation that is completed to obtain baseline information and/or information for the purposes of determining candidacy.

Age Groups Presenting for Cochlear Implant Candidacy Evaluations

Infants (6 to 18 months)

With the advent of universal newborn hearing screenings, the number of children being diagnosed with hearing loss within the first several weeks of life has dramatically increased. The 1-3-6 plan laid out by the Centers for Disease Control (CDC, 2006; Joint Committee on Infant Hearing, 2007) recommends all infants be screened for hearing loss by 1 month of age. If the screening results are positive, diagnostic testing should be completed by 3 months of age and intervention begun by 6 months of age. Following this plan, infants ideally will be referred for an evaluation to determine CI candidacy within the first 6 months of life.

It is unusual that the team would make a decision regarding an infant's candidacy as a CI recipient in only a single day of evaluations. More typically with infants, determination of cochlear implantation candidacy is a decision that occurs across a period of several weeks or even months in order to accommodate the extensive testing that is required across the various disciplines. The time required to complete this testing is lengthened by the developmental confines of infants. By virtue of the developmental restriction of age, infants have a very narrow window of attention. In addition, infants may arrive at the evaluation tired, hungry, sleeping, or for whatever reason, unable to actively interact with the testers. Furthermore, infants are unable to provide the more concrete responses (e.g., pointing, providing verbal or signed responses) that older children are able to provide. Infants' responses are typically much more subtle, if present at all. Thus, evaluation methods must rely on parent report, observation, informal interactions during play, and, when possible, formal test interactions using standardized test measures with normative data from infants who have normal hearing.

The primary goal of the SLP's observations or interactions with the infant is to establish that the child demonstrates communicative intent. The most commonly identified examples of communicative intent include the use of spoken words or signs. However, the infant can demonstrate communicative intent at the prelinguistic stage as well. For example, the combinations of certain gestures or vocalizations with gaze shifts between an object of interest and an adult can clearly demonstrate a variety of communicative intents. The value of assessing communicative intent was supported by the Kane et al. (2004) study mentioned in the section entitled "Pre Cochlear Implant Language Abilities." In this study, the *Communication and Symbolic Behavior Scales* (Wetherby and Prizant, 1992), a test that measures these forms of prelinguistic communication in addition to early linguistic development, was administered to a group of children prior to cochlear implantation. The authors found that children who performed poorly on this measure were very likely to perform poorly on a standardized language measure after cochlear implantation.

In addition to assessing the child's communicative intent and early linguistic development, the SLP will informally assess the family's interactions with their child during the speech and language evaluation. For example, the SLP may observe how the family facilitates the language development of their child, the quality of child-caregiver interactions, and the family's understanding of and ability to reinforce their child's therapy goals. The SLP also determines if there is consistency between what the family reports and the behavior or interactions that are observed.

Toddlers (19 months to 3 years)

Although the number of children being evaluated for candidacy for a CI during infancy is increasing, many children are first evaluated in the toddler years. Some of these children have used hearing aids since infancy and have either made insufficient progress with hearing aids or have had a decline in hearing levels such that they are now potential candidates for cochlear implantation. Other children may have lost their hearing as a result of an accident or illness such as meningitis. Additionally, some of the children undergoing a candidacy evaluation during the toddler years are children who have been diagnosed recently with hearing loss that presumably was present from birth.

Some toddlers may have developed pointing or other response behaviors conducive to interactive testing. However, because of variance in their listening and language experiences, some children will be more communicatively similar to infants. In this latter instance, the clinician may need to rely, either wholly or partially, on parent-report measures, observation, and informal interactions during play. In addition, even if the child demonstrates limited oral communication skill development, some of these children may have established manually supported communication, such as sign language or cued speech (CS). Decisions will need to be made concerning how best to test these toddlers to learn about their skills in their primary modality as well as through the aural modality.

As with infants, when working with toddlers the SLP observes the children to determine if they show clear communicative intent whether formally, through speech or sign language, or via the prelinguistic skills discussed in the section on infants. At the toddler age, the child is expected to be using gestures that are more complex (e.g., gesture combinations) than the gestures they used as infants. At this age, the SLP also can observe the ways in which children play with the objects around them. At this age, children will begin sorting objects by color and shape. They may begin make-believe play.

The SLP will listen carefully to the sounds the child produces to determine if the sounds are consistent with what might be expected from the child's audiometric levels. The SLP determines this by plotting the child's hearing levels on a "speech banana" audiogram (an audiogram with shading in the area in which most speech sounds are audible). If a child demonstrates greater variety in his or her speech sound repertoire than anticipated, it may be an indication that the child's hearing was at one time better and the hearing loss has progressed at some point or, alternatively, that the child's hearing may be fluctuating. For children in the toddler years, parents often have difficulty detecting hearing fluctuations and these children are too young to report changes independently.

If a child uses a manually supported form of communication, the SLP will observe the child's use and understanding of language through that means. The child's skills must be considered in relation to the length of time the family has used the specified means of communication with the child. At these early ages, good language development through sign language or CS can be a positive indicator for implantation because it clearly demonstrates the child's ability to learn and acquire language. It also demonstrates a high level of parental commitment because it suggests that the child has had consistent language input and reinforcement. There may be situations when parents report that their child has been in sign-based therapy for a significant period of time but the child evidences limited sign-skill development. In this situation the SLP would want to determine the consistency of sign modeling provided to the child and the level of expectation that is present for the child to use signs for communication. Additionally, this may raise red flags about the child's general learning patterns.

Preschool-Aged Children (3 to 5 years)

Candidates in the preschool years are often those who are making insufficient progress with hearing aids, have had a progressive hearing loss or who have suddenly lost their hearing as a result of an accident, illness, or medical intervention. Many of these children may have established some form of manually supported communication or have been communicating orally but are reaching a plateau or making very slow progress.

By the time children reach preschool age, it generally is expected that at least some emergent language skills are present, whether manually or orally. These skills can be assessed via a clinician-elicited norm-referenced test measure (NRT, see explanation under the section entitled "Variables to Consider During Test Selection"). If the

child's spoken language skills are nearing the three-year level, vocabulary testing may also be attempted. Similarly, if speech is present, an articulation measure may be attempted. Depending on the child's general abilities, his or her level of participation and cooperation with testing tasks, and the presence or absence of cognitive or learning delays, parent-report measures may be needed. For children who use a manually supported form of communication, the SLP who is not fluent in this modality may opt to use both a parent-report measure to assess the child's manually-based skills and a clinician-elicited NRT measure to establish the baseline by which to compare spoken language progress over time.

In addition to the formal assessment of skills, the SLP will observe the child to determine his or her overall level of communication, evidence of consistent hearing aid use, the degree of reliance on spoken versus manual communication, and the potential the child demonstrates for using the CI for spoken language development. The SLP will observe the families for evidence of consistent interactions with the child promoting language development (whether through sign language, cued speech, or spoken language), a history of appropriate follow through regarding past recommendations, and the presence of realistic expectations of what cochlear implantation may or may not provide.

If the child uses CS or a form of signed English (as opposed to American Sign Language or ASL), the SLP will observe whether the parents use their voice when communicating with the child, or if most interactions occur with cues or signs but without voice. This is because following implantation it would be expected that an emphasis be placed on oral language development. So even if the habilitation plan following implantation included continued use of manual support with spoken language, it would be expected that the family emphasize use of oral language models. That is, they would be encouraged to first present information through the oral modality. Then, if the child does not understand, information can be presented through the TC modality, and finally through the oral modality again. Koch (1999a, 1999b) refers to this technique as an "auditory sandwich." Parents are encouraged to adopt this mindset, even before implantation.

With the goal of oral communication in mind, for children who use manual support, the clinician also observes the child's ability to speechread and understand language in absence of the manual support. As discussed in the section on Pre Cochlear Implant Language Abilities, the presence of at least some oral communication skills in general is a more positive prognosticator for implantation than were a child to evidence no oral skill development. Implantation for children in the four to five year age range is at times counseled against in children showing no evidence of spoken language development.

School-Aged Children (6 to 21 years)

The majority of school-aged children presenting at the House Ear Institute CARE Center for a CI candidacy evaluation are children with established spoken language abilities who have had progressive hearing losses, have recently lost their hearing, have plateaued in their spoken language development or are progressing slowly with hearing aids. Whereas a portion of the children seeking implantation in the school-age years will have established communication that incorporates manual support, many will demonstrate functional, if not age-appropriate, spoken language abilities.

Some of the school-aged children may have been evaluated and determined to not meet candidacy criteria in the past. Implantation candidacy requirements have changed over the years due to research demonstrating the benefits implants can provide even for those with some residual hearing. This, in turn, has resulted in relaxation of previous candidacy criteria that required that CI candidates have a bilateral profound hearing loss. As a result of this change in candidacy criteria, a child might now qualify for implantation even when demonstrating severe (and not profound) hearing loss bilaterally. Similarly, a child might qualify as a candidate for a CI in the worse ear even when there is some usable hearing in the better ear provided that the worse ear meets the appropriate candidacy criteria.

Occasionally, school-aged children born deaf who have grown up using sign language and demonstrate minimal benefit from or use of hearing aids may present for a CI candidacy evaluation. In these circumstances, a child may demonstrate extremely limited oral language development. One situation in which this may occur is for a child who is diagnosed with Ushers syndrome, which includes the prognosis for progressive loss of vision. This situation also might occur when a child meets someone else with a CI and decides to investigate the option for himself or herself. A third circumstance in which this might occur is in the case of individuals in the 18- to 21-year age range. In this situation, the individual may rely primarily, if not exclusively, on manual language to communicate. Then, as a young adult, he or she may make an independent decision to consider the option of cochlear implantation.

Once children reach the school-age years, it is expected that they will be capable of actively participating in the evaluation process. This allows a large amount of information to be gathered in a relatively short period of time. Barring other learning or developmental factors, children in this age group are usually able to complete a full battery of speech and language testing, including assessment of total language, receptive and expressive vocabulary, and articulation skills. In addition, the SLP may have the children provide a written language sample, stating what they know about CIs, the benefits they expect to receive from a CI and why they may or may not wish to have one. In so doing, along with the information gained about the child's written use of English, the writing sample helps the SLP gauge whether the child has realistic expectations or if there are any misperceptions that need to be corrected. In addition, it provides information regarding the child's level of interest in receiving the device. This is a critical component because if the child is not in agreement with the decision to receive an implant, he or she may covertly or overtly undermine the process.

In almost all situations for school-aged children, the SLP's ultimate goal is to ascertain whether the child has the necessary spoken language foundation to benefit from implantation. In less typical circumstances (e.g., the case of a child who is diagnosed with Usher's syndrome and has progressive vision loss, or a young adult who is independently seeking cochlear implantation), a decision in favor of implantation may be agreed upon even without evidence of oral language development. In both the typical and less typical circumstances described, the child must still demonstrate the willingness and motivation to participate in aural (re)habilitation therapy with a CI for an extended period of time after receiving the

implant. Also, in all situations, both family and child expectations should be realistic and both the parents and child must be supportive of the decision to implant. Cochlear implantation would not be recommended unless or until a unified decision to implant is reached between the child and family. An exception may be made in the situation of a young adult of legal age who decides, possibly against his or her parents' expressed wishes, to receive a CI. In this latter situation, every effort would be made to help the family reach consensus, but ultimately, it would be left to the young adult to make the final decision.

Planning and Preparing for the Candidacy Evaluation

Step 1: Chart or Record Review

The SLP typically begins preparing for the candidacy evaluation by reviewing the child's chart. Information that will be helpful includes the child's age, a birth and health history, the child's degree of hearing loss, the duration of hearing loss, the child's history of hearing aid usage, whether other diagnoses are present, and whether the child's hearing levels are better in one ear than the other.

Step 2: Speaking with Other Professionals

Although it is not always possible, it is advantageous to speak with other professionals, in addition to those on the CI team, who have worked with the child, such as the child's educational audiologist, classroom teacher, SLP, TOD, or other early interventionist. The other professionals may be able to provide additional insight as to what motivates the child, the concerns the parents might raise, or the child's general communication interactions. They can also provide information about the family's interactions and whether the family demonstrates or expresses need for additional instruction regarding their child's hearing loss, language development or the child's general learning needs. Along these lines the professionals may be able to identify concerns they have based on their interactions with the child or family with regard to the child's CI candidacy. If there are multiple languages spoken in the home, the other professional may also be able to indicate whether or not the clinician should anticipate need for an interpreter. The information gathered through the chart review and speaking with other professionals is utilized in the last step of the preparations, test selection.

Test Selection (Step 3 of planning and preparing)

There are many tests available to assess the speech and spoken language abilities of children across the age span from infancy to adulthood. CI centers may choose to develop a core set of measurement tools that will best assess the populations served at their center. Whereas most tests are geared to and normed on children who have normal hearing, some are normed and designed specifically for use with children who have hearing loss. A frequent limitation of tests normed on children with hearing loss is that standard deviations may be large because of the variability in skills among this population. So, unless a child is substantially delayed, he or she may still appear similar to the normative sample. Given this consideration, and that a frequent goal of implantation is development

of spoken language, it is common practice in many clinics to use measures designed for use with children who have normal hearing. This is especially the case when the educational goals for the child include the potential for integration into a regular educational classroom in which the implanted child must keep pace with peers who have normal hearing. Be aware, however, whenever tests designed for children with normal hearing are applied to children with hearing loss, test results should be cautiously interpreted and the impact of a child's speech perception abilities should be included in all discussions of results.

Tables 11–1A, 11–1B, and 11–1C list a range of speech and language tests that are used by the authors. The language tests are divided into those based on parent-report (Table 11–1B) versus those that are clinician-elicited (Table 11–1C), requiring direct interactions between the SLP and the child. The clinician-elicited language measures are further divided based on the level of language assessed: vocabulary, total language, or supralinguistic language skills. These tests represent a broad cross-section of the array of speech and language measures available for testing children. Appendix 11–A further elaborates on these measures.

Figure 11–1 shows a flow chart that depicts the decision-making process that the authors use when selecting tests. The graph demonstrates the general flow of test selection by the child's age level. Whereas the flow chart provides general considerations regarding test selection, the SLP also considers specific variables when selecting test instruments. An example of how this flow chart can be used in clinical decision making is provided later in this chapter. First, other test selection considerations are discussed.

TABLE 11–1A. Speech production measures are shown with the age range the test is normalized on or age for which its use is intended. The table shows the speech response that is needed to participate in testing. It also indicates whether the measures are norm-referenced tests (NRT), criterion-referenced tests (CRT) or neither

Test	Age Range	Preferred Speech Response/Accepted Response	NRT, CRT or Neither
Arizona Articulation Proficiency Scale, 3rd Edition (Arizona-3)	1½–18 years	Spontaneous/imitative	NRT
Fundamental Speech Skills Test (FSST)*	Age independent	Spontaneous/imitative	Provides NRT, CRT, and percentage information
Goldman-Fristoe 2 Test of Articulation (GFTA-2)	2;0–21;11	Spontaneous/delayed imitation (immediate imitation as last resort)	NRT
Identifying Early Phonological Needs in Children with Hearing Impairment (Paden/Brown)*	Age independent	Spontaneous/imitative	Neither (percentages are obtained that can be used descriptively)
Khan-Lewis 2 Phonological Assessment (KLPA-2)	2;0–21;11	(Based on responses from the GFTA-2)	NRT
*Picture SPeech INtelligibility Evaluation (Picture SPINE)	School-age	Spontaneous	Neither (percentages are obtained that can be used descriptively)

*Tests designed specifically for use with children who have hearing loss.

TABLE 11–1B. Parent-Report Language Tests for Children

Test	Age Range	NRT or CRT
SKI*HI Language Scales*	Birth–5 years	CRT
MacArthur-Bates Communicative Development Inventories (MCDI)		
• Gestures and Words (MCDI: WG)	8–18 months	NRT
• Words and Sentences (MCDI: WS)	16–30 months	NRT
• CDI: III (MCDI: III)	31–37 months	NRT
Rossetti Infant-Toddler Language Scale	Birth–3 years	CRT

*Tests designed specifically for use with children who have hearing loss. Note: NRT = Norm-referenced test, CRT = Criterion-referenced test.

TABLE 11–1C. Clinician-elicited language tests used in the CARE Center and/or Carle ECHO for evaluating children's language skills. The appropriate age range for use of the test and pertinent variables to consider are also shown. Tests are divided by language level assessed (vocabulary, total language, or supralinguistic language).

Test	Age Range (in years unless otherwise indicated)	Pertinent Variables to Consider
Receptive Vocabulary Measures:		
Carolina Picture Vocabulary Test (CPVT)	4;0–11;6	Choice response, picture pointing, comprehension of signs
Receptive One-Word Picture Vocabulary Test (ROWPVT)	2;0–18;11	Choice response, picture pointing, comprehension of spoken words
Peabody Picture Vocabulary Test, 4th Edition (PPVT-4)	2;6–≥90	Choice response, picture pointing, comprehension of spoken words
Expressive Vocabulary Measures:		
Expressive One-Word Picture Vocabulary Test (EOWPVT)	2;0–18;11	Labeling response
Expressive Vocabulary Test, 2nd Edition (EVT-2)	2;6–≥90	Labeling response, use of synonyms, use of cloze (i.e., fill in the blank)

continues

TABLE 11–1C. *continued*

Test	Age Range (in years unless otherwise indicated)	Pertinent Variables to Consider
Total Language Measures:		
Communication and Symbolic Behavior Scale (CSBS)*	8 months– 24 months developmentally*	Structured and unstructured interactive play
Preschool Language Scales, 4th Edition (PLS-4)	Birth–6;11	Interactive play, choice task, picture pointing, labeling, following directions, use of words and sentences, describing, retelling
Reynell Developmental Language Scales (RDLS)	1;0–6;11	Choice task, following directions, real labeling, defining, describing pictures
Clinical Evaluation of Language Fundamentals-Preschool, 2nd Edition (CELF-P2)	3;0–6;11	Choice task, picture pointing, following directions, labeling, use of cloze sentence procedures, use of words and sentences
Oral and Written Language Scales (OWLS)	3;0–21	Choice task, picture pointing, following directions, use of cloze sentence procedures, use and understanding of abstract language
Clinical Evaluation of Language Fundamentals, 4th Edition (CELF-4)	5;0–21	Choice task, picture pointing, following directions, use of cloze sentence procedures, heavy memory load
Supralinguistic Language Measures:		
Comprehensive Assessment of Spoken Language (CASL)	3;0–21	Choice task, picture pointing, use and understanding of abstract language, use of language for reasoning, logic and higher order thought processing
Listening Comprehension Test, 2nd Edition (LCT-2)	6;0–11;11	Use and understanding of abstract language, ability to use reasoning, logic, and higher order thought processing, heavy memory load, use of cloze
Test of Auditory Processing, 3rd Edition (TAPS-3)	4;0–18;11	Use and understanding of abstract language, good auditory perceptual skills, ability to use language for reasoning, logic, and higher order thought processing.

*Can be used up to ages 5 or 6 years but with children who are functioning developmentally at the 8 to 24 month level.

Variables to Consider During Test Selection

Table 11–1C includes a column labeled "pertinent variables to consider." Although not an exhaustive listing, they are representative of the range of variables that the SLP considers when selecting tests. General considerations include the child's age, overall language and developmental abilities, the amount of benefit the child receives from hearing aids, and the child's length of experience with hearing aids. More specific variables to consider include test design and the skills assessed by the measure in relation to the responses the child most likely is able to provide. All of these factors can influence the child's ability to complete the tests and the outcomes that are obtained.

A variable unique to testing children who have hearing loss is mode of test presentation. For children who use some form of manually supported communication, it is important to assess their oral language abilities without manual support and their language abilities with manual support. For older children who have experienced a sudden hearing loss, even if testing is administered in the child's primary communication mode (i.e., spoken language), test results will be confounded by the child's sudden change in hearing. In this scenario, knowing that the child's receptive language will be severely impacted by his or her sudden hearing loss, the SLP can secure a language sample based on written questions in addition to any other oral language tests that may be administered.

Another consideration, common to testing any child, is whether the assessment measure is a criterion-referenced test (CRT), norm-referenced test (NRT), or neither of the two. Whereas CRT measures simply reflect a child's mastery of skills, NRT measures are intended to compare a child's performance to that of other, similar children across a curve distribution (e.g., bell-shaped curve). Both CRT and NRT measures often provide age-equivalent information to reflect the age at which children typically demonstrate the evaluated skills, or at which half the children in the normative sample attained a higher raw score than the child and half the children attained a lower raw score than the child. Only NRT measures, however, provide distributed score information (e.g., standard scores, percentile ranks, z-scores) that can serve to compare the child being assessed to age-matched children in the normative sample. Whereas parent-report measures are often (but not always) CRT, clinician-elicited measures generally are norm-referenced test measures.

There are some exceptions to these test types, with some tests providing neither criterion-referenced nor normative scores but rather providing percentage correct scores. The resultant scoring information is then used descriptively over time to demonstrate changes in skill development. Many of the speech production measures specifically designed for children with hearing loss are of this nature. Although such measures do not provide a means by which to compare the child being assessed to other age mates, they can serve as a means to compare the child to himself or herself over time. The ability to compare the child to him- or herself can be helpful, especially when testing children whose skills are severely delayed when compared to peers who have normal hearing. Tables 11–1A and 11–1B indicate whether the measures are NRT-based, CRT-based or neither of the two. (All tests in Table 11–1C are norm-referenced.)

Test Selection Flow Chart for Testing Children

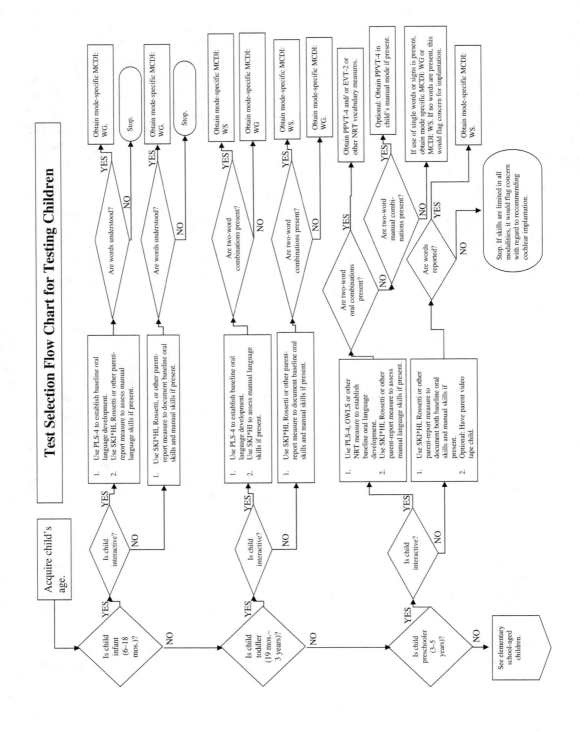

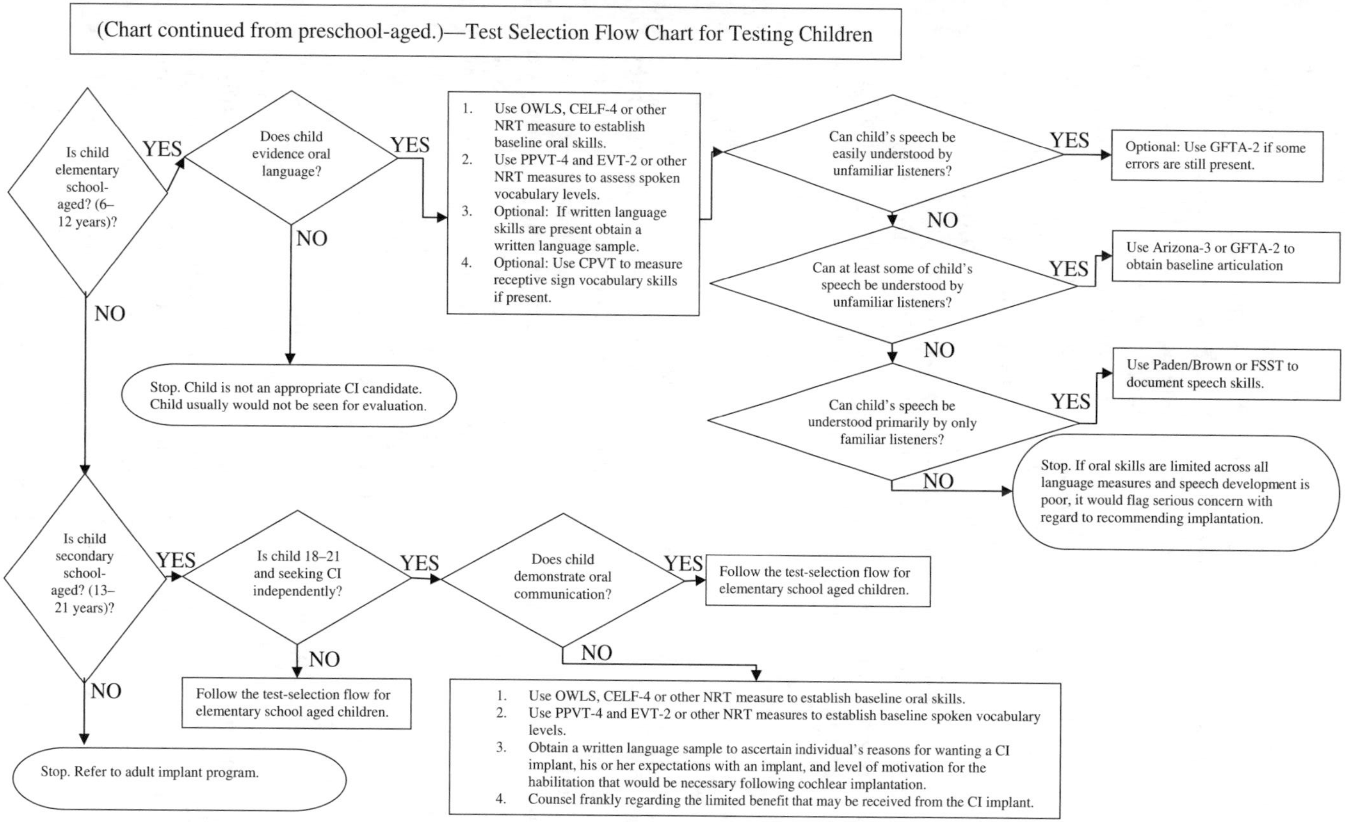

(Chart continued from preschool-aged.)—Test Selection Flow Chart for Testing Children

Figure 11–1. Flow chart depicting the general decision-making process that the SLPs in the CARE Center or Carle ECHO program use when selecting speech and language tests. The decision process starts with acquiring the child's age (*top left corner of the first page*) and takes various routes based on the yes/no answers to the questions posed in the diamond-shaped boxes in the flow chart. Abbreviations used are as follows: PLS-4 = Preschool Language Scales, 4th Edition; SKI*HI = SKI*HI Language Development Scale; Rossetti = Rossetti Infant-Toddler Language Scale; MCDI: WG and MCDI:WS = MacArthur-Bates Communicative Development Inventories: Words and Gestures and Word and Sentences, respectively; OWLS = Oral and Written Language Scales; PPVT-4 = Peabody Picture Vocabulary Test, 4th Edition; EVT-2 = Expressive Vocabulary Test, 2nd Edition; NRT = Norm Referenced Test; CPVT = Carolina Picture Vocabulary Test; GFTA-2 = Goldman Fristoe 2 Test of Articulation; Arizona-3 = Arizona Articulation Proficiency Scale, 3rd Edition; Paden/Brown = Identifying Early Phonological Needs in Children with Hearing Impairment; FSST = Fundamental Speech Skills Test; and CELF-4 = Clinical Evaluation of Language Fundamentals, 4th Edition.

277

Selecting Tests Based on Administration Format

Parent-Report Measures. Clinician-elicited NRT measures are usually the preferred means of assessment across all age groups. At times, however, specific variables are present that cause the SLP to opt for parent-report measures. The most common reason for use of a parent-report measure is that the child is not developmentally ready to participate in clinician-elicited measures. Another circumstance in which parent-report measures may have good utility, depending on the knowledge and ability level of the parent, is for providing a means to assess skill development for children who use CS, some form of manually supported signed English or for children who use ASL.

Two common parent-report measures are the *Rossetti Infant-Toddler Language Scale* (Rossetti, 2006) and the *SKI*HI Language Development Scale* (Tonelson & Watkins, 1979). For both of these measures, the SLP interviews the parents or caregiver regarding the child's comprehension and use of language. Whereas the *SKI*HI* was designed specifically for use with children who have hearing loss, the *Rossetti* was designed for children who have normal hearing.

Although designed for use with children who have hearing loss, the *SKI*HI* is based on the developmental milestones of children who have normal hearing. It is appropriate for use with children from birth through age 5. Unlike most tests designed for children with normal hearing, the *SKI*HI* gives allowances for responses regardless of whether they are obtained through sign language and visual cues or based on oral language and auditory responses. For example, a child receives credit for "babbling" with sign language, not just speech. Similarly, the child may receive credit for responding appropriately to facial expressions, as opposed to vocal tone. For children who use manually supported communication, skill levels can be separately established in the child's preferred language mode and for spoken language. Being that the *SKI*HI* de-emphasizes reliance on auditory-based language skills it may better reflect the child's overall communication capabilities. In addition, because the measure includes skill sets for children up to the age of 5 years, it may provide a means to track progress in a child with multiple disabilities or for children who demonstrate slower language development in general.

Unlike the *SKI*HI*, the *Rossetti* is intended for use with children who have normal hearing and are 36 months of age or younger. It includes items that are heavily reliant on auditory skill development. For example, one item includes, "child turns head toward a voice." A potential drawback of using tests that are too heavily laden with auditory-dependent test items is that they may artificially lower a deaf child's language skills. If there are many auditory-oriented questions within a section, the child may do very poorly in that section causing the SLP to reach the criterion for ending a test earlier than they would have based on language or play skills. Once past the auditory-dependent items, a child may still demonstrate mastery of a number of skills such as use or understanding of natural gestures, ability to match objects and pictures, or other more visually oriented communication abilities. Although using tests that include many auditory-dependent items can pose a challenge, there are also benefits. Such a measure may be more sensitive to the growth of these auditory-dependent language skills after implantation. Also, it provides a means by which to compare the skill sets of the children with hearing loss to those without hearing loss, which is especially useful when the ultimate goals for the child include spoken language development and integration into regular education classrooms.

Another parent-report measure is the *MacArthur-Bates Communicative Development Inventory (MCDI)* (Fenson et al., 2007). The *MCDI* includes three inventories for assessing children ages 8 to 18 months, 16 to 30 months, and 31 to 37 months. As with the *Rossetti*, the *MCDI* is intended for use with children who have normal hearing. Unlike the *SKI*HI* and the *Rossetti*, which are criterion-referenced measures, the *MCDI* is an NRT measure. Thus, in addition to age-equivalent scores, normed scores are provided so that the child's ranking relative to same-age peers who have normal hearing can be established. The *MCDI* provides excellent utility for assessing and tracking early vocabulary development, prelinguistic social behaviors, and the emergence of sentence structures. In addition, Thal, DesJardin, and Eisenberg (2007) found the *MCDI* to be valid instruments for use with children who have CIs and are in the early stages of communication development, even if older than the normative sample of children with whom the test is typically used. For these reasons the inventories are used with infants, toddlers and, at times, preschool-age children who are not yet able to participate in clinician-elicited vocabulary measures.

As stated earlier, the SLP must consider both the general and specific variables involved when selecting tests and then decide which measures are appropriate. To make this less ambiguous, an example, utilizing the flow chart (see Figure 11–1) discussed earlier may help illustrate this process. Consider the story of Anthony, described below.

Anthony is 2 years, 3 months of age. He received hearing aids at 12 months of age but his parents report that he does not respond to others calling his name and only rarely responds to other environmental sounds such as a big dog barking loudly. Anthony's family began using sign language with him as soon as they learned of his hearing loss. He is very interactive with others around him using up to 50 signs, lots of gestures, and occasionally vocalizations. At times, when he is very eager to get his thoughts or needs across to his listener, he uses multiple gestures or a gesture and a sign together. Anthony's family is seeking a CI because they also would like him to learn spoken language if it is possible. Although interactive with the SLP in the waiting area earlier in the day, Anthony's speech and language evaluation occurred late in the day, and Anthony had just fallen asleep as his parents arrived at his appointment, making direct assessment challenging. His parents reported that the SLP could try to wake him but he usually responds unfavorably to being awakened from sleep.

How does the SLP decide which tests to administer in this situation? Utilizing the flowchart, first consider Anthony's age. He is in the toddler age group. Is he interactive? Usually yes, but at the moment he is completely exhausted from his morning appointments and he is sound asleep. His parents report that he is usually very irritable when woken from sleep. Given this information, Anthony is determined to be non-interactive at the moment so a parent report measure is selected. Two questionnaire options considered by the SLP are the *Rossetti Infant Scales* and the *SKI*HI Language Development Scales*. Whereas the *Rossetti* is an option, the *SKI*HI* is ultimately chosen because it can tap into Anthony's sign language abilities. If Anthony awakens from his nap before the session is completed the SLP would test Anthony's spoken language skills with an NRT-based measure, the *PLS-4*. This means the current portion of the assessment would focus on Anthony's language abilities using his primary means of communication, TC. It was decided, based on the explanations provided earlier, that the *SKI*HI* would better capture Anthony's overall communication skills.

Anthony was still asleep when the *SKI*HI* administration was completed. Based on the information his parents reported about his use of words and signs, his parents were provided with the *MacArthur Development Scales* to complete. They were asked to fill out the version for younger children, *MCDI: Words and Gestures* based on his spoken communication skills, and the *MCDI: Words and Sentences* based on his use of signs. As Anthony's parents were completing the MacArthur questionnaires, Anthony woke up. The SLP was then able to complete the *PLS-4* with him when he was awake and interactive, thereby completing Anthony's speech and language testing. As demonstrated in this example, understanding the goals of the evaluation, available tests, what the tests are designed to measure, and how to use them most effectively is important for choosing the most appropriate tests for a given child and set of circumstances.

Clinician-Elicited NRT Measures. As previously mentioned, use of clinician-elicited NRT measures is generally preferred over parent-report measures because NRT measures are based on the SLP's direct interactions with the child. Direct interaction with the child provides the SLP with a more comprehensive understanding of the child's skill levels and his or her general abilities, including the child's ability to comply with tasks and follow directions. Additionally, NRT measures help the SLP to track the child's progress over time relative to peers with normal hearing.

Total Language Measures. At the youngest age levels, the *Preschool Language Scales, 4th Edition* (*PLS-4*) (Zimmerman, Steiner, & Pond, 2002), the *Communica-*

tion and Symbolic Behavior Scale (*CSBS*) (Wetherby & Prizant, 1993), and the *Reynell Developmental Language Scales* (*RDLS*) (Reynell & Gruber, 1990) are examples of NRT measures that may be utilized when testing infants. Whereas normative scores start at birth for the *PLS-4*, such scores start at 8 months and 1 year respectively for the *CSBS* and *RDLS*. At the upper end of the normative limits, the *PLS-4* and *RDLS* extend to 6 years, 11 months but the *CSBS* extends to only 24 months.

Once the child is preschool-aged, measures such as the *Oral and Written Language Scales* (*OWLS*) (Carrow-Woolfolk, 1995), *Clinical Evaluation of Language Fundamentals-Preschool, Second Edition* (*CELF-P2*) (Semel, Wiig, & Secord, 2003), and the *Comprehensive Assessment of Spoken Language* (*CASL*) (Carrow-Woolfolk, 1999) also may be utilized. The norms on these measures begin at age 3 years. For children with sufficient spoken language abilities, the *OWLS* often is selected because it assesses a broad range of skills including pragmatic language abilities and it is efficient to administer. Efficiency is an important consideration because of the short attention span of the preschool population.

When assessing a preschool-aged child who has well-developed spoken language skills and who may be a borderline candidate for implantation, assessment measures that provide more detailed assessment options such as the *CELF-P2* or the *CASL* can be helpful. These tests assess skills more systematically in distinct skill areas and thus may identify areas of subtle difficulty not reflected on the *OWLS*. Age should be considered when making the test selection, however, because the norms for both the *CELF-P2* and the preschool-age portion of the *CASL* extend up to 6 years, 11 months. If the child being tested is currently over 5 years of age, although these measures would serve the purpose of the candidacy evaluation, they may not provide the best means to obtain a measurement of rate of language growth after implantation. By the time the child is implanted and returns for his or her first post-CI speech and language evaluation, a year or more may have elapsed. In this case, the child may be nearing or exceeding the upper limits of the norms on the two measures. Although the child could be transitioned to the upper extensions of the two measures (e.g., the *CELF-4* or the *CASL* for children 7 to 21 years) for the first post-CI assessment, it would not provide the most direct measure of comparison to establish rate of language growth with the CI.

Once children reach school-age, there are a number of tests that can be used including the *OWLS, CELF-4,* and *CASL.* These tests measure the child's development of the fundamental aspects of language achievement, such as word knowledge and the ability to use and understand sentence constructs. These tests are chosen as opposed to tests that are designed to assess higher level language skills (e.g., supralinguistic language skills such as use of language for reasoning and logic, use and understanding of idioms and idiomatic language, etc.) and literacy skills because they are more appropriate for determining whether or not the child possesses sufficient spoken language skill to benefit from a CI.

Vocabulary Measures. Most children who present for a CI candidacy evaluation will have stronger oral vocabulary skills than total language skills due to the decreased impact of speech perception and speech production impairments on single-word measures. Thus, the SLP will often administer clinician-elicited NRT measures to evaluate vocabulary level. Examples of this type of test include the *Peabody Picture Vocab-*

ulary Test, 4th Edition (PPVT-4) (Dunn & Dunn, 2007), the *Receptive One-Word Picture Vocabulary Test (ROWPVT)* (Brownell, 2000b), the *Expressive One-Word Picture Vocabulary Test (EOWPVT)* (Brownell, 2000a), and the *Expressive Vocabulary Test, 2nd Edition (EVT-2)* (Williams, 2007). All of these tests are designed for and normed on children who have normal hearing. The SLP also may administer a sign vocabulary test such as the *Carolina Picture Vocabulary Test (CPVT)* (Layton & Holmes, 1985). The *CPVT* is a measure of receptive sign language vocabulary that is designed for and normed on children who are deaf and use manual signs for communication.

The *PPVT-4* and *EVT-2* are frequently used vocabulary measures that assess the children's oral receptive and expressive vocabulary. These tests are selected together because they are co-normed and thus can indicate when a child's receptive and expressive vocabulary skills are significantly different from one another. Whereas the *PPVT-4* requires that the child have a consistent picture pointing choice task response, the *EVT-2* requires that the child be able to label pictures and, for some items, provide a cloze response (i.e., provide a one-word, fill-in-the-blank response to complete a sentence). This is a challenging test for some children because it requires them to vary their response pattern. That is, for some items the child is simply labeling the pictured item or action and at other times, the child must provide a synonym or complete a sentence using a single-word answer. The normative scores for these two tests begin at 2½ years of age.

If a child demonstrates some spoken words but does not yet have the rich vocabulary necessary to complete this pair of tests then the SLP might consider administering the *ROWPVT* and the *EOWPVT.*

The *ROWPVT* and the *EOWPVT* also are co-normed but the normative scores for the measures extend down to age 2 years. Whereas the child's response varies on the *EVT-2*, the *EOWPVT* requires a redundant naming task so it may be more suitable for very young children or children whose language skills are more limited. If none of these measures is feasible, the SLP would request that the caregiver complete the *MCDI*.

Articulation Measures. Clinician-elicited NRT measures that assess articulation skills include the *Goldman Fristoe Test of Articulation, Second Edition (GFTA-2)* (Goldman & Fristoe, 2000) and the *Arizona Articulation Proficiency Scale, Third Edition (Arizona-3)* (Barker Fudala, 2000). Both measures require the child to provide a labeling response, preferably spontaneously but at least imitatively. The normative scores extend down to 1.5 years of age for the *Arizona-3* and 2 years of age for the *GFTA-2*. Whereas the *Arizona-3* evaluates both consonant and vowel sounds within words, the *GFTA-2* assesses only consonant sounds. The *Arizona-3* also assigns a rating of predicted intelligibility based on the child's total score. The *GFTA-2* has a companion tool, the *Khan Lewis Phonological Analysis, Second Edition (KLPA-2)* (Khan & Lewis, 2002). The *KLPA-2* can be used to further analyze the responses from the *GFTA-2* to determine the types of phonological processes that the child uses.

The *GFTA-2* and the *Arizona-3* are appropriate measures for children who demonstrate consistent use of words or word approximations. They may be inappropriate for use with children who have very limited vocabulary or limited phoneme repertoires. In this latter instance, the SLP may rely on measures designed specifically for use with children who have hearing loss or on descriptive information obtained through observation during the test session. One

NRT speech production measure designed for children with hearing loss is the *Fundamental Speech Skills Test (FSST)* (Levitt, Youdelman, & Head, 1990). Although the *FSST* does broadly sample articulation skills, its main focus is assessing the underlying (i.e., first order) aspects that contribute to intelligible speech. Examples of the skills assessed include breath support, pitch control, use of stress and intonation, syllable accuracy, voicing features and stability of the child's word productions across multiple attempts. Both norm referenced and criterion referenced values can be obtained from this measure. Basic percentages also are calculated.

Other Measures. The parent-report and clinician-elicited tests described so far provide norm- or criterion- referenced information. However, the SLP may also incorporate tests that are clinician-elicited but that are neither CRT nor NRT measures. Instead, as mentioned before, some measures result in a percentage value that can be used to measure progress by comparing the child's performance at one point in time to scores obtained at a later point in time. There are several articulation measures for children with hearing loss of this nature, including the *Identifying Early Phonologic Needs in Children with Hearing Impairment (Paden/Brown)* (Paden & Brown, 1992) and the *CID Picture SPeech INtelligibility Evaluation (Picture SPINE)* (Monsen, Moog, & Geers, 1988). As opposed to scoring responses based on the consonant or vowel accuracy, these measures evaluate first order production characteristics such as those described for the *FSST* in the section above. They also focus more on a child's overall intelligibility as opposed to specific vowel or consonant errors that are present.

The *Paden/Brown* assesses suprasegmental, vowel, and consonant accuracy based on the child's ability to match key features for each as opposed to the child's ability to attain an exact phoneme match. For example, vowel accuracy is based on how well the child matches basic vowel areas—not necessarily the vowel itself. That is, if a child used /ɪ/ for /i/ (e.g., saying "fit" for "feet"), he or she would receive one of three possible points by approximating the proper vowel height and location, even if not achieving an exact match. Similarly, a mild distortion would result in the loss of only one point, so the child would receive two of three possible points on the *Paden/Brown*. Consonant accuracy also is broken down by accuracy of consonant features (e.g., place, manner, voicing) as opposed to phoneme accuracy. In contrast, on measures designed for children with normal hearing, a vowel or consonant distortion would be counted as an error and the child would receive no credit even if the sound was still easily identifiable. The SLP may choose to administer the *Paden/Brown* to a school-aged child who can provide gross word approximations but who still demonstrates a high number of articulation errors.

The *Picture SPINE* (Monsen, Moog, & Geers, 1988) was designed to assess a child's overall speech intelligibility (as opposed to individual phonemes or features of speech). The test consists of 100 pictures grouped into four sets of 25 items. The words used reflect phoneme contrasts that children who have hearing loss often have difficulty producing. Each 25-word set contains words that are phonemically confusable (e.g., words in set A include words such as: pie, pear, bear, bell, belt; words in set B include: cake, coat, goat, car, card). The test is scored based on a listener's ability to accurately determine the word the child produced without seeing the picture the child viewed. The score results in a percent intelligibility score.

At times, the SLP may also have the child provide a written language sample. Although there are guidelines available for analyzing written language samples, more often when they are utilized within CARE Center or Carle ECHO it is to obtain information from the child regarding his or her knowledge of, expectations with and desire for the CI. Although information-seeking is the primary purpose of the written language sample, informally, the SLP attends to the child's use of sentence structures and his or her ability to organize and convey thoughts through written language.

Executing the Candidacy Evaluation

Step 4: Parental Interview

When the family arrives for the formal speech and language evaluation, the first segment of the session is a parental interview that is designed to gain more information about the child and family. In order for the parental interview to be successful, it is important to establish good rapport with the family. This in turn will foster more open communication. Additionally, in order for the later evaluation to be successful, it is important to establish good rapport with the child. Initially, this may involve giving the child age-appropriate toys to play with, thus allowing the child to become accustomed to his or her new surroundings. These toys will also serve to entertain the child during the parental interview. After the child is comfortable in the new surroundings and in the presence of the examiner and after the parental interview is completed, the examiner should be able easily to transition into play and then formal assessment with the child.

Generally, after initial greetings are completed, the family talks about their goals for the appointment and poses their questions. This assists in the rapport building process. Some families will have well-defined goals and questions about the appointment. Other families may be reluctant to ask questions or may report that they do not have any. If testing an older child, the SLP should include the child in these discussions as well. In so doing, the SLP acknowledges to the child that his or her thoughts are important as well.

After addressing the family's questions, if the family has not already provided a case history, the SLP may assist the family in filling out a center-designed parent questionnaire or going over the information on a questionnaire the parents have already filled out. The forms may require the family to report on an array of information such as contact information, basic family information, the child's birth date, birth history, surgeries the child has undergone, major illnesses the child has had, the age at which the child's hearing loss was identified, the age at which the child received hearing aids, the frequency and duration of any therapy the child receives, communication mode, the age at which language and other developmental milestones were reached, and educational placement information.

After gathering this information, the SLP will be in a better position to lead the interview by asking open ended questions based around the information that was attained on the questionnaire or more general questions. For example, the SLP may ask:

"Why are you considering a cochlear implant for your child?"

"How did you choose the aural communication methodology for your child out of all the possible communication options?"

"What are your ultimate goals for your child?"

In addition to helping the SLP learn about the family's goals for their child and their level of understanding with regard to implantation, such questioning also provides an opportunity to identify gaps or misperceptions in the parents' knowledge, or to observe that the parents possess unrealistic expectations. For example, when asking about communication methodologies, the SLP may find that the parents are unaware of other communication options. The parents may see their child's options as being a noncommunicator or being an oral communicator. Similarly, the parents may tell the SLP that their plan for post-CI aural habilitation includes being their child's only interventionist. In addition to developing a good rapport, the goals during this opening dialogue with parents are to correct any misperceptions or fill in any gaps in their knowledge regarding CIs and hearing loss (or point them toward resources, including their audiologist, to fill those gaps) and to help redirect any unrealistic expectations.

When having this conversation with parents, it often is helpful to have a variety of resources at your fingertips. For example, a SLP may choose to have an audiogram available that shows the frequency and intensity levels at which familiar sounds are heard and an audiogram with a speech banana to indicate the frequency and intensity with which different phonemes are generally produced. Parents occasionally tell the SLP that they think their child hears what they say and even that they follow simple spoken directions. These parents are often confused or apprehensive regarding the need for a CI. However, assuming that auditory neuropathy and fluctuating hearing loss have been ruled out, a glance at the child's audiogram often will tell the SLP that the parents' perceptions about what their child is attending to and whether their child is understanding speech are not accurate. The parents who believe their child is able to understand all spoken communication actually may have a child with a hearing loss in the profound range this is unaided and still well below the level where most speech sounds are heard when aided. The familiar sounds audiograms can help the SLP explain to parents why the child is not actually "hearing" and may instead be responding to visual (i.e., lipreading, gestures, or facial expressions) or contextual cues. Similarly, when a child has aided access to some sounds, it is important to point this out to parents who believe their child has no auditory access and to explain the importance of helping their child attend to the sounds they can hear.

Nearing the end of the parental interview, in an effort to begin shifting the focus toward the actual test administration segment of the evaluation, the SLP can discuss the plan for the rest of the evaluation, the tests that will be administered, and how the information obtained from the tests will be used. Also, at this point, if it has not happened earlier during the parental interview, the SLP begins to more directly or actively interact with the child. For instance, the SLP may present a novel toy as a way to invite the child to play at the table or on the floor closer to the SLP. Wind-up toys, bubbles, a spinning top, or a mechanical piggy bank can all work well to draw in the child's attention. Once the child is engaged and interactive, the test instruments are introduced.

Step 5: Testing the Child

By the time the evaluation transitions to actual testing of the child, the SLP has gathered much information about the child. The SLP has now at least observed, if not interacted directly with the child. More is known about the child's communication abilities and general developmental capabilities than at the outset of the evaluation. This additional information is used to make any final changes in test selection or to confirm the use of the measures selected earlier.

If a parent-report measure is being used, then the interview-style format used during the opening of the evaluation session would continue but the interview would be driven by questions posed on the selected parent-report measure. If the child is very young and playing on the floor, the SLP might choose to sit on the floor while completing the parent-report measure with the family. In this fashion the SLP can continue to observe the child's behaviors and the family's interactions with the child. This is also a way to encourage the child's casual interactions with the SLP.

Unless the child is an infant or toddler, testing will probably occur at a table with clinician-elicited NRT measures. Test practices with children who have hearing loss are largely the same as when testing those children who have normal hearing. This includes the need for periodic rewards; verbally, in the form of short breaks, or in a more tangible form such as stickers. Additionally, as with hearing children, parents should be counseled prior to the administration of the first NRT that the SLP will be administering very specific test items and that the parents must refrain from commenting, clueing the child as to whether his or her answers are correct, repeating or rephrasing the test stimuli, or providing any unintentional hints. As in any test situation, proactively setting the expectations will minimize need for such direction of the family while testing the child and reduce the likelihood of compromised test results. The SLP may also let parents know that testing will continue until the items are above the child's ability level; thus, every child will miss many items during the administration of the test. Helping the parents understand that missing items and guessing on items is acceptable may make the testing process go more smoothly. It also can be helpful to explain this latter point to older children who may be sensitive to making errors.

An important difference between testing hearing children and children presenting for a CI candidacy evaluation is the need for the SLP to be cognizant of the child's aided hearing abilities and to sit on the side of the child's best aided ear. Another difference is that tests may be administered in a manual modality in addition to the aural modality, as discussed earlier. When NRT measures are administered through sign language or CS, individuals fluent in the child's mode of communication should complete the testing. In addition, whereas age-equivalent scores may be used descriptively in a diagnostic report, standardized scores are not assigned to scores obtained using manually supported communication.

Step 6: Establishing Closure

The evaluation typically is brought to a close by a discussion of the SLP's preliminary findings. By the time the speech and language testing is completed, the SLP usually has a good impression of the child's candidacy as a CI recipient. Although this is the case, counseling the family regarding these initial impressions must be done very carefully. At the speech and language evaluation, it may appear the child is an appropriate candidate for cochlear implantation from a speech and language perspective. However, the family must be counseled that the decision is based on a variety of information including medical, audiologic, psychological, and educational information. Thus, the candidacy decision is not based solely on speech and language information. Instead, the SLP can only counsel on whether the child is an appropriate candidate from one perspective. Whether the child is or is not a good candidate from the speech and language perspective, the SLP should counsel the parents about the findings. For example, if an older child evidences poor hearing aid use and limited oral skill development, the

SLP may counsel the family on the concern that the child would be considered at high risk for becoming a nonuser of the CI. From a speech and language standpoint, this is a contraindication for implantation. Again, as when results support implantation, the SLP should make it clear that the speech and language outcomes are only one consideration and that the final recommendation will be based on the collective results across all areas of assessment.

On occasion, results of the speech and language evaluation are less clear in one direction or the other. This may happen when a child is a borderline candidate audiologically. In this situation, it may be a child who has developed strong spoken language skills using hearing aids, but who has difficulty with complex language learning. Many higher level language skills are learned through children overhearing those around them interact. When a child has a severe or profound hearing loss, their ability to benefit from these learning opportunities is limited. In this situation, it may be unclear if the child will obtain sufficient added benefit from a CI (over continued use of hearing aids) to justify cochlear implantation. The conversation with the family in this situation often involves discussing the potential benefits or limitations of cochlear implantation from a speech and language perspective, acknowledging that the findings are not clear-cut.

Step 7: Reporting Results to the Team

When reporting results to the team, the SLP presents the scores the child obtained on the speech and language measures and makes a formal recommendation supporting or opposing the child's candidacy for cochlear implantation. The SLP also summarizes the reasons for the recommendation. The information reported by the SLP is referenced against information gathered about the child from each of the other team members. Comparing outcomes across disciplines allows the team to establish a more comprehensive understanding of the child and his or her family system. In addition, by comparing information across the disciplines, determinations can be made regarding whether or not the outcomes support each other. That is, it should be determined whether the results from the speech and language evaluation are consistent with what would be expected based on the degree of hearing loss that is documented through audiometric testing. Through this process, team members gain a better ability to ascertain the benefits a CI might provide and then make a decision accordingly.

If any of the team members has specific concerns or if opinions vary with regard to the recommendation to implant, the team members discuss the concerns and differences of opinion. In this situation, it is often useful for the team members to each complete a CI candidacy scale such as the ones discussed in the section entitled "General Candidacy Considerations of the Cochlear Implant Team." Use of a scale provides both a means to document the concerns and recommendations of each of the team members and a framework for team discussions designed toward reaching a unified team decision. In most cases these discussions lead to a final candidacy determination. If the decision remains unclear following these discussions, a recommendation for diagnostic therapy or use of a contract might be recommended before a final candidacy determination is rendered.

When the Cochlear Implant Candidacy Decision Is Unclear

Diagnostic Therapy

Occasionally, the SLP is presented with a situation in which the necessary information for determining whether a child is a candidate for a CI from a speech and language perspective cannot be determined within the context of the conventional evaluation. Findings from other discipline areas may also be unclear or ambiguous in these situations. For example, this may occur when a child presents with multiple handicaps and there are questions about the child's ability to make use of the auditory signal from a CI for learning. Another example is when a child is not performing as well as expected with his or her current amplification. In this situation, more needs to be learned about the causes for the discrepancy between the child's demonstrated audiometric abilities and the language or perception skills. It may be that there is still untapped potential with hearing aids that should be maximized before making a final decision with regard to CI candidacy. When there is uncertainty related to developmental factors, a period of diagnostic therapy can be instrumental.

The purpose of diagnostic therapy is to target focused goals that will yield information about the child's ability to learn with and to benefit from a CI. As opposed to traditional speech therapy in which the goals are geared toward developing speech sounds, language concepts, or specific listening skills, the aim of diagnostic therapy is to determine the child's potential for skill development in general, and with a CI specifically. Because diagnostic therapy targets specific goals with well-defined questions, it typically is of very short duration, often for a period of 3 to 6 months. Decisions with regard to a child's candidacy for cochlear implantation would be delayed until the additional information is obtained through diagnostic therapy.

If a child demonstrates cognitive delays and at 18 months of age is not yet sitting or walking, uses a feeding tube, and does not yet demonstrate speech, even a CI team who is willing to implant children with additional disabilities may be very hesitant to proceed with cochlear implantation. The hesitancy occurs because the team may be unsure how these developmental delays will affect the child's ability to use the auditory information from a CI in a meaningful way. In such a situation, a period of diagnostic therapy can be useful. Goals for therapy would be to determine the child's responsiveness to general social and environmental stimuli. If no overt responses are demonstrated, the first step would be to determine if such responses can be developed. For example, if a child responds to touch by smiling or looking, the goal will be to determine if those responses can be developed into a visually reinforced or conditioned response so that when a child perceives tactile stimulation, he or she smiles or looks toward the caregiver. If such a response can be generated to tangible stimuli like touch, it is a positive indicator that the child is perceiving and reacting to at least some external stimuli and, therefore, may be able to learn to do the same with auditory information. If the child continues to demonstrate no response to any stimuli, even after six months of diagnostic therapy, it would be difficult to justify implantation.

In the scenario where a child's speech perception abilities or language abilities differ greatly from what might be expected based on the child's audiometric levels, the goal of diagnostic therapy would be to establish goals that will help identify the factors that may be contributing to the discrepancy. It may be found that with increased emphasis on auditory skill development, the child begins to develop skills not previously demonstrated. This would suggest that more focused therapy can yield the desired outcomes without a CI. Alternatively, it may be determined that there are other subtle language or learning factors that limit the child's progress and would still be present even with a CI. It may also be determined

that although the child's audiometric levels appear adequate the child seems to receive a very poor quality auditory signal that limits his or her progress. Cochlear implantation may help in this latter situation.

Use of Contracts

In addition to uncertainty that may arise due to developmental factors, ambiguity about the decision to implant may also occur when a family demonstrates poor ability to comply with previously recommended care or if they have a history of repeatedly missed or canceled appointments. Resistance on the family or child's part toward compliance with therapy also is problematic and must be addressed before a final decision to implant can be made. In these situations, diagnostic therapy is not appropriate because it is believed that the child is an appropriate candidate, provided that other overriding concerns can be alleviated. In this latter circumstance, a contract may be established between the family and the CI center that clearly outlines the goals and expectations that must be met as part of the CI candidacy evaluation. Consistent attendance and participation in weekly therapy for a period of up to three months may be a component of such a contract. At other times, the contract may be based strictly on the family's ability to attend key appointments or complete specific tasks. In the instance that a period of speech-language therapy is included in the contract, the primary goal is to establish basic communication goals for the child and family to work toward. At each appointment, progress checks are completed and new goals are established as appropriate. A significant portion of goal attainment is that the family attends each of the scheduled appointments, at the scheduled time, with the child and family having completed any weekly "homework" requirements. If a positive history of follow-through can be established, it would better support a decision to implant than would a continued history of missed appointments and lack of compliance with established goals.

Post-Cochlear Implant Speech and Language Evaluation

At the House Ear Institute CARE Center, each child participates in a full speech and language assessment annually following cochlear implantation. Children and parents also meet with the SLP at the 6-month post-CI follow-up interval for a counseling session. Additionally, annual evaluations can be supplemented with semi-annual evaluations if the CI team has concerns about a child's speech and language progress. Evaluations can also be reduced in frequency in the middle to high school years if the SLP and the parents feel this is advisable, as discussed later in this section.

6-Month Post-Cochlear Implant Counseling Session

The format of the 6-month post-CI counseling session is different than the other post-CI speech and language evaluations because of the lack of formal testing. For this reason, it is described independently of the evaluation section. The reason that a full speech and language assessment is not completed at the 6-month post-CI time point at the CARE Center is two-fold; the first is due to timing and scheduling challenges. Many test measures require that the assessment not be administered more frequently than once every 6 or 12 months. Thus, if scheduling difficulties result in a child coming in shortly after the actual 6-month date and then at or before the 1-year date, the mea-

sure cannot be readministered at the 1-year post-CI evaluation. The second reason to avoid formalized assessments at 6 months post-CI is that the results of such an evaluation can be discouraging to parents. Although children often make significant auditory progress during the first 6 months following implantation, the progress is often not measurable on standardized language assessments. Despite these difficulties, completely eliminating the 6-month post-CI appointment with the SLP is not advisable. During this interval, parents have often formulated many questions about their child's auditory, speech, and language development. Thus, a counseling session at 6 months post-CI allows the SLP to answer any questions the family has formulated or address any concerns they may have. Additionally, it allows the SLP to ensure that the child is receiving appropriate aural habilitation services, that the parents have realistic expectations, and that the parents understand and feel empowered in their role as facilitators of their child's auditory and spoken language development. Certainly, every attempt is made to cover these topics during the CI candidacy process; however, it is helpful for parents to receive this information again and to ask questions after they have had a chance to watch their child's response to the auditory information provided by the CI.

The beginning of the counseling session typically is informal and serves as a time for the SLP to discuss with the parents the child's progress and current educational services. Parents should also be encouraged to ask the SLP questions during this time. If there are concerns about the child's aural habilitation services or educational placement, this time can be used for devising a plan to help the family attain more appropriate services and for discussing the child's educational needs. This may include discussions of services and educational placements available in the family's area, how the individualized family service plan (IFSP) or individualized education plan process can be used to request these services, and brainstorming other ways services may be secured (e.g., through private insurance, available community resources, etc.). Families are given so much information prior to their child receiving a CI that they often become overwhelmed and have difficulty recalling what was discussed or recommended. The 6-month post-CI counseling session provides an opportunity to review goals and expectations and to ensure any potential obstacles to achieving the goals are identified and addressed at the earliest point possible.

After this initial discussion, the SLP must find a way to move into a directed discussion designed to garner more specific information about the child. One tool that can aide in facilitating such a discussion is the *Auditory Skills Checklist* (Caleffe-Schenck, 2006). This checklist reviews 27 skills ranging from awareness of sound to understanding language when background noise is present. Most items can be marked as having been demonstrated never, sometimes (25%), often (50%), or always (75% or more). This checklist allows the SLP to ask very specific questions about the child's auditory, speech, and language development. It also serves as a tool to help parents understand the auditory hierarchy that their child will move through. In the early months of cochlear implantation, parents may be more focused on the development of skills that are midway through the auditory hierarchy as opposed to more appropriate earlier skills. As a result, they may be concerned or discouraged regarding their child's progress. For example, parents may only focus on whether their child can imitate or spontaneously produce words and not the skills that build up to word recognition such as the child's ability to detect sounds or notice

when a sound begins and ends (e.g., when a phone starts and stops ringing). Using the *Auditory Skills Checklist* helps families become more familiar with the auditory skills hierarchy so that they better understand the normal progression of skill development and how to systematically develop the skills that will lead to their child's ability to produce words. The SLP marks where a child appears to be functioning on the *Auditory Skills Checklist* and identifies the next steps that parents can work toward facilitating with their child. The SLP also can brainstorm with parents regarding games or activities that they can play with their child to facilitate these targeted skills. Conversation generated from using the *Auditory Skills Checklist* with the family gives the SLP information about the child's current state of auditory, speech, and language development that can be used for descriptive comparison at the 12-month post-CI evaluation, helps the parents understand the hierarchy of skill development, and instills confidence in the parents by giving them concrete goals to work toward.

Additional resources that can be recommended vary greatly depending on the goals that were established and the child's age. At the CARE Center, the families of children under the age of 6 years and the families of children who are deaf-blind are given information about the John Tracy Clinic Correspondence Courses. These courses are offered free to families both in the United States and other countries who speak Spanish or English. Information on these courses can be found at www.jtc.org or by calling 800-522-4582. These courses can also be helpful for professionals as they learn how to work with young children with hearing loss. Other common resources to recommend for parents are included with resources for professionals in Table 11–2.

TABLE 11–2. Aural Habilitation Resources

Caleffe-Schenck, N. (2006). *Auditory skills checklist.* Durham, NC: MED-EL Corp.

Description: This checklist can be used to establish auditory goals or to keep track of progress in the area of audition.

Caleffe-Schenck, N., & Baker, D. (2008). *Speech sounds: A guide for parents and professionals.* Englewood, CO: Cochlear Corporation.

Description: This guide was designed for use with children who are ages 1 to 5 years, but it can also be adapted for older children. It is used to assist in stimulating the development of speech through listening. There are units for 20 English consonant speech sounds with suggested activities and books to target each consonant. Additionally, there are ideas for planning therapy sessions and activities in the classroom. Parents can use this guide as a resource for carryover in the home. There is an online version for parents at www.cochlear.com

Estabrooks, W. (1994). *Auditory-verbal therapy for parents and professionals.* Washington, DC: AG Bell Association for the Deaf.

Description: This book explains and supports the auditory-verbal approach. It was written for parents of children who are deaf and hard of hearing and for therapists and educators who provide services to children who are deaf or hard of hearing.

Estabrooks, W. (1998). *Cochlear implants for kids.* Washington, DC: AG Bell Association for the Deaf.

Description: This book provides information about cochlear implant surgery, the history and ethical issues related to cochlear implantation, the importance of therapy, and the roles of parents and professionals. It also includes information on professional approaches to therapy and personal narratives written by parents.

Kiernan, K., & Zentz, B. (1986). *Contrastive word pairs.* Baltimore, MD: KZ Associates.

Description: This is a therapy tool that can be used toward developing discrimination of the sound units of language (e.g., bite-bike). Each of the six booklets has line drawings for initial sound contrasts, final sound contrasts, open-closed contrasts, cluster contrasts, and vowel contrasts. Considering the wide variety of line drawings used to represent objects, it is important that this tool be used with children who have a foundation in language.

Pollack, D., Goldberg, D., & Caleffe-Schenck, N. (1997) *Educational audiology for the limited-hearing infant and preschooler: An auditory-verbal program* (3rd ed.). Springfield, IL: Charles C. Thomas.

Description: The third edition of this book provides up-to-date materials from the previous editions. Topics include audiologic screening and evaluation, developing listening, speech, and language abilities, the role of parents, and educational placements and supports.

Sindrey, D. (1997). *Cochlear implant auditory training guidebook.* Ontario, Canada: Wordplay Publications.

Description: This is an auditory training guidebook for parents and for professionals working with children with cochlear implants that are 4 years of age and older.

continues

TABLE 11–2. *continued*

Sindrey, D. (1997). *Listening games for littles.* Ontario, Canada: Wordplay Publications.

Description: This book provides parents with information on auditory development. It also provides parents with very specific activities to target listening and language in young children.

Srinivasan, P. (1996). *Practical aural habilitation for speech-language pathologists and educators of hearing impaired children.* Springfield, IL: Charles C. Thomas.

Description: This book was written for therapists and educators who provide intervention to hearing impaired children. The book provides information regarding the development of spoken language in children with hearing losses. It also provides extensive examples of activities to do with children to promote their integrated use of speech, language, and listening.

www.hearingjourney.com

Description: The Listening Room provides activities and ideas to support the development of listening and language skills in children, adolescents, and adults. The website is sponsored by Advanced Bionics, and the activities and ideas on this site were developed by Dave Sindrey, certified Auditory-Verbal Therapist.

www.cochlear.com/HOPE

Description: The Web site for Cochlear Corporation, manufacturer of the Nucleus Freedom Cochlear Implant System and the Baha System, provides information about Cochlear Corporations' products, services, and about the Habilitation Outreach for Educators, Parents, and Adults (HOPE), a program that provides online training as well as products and services on (re)habilitation and educational issues.

www.listen-up.org

Description: The Listen-Up Web provides information, answers, help, ideas and other useful resources related to hearing loss. This Web site also includes a free downloadable module from the Listen Up and Talk It Up! Aural Habilitation Programs. The module provides information on how to work with children using sound-object association. Printable cards with pictures for each sound-object association are included in the free module.

www.bionicear.com

Description: The Web site for Advanced Bionics, the manufacturer of the Harmony Cochlear Implant System, provides information about Advanced Bionics' products and services among other information.

www.agbell.org

Description: The Web site for the Alexander Graham Bell Association (AG Bell) is a national organization that provides information on pediatric hearing loss, the auditory-oral approach, technological advances for the deaf and hard of hearing, and advocates legislation.

www.medel.com

Description: The Web site for Medical Electronics (MED-EL), manufacturer of the Maestro Cochlear Implant System, provides information regarding MED-EL products and services. On this site, there is a link to information about the Bridge to Better Communication, a resource program that has a variety of products, resources, assessments, and tools for adult and pediatric habilitation.

Planning and Preparing for the Post-Cochlear Implant Evaluation

Step 1: Chart or Record Review

In terms of carrying out the post-CI speech and language evaluation, many of the steps are the same or similar to the steps carried out during the CI candidacy evaluation. For example, the SLP will always begin with a record review, although the information to be gathered will differ slightly. Following implantation, the SLP is looking for information about the child's chronologic age, age at implantation, length of CI use, the device that the child received, and any information about communication modality. Additionally, the SLP will want to note which side was implanted, or, if the child received sequential bilateral implants, which side was implanted first. This allows the SLP to determine where to sit in relation to the child during the evaluation. The SLP will also note the last known information about the child's post-CI educational placement, aural habilitation, and any significant recommendations that were made at the child's previous evaluation. Finally, the SLP will want to know which tests were administered at the child's last speech and language evaluation and how the child performed on those tests. This may have been the child's CI candidacy evaluation or this may have been a previous post-CI speech and language evaluation.

Step 2: Speaking with Other Professionals

Another step that remains similar between the CI candidacy evaluation and the post-CI evaluations is the process of speaking to other professionals who work with the child. Speaking with those who work daily with the child and family can provide information regarding the child's CI use, such as whether or not the device is appropriately set and functioning when the child arrives at school and if the child alerts the teacher or others if having difficulty hearing. Speaking with other professionals also allows the professionals to report about recent testing they have done with the child (so that tests are not repeated too soon, rendering the test results invalid), the child's strengths or weaknesses, any changes they think need to be made in the child's educational placement or services, and specific skills or concepts that they are working to develop with the family and child.

Step 3: Test Selection

The process of selecting tests for post-CI evaluations also is very similar to the test selection process during the CI candidacy evaluation. The SLP will consider whether the tests are parent report measures or clinician-elicited measures and whether the measures are CRT or NRT. Additionally, the SLP will consider the level of language assessed. With children who are old enough to complete multiple NRT, the SLP will utilize at least one measure for each of the following areas: total language, speech production, receptive vocabulary, and expressive vocabulary.

The Test Selection Flow Chart for Testing Children (see Figure 11–1) can be used not only for the CI candidacy evaluation, but also for post-CI speech and language evaluations. The SLP will continue to consider important factors, such as whether the child is interactive, whether the child is using words or two-word combinations, and whether the child's speech can be easily understood by unfamiliar listeners. The tests mentioned on the flow chart are the tests that will be utilized for the majority of children during the post-CI language evaluations. Although not included on the flow chart, the SLP may also choose to use additional tests to assess literacy or higher-level linguistic abilities.

Unlike the candidacy evaluation, for the post-CI evaluation, the SLP must consider which tests were administered at the previous evaluation This is the case whether that evaluation was the CI candidacy evaluation or a previous post-CI evaluation. Because the goal of the post-CI evaluation is to track progress over time, it is important that one measure remain constant from one evaluation to the next. For example, if a child was seen for a CI candidacy evaluation and the *PLS-4* and the *SKI*HI* were administered because of the child's age, at the next evaluation at least one of the measures from the previous evaluation should be administered, even if the child is old enough to complete a measure designed for older children (such as the *OWLS*). Thus, the SLP might choose to administer the *PLS-4* in addition to the *OWLS*. Then, at the following evaluation, the SLP could discontinue administering the *PLS-4* and administer the *OWLS* in conjunction with other tests such as vocabulary measures. The continuous use of at least one measure from year to year will be critical when discussing results with parents and other professionals.

When time permits and a child is able to continue participating in testing, the SLP may test additional areas of the child's language development, such as the child's literacy and higher level linguistic abilities. For preschool-aged children, the *Test of Preschool Early Literacy* (Lonigan, Wagner, & Torgesen, 2007) can be utilized to test emergent literacy abilities. The results of this test may result in recommendations that emphasize the development of print knowledge or phonological awareness. For children above the age of 5 years, a variety of NRTs are available to test literacy skills. These include the *Comprehensive Test of Phonological Processes* (Wagner, Torgesen, & Rashotte, 1999), the *Written Expression Scale* of the *Oral and Written Language Scales* (Carrow-Woolfolk, 1996), the *Woodcock Reading Mastery Tests-Revised* (Woodcock, 1998), and selected tests from the *Woodcock-Johnson III NU Tests of Achievement* (Woodcock, McGrew, & Mather, 2001). The latter of these tests is especially inclusive. An SLP may choose to administer specific tests to assess reading ability, written language, or listening comprehension. It is important to note that several of these tests include the presentation of stimuli via audio recording. In these instances, it will be difficult to parse out whether weaknesses in a child's performance are due to the presentation of stimuli without visual cues or due to a child's difficulty with the content of the stimuli. For more on this topic and on the assessment of the phonological processing skills of children with CIs, see Spencer and Tomblin, 2008.

In addition to literacy skills, the SLP may choose to assess other linguistic skills. For example, the *CASL* can be utilized for testing a child's pragmatic skills and/or comprehension of nonliteral or idiomatic language (Carrow-Woolfolk, 1999). The *Test of Auditory Processing, 3rd Edition* (*TAPS-3*) (Martin & Brownell, 2005) can be used to assess basic auditory skills (e.g., word discrimination, sound segmentation, and sound blending), auditory memory, and auditory cohesion (e.g., auditory comprehension and the ability to use reason). Similarly, the *Listening Comprehension Test-2* (*LCT-2*) (Huisingh, Bowers, & LoGiudice, 2006) can be utilized to assess how students are attending to, processing, and extracting meaning from what they hear. Although the SLP should not interpret the results of these tests in the same manner as he or she would for a hearing child, the results still can be very helpful in pointing out weaknesses in a child's linguistic development that can and should be addressed in intervention assuming the child's other language skills are progressing appropriately.

Executing the Post-Cochlear Implant Evaluation

Step 4: Parental Interview

Whenever possible, the same SLP who completed the CI candidacy evaluation should complete the post-CI evaluations. This allows the family to develop a trusting relationship with the SLP and for the child to become more familiar with the examiner. This also allows the parental interview portion of the evaluation to differ from the CI candidacy evaluation because the SLP will already be familiar with the family's goals for their child and with the child's history and, thus, will not have to focus on questions designed to attain this information. Instead, the interview portion may be much briefer than in the CI candidacy evaluation, with questions focusing on what concerns have arisen for the family since their most recent speech and language evaluation. Questions may also focus on what the family is doing at home to facilitate language and on what level of knowledge the family has about the goals being implemented in the child's aural habilitation sessions.

Step 5: Testing the Child

This step differs very little from the CI candidacy evaluation to the post-CI language evaluations. However, one important point to note is that, although the examiner should still sit on the side of the child's "better hearing ear," the "better hearing ear" may no longer be the best aided ear, as during the CI candidacy evaluation. Instead, the SLP should position himself or herself on the side of the child closest to his or her CI. For children with sequential bilateral implants, the SLP should position himself or herself next to the CI the child received first. If a child received bilateral simultaneous CIs, often the child will not have a "stronger" side. However, for older children, the SLP may ask the child if he or she has a preferred side for listening. The SLP may also look at the detection audiogram or speech perception scores for the child, especially for children who have partial insertions, cochlear malformations, or electrodes that are not functioning on either of the implants.

A new issue that may arise, which typically is not present during the CI candidacy evaluation, is that parents may want to write down the items that their child misses so these words or skills can be taught at home. This is certainly a natural desire and, indeed, likely arises from the fact that the goal of the SLP and the child's intervention team has been to teach parents to be highly involved in their child's speech and language development. However, the SLP must not allow the parent to do this, because it will render the following year's test results invalid. This is especially problematic with vocabulary tests. Thus, before testing, the SLP can assure the parents that, following the evaluation, the SLP will analyze the types of items the child missed and will include this information in the upcoming report.

Step 6: Establishing Closure: Presenting Results and Making Recommendations

As previously discussed, the general goal of post-CI evaluations is to assess the child's speech and language development in order to determine whether the child is fully reaching his or her potential in these areas. A reasonable goal is for a child to make 12 months of language progress for each 12 months the child has been wearing his or her CI. Thus, for children who received their CI prior to developing language, it is a reasonable goal for the child's age-equivalent scores on language measures to be similar to their "hearing age" (i.e., the amount of time that has elapsed since the initial stimulation of the CI) at each evaluation. However, this formula of 12 months of progress during each 12-month period may not be reasonable for all children. For example, for children with additional disabilities a slower rate of progress may be inevitable.

During the annual post-CI speech and language evaluation, the SLP must use test results in addition to information from the child's educational team, family, and audiologist to decide whether the child's rate of progress is appropriate for that particular child. In order to do this, the SLP must consider the child's school placement, the family's goals for their child, whether the child has learning disabilities, and so on. After considering the child's results in the context of other information, the SLP may come to one of several conclusions and thus may make any number of recommendations to the parents. During the first year to two years following the child's receipt of a CI, the SLP may find that functional spoken language is still in the early stages of development and that efforts need to be made to continue facilitating that development. Later, one of the most positive conclusions

the SLP can reach is that the child has achieved age-appropriate language abilities and the child needs simply to maintain a steady rate of month-for-month language growth. Another potential conclusion is that the child has developed functional communication abilities, but that gaps in language development are still present which require continued attention. Finally, the SLP may reach the conclusion that the child is struggling to develop spoken language abilities that are sufficient for social interactions or academic learning, raising a strong flag of concern about the child. These scenarios and the resulting recommendations that the SLP may make are each discussed in the following sections.

It should be noted that these recommendations are not always made during the speech and language appointment. Instead, in some instances the SLP will need to obtain more information after the appointment in order to make final conclusions about the child's progress or to make specific recommendations to the family. This is especially the case if the SLP has concluded that the child is struggling to develop sufficient spoken language abilities. At the CARE Center, if the speech and language evaluation happens before the annual speech perception testing, the SLP will wait to consider the speech perception results before any changes are recommended to the family. It is important to consider speech perception information because a child's progress in auditory skill development can precede a leap in language development. Additionally, the SLP typically will confer with the CI team and the child's educational team before making recommendations for significant changes for the child. In these situations, the SLP may choose to make recommendations at a later appointment with the family or via a written report.

When Children Have Achieved Age-Appropriate Language Abilities

The optimal outcome following an evaluation is that the SLP comes to the conclusion that the child is developing speech and language abilities at an appropriate pace and no significant changes are needed to the child's intervention, education, or home environment. In this instance, recommendations may be as straightforward as continuing with the child's current educational placement with their current classroom modifications and level of aural habilitation. For these children, if they have already made the successful transition into middle school, it may be reasonable to switch from annual speech and language evaluations to evaluations on a biennial basis. This decision typically is made with the parents, with the understanding that if the child has any changes in functioning or educational achievement, a speech and language evaluation can and should be scheduled before the 2-year time window has elapsed. Parents of students in high school may choose to have even larger time windows between evaluations. However, for these students, it is typically helpful to have at least one evaluation during their senior year of high school if the student is considering attending college or other secondary learning institutions. This allows the SLP to make recommendations about the communication needs or classroom modifications the student may require in the specified setting, such as a note taker or extended test-taking time.

When Language Gaps Exist Following the Development of Functional Communication

Once children have developed a basic language foundation and can answer questions, express their thoughts and ideas and speak generally about daily events, parents may relax their vigilance in monitoring and facilitating their child's spoken language development. Many children reach a point at which they may score within the range of normal limits on total language measures such as the *OWLS* or *CELF-4* but demonstrate delayed scores on measures that assess a child's use or understanding of high-level skills such as inference, logic, verbal reasoning or idiomatic language. An evaluation indicating a slowed rate of progress or substantially poorer performance relative to previously obtained scores can be a shock to parents. When sharing results of such an evaluation, the SLP should discuss the changing communication needs of children and the necessity of a continued emphasis on facilitating advanced language skills in the home and in the school and intervention settings. This discussion should also examine whether any changes over the past year may have had an impact on the child's progress. One area to explore is the elimination of or changes to aural habilitation and speech and language services. These might include changes in the frequency or duration of therapy sessions, the interventionist, expectations, or changes in therapy goals. Other areas to consider include the presence of a new classroom teacher, an increase in the number of students in the classroom, a move to a new classroom with poor acoustics, a child's independent decision to discontinue use of an FM system, or a change in the mode of communication used for classroom instruction. In many instances, no cause can be identified outside the increased language demands being placed on the child. Nonetheless, the SLP and family must work together to understand the reasons for the finding and to develop a plan with the goal of increasing the child's rate of progress or addressing any areas of language weakness identified during the evaluation.

Being able to view the child's IEP is especially helpful when developing this plan. For example, if the IEP indicates that the child is receiving traditional articulation therapy despite significant lags in language development, the SLP may suggest alternative broad goals for the interventionist working with the child to target. Additionally, the SLP should note whether the goals are sufficiently challenging for the child or if the goals are too limited to fully address the child's language needs. Furthermore, the SLP may suggest specific educational strategies that can be implemented by a classroom teacher or, in some instances, an itinerant TOD, resource teacher, or SLP. These recommendations may include:

1. Having a professional responsible for completing daily listening checks using Ling sounds (Ling, 1976, 1989) with the child to make sure the child's CI is functioning correctly.

2. Providing the child with a Frequency Modulated (FM) system to improve the signal-to-noise ratio, thus ensuring that the teacher's voice will be louder than the background noise. For older children, a hand-held microphone that can be passed around the room during group discussions should accompany the FM system.

3. Completing comprehension checks after directions or lessons to make sure the child understands the information.

4. Previewing or preteaching vocabulary and concepts to the student prior to a lesson and reviewing vocabulary and concepts with the student after the lesson.

5. Giving the parents information on vocabulary and concepts that will be taught in the classroom during the upcoming week.

6. Writing assignments and instructional information on the board to make sure the information is clear and accessible to the child.

7. Having another child in the classroom use carbon paper for his or her notes to share with the student or allowing the child to use the teacher's lecture notes so the child can be watching the teacher as opposed to looking down while taking notes.

8. Using captioning on all movies and television programs shown in the classroom.

9. Giving the student preferential seating to improve the signal-to-noise ratio, allowing the student to see the teacher's face, and allowing the student to observe other students so that he or she can follow the cues of students around him or her.

10. Providing the child with an oral interpreter. Oral interpreters use silent lip movements to repeat the words that are spoken by the teacher and classmates giving the student greater access to speechreading information. Oral interpreters can rephrase sentences to eliminate words that are hard to lipread. They can also add facial expressions and gestures to help clarify meaning and convey the tone with which the speaker is conveying information.

11. Providing the child with a real-time captionist in the classroom to allow the child to follow classroom instruction without having to rely on auditory information and speechreading alone.

When the Goal is Facilitating Spoken Language Development

In the first one or two years following a child's receipt of a cochlear implant, a child who was implanted prior to the development of any spoken language will likely still be in the process of developing spoken language abilities. In these instances, the recommendations to the parents will look very similar to those discussed in the section on the 6-month post-CI counseling session. The primary difference is that whereas at the 6-month counseling session a listening checklist is used to generate discussion, at subsequent annual evaluations recommendations are generated through formal test results with or without the use of a listening checklist. However, the remainder of the evaluation will be very similar, with the SLP helping the family understanding how to facilitate spoken language and how to access appropriate resources to help in that process.

When Spoken Language Skills Are Not Sufficient for Social Interactions or Academic Learning

There are times when, after the SLP has considered all of the information available regarding a child, including the audiologist's speech perception assessment results, the results of the speech and language assessment, and information from a child's family and educational team, the SLP will conclude that the child does not have spoken language skills that are sufficient for social interactions and/or academic learning. Some families will come to the assessment having already reached this conclusion. They may have tired of struggling to convey important information to their child and they may have witnessed their child's frustration with communicating with those around him or her increase. Other families will have been prepared for this conclusion due to the information they received during previous speech and language evaluations and their own observations of the limited changes

in their child's language abilities over the intervening time. In these instances, it may be relatively easy to move into a discussion of the factors that may be contributing to this limited progress, including an open discussion of the family's options regarding communication mode. However, for other families, hearing the conclusion the SLP has reached can be very difficult and overwhelming despite ongoing discussions about their child's progress and the CI team's concerns at each evaluation point. The conclusion can be met with denial or anger. In instances where this may occur, the SLP must be very cautious with sharing his or her conclusions and, whenever possible, should help the parents consider all the available information in order to come to such a conclusion on their own.

In regard to testing results, the SLP may help the parents draw natural conclusions from the data by asking the parents to consider what it will mean for their child if the child's rate of progress remains steady at its current rate. For example, if a prelingually deafened child received his or her CI at four years of age and has made approximately 6 months of progress or less during each of the first two years that the child has been utilizing his or her cochlear implant, the SLP can walk the family through what the child's language abilities will look like in another 2 or 4 years if this rate of progress does not increase. If the child is currently 6 years old with language skills at approximately the 1-year level, 6 months of progress each year would result in this child having the language abilities of a 2-year-old when the child is 8 years old and the language abilities of a 3-year-old when the child is 10 years old.

In order to move away from test results and instead tap into the family's interactions with the child, the SLP may ask the parents to consider the many functions of language and how their child can use language to serve those functions. For example, a primary function of language is for general safety. The SLP can talk about the importance of being able to answer "wh" questions that are critical for safety such as "What is your name?" "Where do you live?" and "Who are your parents?" The SLP can then encourage the family to consider how well their child can share personal information such as their address and phone number if they were to get lost, or explain if they were hurt or in pain. In addition to using language for safety, we also use language to help us relate to one another. The SLP can talk with the family about their observations of their child interacting with age level peers and how they envision that changing as their child grows older.

Additionally, the SLP may talk with parents specifically about their academic goals for their child. It may be helpful to have copies of standards for subjects such as math and science for the child's grade in the state where the child attends school. The SLP and parents can talk about whether reaching these standards is something that the child will be able to do in the near future. The SLP should avoid overwhelming the parents with this type of information, but should allow the parents as much information as necessary to help them consider their child's language needs in regard to social situations and academic learning.

After helping the parents understand the necessity for their child to develop language abilities that will be sufficient for social interactions and academic achievement as soon as possible, families should be encouraged to evaluate and identify factors that they feel may be contributing to their child's slow rate of progress. With the parents and separately with the CI team, the SLP will discuss any factors that he or she

thinks may be contributing to the child's limited rate of progress and any recommendations that may be warranted. Such recommendations might include diagnostic testing for other behavioral or learning factors that may be impacting the child's rate of progress, changes in the type or frequency of the child's therapy or educational services, and/or consideration of whether changes in the child's communication modality may benefit the child. The SLP also should discuss the child's strengths with the family in order to come to a better understanding of how the child learns best. This, in turn, may be used to segue into a discussion about how the child's therapy and educational planning can be modified to work toward these strengths.

If referrals are not made for further diagnostic testing and if no changes in the type and frequency of the child's educational services can be made that would be expected to increase the child's rate of progress, the discussion may center around the third consideration, a change in communication mode. Changes in a child's communication modality are not uncommon for children with cochlear implants. Many children are enrolled in TC programs prior to receiving a CI and switch to programs with a stronger emphasis on spoken language upon receiving a cochlear implant. Similarly, some children begin learning CS prior to implantation but then once implanted, the focus shifts to more auditorily based learning. For other children, parents may avoid an immediate change in communication mode after implantation and instead may transition their child to an AO option once the child begins to evidence some functional spoken language abilities.

Changing from oral to manual communication can occur for several reasons as well. For some children, the parents decide to switch from oral to manual communication in an effort to improve their child's rate of language development. For other children, especially those who have poor ability to perceive speech with their cochlear implant, sign language or CS provides more reliable language input in that the child both sees and hears what is being said. This pairing of unclear auditory information with clear visual input may help some children more effectively learn to decipher the previously ambiguous auditory infor-mation. That is, it provides the underlying language framework from which the child then begins to advance in oral skill de-velopment as well. For whatever reason, even with an implant, some children continue to receive poor speech perception benefit and will continue to benefit from sign language or CS for academic language growth and social interactions. Another instance in which the addition of sign language may be beneficial is for children who may begin with a strong increase in language growth, but then plateau in their skills at a later time. Additionally, it may benefit children who have relatively strong receptive AO language skills, but who have limited speech intelligibility. In this instance, the use of sign language may assist the child greatly in expressive communication.

When it is evident that a child may benefit from a change in communication mode, it is best to discuss additional communication options sooner rather than later. First, having such discussions as soon as concerns arise gives the child the best opportunity to reach his or her full potential because timely decisions can be made. Conversely, waiting on such discussions may result in the child developing such large gaps in language development that the child is placed at severe risk for academic failure and social isolation. Throughout all discussions, the SLP should maintain the focus of the conversation on identifying how the child learns best and how changes in communication mode may take better advantage of the child's learning strengths. Families should never be given the impression that a change in communication mode indicates a failure on their part or their child's.

Young Adults Who Use ASL

For the group of young adults who are fluent ASL users, the annual appointment with the SLP may include more counseling than formal assessment. During this time, the SLP will address any questions regarding learning to listen with the implant. The SLP may also share resources with the young adult. Many of the resources available for young adults are available through the CI companies (educational products from each company can be used for all students with cochlear implants, regardless of the device they use). For example, MED-EL offers a wide range of rehabilitation resources through their BRIDGE to better communication. Both Cochlear Corporation and Advanced Bionics offer a number of resources, including CDs with listening exercises for preteens and teenagers and free on-line seminars for parents and professionals working with children with CIs. Additionally, Advanced Bionics' Web site includes a list of listening websites that can be used by older children and adults for independent listening practice. The Listening Room, provides practice activities for older children with CIs.

In addition to answering questions and sharing resources with the young adult, assessments may also be completed, but the

SLP should focus on presenting the results by indicating what progress has been made since the CI candidacy evaluation. Sharing age-equivalents or percentiles with these young adults can prove to be discouraging if the results are not presented in a delicate manner. The decision on the frequency of the speech and language sessions or evaluations should be determined with input from the audiologist and the young adult. For many young adults, it is not necessary to complete both a 6-month post-CI counseling session and a 12-month post-CI speech and language evaluation. Instead, the evaluation schedule may include a 6-month post-CI counseling session, an 18-month post-CI speech and language evaluation, and an additional evaluation immediately before the young adult pursues higher education.

Step 7: Reporting Results to the Team

For most CI teams, each child's test results are generally presented in a regular team meeting. Whenever possible, the SLP presents this information at the same time that the audiologist presents information on the child's auditory progress. This assists the team in developing a comprehensive understanding of each child, incorporating how speech perception, speech production, and language are interrelated for the child. The information presented for each child should include not only the child's scores on the test, but also the amount of progress the child has made over the past year. During this time, the team may brainstorm on whether changes are necessary in the child's aural habilitation services, communication mode, or educational placement. A discussion of the recommendations to be made for the family is important so that the report from the audiologist and SLP can include similar recommendations.

Aural Habilitation

As mentioned previously, some SLPs on the CI team may also serve as an interventionist for implanted children. Although step-by-step guidelines for implementing an aural habilitation plan is beyond the scope of this chapter, even SLPs who do not directly participate in intervention need to know fundamental information about aural habilitation. For those interventionists with little knowledge in this area who will be working with children with CIs, additional information is available via several auditory curricula that are available for children with hearing loss. Table 11–3 lists examples of auditory curricula that can be used by SLPs when developing auditory goals and activities to be used for each child. The SLP on a CI team should have a number of these resources readily available to share with families and any members of an educational team that will be working with a child with a CI for the first time.

Auditory Hierarchy

The basics of aural habilitation can be conceptualized as an auditory hierarchy through which the interventionist must help the child progress. The auditory hierarchy of detection, discrimination, identification, and comprehension serves as a framework for setting goals for children with CIs. Each level of the auditory hierarchy is built upon the earlier level. Although it presents as a framework, it is not the case that these skills develop in a uniform manner. For example, the child may be at a detection level for one skill, but at an identification level or comprehension level for another skill. Within these areas, therapy should not be compartmentalized, but rather

TABLE 11–3. Auditory Curricula

Name	Ordering Information	Description
Bringing Sound to Life: Principles and Practices of Cochlear Implant Rehabilitation (Koch 1999b)	Advanced Bionics Corp www.bionicear.com	Provides a systematic approach to learning spoken language. Includes four videos, a manual, and the Word Associations for Syllable Perception program.
Speech Perception Instructional Curriculum and Evaluation (SPICE)	Central Institute for the Deaf 4560 Clayton Avenue St. Louis, MO 63110 www.cid.wustl.edu	A curriculum for developing speech, listening, and processing skills. Includes a manual, set of toys, picture cards, and a video.
Cottage Acquisition Scales for Listening, Language, and Speech	Alexander Graham Bell Association 3417 Volta Place, NW Washington D.C 20007 www.agbell.org	Includes a set of scales that follow the development of language, listening, cognition, and speech. Suggestions are provided to use the tool for instruction. An assessment component is available.
The Miami Cochlear Implant, Auditory & Tactile Skills Curriculum (CHATS)	Alexander Graham Bell Association 3417 Volta Place, NW Washington D.C 20007 www.agbell.org	Includes a sequence of goals to facilitate auditory development for all ages. Receptive and expressive goals are the target areas. Objectives and activities are provided for each area.
St. Gabriel's Curriculum for the Development of Audition, Language, Speech, and Cognition	Alexander Graham Bell Association 3417 Volta Place, NW Washington D.C 20007 www.agbell.org	Provides a developmental sequence for audition, speech, language, and cognition.

should be comprehensive so that audition, language, speech, and cognition are being integrated simultaneously.

Detection

Detection refers to the child's ability to respond to the presence of sound. For a younger child, detection of sounds can be accomplished by working on the conditioned play response to a variety of sounds (e.g., speech sounds, environmental sounds, and noise-making toys). Typically, when children are between 2 and 3 years of age, they can be taught to perform a conditioned play task (e.g., putting a block in a bucket or putting a peg in a hole whenever a sound is heard). Another detection activity that can be used with a younger child is having the child begin participating in an activity, such as coloring, when music is turned on. The child can also be taught to stop participating (e.g., stop coloring) when the music stops. For an older child, detection of sounds can be accomplished by presenting a variety of sounds and then having the child indicate the presence or absence of sound by verbalizing "I heard that" or by raising a hand. Older children can also participate in detection tasks by listening to music or listening for a cell phone ring and indicating when the sound begins or ends.

At the beginning of each therapy session, it is important to utilize the Ling sounds (Ling, 1976, 1989) in a detection task (ah, oo, ee, sh, s, m) because detection of these speech sounds assists in evaluating the functioning of the CI. Additionally, during this exercise, the "absence of sound" can be added as a distracter to ensure careful listening on the part of the child. In addition to having the child indicate when he or she hears a sound or when there is an absence of sound, it is important for the SLP to integrate higher-level language concepts and cognitive skills. Language and cognition can be integrated into detection tasks, for both a young child and older child, by providing the labels, descriptions, and actions associated with the sounds the child detects.

Discrimination

Discrimination refers to the child's ability to know whether two separate sounds are the same or different. At the level of discrimination, activities can become more complex. Thus, it is necessary to have control over the number of factors that may be affecting the child's choices. With an early listener, it is important to begin with small closed sets using high acoustic contrasts, such as differences in intensity, duration, and pitch. For targeting duration of speech with a new listener, the SLP can contrast a one syllable continuous sound (e.g., "ahhhh" for a toy airplane) with a three syllable short sound (e.g., "bah bah bah" for a toy sheep). For listeners with a bit more experience, the SLP can contrast a single syllable long duration sound (e.g., "ahhhh" with a toy airplane) with a two syllable short duration sound (e.g., "beep beep" with a toy car). At the

next level, the SLP can have the child contrast all three (e.g., "ahhhh" vs. "beep beep" vs. "bah bah bah"). For discrimination of pitch using environmental sounds, the SLP can use a drum for a low pitched sound, a toy trumpet for a mid pitched sound, and a whistle for a high pitched sound. When progress is demonstrated, the tasks can be made more difficult by widening the set and keeping the same level of acoustic contrast, and then by making the choices increasingly more similar acoustically.

Mary Koch provides a table, "Challenge Factors," in her aural habilitation manual, *Bringing Sound to Life* (1999b). This table can be useful for the SLP in determining the content and presentation factors for listening activities. Content factors include familiarity of the vocabulary, the number of items in a choice set, the acoustic contrast of items, and the number of critical elements. Presentation factors include the rate of presentation, the presence of acoustic highlighting (i.e., a strategy used to draw a child's attention to targeted words or sounds by slightly prolonging the key word or sound or saying the word or sound with a slight emphasis), the presence of a carrier phrase, and the number of repetitions provided. Dave Sindrey provides a useful tool called the "Listening Ladder" in the book, *Listening Games for Littles* (Sindrey, 1997). The "Listening Ladder" can be helpful in providing information about the ten-step hierarchy to discriminating sounds. If the child is making slow or inconsistent progress or is demonstrating frustration, then the "Listening Ladder" allows the SLP to see which step to go back and address.

Discrimination activities should be highly motivating for a younger child and should incorporate the use of speech sounds with real objects. For an older child, discrimination activities should be modified to make the activity more appropriate for the child's age. For example, if the goal is to discriminate the duration of speech, specifically a continuous sound, the SLP can provide a continuous speech sound such as "ahhhhh," and then the older child can indicate whether the sound he or she heard was a long sound or a short sound verbally or by pointing to line drawings to represent duration (e.g., a long line to represent long duration and a short line to represent short duration, or several dashes to represent short-short-short duration). *Contrastive Word Pairs* developed by Kiernan and Zentz (1986) can be used for older children who are working on developing finer discrimination of the sound units (e.g., bite-bike). There are a series of six booklets with contrastive word pairs. Each booklet has line drawings for Initial Sound Contrasts, Final Sound Contrasts, Open-Closed Contrasts, Cluster Contrasts, and Vowel Contrasts. The goals addressed in these booklets regarding discrimination are to discriminate words, phrases, and sentences within closed set listening tasks (in which the child has a limited number of choices) and then to generalize these skills into open set listening tasks (in which choices are limitless).

Identification

Identification refers to the child's ability to correctly associate a sound with an object, picture, word, or action when presented with various possibilities. For a younger child, identification tasks should be simple, using real objects rather than pictures. This allows the objects to be incorporated into play activities and manipulated in a variety of ways. Identifying sound-object associations is an easier listening task than word-object association, so teaching animal sounds rather than the names of animals is an appropriate first step. After the child shows consistent identification of the animal sounds then it is appropriate to move on to word-object association. Activities such as hide and seek with the objects can be used to accomplish sound-object identification tasks (e.g., SLP: "I have something in my room that is furry, has four legs, and it says, *'ruff, ruff'"*). It is important to emphasize the targeted sound by using the technique "acoustic highlighting."

Within identification tasks, it is important to have the child attempt to imitate the sound. The SLP should encourage close sound approximations, but exact articulation should not be the focus. The aforementioned activities can be useful in reinforcing previously learned vocabulary and for expanding vocabulary. For a younger child, teaching novel vocabulary can continue the process of incorporating listening, language, and cognition into one activity. An identification task used for a younger child can be adapted for an older child to make the task more age appropriate. For example, four pictures or drawings can be placed on the table and the SLP can ask the child to pick up the targeted item. It is important to provide descriptions of each toy before it is presented to the child (e.g., SLP: "I have something in my bag that is pink, it lives on a farm, and it says *'oink, oink'"*). This technique encourages listening first rather than being provided with the visual cue first. The goal for identification tasks is to identify words, phrases, and sentences within closed set listening tasks (in which the child has a limited number of choices) and then to generalize these skills into open set listening tasks (in which choices are limitless).

Comprehension

Comprehension is the highest level of the auditory hierarchy at which the child is able to comprehend spoken language. At this point, the focus in therapy is on sustaining the child's auditory attention as the length and complexity of the auditory message increases. All activities at this level are open set. Following multipart directions, retelling stories in the correct sequence, or memorizing songs and nursery rhymes are appropriate activities at this level. The SLP should choose stories, songs, and directions that are appropriate for the child's age, interests and developmental abilities.

Speech Production

The development of speech production skills can be included as an incidental part of therapy, but should not be drilled, especially at the expense of auditory and language activities. In the earlier stages of listening, speech errors should be corrected through audition and not through visual means. Many errors the child is producing may be developmental in nature because a child's hearing age may be several years behind his or her chronologic age. These errors may also be due to difficulty perceiving the sound as opposed to producing the sound.

With increased auditory experiences, a child's speech errors often spontaneously correct. When the child has established sufficient auditory and language abilities then traditional speech therapy may be indicated, if speech patterns are clearly deviant. If speech production problems are noted, it would be necessary to obtain an analysis of the child's articulation patterns before determining if therapy focused on articulation is indicated. If therapy is indicated for a younger child then a phonological approach may be appropriate. A phonological approach enables the child to distinguish correct production of the error pattern (e.g., pairing the word "bite" with the word "bike").

Aural Habilitation Resources

Table 11–2 provides a list of additional resources that may be helpful to professionals as they begin to develop their aural habilitation skills. The resources may also be helpful for parents who are considering different communication modalities or who have made the decision to raise an oral deaf child.

Summary

This chapter has depicted the responsibilities of the speech-language specialist on a CI team and explained the various methods for fulfilling these responsibilities. However, it must be emphasized that different CI centers function in very different ways in relation to the role of the SLP on the team, how decisions are made about CI candidacy, and how or whether post-CI speech and language evaluations are conducted. Indeed, how any one specialist carries out his or her role is dependent on training, the CI program's service philosophy, the clinical intuition, and how he or she integrates and generalizes information from research literature. It is our intention that this chapter will serve as a resource for SLPs as they determine the best ways to manage the speech and language needs of children with CIs.

References

Barker Fudala, J. (2000). *Arizona Articulation Proficiency Scale* (3rd ed.). Los Angeles: Western Psychological Services.

Brownell, R. (2000a). *Expressive One Word Picture Vocabulary Test (EOWPVT)*. Los Angeles: Western Psychological Services.

Brownell, R. (2000b). *Receptive One Word Picture Vocabulary Test (ROWPVT)*. Los Angeles: Western Psychological Services.

Calandrella, A. M., & Wilcox, M. J. (2000). Predicting language outcomes for young prelinguistic children with developmental delay. *Journal of Speech, Language, and Hearing Research, 43*(5), 1061–1071.

Caleffe-Schneck, N. (2006). *Auditory Skills Checklist*. Durham, NC: MED-EL Group.

Carrow-Woolfolk, E. (1995). *Oral and Written Language Scales (OWLS): Listening Comprehension and Oral Expression Manual*. Circle Pines, MN: America Guidance Service.

Carrow-Woolfolk, E. (1996). *Oral and Written Language Scales (OWLS): Written Expression Scale Manual*. Circle Pines, MN: America Guidance Service.

Carrow-Woolfolk, E. (1999). *Comprehensive Assessment of Spoken Language Manual*. Circle Pines, MN: America Guidance Service.

Centers for Disease Control and Prevention's (CDC, 2006, October 27). *National goals, program objectives, and performance measures for the Early Hearing Detection and Intervention (EHDI) tracking and surveillance system*. Retrieved October 1, 2008 from the CDC website at http://www.cdc.gov/ncbddd/ehdi/nationalgoals.htm

Colletti, V., Carner, M., Miorelli, V., Guida, M., Colletti, L., & Fiorino, F. G. (2005). Cochlear implantation at under 12 months: Report on 10 patients. *Laryngoscope,115*(3), 445–449.

Connor, C. M., Hieber, S., Arts, H. A., & Zwolan, T. A. (2000). Speech, vocabulary, and the education of children using cochlear implants: Oral or total communication? *Journal of Speech, Language, and Hearing Research, 43*(5), 1185–1204.

Connor, C. M., & Zwolan, T. A. (2004). Examining multiple sources of influence on the reading comprehension skills of children who use cochlear implants. *Journal of Speech, Language, and Hearing Research, 47*(3), 509–526.

Daya, H., Ashley, A., Gysin, C., & Papsin, B. C. (2000). Changes in educational placement and speech perception ability after cochlear implantation in children. *Journal of Otolaryngology, 29*(4), 224–228.

Daya, H., Figueirido, J. C., Gordon, K. A., Twitchell, K., Gysin, C., & Papsin B. C. (1999). The role of a graded profile analysis in determining candidacy and outcome for cochlear implantation in children. *International Journal of Pediatric Otorhinolaryngology, 49*(2), 135–142.

Dettman, S. J., Pinder, D., Briggs, R. J., Dowell, R. C., & Leigh, J. R. (2007). Communication development in children who receive the cochlear implant younger than 12 months: Risks versus benefits. *Ear and Hearing, 28*(Suppl. 2), 11S–18S.

Dorman, M. F., Sharma, A., Gilley, P., Martin, K., & Roland, P. (2007). Central auditory development: Evidence from CAEP measurements in children fit with cochlear implants. *Journal of Communication Disorders, 40*(4), 284–294.

Dunn, L. M., & Dunn, L. M. (1997). *Peabody Picture Vocabulary Test-III*. Circle Pines, MN: American Guidance Service.

Dunn, L. M., & Dunn, D. M. (2007). *Peabody Picture Vocabulary Test, Fourth Edition (PPVT-4)*. Minneapolis, MN: NCS Pearson.

Edwards, L. C. (2003). Candidacy and the Children's Implant Profile: Is our selection appropriate? *International Journal of Audiology, 42*(7), 426–431.

Fenson, L., Marchman, V. A., Thal, D., Dale, P. S., Reznick, J. S., & Bates, E. (2007). *MacArthur-Bates Communicative Development Inventories: User guide and technical manual* (2nd ed.). Baltimore: Paul H. Brookes.

Francis, H. W., Yeagle, J. D., Bowditch, S., & Niparko, J. K. (2005). Cochlear implant outcome is not influenced by the choice of ear. *Ear and Hearing, 26*(Suppl. 4), 7S–16S.

Geers, A. E. (2002). Factors affecting the development of speech, language, and literacy in children with early cochlear implantation. *Language, Speech, and Hearing Services in Schools, 33*(3), 172–183.

Geers, A. E. (2004). Speech, language, and reading skills after early cochlear implantation. *Archives of Otolaryngology-Head and Neck Surgery, 130*(5), 634–638.

Geers, A. E., Nicholas, J. G., & Sedey, A. L. (2003). Language skills of children with early cochlear implantation. *Ear and Hearing, 24*(Suppl. 1), 46S–58S.

Goldman, R. & Fristoe, M. (2000). *Goldman Fristoe 2 Test of Articulation manual*. Minneapolis, MN: NCS Pearson.

Hellman, S. A., Chute, P. M., Kretschmer, R. E., Nevins, M. E., Parisier, S. C., & Thurston, L. C. (1991). The development of a children's implant profile. *American Annals of the Deaf, 136,* 77–81.

Holt, R. F., & Svirsky, M. A. (2008). An exploratory look at pediatric cochlear implantation: Is earliest always best? *Ear and Hearing, 29*(4), 492–511.

Huisingh, R., Bowers, L., & LoGiudice, C. (2006). *The Listening Comprehension Test-2*. East Moline, IL: LinguiSystems.

Joint Committee on Infant Hearing. (2007). Year 2007 position statement: Principles and guidelines for early hearing detection and intervention programs. *American Academy of Pediatrics, 120*(4), 898–921.

Kane, M. O. L., Schopmeyer, B., Mellon, N. K., Wang, N. Y., & Niparko, J. K. (2004). Prelinguistic communication and subsequent language acquisition in children with cochlear implants. *Archives of Otolaryngology-Head and Neck Surgery, 130*(5), 619–623.

Khan, L. M., & Lewis, N. P. (2002). *Khan-Lewis 2 Phonological Analysis*. Circle Pines, MN: American Guidance Service.

Kiernan, K., & Zentz, B. (1986). *Contrastive Word Pairs*. Baltimore: KZ and Associates.

Kirk, K. I., Diefendorf, A. O., Pisoni, D. B., & Robbins, A. M. (1997). Assessing speech perception in children. In L. L. Mendel & L. J. Danhauer (Eds.), *Audiologic evaluation and management and speech perception assessment* (pp. 101–132). San Diego, CA: Singular.

Koch, M. (1999a) *Bringing sound to life*. Timonium, MD: York Press.

Koch, M. (1999b). *Bringing sound to life: Principles and practices of cochlear implant rehabilitation [Manual]*. Baltimore: York Press.

Layton, T. L., & Holmes, D. W. (1985). *Carolina Picture Vocabulary Test*. Austin, TX: Pro-Ed.

Levitt, H., Youdelman, K., & Head, J. (1990). *Fundamental Speech Skills Test*. Englewood, CO: Research Point, a division of Cochlear Corporation.

Ling, D. (1976). *Speech and the hearing-impaired child: Theory and practice*. Washington, DC: Alexander Graham Bell Association for the Deaf.

Ling, D. (1989). *Foundations of spoken language for the hearing-impaired child*. Washington, DC: Alexander Graham Bell Association for the Deaf.

Lonigan, C. J., Wagner, R. K., Torgesen, J. K., & Rashotte, C. A. (2007). *Test of Preschool Early Literacy*. Austin, TX: Pro-Ed.

Manrique, M., Cervera-Paz, F. J., Huarte, A., & Molina, M. (2004). Advantages of cochlear implantation in prelingual deaf children before 2 years of age when compared with later implantation. *Laryngoscope, 114*(8), 1462–1469.

Martin, N. A., & Brownell, R. (2005). *Test of Auditory Processing Skills, Third Edition (TAPS-3)*. Novato, CA: Academic Therapy.

McConkey Robbins, A., Green, J. E., & Waltzman, S. B. (2004). Bilingual oral language proficiency in children with cochlear implants. *Archives of Otolaryngology-Head and Neck Surgery, 130*(5), 644–647.

Monsen, R., Moog, J. S., & Geers, A. E. (1988). *CID Picture SPINE: Speech INtelligibility Evaluation*. St. Louis, MO: Central Institute for the Deaf (CID).

Nicholas, J. G., & Geers, A. E. (2006). Effects of early auditory experience on the spoken language of deaf children at 3 years of age. *Ear and Hearing, 27*(3), 286–298.

Nikolopoulos, T. P., Dyar, D., & Gibbin, K. P. (2004a). Assessing candidate children for cochlear implantation with the Nottingham Children's Implant Profile (NChIP): The first 200 children. *International Journal of Pediatric Otorhinolaryngology, 68*(2), 127–135.

Nikolopoulos, T. P., Gibbin, K. D., & Dyar, D. (2004b). Predicting speech perception outcomes following cochlear implantation using Nottingham children's implant profile (NChIP). *International Journal of Pediatric Otorhinolaryngology, 62*(2), 137–141.

Osberger, M. J., Todd, S. L., Berry, S. W., Robbins, A. M., & Miyamoto, R. T. (1991). Effect of age at onset of deafness on children's speech perception abilities with a cochlear implant.

Annals of Otology, Rhinology, and Laryngology, 100(11), 883–888.

Paden, E., & Brown C. (1992). *Identifying Early Phonological Needs in Children with Hearing Loss.* Durham, NC: MED-EL Group.

Reynell, J. K., & Gruber, C. P. (1990). *Reynell Developmental Language Scales* (US ed.). Los Angeles: Western Psychological Services.

Robbins, A. M., Bollard, P. M., & Green, J. (1999). Language development in children implanted with the Clarion® Cochlear Implant. *Annals of Otology, Rhinology, and Laryngology, 108*(Suppl. 177), 113–118.

Rossetti, L. (2006). *The Rossetti Infant-Toddler Language Scale.* East Moline, IL: LinguiSystems.

Semel, E., Wiig, E. H., & Secord, W. A. (2003). *Clinical Evaluation of Language Fundamentals-Fourth Edition (CELF-4).* San Antonio, TX: Pearson Education.

Sharma, A., Dorman, M. F., & Spahr, A. J. (2002). A sensitive period for the development of the central auditory system in children with cochlear implants: Implications for age of implantation. *Ear and Hearing, 23*(6), 532–539.

Sindrey, D. (1997). *Listening games for littles* (2nd ed.). London, Ontario, Canada: Word Play.

Spencer, L. J., & Tomblin, J. B. (2008). Evaluating phonological processing skills in children with prelingual deafness who use cochlear implants. *Journal of Deaf Studies and Deaf Education Advance Access*; doi: 10.1093/deafed/enn013. Retrieved September 26, 2008, from http://jdsde.oxfordjournals.org/cgi/content/abstract/enn013 .

Svirsky, M. A., Teoh, S. W., & Neuburger, H. (2004). Development of language and speech perception in congenitally, profoundly deaf children as a function of age at cochlear implantation. *Audiology and Neuro-otology, 9*(4), 224–233.

Szagun, G. (2001). Language acquisition in young German-speaking children with cochlear implants: Individual differences and implications for conceptions of a "sensitive phase." *Audiology and Neuro-otology, 6*(5), 288–297.

Thal, D., Desjardin, J. L., & Eisenberg, L. S. (2007). Validity of the MacArthur-Bates Communicative Development Inventories for measuring language abilities in children with cochlear implants. *American Journal of Speech-Language Pathology, 16*(1), 54–64.

Thomas, E., El-Kashlan, H., & Zwolan, T. A. (2008). Children with cochlear implants who live in monolingual and bilingual homes. *Otology and Neurotology, 29*(2), 230–234.

Tobey, E. A., Geers, A. E., Douek, B. M., Perrin, J., Skellet, R., Brenner, C., & Toretta, G. (2000). Factors associated with speech intelligibility in children with cochlear implants. *Annals of Otology, Rhinology, and Laryngology, 109*(Suppl. 185), 28–30.

Tomblin, J. B., Barker, B. A., Spencer, L. J., Zhang, X., & Gantz, B. J. (2005). The effect of age at cochlear implant initial stimulation on expressive language growth in infants and toddlers. *Journal of Speech, Language, and Hearing Research, 48*(4), 853–867.

Tonelson, S. & Watkins, S. (1979). *SKI*HI Language Development Scale.* North Logan, UT: Hope.

Wagner, R. K., Torgesen, J. K., & Rashotte, C. A. (1999). *Comprehensive Test of Phonological Processes: CTOPP.* Austin, TX: Pro-Ed.

Waltzman, S. B., & Roland, J. T. Jr. (2005). Cochlear implantation in children younger than 12 months. *Pediatrics, 116*(4), e487–e493.

Watt, N., Wetherby, A., & Shumway, S. (2006). Prelinguistic predictors of language outcome at 3 years of age. *Journal of Speech, Language, and Hearing Research, 49*(6), 1224–1237.

Wetherby, A. M., & Prizant, B. M. (1992). Profiling young children's communicative competence. In S. Warren & J. Reichle (Eds.), *Causes and effects in communication and language intervention* (pp. 217–253). Baltimore: Paul H. Brookes.

Wetherby, A. M., & Prizant, B. M. (1993). *Communication and Symbolic Behavior Scales.* Baltimore: Paul H. Brookes.

Wetherby, A. M., & Prizant, B. M. (2002). *Communication and Symbolic Behavior Scales Developmental Profile (CSBS-DP).* Baltimore: Paul H. Brookes.

Wiig, E. H., Secord, W. A., & Semel, E. (2004). *Clinical Evaluation of Language Fundamentals-Preschool* (2nd ed.) *(CELF-P2)*. San Antonio, TX: Pearson Education.

Williams, K.T. (2007). *Expressive Vocabulary* (2nd ed.). Minneapolis, MN: Pearson Education.

Winter, M., Johnson, K. C., & Vranesic, A. (2004). Performance of implanted children with developmental delays and/or behavioral disorders: Retrospective analysis. In R. Miyamoto (Ed.), *Proceedings of the 8th International Cochlear Implant Conference. International Congress Series, Vol. 1273* (pp. 277–280). Netherlands: Elsevier.

Woodcock, R. W. (1998). *Woodcock Reading Mastery Tests-Revised: Normative update*. Minneapolis, MN: Pearson Education.

Woodcock, R. W., McGrew, K. S., & Mather, N. (2001). *The Woodcock-Johnson III*. Itasca, IL: Riverside.

Zimmerman, I. L., Steiner, V. G., & Pond R. E. (2002) *Preschool Language Scales (4th ed.) (PLS-4)*. San Antonio, TX: Pearson Education.

APPENDIX 11–A
Detailed Test Descriptions

PARENT-REPORT LANGUAGE MEASURES

MacArthur-Bates Communicative Development Inventories: Words and Gestures (MCDI: WG)

Authors: Fenson, L., Marchman, V. A., Thal, D., Dale, P. S., Reznick, J. S., & Bates, E. (2007)

Administration Time: Parents can usually complete the form in 20–40 minutes

Ages: 8–18 months (first edition provides norms up to 16 months of age)

Areas Assessed: Through parent-report, the *MCDI:WG* evaluates early communication skills including the infant's first indications of language comprehension, his or her understanding of early routine phrases, and the child's use and/or understanding of 396 common early words across 19 semantic categories (e.g., object labels, actions, prepositions, quantifiers, question words, etc.). In order to evaluate skills not reliant on verbalizations, parents are also asked about the spontaneous and imitative actions and gestures their infant uses.

Comments: Thal et al. (2007) found the *MacArthur Communicative Development Inventories* to be valid instruments for use with children who have CIs and are in the early stages of communication development, even if older than the normative sample of children with whom the test is typically used. This test has English and Spanish versions.

Ordering Information: Paul H. Brookes Publishing; www.brookespublishing.com; Phone: 800-638-3775

MacArthur-Bates Communicative Development Inventories: Words and Sentences (MCDI: WS)

Authors: Fenson, L., Marchman, V. A., Thal, D., Dale, P. S., Reznick, J. S., & Bates, E. (2007)

Administration Time: Parents can usually complete the form in 20–40 minutes

Ages: 16–30 months (There is also a 1-page extension of the MCDIs for children 30–37 months of age, the MCDI-III.)

Areas Assessed: Through parent-report, the *MCDI: WS* evaluates 680 expressive vocabulary items across 22 semantic categories. In addition, it assesses how frequently the child uses words to refer to past or future events or objects that are absent from immediate view. In order to evaluate emergence of sentence-level skills, parents are also asked questions about grammatical or sentence patterns their child uses.

Comments: This test has English and Spanish versions.

Ordering Information: Paul H. Brookes Publishing; www.brookespublishing.com; Phone: 800-638-3775

SKI*HI Language Development Scale (SKI*HI)

Authors: Tonelson, S., & Watkins, S. (1979)

Administration Time: 15–40 minutes

Ages: Birth–5 years

Areas Assessed: The *SKI*HI* is a criterion-referenced measure. It was originally designed for use with children who have hearing loss as part of parent-infant programs that followed the SKI*HI Model of intervention. It uses typically developing milestones and gives credit for the child's use of signs or voice. To the extent possible, the measure avoids inclusion of auditory-dependent milestones that may be lacking when hearing loss is present.

Comments: N/A

Ordering Information: Hope Publishing, Inc; http://www.hopepubl.com; Phone: 435-245-2888; or SKI*HI Institute; www.skihi.org; Phone: 435-797-5600

The Rossetti Infant-Toddler Language Scale (Rossetti)

Author: Rossetti, L. (2006)

Administration Time: 15–40 minutes

Ages: Birth–3 years

Areas Assessed: The *Rossetti* is a criterion-referenced measure. It uses a combination of parental interview, observation, and elicited play interactions to obtain an age-score performance profile across the communication areas of attachment, pragmatics, gestures, play, language comprehension and language expression. A spontaneous language sample is obtained with the older toddlers.

Comments: Some items are dependent on a child's auditory abilities (e.g., turns head toward voice, searches for speaker, responds to sounds when source is not visible, etc.). This test is available in English and Spanish versions.

Ordering Information: LinguiSystems, Inc.; www.linguisystems.com; Phone: 800-776-4332

CLINICIAN-ELICITED VOCABULARY MEASURES

Carolina Picture Vocabulary Test (CPVT)

Authors: Laton, T. L., & Holmes, D. W. (1985)

Administration Time: 10–15 minutes

Ages: 4;0–11;6

Areas Assessed: The *CPVT* evaluates receptive sign vocabulary skills through a four-choice picture-pointing task.

Comments: Testing can take up to 30 minutes if the child is unable to establish standard basal or ceiling criteria.

Ordering Information: Stoelting Co.; http://www.stoeltingco.com; Phone: 630-860-9700

Peabody Picture Vocabulary Test, 4th Edition (PPVT-4)

Authors: Dunn, L. M., & Dunn, D. M. (2007)

Administration Time: 10–15 minutes generally, but up to 20 minutes

Ages: 2;6–90+

Areas Assessed: The *PPVT-4* evaluates receptive vocabulary skills through a four-choice picture-pointing task.

Comments: The test manual provides Growth Scale Value (GSV) scores that allow growth performance to be measured over time and to provide a means for measuring progress from the *PPVT-3* to the *PPVT-4*. This test is co-normed with the *EVT-2*.

Ordering Information: NCS Pearson, Inc.; http://ags.pearsonassessments.com; Phone: 800-627-7271

Receptive One-Word Picture Vocabulary Test (ROWPVT)

Author: Brownell, R. (2000b)

Administration Time: 15–20 minutes

Ages: 2;0–18;11

Areas Assessed: The *ROWPVT* evaluates vocabulary comprehension skills. It requires the child to point to a picture that corresponds to a word that is said.

Comments: The test is co-normed with the *EOWPVT*. A Spanish-Bilingual Version of the test is also available for use with children ages 4–12;11. The Spanish-Bilingual Version uses the English picture plates with Spanish word translations.

Ordering Information: Pearson Education, Inc.; www.pearsonassess.com; Phone: 800-211-8378, or Western Psychology Services; http://portal.wpspublish.com; Phone: 800-648-8857

Expressive Vocabulary Test, 2nd Edition (EVT-2)

Author: Williams, K. T. (2007)

Administration Time: 15 minutes

Ages: 2;6–90+

Areas Assessed: The *EVT-2* evaluates expressive vocabulary skills. Unlike many vocabulary measures that simply require children to label a pictured object or action, the *EVT-2* requires the children to provide one-word responses to label, provide a synonym, or to complete a sentence that is read to them.

Comments: The test manual provides Growth Scale Value (GSV) scores that allow growth performance to be measured over time and to provide a means to measure progress from the *EVT* to the *EVT-2*. The test is co-normed with the *PPVT-4*.

Ordering Information: NCS Pearson, Inc.; http://ags.pearsonassessments.com; Phone: 800-627-7271

Expressive One-Word Picture Vocabulary Test (EOWPVT)

Author: Brownell, R. (2000a)

Administration Time: 15–20 minutes

Ages: 2;0–18;11

Areas Assessed: The *EOWPVT* evaluates expressive vocabulary skills. It requires the child to label pictured objects, actions or concepts.

Comments: The test is co-normed with the *ROWPVT*. A Spanish-Bilingual Version of the test is also available for use with children ages 4–12;11. The Spanish-Bilingual Version uses the English picture plates with Spanish word translations.

Ordering Information: Pearson Education, Inc.; www.pearsonassess.com; Phone: 800-211-8378, or Western Psychology Services; http://portal.wpspublish.com; Phone: 800-648-8857

CLINICIAN-ELICITED TOTAL LANGUAGE MEASURES

Communication and Symbolic Behavior Scale (CSBS)

Authors: Wetherby, A. M., & Prizant B. M. (1993)

Administration Time: 50–75 minutes (with an additional 65–75 minutes needed for scoring)

Ages: 18 months–24 months developmentally*

Areas Assessed: The *CSBS* consists of 22 rating scales that evaluate seven early developing behaviors or skills that are predictive of later language development including communicative functions, communicative gestures, means of vocal communication, means of verbal communication, reciprocity with communication partner, social-affective signaling and symbolic play. A child's pattern of errors can be an indicator of the presence of language or developmental disorders. Additional information about the child is collected through a caregiver questionnaire survey.

Comments: *This test can be used up to ages 5 or 6 years, but with children who are functionally at a developmental level of 8-24 months. Given the length of time required to administer and score this measure, use of this test may not be feasible in some clinical settings. A shorter screening and testing tool, the ***Communication and Symbolic Behavior Scales Developmental Profile*** (CSBS DP, Wetherby & Prizant, 2002) is also available.

Ordering Information: Paul H. Brookes Publishing; www.brookespublishing.com; Phone: 800-638-3775

Preschool Language Scales, 4th Edition (PLS-4)

Authors: Zimmerman, I. L., Steiner, V. G., & Pond, R. E. (2002)

Administration Time: 20–45 minutes

Ages: Birth—6;11

Areas Assessed: The *PLS-4* consists of two subscales: Auditory Comprehension (AC) and Expressive Communication (EC). It uses a combination of play interactions and direct questioning using real objects or pictures for assessment. Receptively the test evaluates precursors for language development such as attention to speakers and appropriate play with objects. At a linguistic level it assesses basic vocabulary, concepts, grammatical markers, and a range of sentence structures. At older ages, it also assesses a child's ability to make comparisons and inferences. Expressive skills assessed include early vocal development, social communication, naming of common objects, use of concepts that describe objects and express quantity, use of prepositions, use of grammatical markers, use of varying sentence structures, phonological awareness, sequencing skills, and the use of language to define words and retell short stories.

Comments: The *PLS-4* is also available in a Spanish version.

Ordering Information: Pearson Education, Inc.; www.pearsonassess.com; Phone: 800-211-8378

Reynell Developmental Language Scales (RDLS)

Authors: Reynell, J. K., & Gruber, C. P. (1990)

Administration Time: 25–30 minutes

Ages: 1–6;11

Areas Assessed: The *RDLS* is composed of two sections, a verbal comprehension portion and an expressive language portion. It uses a combination of real objects and pictures for assessment. Receptively, it assesses a child's understanding of common object labels, action labels, object attributes, functions of objects and ability to follow directions using simple animal or people props. It also assesses a child's ability to follow longer, multi-element directions and abstract language. Expressively, the measure evaluates a child's vocabulary, use of sentence structures, and, through a picture description task, evaluates the child's ability to use language to express connected thoughts and ideas.

Comments: The *RDLS* has been used widely with children who have hearing loss. The scoring manual includes a chapter on the use of the measure with children who are deaf or hard of hearing. For the verbal comprehension section, alternative test administration instructions utilizing eye gaze are provided for children who are unable or unwilling to use their hands to manipulate or select test items. The test originated in the UK but a US version is also available. Some may consider isolated test content inappropriate (e.g., one test item queries, "Which one shoots the rabbit?"). One section of the test uses stimuli that may be auditorily challenging for newer listeners because of their acoustic similarity (e.g., child must discriminate Mommy, Bobby, Baby and Mary, all which look visually similar if speech reading and which require minimal pair discrimination).

Ordering Information: Western Psychology Services; http://portal.wpspublish.com; Phone: 800-648-8857

Oral and Written Language Scales (OWLS)

Author: Carrow-Woolfolk, E. (1995, 1996)

Administration Time: 15–40 minutes

Ages: 3–21

Areas Assessed: The *OWLS* is composed of three evaluative scales: oral expression, listening comprehension, and a written language scale. Collectively, the three scales, either through oral language or print, measure a broad range of lexical (word), syntactic (grammar) and pragmatic (social) connected language abilities. In addition, the scales assess a child's use and understanding of supralinguistic language (e.g., comprehension or use of idioms, inference, figurative language and higher-level thinking skills). Although the three scales can be used together in a single evaluation, more commonly, the written scale is used independently of the two oral language scales.

Comments: For the Listening Comprehension portion of the *OWLS*, the correct answer is pictured on the tester's side of the easel. This may create a challenging testing situation at times (e.g., in rooms with one-way observation mirrors, for children who are drawn toward looking at what the tester is doing/seeing, etc.).

Ordering Information: American Guidance Services; http://ags.pearsonassessments .com; 800-627-7271, or Western Psychology Services; http://portal.wpspublish.com; Phone: 800-648-8857.

Clinical Evaluation of Language Fundamentals-Preschool, 2nd Edition (CELF-P2)

Authors: Wiig, E. H., Secord, W. A., & Semel, E. (2004)

Administration Time: 15–20 minutes for core tests, up to an hour if additional subtests are administered

Ages: 3;0–6;11

Areas Assessed: The *CELF-P2* provides four levels of testing. At the first level, the SLP can administer core subtests to assess the child's overall language functioning. Level two provides supplemental tests that can be used for more detailed diagnostic purposes. Levels three and four provide rating scales or checklists to evaluate preliteracy skills and social language development.

Comments: Some subtests may be challenging for children who have limited auditory memory skills or poor auditory acuity.

Ordering Information: Pearson Education, Inc.; www.pearsonassess.com; Phone: 800-211-8378

Clinical Evaluation of Language Fundamentals, 4th Edition (CELF-4)

Authors: Semel, E., Wiig, E. H., & Secord, W. A. (2003)

Administration Time: 30–60 minutes

Ages: 5;0–8;11; 9;0–21;11

Areas Assessed: The *CELF-4* as with the *CELF-P2* provides four levels of testing, mirroring the levels of the *CELF-P2*. In addition to preliteracy skills for level 3, the *CELF-4*

includes tests to assess underlying clinical behaviors that can be associated with language deficits such rapid automatic naming and number repetition skills.

Comments: Test may be challenging for children who have limited auditory memory skills or poor auditory acuity.

Ordering Information: Pearson Education, Inc.; www.pearsonassess.com; Phone: 800-211-8378

ARTICULATION AND SPEECH INTELLIGIBILITY MEASURES

Arizona Articulation Proficiency Scale, Third Edition (Arizona-3)

Author: Barker Fudala, J. (2000)

Administration Time: Approximately 3 minutes

Ages: 1;6—18

Areas Assessed: The *Arizona-3* is a tool that measures the articulatory proficiency of children at the single word level. Children are shown picture cards and asked to label the pictures. At older ages, the children can read the target word from a printed script. Responses are judged for articulatory proficiency for targeted consonant or vowel sounds in various positions within words. The measure generates an impairment rating that gives a general indication of speech intelligibility.

Comments: This assessment tool can be used with individuals above age 18 but normative scores are not available beyond 18 years of age. The measure also provides optional assessment tasks to evaluated conversational/connected speech skills. The optional assessments yield descriptive information and not normative scores.

Ordering Information: Western Psychology Services; http://portal.wpspublish.com; Phone: 800-648-8857

Fundamental Speech Skills Test (FSST)

Authors: Levitt, H., Youdelman, K., & Head, J. (1990)

Administration Time: 25 minutes or less

Ages: Age independent

Areas Assessed: The *FSST* is specifically designed for use with children who have hearing loss. It is designed to assess fundamental aspects of voice control or production such as timing, stress and intonation patterns. It also assesses production of targeted vowels or consonant within words.

Comments: Both norm-referenced and criterion-referenced values can be obtained. The test has been normed on 250 children with hearing loss who live in the New York area. The children's backgrounds vary, representing both aural and total communication modes.

Ordering Information: NCS Pearson, Inc.; http://ags.pearsonassessments.com; Phone: 800-627-7271

Goldman-Fristoe 2 Test of Articulation (GFTA-2)

Authors: Goldman, R., & Fristoe, M. (2000)

Administration Time: 15 minutes

Ages: 2;0–21;11

Areas Assessed: The *GFTA-2* evaluates a child's ability to produce consonant sounds within the context of common early childhood words. Whereas the preferred response format is spontaneous productions, delayed imitation productions are acceptable. The test evaluates the targeted consonants in various positions within words (at the beginning, middle and/or end of words). Some consonants are also assessed within consonant clusters at the beginning of words (e.g., "*sl*ide").

Comments: This assessment tool also has a section to assess sounds in sentences but this section places a heavy load on the child's auditory memory. In addition, some words are used that may not be in a young child's vocabulary, especially if language delays are also present (e.g., "His daddy *covers* him with the sheet."). For these reasons, this portion of the measure becomes effectively reduced to a word-level task for some children.

Ordering Information: NCS Pearson, Inc.; http://ags.pearsonassessments.com; Phone: 800-627-7271

Khan-Lewis 2 Phonological Analysis (KLPA-2)

Authors: Khan, L., & Lewis, N. (2002)

Administration Time: (Based on responses from GFTA-2)

Ages: 2;0–21;11

Areas Assessed: The *KLPA-2* uses the responses from the *GFTA-2*, analyzing them further to assess 10 developmental phonological processes that may be present. The phonological processes evaluated fall into one of three process areas: reduction processes (e.g., cluster simplification), place and manner processes (e.g., velar fronting) and voicing processes (e.g., voicing of unvoiced initial consonant sounds).

Comments: It can take 10–30 minutes to score the analysis.

Ordering Information: NCS Pearson, Inc.; http://ags.pearsonassessments.com; Phone: 800-627-7271

Identifying Early Phonological Needs in Children with Hearing Impairment (Paden/Brown)

Authors: Paden, E., & Brown, C. (1992)

Administration Time: 15 minutes

Ages: Age independent

Areas Assessed: The *Paden/Brown* was designed for use with children who have hearing loss. Vocabulary is controlled to include words common to the vocabulary of this population. Productions are rated based on first level phonological patterns including suprasegmental features (e.g., accuracy of stress patterns and syllable number), vowel accuracy and accuracy of consonant place, manner and voicing features. Percent accuracy scores are obtained, not normative scores. The test allows either spontaneous or imitative responses.

Comments: Children may have the vocabulary necessary for spontaneous productions sooner on this measure than on tests designed for and normed for children who have normal hearing (e.g., the GFTA-2). Test may give better indication of early speech production development by focusing on first level phonological patterns as opposed to consonant or vowel accuracy per se.

Ordering Information: NCS Pearson, Inc.; http://ags.pearsonassessments.com; Phone: 800-627-7271

CID Picture SPINE Speech Intelligibility Evaluation (Picture SPINE)

Authors: Monsen, R., Moog, J. S., & Geers, A. E. (1988)

Administration Time: 20–30 minutes (approximately 10 minutes to score)

Ages: School-aged (need to be able to name pictured items)

Areas Assessed: The *Picture SPINE* was designed for use with children who have hearing loss to measure intelligibility. Vocabulary was chosen based on its ability to reflect characteristics of speech production that are often problematic for children with significant hearing loss. In addition, words are based on those that are common to the vocabulary of children with hearing loss. As opposed to normative scores, percent of words understood by a listener is obtained.

Comments: Testing can become lengthy if the child needs to be repeatedly familiarized with the vocabulary. Validity of test is reduced if items must be removed as a result of the child being unfamiliar with the vocabulary.

Ordering Information: CID Publications; http://www.cidedu.com; Phone: 314-977-0133

CLINICIAN-ELICITED SUPRALINGUISTIC-LEVEL LANGUAGE MEASURES

Comprehensive Assessment of Spoken Language (CASL)

Author: Carrow-Woolfolk, E. (1999)

Administration Time: Varies based on the age-level of child and whether or not supplementary tests are being given. For children up to five years of age, the core battery generally takes about 25 minutes. For older children it may take up to 60 minutes for the core battery.

Ages: 3;0–21;11

Areas Assessed: The *CASL* is composed of 15 test measures divided into four language categories to assess a child's comprehension of language, expression of language and language retrieval abilities. The four categories of language assessed include lexical/semantic, syntactic, supralinguistic and pragmatic abilities. There is a suggested core battery dependent on the child's age. Additional test sections can be given to supplement findings of the core battery.

Comments: Although response exemplars are provided to ease scoring (so that the tester can circle response item that most closely resembles the child's response) for sections that elicit open-ended replies, if the child's exact responses are desired the tester must hand record them. In this situation, testing becomes more tedious (and time consuming) because of the amount of time needed for transcription.

Ordering Information: American Guidance Services; http://ags.pearsonassessments .com; 800-627-7271, or LinguiSystems, Inc.; www.linguisystems.com; Phone: 800-776-4332

Listening Comprehension Test 2 (LCT-2)

Authors: Huisingh, R., Bowers, L., & LoGiudice, C. (2006)

Administration Time: 35–40 minutes

Ages: 6–11;11

Areas Assessed: The *LCT-2* assesses a child's ability to process and ascribe meaning to short passages that are read aloud. The passages are based on realistic learning and life experiences and require the child to identify the main idea or details, to follow reasoning, to understand higher-level vocabulary, and to demonstrate comprehension of messages.

Comments: This test may be challenging for children who have poor auditory memory skills.

Ordering Information: LinguiSystems, Inc.; www.linguisystems.com; Phone: 800-776-4332

Test of Auditory Processing, Third Edition (TAPS-3)

Authors: Martin, N.A., & Brownell, R. (2005)

Administration Time: 60 minutes if administering all subtests

Ages: 4-18; 11

Areas Assessed: The *TAPS-3* assesses a child's ability to auditorily process language in three general domains: (1) basic auditory skills including word discrimination, sound segmentation and sound blending, (2) auditory memory including words, sentences and numbers forward and reversed, and (3) auditory cohesion including auditory comprehension and ability to use reason.

Comments: The information gained from this measure should be used as an adjunct to other measures. Use of this test requires excellent auditory perceptual skills, thus, it should be used very cautiously with children who use hearing aids or implants and only with children who are making good progress on most other spoken language measures.

Ordering Information: LinguiSystems, Inc.; www.linguisystems.com; Phone: 800-776-4332

LITERACY MEASURES

Comprehensive Test of Phonological Processing (CTOPP)

Authors: Wagner, R., Torgesen, J., & Rashotte, C. (1999)

Administration Time: 30 minutes

Ages: 5-24

Areas Assessed: Phonological awareness, phonological memory, and rapid naming

Comments: This test has two versions, one for children ages five and six, another for children ages seven through 24. For both versions, supplemental tests are provided that allow the examiner to assess specific strengths and weaknesses.

Ordering Information: PRO-ED Inc.; www.proedinc.com; Phone: 800-897-3202

Test of Preschool Early Literacy (TOPEL)

Authors: Lonigan, C. J., Wagner, R. K., & Torgesen, J. K. (2007)

Administration Time: 25 to 30 minutes

Ages: 3-5; 11

Areas Assessed: Print knowledge, definitional vocabulary, phonological awareness

Comments: This test is the only available NRT that examines phonological awareness skills in children as young as three years of age. Use of the phonological awareness subtest requires excellent auditory perceptual skills.

Ordering Information: PRO-ED Inc.; www.proedinc.com; Phone: 800-897-3202

Woodcock-Johnson III Normative Update Tests of Achievement (WJ III NU TA)

Authors: Woodcock, R. W., McGrew, K. S., & Mather, N. (2001)

Administration Time: Approximately five minutes per test

Ages: Depends which tests are administered.

Areas Assessed: Oral expression, listening comprehension, written expression, basic reading skills, reading comprehension, reading fluency, math calculation skills, math reasoning.

Comments: The SLP typically does not administer the full test. Selected oral language literacy tests can be chosen based on the child's age and language abilities. This test includes some audio-recorded measures, the results of which should be interpreted with caution considering the effects of the auditory only presentation.

Ordering Information: Riverside Publishing; www.riverpub.com; Phone: 800-323-7000

Woodcock Reading Mastery Tests-Revised-Normative Update (WRMT-R/NU)

Authors: Woodcock, R. W. (1998)

Administration Time: 10–30 minutes for each grouping of tests

Ages: 5–75+

Areas Assessed: Reading readiness and reading achievement. Subtests include Visual-Auditory Learning, Letter Identification, Word Identification, Word Attack, Word Comprehension, and Passage Comprehension.

Comments: N/A

Ordering Information: NCS Pearson, Inc.; http://ags.pearsonassessments.com; Phone: 800-627-7271

CHAPTER 12

Prelexical Infant Scale Evaluation: From Vocalization to Audition in Hearing and Hearing-Impaired Infants

LIAT KISHON-RABIN
RIKI TAITELBAUM-SWEAD
OSNAT SEGAL

Introduction

The population of early implanted deaf infants is increasing substantially because of broadening candidacy criteria and because hearing loss can be detected in the first months of the newborn's life due to advanced hearing diagnostic and screening techniques (Joint Committee on Infant Hearing, 2000; Yoshinaga-Itano, 2000). Furthermore, the trend to detect and identify hearing loss and to intervene at younger ages is driven by what used to be a general belief and now substantiated by considerable data showing that the earlier in development a child has access to hearing, the better the chances that he or she will acquire spoken language skills that are comparable to normal hearing peers (Miyamoto, Kirk, Svirsky, & Seghal, 1999; Svirsky, Teoh, & Neuburger, 2004; Yoshinaga-Itano, Sedey, Coulter, & Mehl, 1998). Specifically, early auditory habilitation, younger than 6 months of age, was found important for the later development of speech, language and scholastic achievements in young hearing-impaired (HI) children (e.g., Fryauf-Bertschy, Tyler, Kelsay, & Gantz, 1997; Kirk, Miyamoto, Lento, Ying, O'Neill, & Fears 2002; Waltzman & Cohen, 1998). On this background, assessing auditory perception skills in HI infants for diagnosis and evaluation of appropriate intervention methods and hearing devices is considered a crucial first stage to ensure that they will receive all the intervention that is needed to develop age-appropriate speech and language skills. Unfortunately, assessing auditory perception in young infants is not a simple task. Due to lack of cooperation and limited cognitive, linguistic, and motoric skills, many clinicians refer to objective-electrophysiologic measures for estimating audiometric thresholds. Although these measures provide good estimation for audiometric thresholds, they do not provide a measure of "hearing" percept (Cone-Wesson, 2003). Auditory behavior assessment tools that are practical to administer include parent questionnaires, such as the Infant-Toddler Meaningful Auditory Integration Scale (IT-MAIS), which evaluates gross auditory behavioral skills by means of parent interview (Kishon-Rabin, Taitelbaum-Swead, Ezrati-Vinacour, & Hildesheimer, 2005; Robbins, Koch, Osberger, Zimmerman-Phillips, & Kishon-Rabin, 2004). In the present chapter, we suggest supplementing existing information by evaluating the infant's *preverbal production skills*. We hypothesize that the intrinsic relation between auditory perception and production will manifest itself in strong predictive values between auditory perception and preverbal vocalizations, thus allowing the production test to be an indirect measure of auditory perception. The purpose of the present chapter is to introduce in detail the Production Infant Scale Evaluation (PRISE) parent questionnaire and to discuss the rationale that led to its development (Kishon-Rabin et al., 2005). The chapter is divided into three major sections. The first discusses the theoretical and empirical basis for the relationship between auditory perception and speech production and provides the theoretical background for developing the PRISE. The second part is a detailed

elaboration of each of the PRISE questions, whereas the third part is devoted to describing the PRISE data in normal-hearing and HI infants and its validation with direct measures of hearing. We argue that the PRISE is a clinically feasible tool for assessing prelexical vocalizations in infants younger than 1 year of age and that it is sensitive to the effects of auditory deprivation, auditory feedback, age at implantation, unilateral hearing loss and premature birth.

The issue of assessing speech perception skills has been discussed extensively, especially for children 2 to 3 years of age and older (e.g., Boothroyd, 1991; Eisenberg, Martinez, & Boothroyd, 2007; Mendel & Danhauer, 1997). Evaluating speech perception skills in infants younger than 1 year of life, however, is more complicated and presents a considerable challenge to the clinician and experimenter (Houston, Pisoni, Kirk, Ying, & Miyamoto, 2003). As mentioned above, it is difficult to test auditory behavior in infants at this age due to short attention span, highly variable levels of compliance, and very limited skills in understanding and using language (e.g., Robbins et al., 2004; Weber, Hahne, Friedrich, & Friederici, 2004). Thus, any evaluation methods should consider these issues and yet provide valid and reliable information that can predict auditory performance in realistic listening situations (Mendel & Danhauer, 1997).

In practice, clinicians often use electrophysiologic methods to evaluate the integrity of the auditory system, thus assessing the degree of hearing loss and aiding in the fitting of hearing devices. Otoacoustic emissions are widely used in newborn screening programs for diagnosing hearing loss of cochlear origin, whereas auditory evoked potential (AEP) methods such as compound nerve action potential (CAP), auditory brainstem response (ABR), and auditory steady state response (ASSR) are used to establish responses higher along the auditory pathway. One advantage of these methods is that they can be conducted while the infant sleeps. In many cases, the obtained results are in good correlation with behavioral audiometric thresholds. A major limitation of these tests, however, is that they do not test "hearing," thereby implying perception. Rather, they depend on neural synchrony activated in response to sound. Although perceptual thresholds and neural synchrony are correlated, it is possible to have good neural synchrony and poor perception, and vice versa (Cone-Wesson, 2003). Recently, researchers have attempted to utilize electrophysiologic methods to assess passive auditory discrimination abilities of infants (e.g., mismatch negativity response, Weber et al., 2004; Weber, Hahne, Friedrich, & Friederici, 2005). Although these techniques provide more specific information regarding the infant's brain response to stimuli at different "stations" along the auditory pathways (including the auditory cortex), they are currently time consuming, require special equipment and very carefully controlled stimuli, and the variability in responses is very large (Conboy, Rivera-Gaxiola, Silva-Pereyra, & Kuhl, 2008). Furthermore, today their prognostic value for predicting auditory perception is limited and the relationship between the brain's electrical response and the behavioral speech perception has yet to be established. Unless a strong correlation between the two is found, electrophysiologic measures cannot *substitute* for evaluation of overt behavioral responses.

Behavioral assessment of auditory function for children and infants has always been the foundation of clinical audiology (Katz, 1994). Responses such as eye blinks, changes in sucking rate, body movements and, by 6 months of age, head turning, have been used for evaluating sound thresholds in infants for the last few decades (Eilers,

Wilson, & Moore, 1977; Kuhl, 1985; Werker et al., 1998). The growing body of evidence suggesting that language acquisition depends on speech perception skills, which develop through the first year of life, and that early intervention is crucial for developing spoken language (Kirk et al., 1998) has led to new behavioral methods using advanced technology (Houston et al., 2003; Houston, Horn, Qi, Ting, & Gao, 2007). These paradigms include the ***Conditioned Head Turn (CHT)***, the ***Visual Habituation Procedure (VHP)*** and the ***Headturn Preference Procedure (HPP)***. They are based on the use of universal nonverbal behavior such as head-turning and looking, on the tendency of infants to be interested in novel stimuli, and on the preference of listening to familiar stimuli (Kemler-Nelson, Jusczyk, Mandel, Turk, & Gerken, 1995, Kuhl, 1985; Werker et al., 1998). Their advantage is that they enable assessment of suprathreshold speech perception processes including discrimination and recognition in infants. Because the paradigm includes coding the infant's responses during testing as well as video recording, the experimenter can validate his or her coding of infant's behavior by using an independent tester which examines the video recording only.

Recently, there have been attempts to use special infant testing paradigms (as described above) for assessing auditory speech perception of infants with hearing loss before and after cochlear implantation. Houston et al. (2003), for example, tested infants' ability to discriminate between a continuous ("ahhhh") sounds versus discontinuous ("hop hop hop") sound patterns. Both normal-hearing infants and HI infants with cochlear implants were able to discriminate these sound patterns. Additionally, Horn, Houston, and Miyamoto (2007) showed that prelingually deaf infants within three months after cochlear implantation were able to discriminate non-meaningful words based on segmental differences when presented audiovisually. Overall, these results suggest an improvement in speech discrimination skills following cochlear implantation in deaf infants. In order to evaluate the perception of phonological contrasts in young infants and toddlers, Eisenberg et al., (2007) developed the Visual Reinforcement Assessment of the Perception of Speech Pattern Contrasts (VRASPAC) using the Conditioned Head-turn Procedure. They found that normal-hearing infants as well as hearing-impaired (HI) infants with moderate hearing loss were able to discriminate mainly the vowel contrasts. This is further detailed in Chapter 9 by Arthur Boothroyd. Most of these methods, however, are limited in their clinical use. They require some cooperation from the infant which was found to be lacking in 28 to 50% of the infants (depending on the study and method) (Best, Sithole, & McRoberts, 1988; Houston et al., 2007; Nittrouer, 2001; Werker et al, 1998). Furthermore, these techniques require equipment and personnel highly trained in behavioral infant testing.

The few existing clinically useful measures for evaluating auditory behavior in infants and toddlers motivated clinicians to develop an interview questionnaire for parents which yields a quantitative value for the auditory behavior of their children as young as newborns regardless of whether they have impaired or normal hearing (Zimmerman-Phillips, Robbins, & Osberger, 2000). This questionnaire, known as the Infant-Toddler Meaningful Auditory Integration Scale (IT-MAIS), is a structured interview schedule that queries parents about their child's spontaneous listening behaviors in everyday situations (Zimmerman-Phillips et al., 2000). It is based on interview elicitation techniques that are widely used in developmental psychology and are similar to those used with the Vineland Adaptive Behavior Scales (Sparrow, Balla, & Cicchetti, 1984). Among the advantages of such structured interview tools are that clinicians may obtain information without requiring a young child's compliance or attention and they are not considered language specific. Moreover, the reliability of parent report on infant babbling is known to be high (Oller, Eilers, Neal, & Schwartz, 1999). In the IT-MAIS, 10 questions are posed to parents that sample three different areas of auditory skill development. These three areas include changes in vocalization associated with device use (Questions 1 and 2); alerting to sounds in everyday environments (Questions 3, 4, 5, 6); and deriving meaning from sound (Questions 7, 8, 9, 10). Using information provided by the parent, the examiner scores each question based upon the frequency of occurrence of a target behavior. Scores for each question range from 0 ("never demonstrates the behavior") to 4 ("always demonstrates the behavior").

The IT-MAIS has been used primarily to evaluate the benefit of cochlear implants in infants and toddlers with hearing loss and to assess the effect of age at implantation on the outcome of auditory behavior (Robbins et al., 2004). In this study, 107 infants and toddlers, implanted between 12 and 36 months of age, showed rapid improvement in their auditory skills during the first year of device use, regardless of age at implantation. Younger implanted children, however, achieved higher scores. When comparing the implanted data to those of 109 normal-developing infants between 0.5 and 36 months of age, it was found, that children who were implanted at a younger age acquired auditory skills nearer to their normal-hearing peers in comparison to older children. The mean rate of acquisition of auditory skills was found to be similar to normal-hearing infants and toddlers regardless of age at implantation. These data support the sensitivity of the IT-MAIS for demonstrating increased auditory abilities after cochlear implantation compared to their hearing status preimplant.

In the absence of easily administered auditory evaluation tests for young infants, the IT-MAIS provides valuable information regarding the auditory behavior of young infants with cochlear implants and therefore was adopted for use in clinics throughout the world (Tailtelbaum-Swead et al., 2005; Kubo, Iwaki, & Sasaki, 2008). The IT-MAIS however, has a few caveats that necessitated the development of additional measures of auditory behavior. One of its limitations is that one of the 10 questions is related to device use and, therefore, for assessing auditory behavior in populations that do not use listening assistive devices, the questionnaire is based on only nine questions. Another limitation of this tool is that it was not found to be sensitive to certain hearing losses such as infants with unilateral hearing loss (see later in this chapter). Thus, the rising population of very young infants (less than 1 year old) who were diagnosed with hearing loss at the Sheba Medical Center at Tel-Hashomer (Israel) and the immediate need to evaluate behaviorally their hearing status for appropriate intervention, motivated us to develop an additional evaluation test that would supplement the information provided by the current tests (i.e., electrophysiologic tests and IT-MAIS).

There were several requirements that guided us in the development of an additional evaluation test for young infants. The first is that it should be easily administered in the timeframe allocated in clinics. The experience we accumulated with the IT-MAIS supported using a parent interview questionnaire technique (Kishon-Rabin et al., 2005; Taitelbaum-Swead et al., 2005). It is quick to administer and highly reliable among interviewers (i.e., clinicians[1]). Another important issue is the relevance of this test to linguistically diverse populations. Israel is considered a "melting pot" of many cultures due to immigration from many countries around the world (Leshem & Shuval, 1998). Demographically, the majority of the adult population speaks Hebrew (6 million speakers). Only half of them, however, are native speakers of Hebrew. A second official language of Israel is Arabic, which is considered the dominant language in 23% of the population (1,400,000 speakers). Additionally, there are 16% (about 1,000,000) Russian speakers. Other spoken languages in Israel include Yiddish, English, Amharic, and French. Thus, from a clinical point of view, it was preferable that this new test be applicable to all of populations of diverse linguistic background.

To meet the above requirements, we raised the possibility that the *evaluation of preverbal vocalizations* may be a good predictor of functional hearing in young infants. This assumption had a theoretical and empirical premise. Theoretically, many advanced theories of speech perception support the intrinsic relation between auditory perception and production. Empirically, there have been many studies which examined the effect of hearing loss on the quality and quantity of the child's verbal productions, as well as on the preverbal babbling behavior of infants with hearing

---

[1]Note that in the present context, the term "clinicians" is used to refer to speech-language pathologists and/or audiologists. In Israel, most professionals are dually certified and are therefore termed "clinicians."

loss. Recent research also shows the effect of restored hearing via cochlear implants on the child's verbal productions.

One of the most influential theories of speech perception, the *Motor Theory*, assumes that the phonemes are associated with the movements that produce speech (Liberman, Cooper, Shankweiler, & Studdert-Kennedy, 1967). Specifically, it suggests that the vocal tract movements themselves are reconstructed when the auditory pattern is decoded. In the later *Revised Motor Theory*, listeners are assumed to reconstruct the talker's *intended gestures* for phonetic categories such as tongue backing, lip rounding, and jaw/tongue raising (Liberman & Mattingly, 1985). In other words, the listener perceives the articulatory plans that control the vocal tract movements that would produce a perfect exemplar on the talker's intended utterance. These intended gestures are assumed to be the only invariant property that unites the phonemic message through differences in rate of speech, talker, dialect or other speaker characteristics. It is, therefore, the only invariant property the child can pick up from the signal. The Motor Theory also argues that the speech percept is nonhomomorphic with the auditory signal (i.e., the percept does not have the same form as the signal), because we use our innate knowledge of how to make sounds in order to understand speech. The percept of the nonspeech auditory signal, on the other hand, is homomorphic and the percept has the same form as the signal. Moreover, the theory assumes that the human vocal tract evolved to its present state partly to make speech possible, and that the brain's perceptual abilities developed in tandem, and in response to, its productive abilities. The consequence is that, according to this theory, speech production and perception share a common link and a common processing strategy (Hawkins, 1999). Early

motor theorists assumed that infants first learn the connection between movement and sound from their sound play and then learn to discriminate sounds in the speech of others by reconstructing the motoric gestures that would be needed to make those sounds. This notion was questioned after Eimas and colleagues (1971) demonstrated that babies perceive voice-onset time (VOT) categorically, thus not supporting the idea that perception follows production (because infants discriminate between sounds that they cannot produce). An alternative explanation to Eimas et al.'s (1971) infant data is that there is a universal, nonspeech auditory sensitivity area that influences category boundaries in categorical perception (Kishon-Rabin, Rotshtein, & Taitelbaum, 2000; Kuhl & Miller, 1978; Steinschneider, Schroeder, Arezzo, & Vaughan, 1995), thus not necessarily contradicting the Motor Theory.

Recent studies provide neurobiological evidence to the connection between speech perception and production. Transcranial magnetic stimulation of the motor cortex demonstrated activation of speech-related muscles during the perception of speech (Fadiga, Craiqhero, Buccino, & Rizzolatti, 2002). FMRI studies have demonstrated that there is overlap between the cortical areas that are active during speech production and those active during passive listening to speech (Pulvermuller et al., 2006; Wilson et al., 2004).

Although the Motor Theory of Speech assumes an innate link between perceptual and production parameters, a developmental account is given by the Articulatory Filter Hypothesis (Vihman, 1993). According to this hypothesis, experiences with speech patterns in the ambient language highlight the corresponding motor-sound pairs that have been learned through babbling. The theory suggests that the experience of frequently self-producing consonant-vowel (CV) syllables sensitizes infants to similar patterns in their ambient language, making these forms more salient as potential building blocks for first words. Westermann and Reck Miranda (2004) suggest a simple mechanism as the basis for phonological development in the infant babbling phase. That is, a coupling between the representations of articulatory parameters and auditory perception develops in an experience-dependent way. During this process both perceptual and motor representations may occur. This model is based on neurobiologically plausible principles, such as the emergence of mirror neurons for acoustic stimuli. Auditory mirror neurons are thought of as an extension to visual mirror neurons which were found to fire both when the animal acts and when it observed the same action performed by others (Galantucci, Fowler, & Turvey, 2006). The neuron "mirrored" the behavior of another animal, as though the observer itself was acting. It is assumed that mirror neurons perform for actions that are either seen or *heard* (Galantucci et al., 2006). Based on this model, it is assumed that by producing babbling sounds, Hebbian connections[2] start to develop between the motor and auditory map based on the co-variance between the articulatory parameters and the auditory consequences. A subsequent external sound directly activates only the auditory map. However, some motor units receive activation through the developing Hebbian connections from the active auditory units. As a consequence, auditory and motor units are active simultaneously and the Hebbian weights are strengthened.

In this way, sounds from the ambient language selectively reinforce these sounds from the infant's babbling inventory. This mechanism also suggests how mirror neurons develop in the motor area that responds when an external sound is heard. These are the same units that would be active when the model produces the sound independently. Thus, based on these theories, it is suggested that the vocalizations of young infants reflect the use of auditory information. Alternatively, lack of certain vocalizations may imply inability to either use or hear auditory information (Westermann & Reck Miranda, 2004).

Another significant implication of the model is that motor practice should have an effect on auditory perception, and vice versa. For example, infants that were prevented from normal babbling due to tracheotomy showed abnormal patterns of vocal expressions that persist even one year after the tracheostomy was removed (Bleile, Stark, & McGowan, 1993; Locke & Pearson, 1990). In the absence of the ability to couple perception and production of syllables during babbling, these infants showed delayed speech in the presence of normal hearing even though their motor limitation (the tracheostomy) no longer existed. Additionally, individuals with cerebral palsy and speech deficits showed difficulties in discriminating strings of nonsense words (Bishop, Brown, & Robinson, 1990). These findings suggest a close relationship between speech production and perception.

The coupling between auditory perception and motor production is closely linked to the ability of the infant to imitate speech

---

[2]Hebbian connections are connections that develop when any two cells or systems of cells that are repeatedly active at the same time will then tend to become "associated," so that activity in one facilitates activity in the other. Hebbian theory describes a basic mechanism for synaptic plasticity wherein an increase in synaptic efficacy arises from the presynaptic cell's *repeated* and *persistent* stimulation of the postsynaptic cell—thus forming the basis of learning and memory.

sounds. Vocalizations in babbling move from a language universal pattern to one that is specific to the ambient language of the child (de Boysson-Bardies, Halle, Sagart, & Durand, 1989; de Boysson-Bardies & Vihman, 1991). The ability to imitate vowel sounds seems to emerge between 12–20 weeks of age (Kuhl & Meltzoff, 1996). The prelinguistic ability to produce sounds of the ambient language is seen as an important step in the development of a phonological inventory, first words and more complex linguistic structures (Westermann & Reck Miranda, 2004).

The empirical evidence in support of the strong relationship between auditory perception and speech production can also be found in studies investigating the role of audition for normal preverbal vocalizations, or babbling, in infants with impaired auditory feedback. In general, infants with hearing loss demonstrate different babbling behavior than infants with normal hearing, especially at 6 months and older (Moeller et al., 2007; Schauwers, Gillis, Daemers, De Beukelaer, & Govaerts, 2004). It is assumed that the vocalizations of hearing infants in the first six months of their lives are primarily influenced by innate development and maturation of the vocal system (Fletcher, 1992; Koopsman-van Beinum, Clement, & van den Dikkenberg-Pot, 2001). Anatomic, physiologic, and neurologic changes, such as the increasing size of the oral cavity, lowering of the larynx, elongation of the vocal tract, and nerve myelination, result in greater maneuverability of the tongue and other speech organs thus enabling the infants to produce a greater variety of sounds (Fletcher, 1992). Only at approximately 6 to 7 months of age, hearing infants start canonical babbling, (i.e., produce consonant-vowel sequences that are part of the phonetic system of their language). These phonetic syllables, known as "phonetic building blocks of words" (Oller & Eilers, 1988), are considered

crucial for speech and language development and are assumed to be directly influenced by auditory input (Koopsman-van Beinum et al., 2001). Furthermore, Koopsman-van Beinum et al. (2001), in their sensorimotor approach for the classification of early infant vocalizations, stated that " . . . infants' auditory perception and feedback are a prerequisite for the coordination of the movements in the phonatory and articulatory systems necessary in canonical babbling. As canonical babbling contains all basic elements of (adult) speech, it is a strong cue in the normal speech developmental processing" (p. 69).

Indeed vocal behavior of infants with severe-to-profound hearing loss show normative vocalization behavior in the first 6 months of life. This finding supports the hypothesis that very early vocalizations are mediated primarily by anatomic and physiologic growth (and not audition). At 6 months of age, however, the vocalizations of hearing-impaired (HI) infants deviate from normal behavior, coinciding with the same age that hearing babies start babbling (Koopsman-van Beinum et al., 2001; Oller & Eilers, 1988). It has been shown that profound hearing loss results in delays of 5 to 19 months in the onset of babbling in HI infants (Oller & Eilers; 1988; Oller, Eilers, Bull, & Carney, 1985). Koopsman-van Beinum et al. (2001), for example, reported that none of their profoundly HI infants babbled before the age of 18 months. Finally, when the HI infants started babbling, their phonemic repertoire was usually limited and restricted to those language sounds that were visible (e.g., bilabials), acoustically salient (e.g., vowels) and/or provided tactile feedback (e.g., laryngeal) (Fletcher, 1992). It also has been shown that certain stages in vocalization development, such as reduplicated babbling, were absent in profound HI infants (Moeller et al., 2007; Oller et al., 1985).

Thus, the finding that speech production of HI infants deviates from normal development as early as 6 months of age emphasizes the importance of early audition on the formation of subsequent speech and language production.

Our working premise is that evaluation of the early vocalizations of infants, especially at 6 to 12 months of age, may provide valuable information regarding their hearing status. Furthermore, we suggest that the quality and quantity of the infant's preverbal vocalization at ages 6 to 12 months is related to their audition, and therefore may be an indirect measure of auditory sensitivity and resolution. We therefore have developed a parental questionnaire for the purpose of assessing the development of major milestones in preverbal vocalizations in infants following the hierarchy proposed by Oller and Eilers (1988). According to Oller and Eilers (1988), as well as other researchers in the field of prelinguistic vocal development (Stark, 1986), normally developing infants show several stages of vocal development. During the "phonation stage" (0 to 2 months), infants produce "comfort sounds" with normal speechlike phonation. These sounds (also called quasiresonant nuclei or quasivowels) appear to be precursors to vowel production. More advanced speech sounds, such as syllables, are rare at this stage. By 2 to 3 months the infant enters the "gooing" stage (also called "cooing stage"), producing quasivowels as well as articulated sounds in the back of the vocal cavity. These sounds are precursors to consonant production, but are not well formed syllable productions. During the "expansion stage" (4 to 6 months) infants produce a variety of speechlike sounds including raspberries (labial thrills and vibrants), squeals, growls, yells, whispers, vowel-like sounds, and syllable precursors that have been termed "marginal babbling."

Mature syllables, however, are hardly heard during this period. Controlled productions of syllables appear in the canonical stage (7 to 10 months). This stage is characterized by production of reduplicated sequences, such as, [mamama], [dadada], or [bababa] followed by nonreduplicated or variegated babbling period in which variation in both consonants and vowels may appear from syllable to syllable. An example of this is [gadu]. Most infants continue to babble into the time when they say their first words. Close to the appearance of first words, children frequently use "invented words" (also called proto-words, phonetically consistent forms, vocables or quasiwords) (Dore, Franklin, Miller, & Ramer, 1976; Locke, 1983; Menn, 1978; Stoel-Gammon & Cooper, 1984). These are constant productions of syllables in the context of a reference. For example, the child may say [dodo] when being shown a ball. However, these productions do not necessarily resemble the adult-like word in the particular language and thus are not considered real words. Only when the child's productions become more similar to the adult form (e.g., [ba] for a "ball") are they considered words. Around the first birthday, the child starts to produce the first meaningful word, starting a new era: the linguistic stage. The PRISE is constructed on the developmental hierarchy described here.

PRISE: Producton Infant Scale Evaluation Questionnaire

The PRISE is a questionnaire that employs a structured interview technique to obtain information from parents about the inventory and frequency of 11 speech production behaviors demonstrated by their infant in everyday situations (Kishon-Rabin et al., 2002; 2005). It assesses production abilities of normal-hearing as well as HI infants and toddlers during the prelinguistic period, from the first month of life until the appearance of first words. Using a scale of 0 (lowest) to 4 (highest) for rating the frequency of occurrence of target behavior for each question, the clinician assigns a rating based on the parents' answers (similar to the IT-MAIS questionnaire). Performance is scored in terms of the total number of points obtained out of 44 possible points. The probes are worded so that in normally developing infants, scores are accumulated monotonically with age. So far, we have accumulated PRISE data on more than 260 normal-hearing and above 200 HI infants.

As mentioned earlier, infants' vocalizations in the first 6 months of their lives are primarily influenced by innate developmental and maturational characteristics of the vocal and motor systems. Anatomic, physiologic and neurologic changes, such as increases in size of the oral cavity, lowering of the larynx, prolongation of the vocal tract, changes in the ribcage, postural control, and nerve myelination, gradually enable greater maneuverability of speech organs resulting in increased variability of speech sounds. Therefore, the first six questions of the PRISE reflect initial vocal stages (phonation, cooing and expansion) that are determined by these anatomic and physiologic constraints, as well as general vocalization type and quality. The continuing vocal development and expansion of speech sound inventory that occur between the ages of 6 to 12 months are highly dependent on the intactness of the auditory system and auditory feedback. Therefore, the remainder of the questions reflect more advanced vocal stages (canonical and variegated babbling) (questions 7 to 9) and the beginning of one-word stage—the appearance of words (ques-

tions 10 to 11) in which auditory acuity and speech perception influence vocalization.

PRISE Questions

Each of the 11 questions of the PRISE, accompanied with a short rationale for each question, is detailed below.

Question 1. Does the child's voice sound pleasant?

The purpose of this question is to rule out significant voice abnormalities that may imply any neurologic, anatomic, or physiologic abnormalities reflected in voice production (Raes, Michelsson, Dehaen, & Despontin, 1982). Atypical voice quality of newborns may characterize some syndromes. For example, high-pitched cry (identified as cat-like cry) is associated with Cri Du Chat syndrome (Hirschberg, 1999). Voice features, such as, volume, hyponasality, hypernasality, breathiness and hoarseness are assessed in order to establish initial basic assessment of developmental difficulties, other than hearing impairment alone.

Question 2. Does the child produce sounds other than crying?

The purpose of this question is to assess whether any vocal behavior other than crying is manifested in the repertoire of the infant's vocal productions. Reflexive crying is the first vocal behavior of newborns. However, even newborns can produce other reflexive vocalizations such as coughs, grunts, and burps, reflecting the physical state of the infant. Although later vocal behavior can be identified into one of the more structured vocalization stages (e.g., cooing, vocal play, canonical babbling, or first word production), productions of infants with developmental deficiencies may not be identified clearly into one of these stages. This question considers vocalizations that are not yet classified in the classical division of vocal development (Oller, 1986; Oller et al., 1999), although they may resemble it in some manners.

Question 3. Sound Production in Response to Auditory Stimuli. Does the infant produce sounds in reaction (or as a response) to auditory stimuli (both speech and non speech)?

The purpose of this question is to find out whether the infant has developed any initial, basic *auditory-vocal* associations. Auditory perception and vocal production are closely related in normal-hearing infants. For example, one basic response of young infants to loud surprising noises may be crying. Other responses to sound, music or speech may include motor as well as vocal responses. This association is considered essential for the development of speech and language and its existence indicates both awareness to sound and motor control sufficient for producing some type of vocal response. It should be noted that older infants tend not only to respond to but also to imitate speech sounds they hear. The ability to imitate vowel sounds, for example, emerges between 12 and 20 weeks of age (Kuhl & Meltzhoff, 1996).

Question 4. Intonation. Does the infant produce sounds of varying intonation?

The purpose of this question is to find out whether the infant is in the process of acquiring control of basic suprasegmental skills as manifested by changes in intona-

tion. HI infants might show this ability at 4 to 6 months of age (Oller & Eilers, 1988; Oller, et al., 1985) but may reduce it later due to the lack of auditory input. Suprasegmental development in the pre-linguistic stage includes the production of changes in loudness, duration, and fundamental frequency during vocal behavior. The ability to change intonation is shown clearly between 4 to 6 months when infants enter the stage of vocal play. It is during this stage that the infant often produces extreme, and in many cases, uncontrolled variations in loudness and pitch. Usually, vocal play appears during motor activities in which the infant explores his motor and vocal abilities (Alexander, Boehme, & Cupps, 1993). Later in the linguistic development, prosodic features in their variation of pitch, loudness and duration can be used deliberately to signal attitude and emotions and point on different lexical and grammatical meaning. Infants with other developmental deficiencies may not be able to use varying intonation because of structural and/or motor constraints (Mueller, 1997).

Question 5. Vowel-Like Production. Does the infant produce vowel-like and vowel sounds, such as /a/, /e/, /i/?

The purpose of this question is to determine whether the infant uses vowel sounds separately or within syllables or words. Segmental development in the pre-linguistic stage begins with the appearance of vowel-like sounds. Vowel-like sounds emerge during the cooing or gooing stage (2 to 4 months). These sounds resemble vowels and consist of quasiresonant nuclei, usually produced with nasalized resonance (Stark, 1986). By the fourth month, however, anatomical-physiological changes that result in an increase of intraoral space, elongation of the pharyngeal cavity, downward shift of the larynx and hyoid, and separation of the epiglottis and the soft palate, as well as the development of postural stability in various positions against gravity, give rise to more vocalic sounds. At this stage, prolonged, less nasal, anterior vowels appear. Later in development, during the vocal play (4 to 6 months) and canonical babbling (6 months and older) stages, prolonged vowels in combination with anterior consonants serve as a syllable's nuclei for producing babbling and words. These are the stages during which infants are thought to imitate what they hear. Thus, the use of vowels prior to 6 months of age may reflect basic physiologic-motor skills needed for speech, whereas later use of these sounds may suggest use of auditory input as well as increased motor control.

Question 6. Producing Syllable-Like Consonant-Vowel Combinations. How often does the infant produce different consonant-vocal combinations?

Toward the end of the vocal-play stage and the beginning of babbling (5 to 7 months), infants increasingly produce a number of syllables by adding initial consonants to the vowels (Oller, 1986; Stark, 1986). The consonant added may be influenced by visual information (e.g., /baba/), motoric ease (e.g., /ba, ma/), frequency of use in the language or in the immediate surrounding of the child, tactile and proprioceptive feedback (e.g., the feeling of lips closure for bilabials consonants such as /ba/) or by general interest of the infant (Davis & MacNeilage, 2000; Davis, MacNeilage, & Matyear, 2002; Westermann & Reck Miranda, 2004). This fundamental use of syllables is an extremely important step toward speech, as syllables are the building blocks of spoken language. Furthermore, the ability to use syllables with

various consonants increases the diversity of syllable combinations used for words and fluent speech. The purpose of this question is not only to assess the infant's ability to produce the basic unit of speech (i.e., the syllable), but also to evaluate the ability to produce syllables with different consonants. Therefore, the parent is asked to quantify the number of different consonants attached to the vowel. The use of various consonants for the CV combination indicates auditory detection and discrimination between speech sounds differing in frequency, duration, and loudness as well as the developing of fine motor-articulatory control. This is the stage in which HI infants tend to diverge from normal production behavior (Kishon-Rabin et al., 2005). For example, the consonants used in CV combinations by HI infants are usually based on limited information provided either by visual (/ba, ma/) or on tactile/proprioceptive (e.g., glottal stops) feedback (Dromi & Ringwald-Frimerman, 1996). Other pathologic populations (e.g., dyspraxia, cerebral palsy) also may show limited consonant inventory due to motor control deficits.

Question 7. Producing Syllable-Like Consonant-Vowel Combinations. How often does the infant produce different consonant-vowel combinations?

This question is based on the same rational as question 6. It is meant to assess the occurrence in which an infant uses canonical syllables. Most profound HI infants produce some CV combinations based on limited sources of information as mentioned previously (e.g., visual, tactile). However, although audition allows hearing infants to detect and acquire various consonants and produce them frequently within syllables, HI infants usually produce a limited number of consonants and reduce the occurrence of syllable production in the absence of sufficient auditory feedback. Thus, this question may assist in evaluating HI infants' vocal behavior before and after cochlear implantation or in evaluating the efficacy of hearing aids or other sensory devices. It also can serve to assess other pathological populations in which motor, structural or any other factor may limit the production of canonical syllables.

Question 8. The Canonical Stage (Lalling). Does the infant reduplicate syllables?

Canonical babbling is a collective term for reduplicated and non-reduplicated or variegated babbling. It usually begins around 6 months of age and continues until the appearance of the first words. Reduplicated babbling is marked by similar strings of CV productions (e.g., /mamama/) while variegated babbling demonstrates changes from syllable to syllable (e.g., /gadu/). Most researchers agree that these two stages are sequential in order (Elbers, 1982; Oller, 1980; Stark, 1986) and that variegated babbling reflects increasing ability to produce speechlike strings. It also is suggested that the infants' repetition of their own babbling and use of internal auditory feedback contributes to fine tuning as well as the continuance of this vocal behavior (Westermann & Reck Miranda, 2004). Thus, the purpose of this question is to evaluate the extent to which the infant uses reduplicated or variegated babbling. The results may provide information as to the stage of the infant's vocal behavior (i.e., the beginning or ending of the canonical stage). They also indicate the use of auditory input and advanced motor ability to produce changing strings of sounds that eventually will lead to the production of words. Although HI infants might show less use of variegated babbling because of limited access to sound and processing deficiencies of speech, infants with other (e.g., motor) developmental problems may show limited variation in babbling due to poor sensory-motor abilities.

Question 9. The End of the Canonical Stage. Does the infant try to repeat the word he heard or part of it?

Toward the end of the canonical stage, infants start repeating words or part words in imitation games and communication interactions with family members (Stark, 1986). The ability to combine motor-sound pairs, first experienced through the babbling period, is further refined to an improved form of imitation. The imitation is considered an indication that the infant treats the production of others as meaningful and therefore repeats the sound pattern (a word or part of it) based on auditory-visual input. Only partial understanding of the word meaning and limited production accuracy are required for this behavior. The prelinguistic ability to produce sounds of the ambient language is considered crucial for learning word structures, developing a productive lexical storage and further combining acquired words into phrases and sentences (Vihman, 2002; Westermann & Reck Miranda, 2004). Hence, the purpose of the present question is to determine the infant's imitation capacity as a first step toward word acquisition. Hearing-impaired infants might show reduced imitation behavior due to limited awareness to speech or reduced ability to couple auditory-motor association. Infants with other developmental disabilities, however, might show reduced imitation behavior due to motor-control deficiencies, difficulties in sensory integration, or reduced communication interest.

Thus, the improvement of this behavior during habilitation and therapy programs may be an indication of progress.

Question 10. The One-Word Stage. Does the child use a permanent sequencing of sounds in relation to a certain object?

The use of permanent sequencing of sounds to address objects, people or situations appears during the last period of babbling but before the appearance of real words. During this stage, the infant may use consistent phonetic forms which are also termed as "invented words," "proto words," "phonetically consistent forms," or "quasiwords" in specific situations. These forms of words, however, may not necessarily resemble the adult production of the words (Dore et al., 1976; Locke, 1983; Menn, 1978; Stoel-Gammon & Cooper, 1984). The purpose of the present question is to determine whether the child begins to combine any defined vocal template(s), related or not to the adultlike word form, with any aspect of permanent lexical meaning. This ability is typical at the very start of the one-word stage and precedes the beginning of the linguistic period in which consistent acoustic-vocal sequences reflect and indicate permanent meaning. HI infants often show reduced use of "quasiwords" because of limited speech perception abilities and verbal communication experience. However, after about 6 months of CI use, producing permanent sequences of sounds for a certain object is common. Thus, this question is important for evaluating HI infants before and after implantation. In addition, this question is important for assessing infants with other developmental disabilities that may show reduced ability to produce these "quasi words" because of cognitive or motor constraints.

Question 11. The One-Word Stage. Does the child use a number of permanent sequences of sounds in relation to certain objects?

This question is an extension of the previous one and addresses the infant's use of several permanent sequences of sounds for specific objects, people or actions. For example, the infant may refer to a ball as /dodo/, to mommy as /ma/ and to eat as /uhm/. In this example, the inventory of more than one word would be given credit on this question. The number of words infants produce increases during the second year of life and the acquisition of 10 first words is expected during the first months after their first birthday (Fenson et al., 1994). Thus, the purpose of this question is to describe and evaluate how many words the infant uses. This information may reflect the benefit of cochlear implants, hearing aids, sensory devices and other auditory and/or language habilitation strategies used with infants. It also can assist in evaluating high-risk populations as well as infants with suspected dyspraxia, motor and/or communication delays.

More details on the general administration of the PRISE can be found in Appendix 12–A. Appendix 12–B includes examples of two questions from the PRISE (6 and 11) with the additional prompts used by the interviewers to elicit information from the parents. Also included are examples of parents' responses and subsequent scoring.

Studies with the PRISE

We have conducted a set of experiments aimed at validating the questionnaire and its usefulness as a predictor of auditory capabilities and as a measure of normal auditory development. Specifically, we set to answer the following questions:

1. How do preverbal vocalizations of infants develop over time using the PRISE questionnaire? Can it be predicted by age?
2. Are PRISE scores influenced by the language(s. to which the infant is exposed?
3. Are PRISE scores related to normal auditory development?
4. Is the PRISE sensitive to early vocalization delays due to hearing loss? Is it sensitive to the changes resulting from aural habilitation with cochlear implants?
5. Is the PRISE sensitive to detect any vocalization delays that may result from unilateral deafness?
6. Is the PRISE sensitive to developmental delays of infants who are born prematurely?
7. Can the PRISE be validated with a direct behavioral auditory test?
8. How reliable is parent report?
9. How sensitive is the PRISE to abnormalities not related to hearing?

Question 1. How does the PRISE develop with age?

The PRISE questionnaire was administered to 260 normal-developing infants between the ages 2 weeks to 22 months. The ages of the infants were distributed quite evenly especially between the ages of 6 to 12 months. Normal development was determined on the basis of reports by well-baby clinics and parents and results of newborn hearing screening testing (the majority of the babies). Infants who were considered at risk for hearing impairment according to the Joint Committee on Infant Hearing (2000) were excluded from testing. PRISE data were obtained via parent interviews as described above. For each infant, a single

score (in percent) was obtained based on the results of the 11 questions. Figure 12–1 shows the individual results of the tested sample as a function of age (in months). Also shown is the best-fitting function to the data (solid line) and ±2 standard deviations (SD) (in the dotted lines). Several observations can be noted. First, preverbal vocalizations as measured by the PRISE increases with age in a monotonic way until they reach a maximum of 100% at approximately 18 months. Performance over time can be described by an exponential function and increases between 6 and 13 months by an average rate of 10% per 1.5 months. This rate also can be viewed as an increase of mastering one vocal behavior (as manifested in one question) each 1.5 months over a range of 18 months. It also supports the use of the PRISE as a sensitive measure for assessing the major milestones of preverbal vocalization. This is further substantiated by the second finding that approximately 87% of the variance in the PRISE scores can be explained by age in infants with normal hearing. This supports the assertion that vocal development follows a regular sequence of stages from birth to the emergence of words (Oller, 1986; Stark, 1986). The best-fitting function predicts that hearing infants reach a PRISE score of 50% at approximately 6 months of age, suggesting that their vocal development progressed through the first half of the questionnaire (i.e., first 5 to 6 questions) which relate to precanonical behavior. Hearing infants 8 months and older were found to demonstrate either often or always reduplication of syllables, and infants of 14 months and older were found to use a permanent sequence of sounds in relation to a specific object. These stages of vocal development are in agreement with the data on prelexical vocal development cited in the literature (Oller, 1986; Oller et al., 1985;

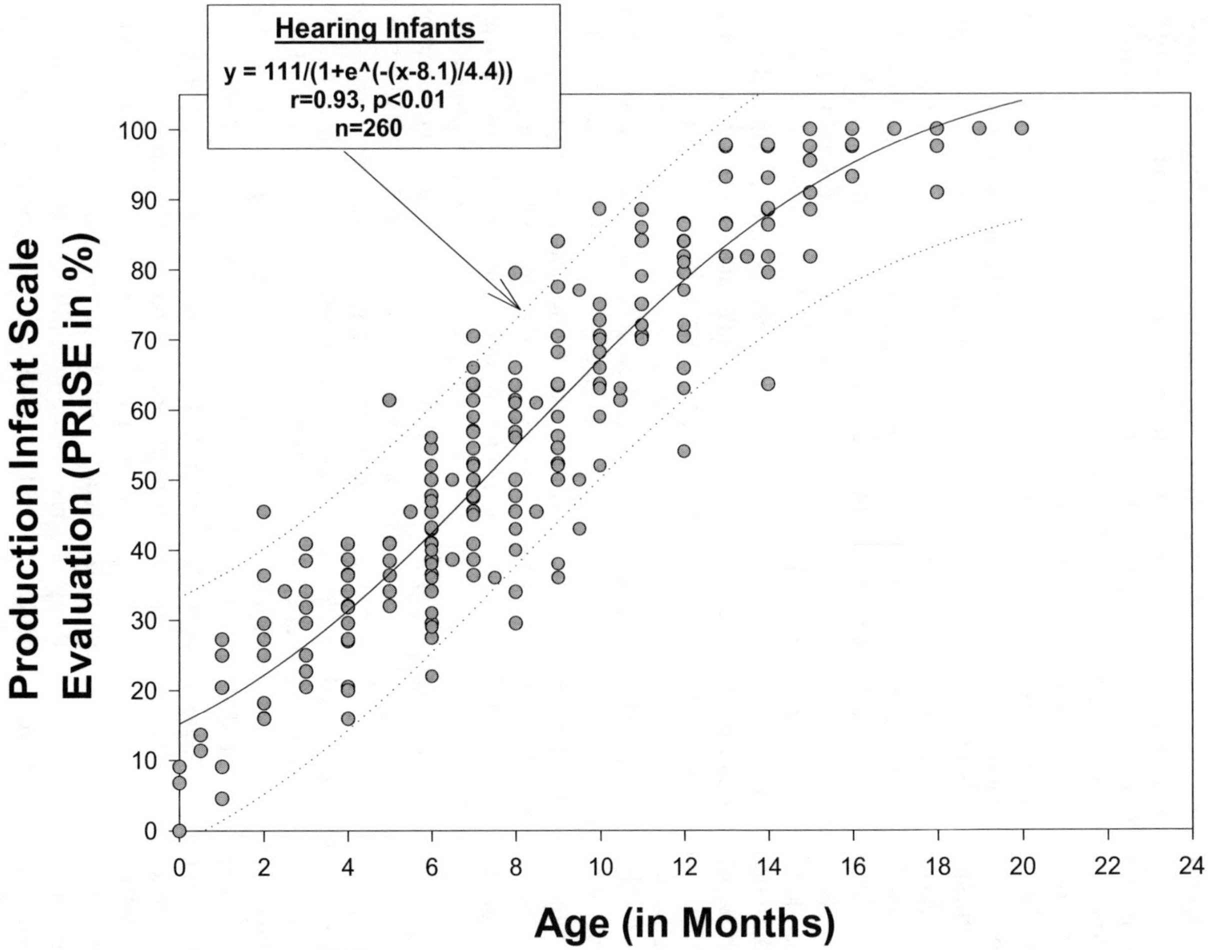
Hearing Infants
y = 111/(1+e^(-(x-8.1)/4.4))
r=0.93, p<0.01
n=260
Production Infant Scale
Evaluation (PRISE in %)
0
10
20
30
40
50
60
70
80
90
100
0
2
4
6
8
10
12
14
16
18
20
22
24
Age (in Months)

Figure 12–1. PRISE performance (in %) of 260 infants as a function of age (in months). Each symbol represents the average PRISE score of one infant. Solid line shows the best-fitting function to the data (indicated in the box at the top-left corner of the graph). Also shown are ± 2 SD in the dotted lines.

Stark, 1980, 1986). Finally, there is substantial variability in the data particularly at 6 to 10 months. For example, scores can vary from 30 to 80% at 8 months of age. This range of scores at these ages is not surprising considering this is the age range at which infants' vocal organs mature for the vocalization of speech sounds as well as the age at which they loose sensitivity to sounds that are not part of their native language (e.g., Best et al., 1988). This is important to consider when evaluating preverbal vocalizations of infants with developmental delays.

In sum, the data reported here on hearing infants provide an important contribution to the validation of the PRISE questionnaire and its sensitivity to the different stages of early vocal development.

Question 2. Is performance on the PRISE influenced by language?

Our next goal was to test whether preverbal vocalization skills as measured by the PRISE are influenced by the language to which the child is exposed. As mentioned earlier, the development of speech production skills during the first year of life is thought to follow hierarchical and universal stages (Oller, 1980; Stark, 1986). During the first year of life, infants progress from the production of reflexive sounds (e.g., crying and discomfort sounds) to cooing/gooing (voluntary productions of comfort and discomfort sounds in the velar area), to vocal play (sounds showing increased control of phonation and articulation), to babbling of repeated and variegated syllables and finally to the production of first words. It is possible that the actual speech sounds, such as the type of consonants produced, are influenced by the ambient language to which the infant has been exposed. Studies from many languages report that intonation develops around 4 months and that the development of vowels precedes that of consonants. Thus, the milestones of infants' vocal development are considered universal and are assumed to depend primarily on physiologic and anatomic changes of the organs producing speech, audition and auditory feedback irrespective of the language. It is, therefore, expected that the PRISE will be similar for infants exposed to different languages.

The multicultural and multilingual society in Israel allowed for testing the hypothesis that language does not influence the hierarchy and quantity of preverbal vocalizations of infants from different ambient languages. Specifically, we tested the Arabic version of the PRISE (ArPRISE) in 60 normal-developing infants of Arabic speaking parents. Normal development was determined on the basis of reports by well-baby clinics, parents, and results from newborn hearing screening testing (when available). Infants who were considered at risk for hearing impairment according to the Joint Committee on Infant Hearing (2000) were excluded from testing, as well as those with middle-ear problems. The ages of the infants varied between 2 weeks and 18 months. The number of infants was distributed quite evenly within that range. It should be noted that the infants were exposed exclusively to the Arabic language at home and at their daycare centers. The interview process was similar to the one described above. In Figure 12–2, the individual ArPRISE data of the Arab infants are plotted (in black symbols) against PRISE scores of 213 infants of Hebrew-speaking parents (open symbols). Also shown in the graph is the best-fitting function to the data (solid line) with ±2 SD (dotted lines). It can be seen that for all but one infant, ArPRISE scores fall within the 2 SD of the Hebrew-speaking infants and that the data follow the predictive function.

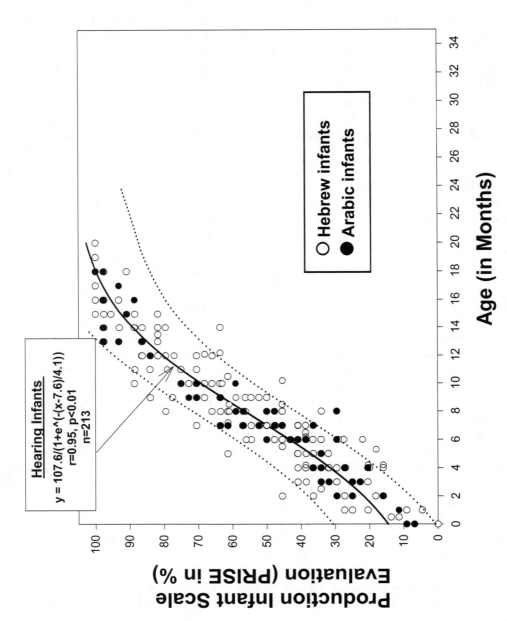

Figure 12–2. PRISE scores for 60 infants of Arabic-speaking parents using the ArPRISE (*black circles*) compared to infants of Hebrew-speaking parents (*open symbols*) as a function of age (in months). Also shown is the best-fitting function to the data (*solid line*) and ±2 SD.

We have developed the PRISE in French, Russian, and English. Preliminary data with normal-developing infants show similar developmental curves as that of infants of Hebrew-speaking parents. In addition, the PRISE has been developed in Italian (Cippone, Cuda, Benvenuti, Murri, & De Fillipis, 2006), Turkish, and German [personal communication: Lu-Ming Joffo (Advanced Bionics Europe), July 2008]. The use of an assessment test that is not influenced by language and used across languages in young infants may allow for a significant impact when pooling data of specific tested populations (such as HI infants with cochlear implants) from different habilitation centers around the world. The resulting increase of data may allow drawing conclusions regarding auditory habilitation issues. Additional research is needed with normal-hearing infants exposed to different ambient languages. The contribution of such data is of both theoretical and clinical relevance.

Because Israel is a "melting pot" of a diversity of cultures and languages of many Jewish immigrants, there are many families in which the infant is exposed from birth to more than one language (sometimes even three or four depending on the origin of the grandparents). Thus, the issue of the effect of bilingualism and babbling is of great interest. Both parents and clinicians raise concerns regarding the acquisition of major milestones and rate of vocal development when the infant is exposed to more than one language compared to monolingual infants. Several studies have focused on the emergence and use of vocabulary and syntax in bilingual infants (Fennell, Byers-Heinlein, & Werker, 2007; Petitto et al., 2001). Although it has been assumed that there is a delay in the acquisition of language in bilingual children compared to monolingual children, most published studies did not find evidence

to this effect (Paradis & Genesee, 1996). Only few studies, however, addressed the issue of the influence of exposure to several languages on the vocalization stage (Oller, Eilers, Urbano, & Cobo-Lewis, 1997). The results showed no delay in vocalizations in bilingual infants aged 4 to 18 months.

Recently, we have collected developmental data from preverbal vocalizations of 22 normal-developing infants who were exposed from birth to the Hebrew and French languages. That is, parents spoke both Hebrew and French at home, or only French, but the infants attended daycare centers where only Hebrew was spoken. Normal development was determined on the basis of reports by well-baby clinics and parents and results of newborn hearing screening testing (when available). Infants who were considered at risk for hearing impairment according to the Joint Committee on Infant Hearing (2000) were excluded from testing, as well as those with middle-ear problems. Mean chronologic age of the infants was 10.3 months (range of 1 and 22 months). Parents were interviewed with the PRISE and IT-MAIS questionnaires. Note that when both Hebrew and French were spoken at home, parents were interviewed separately in their respective language for subsequent validation of the results. Figure 12–3 displays the PRISE scores of the infants exposed to two languages (gray symbols) compared to data of infants exposed to only one language, Hebrew (open symbols). It can be seen that the exposure to two languages did not influence significantly data of preverbal vocalizations. Similar results were found with the IT-MAIS. These results confirm the finding that the age of onset for canonical babbling and the quantitative measures of vocal performance are similar in bilingual and monolingual infants (Oller et al., 1997, Petito et al., 2001).

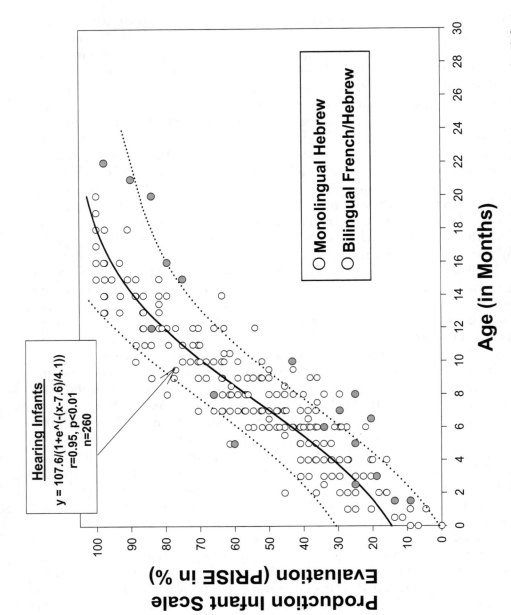

Figure 12–3. PRISE scores of 22 infants exposed to French *and* Hebrew (*gray circles*) compared to infants of Hebrew-speaking parents (*open circles*) as a function of age (in months). Also shown is the best-fitting function to the data (*solid line*) and ±2 SD.

Question 3. How does the PRISE relate to normal auditory development?

Our next goal was to determine whether the PRISE is related to a measure of auditory skills. For this purpose, we examined the relationship between the PRISE score and the IT-MAIS score in infants with normal hearing. Parents of 143 infants with normal hearing were interviewed with the PRISE and IT-MAIS. The results (in gray symbols) are plotted in Figure 12–4. It can be seen that the best-fitting function to the data is linear and that the PRISE score can be predicted from the IT-MAIS. In fact, approximately 87% of the variance of the PRISE can be explained by the IT-MAIS score, and that the PRISE score is almost the same as the absolute value of the IT-MAIS score. This relationship is important for two main reasons. First, it contributes to the validation of the PRISE as an indirect measure of hearing capabilities. This strong relationship in infants with normal hearing suggests that development of preverbal vocalizations can occur only with increases in functional hearing skills. Second, the relationship suggests that reduced auditory input as in the case of HI infants can be monitored by preverbal vocalization as was the original intention. Indeed, the next sections further validate this conclusion when showing that infants with absent or reduced auditory input demonstrate a decrease in their preverbal vocalizations.

Question 4. Is the PRISE sensitive to hearing impairment?

As mentioned in the Introduction, a major incentive for developing the PRISE was to incorporate a behavioral assessment tool (to the very limited existing test battery) for evaluating progress of infants with hearing loss before and after aural habilitation. Thus, our next goal was to examine whether the PRISE taps into early vocalization delays that result from hearing loss and is sensitive to changes in infants' vocalization due to use of hearing devices, such as cochlear implants. Figure 12–5 displays PRISE data of 15 aided infants with severe-to-profound hearing loss between 8 and 15 months of age. All infants were at the preverbal stage and did not exhibit problems or delays other than their hearing loss. The data are plotted as a function of their chronologic age. Also shown on the graph for comparison are data of 213 infants with normal hearing between 0.5 and 20 months (open symbols). It can be seen from the graph that the aided infants (prior to implantation, gray triangles and open diamonds) obtained a PRISE score of 50% or less regardless of their chronologic age. This score was comparable to that of hearing infants who are 6 to 7 months of age and corresponded to the first few questions that related to performance in the precanonical stage. These findings support the assertion that onset of babbling is determined by auditory perception and feedback (Koopsman-van Beinum et al., 2001; Schauwers et al., 2004) and that the PRISE was able to demonstrate the negative outcomes related to auditory deprivation. The PRISE data of the implanted infants also were examined based on the age at which hearing loss was identified and intervention with hearing aids (prior to cochlear implants) was provided (not shown in Figure 12–5). Nineteen of the infants (80%) were fitted with hearing aids by the age of 12 months, of which eight infants were fitted by the age of 6 months. These early identified infants also performed better with their cochlear implants than the 12 children with profound hearing loss who were identified between 2 and 3 years (Kishon-Rabin et al., 2005). These findings supplement the

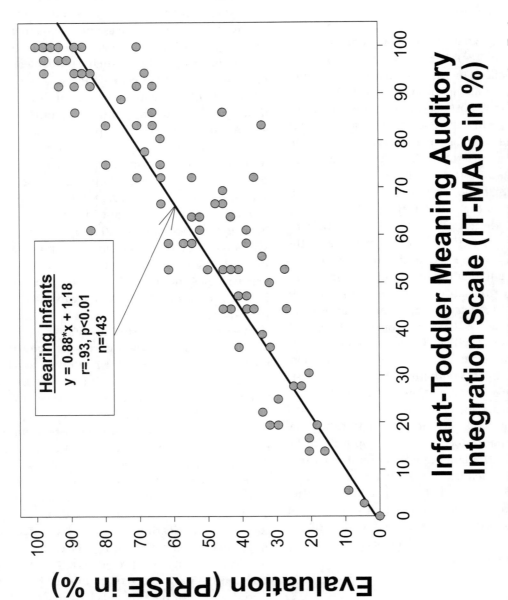

Figure 12–4. The relationship between PRISE and IT-MAIS scores of 143 infants with normal hearing. Each round symbol represents data of one infant. The solid line shows the best-fitting function to the data.

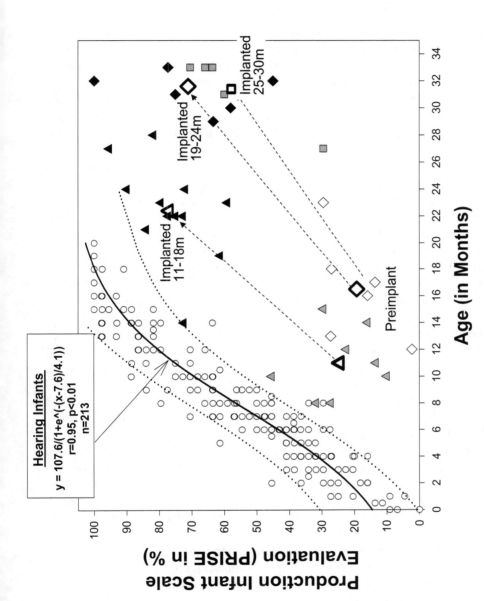

Figure 12–5. Individual PRISE scores of hearing infants (*open circles*), aided infants (*gray triangles*), and implanted infants (*black triangles, black diamonds, and gray squares*) as a function of age at implantation (implanted ≤18 months, implanted 18–24 months, and implanted 24–30 months, respectively) and chronologic age (for the hearing infants). Note that the bold empty large symbols display the average group scores for each range of age at implantation. Also shown is the best-fitting exponential function to the data of the normal-hearing infants (*solid line*) and the ±2 SD (*dotted lines*). The broken arrows show the trajectory of improvement from the mean group aided infants prior to implantation to the mean group score postimplantation.

increasing body of evidence showing the importance of early diagnosis and intervention on subsequent linguistic skills (Apuzzo & Yoshinaga-Itano, 1995; Robinshaw, 1995; Yoshinaga-Itano et al., 1998).

Figure 12–5 also shows PRISE data of 24 HI infants who use cochlear implants grouped by the age at which they were implanted. Twelve were implanted between 11 and 18 months of age, 7 infants were implanted between 19 and 24 months of age, and five implanted between 24 and 30 months of age. All three of the major cochlear implant systems were represented in this sample (Cochlear Corporation, Advance Bionics, and MED-EL). The results show that for all but two implanted infants, PRISE scores postimplantation increased to the range of 60 to 100%. Interestingly, when data are plotted as a function of implant use, nearly all infants achieved scores comparable to or better than those of the infants with normal hearing (Kishon-Rabin et al., 2005). Thus, once infants are provided with access to speech sounds via the cochlear implants, they seem to follow a similar trajectory of development of preverbal vocalization as their normal-hearing peers. The fact that they may appear to perform better (when analyzed by duration of device use) is probably due to their older age.

In terms of the effect of age at implantation on preverbal vocalizations, it can be seen that on average, the two younger implanted groups performed similarly. It should be noted, however, that because the infants in the youngest implanted group also were the youngest in chronologic age, there were more implanted infants from that group that performed closer to their normal-hearing peers when compared by age. The infants from the second group were older and did not appear to close the gap in performance with their normal-hearing

peers (of the same age). The third group (those implanted between 24 and 30 months of age) performed poorly compared to the younger implanted group and also was considerably poorer than the normal-hearing group. Note also the mean rate of improvement over time of the first two implanted groups (as indicated by the broken-line arrows in Figure 12–5) was similar to the rate of development of the infants with normal hearing. In contrast, the rate of improvement of the later implanted infants seemed to be slower compared to the early implanted infants as well as the normal-hearing. These results can be explained in part by the auditory skills of the implanted children using the IT-MAIS questionnaire.

Figure 12–6 displays individual IT-MAIS scores of the implanted infants before and after implantation. It can be seen that the aided infants prior to implantation (open triangles) showed very limited auditory capabilities. After implantation, however, IT-MAIS scores increased significantly. In fact, the data of most infants who were implanted prior to 24 months (black and grey diamonds) were within the ±2 SD of the normal-hearing data. In contrast, those implanted between 24 to 30 months of age (half-filled diamonds) did not reach normal auditory behavior. Thus, the data in Figures 12–5 and 12–6 reinforce the strong link between auditory perception and speech production. These data also support the notion that "earlier is better" (Apuzzo & Yoshinaga-Itano, 1995; Schauwers et al., 2004; Yoshinaga-Itano et al., 1998). Finally, the PRISE demonstrated the effect of hearing loss, the change due to cochlear implantation and the influence of age of cochlear implantation, thus contributing to its validity in special populations. It also showed the strong relationship with functional audition (see Figure 12–4).

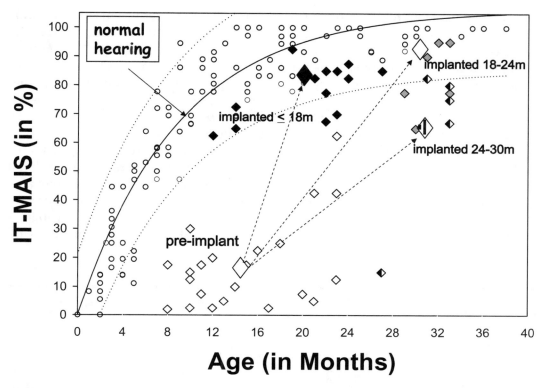

Figure 12–6. Individual IT-MAIS scores of hearing infants (*open circles*), aided infants (*open diamonds*), and implanted infants (*filled diamonds*) as a function of age at implantation and chronological age. Note that the big diamonds display the average group score for each range of age at implantation. Also shown is the best-fitting exponential function to the data of the normal-hearing infants (*solid line*) and the ±2 SD (*dotted lines*). The broken arrows show the trajectory of improvement from the mean group aided infants prior to implantation to the mean group score post implantation.

Question 5. Is the PRISE sensitive to the impact of unilateral deafness in infants at the preverbal stage?

Until the implementation of the universal newborn hearing screening program, many children with unilateral hearing loss (UHL) were identified only at school age (Brookhouser, Worthington, & Kelly, 1991; Johnson, White, & Widen, 2005; Tharpe, 2008). These children were found to be at higher risk for poor academic achievements, speech-language delays, and social-emotional difficulties compared to their normal-hearing peers (Bess, 1986; Bess & Tharpe, 1986; Cho Lieu, 2004; Davis, Elfenbein, Schum, & Bentler, 1986; Kiese-Himmel, 2002; McKay, Gravel, & Tharpe, 2008; Tharpe, 2008). It has been suggested that the loss of binaural advantages (e.g., localization, binaural summation, the head-shadow effect and binaural release from masking) results in difficulties in detecting and recognizing speech in noise which in turn reduces the ease of listening and incidental learning which are considered crucial for normal development of speech and language. Today, the identification of UHL is determined in infancy due to newborn hearing screening programs. We set out to test whether these infants will show any delay in preverbal vocalizations and/or gross auditory skills in their first 18 months of their life compared to their hearing peers. Thirteen infants with moderate (*n* = 5), severe (*n* = 3), and pro-

found (*n* = 5) sensorineural UHL were evaluated using the PRISE and the IT-MAIS. Their ages ranged from 4 to 17.5 months of age (mean 11.5 months). Etiology for hearing impairment was low-birth weight and premature birth (*n* = 7), Cytomegalovirus (CMV) (*n* = 2), unknown etiology (*n* = 3), and familial (*n* = 1).

Figures 12–7 and 12–8 display the IT-MAIS and PRISE scores, respectively, of infants with UHL (black circles) compared to their normal-hearing peers. It can be seen that the data reflecting hearing capabilities using the IT-MAIS of most infants with UHL

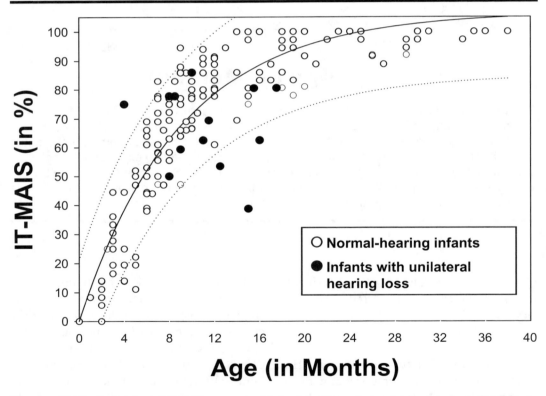

Figure 12–7. Individual IT-MAIS scores of infants with unilateral hearing loss (*black circles*) and hearing infants (*open circles*) as a function of chronologic age. Also shown is the best-fitting exponential function to the data of the normal-hearing infants (*solid line*) and the ±2 SD (*dotted lines*).

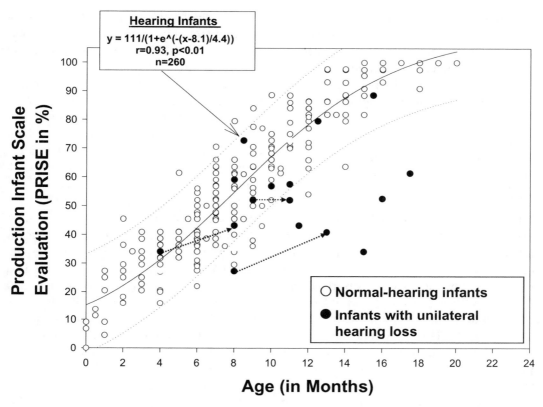

Figure 12–8. Individual PRISE scores of infants with unilateral hearing loss (*black circles*) and hearing infants (*open circles*) as a function of chronologic age. The three infants for whom the PRISE was administered a second time are indicated by the arrows. Also shown is the best-fitting exponential function to the data of the normal-hearing infants (*solid line*) and the ±2 SD (*dotted lines*).

were within ±2 SD of the performance range of the infants with normal hearing. The PRISE data, however, suggested a greater number of infants performed outside the normal range (6/13). Note that the PRISE was administered for the second time after 2 to 3 months for three infants (shown in arrows). Approximately at 2 years of age, these same infants underwent formal speech and language assessment performed by a speech-language pathologist as part of a routine protocol for children at risk for developing speech and language delays. The clinicians performing the evaluation were blind to the results of the questionnaires administered a few months earlier. Comparison between the PRISE results with those of the formal speech and language assessment resulted in a 100% match. That is, infants with UHL who performed poorer than expected relative to normal-hearing infants were the same infants diagnosed as having developmental delays with recommendations for intervention. These data emphasized the power that the PRISE has as a predictive measure for language and speech delays. Thus, the PRISE can assist in early detection and subsequent intervention of infants with ULH who may be at risk for developing future developmental delays.

Question 6. Is the PRISE sensitive to developmental delays of infants who are born prematurely?

Improvements in neonatal medicine and care have resulted in increased survival of infants who were born at a gestational age of less than 37 weeks (infants born prematurely) and who often have low birth weight. It has been shown that most growth in cortical connections and complexity occurs after 25 weeks. This growth results in a substantial increase in surface area. During this period, however, preterm infants are exposed to many potentially damaging factors such as infection, chronic hypoxia, and undernutrition. These factors may lead to neurocognitive impairments such as delays in developing speech, language and hearing (Dyet et al., 2006; Inder, Wells, Mogridge, Spencer, & Volpe, 2003; Woodward, Anderson, Austin, Howard, & Inder, 2006). We, therefore, set out to test whether the parental questionnaires PRISE and IT-MAIS are sensitive to detecting delays in the development of preverbal vocalizations and hearing perception abilities in infants born prematurely compared to full-term infants during the first year of life. Questionnaires were administered to parents of 21 infants born prematurely whose mean gestational age was 31 weeks (range: 24 to 36 weeks, SD = 4.3 weeks). Birth weight ranged between 500 and 2760 grams (mean of 1658 grams, SD = 738 grams). All infants passed newborn hearing screening tests.

Figures 12-9 and 12-10 show the data of the infants born prematurely (black circles) on the PRISE and the IT-MAIS (respectively) as a function of gestational age. Also shown in each graph for comparison are the data of the normal-developing infants. It can be seen that PRISE data of almost half the infants born prematurely (10/21) fell outside the normal range. Of these infants, three showed a significant delay in vocalization. Data were then replotted for the 21 infants based on their age, corrected for prematurity. When plotted in this manner, all but the three infants showing significant vocal delays were within the normal range. The IT-MAIS, on the other hand, was less sensitive in detecting delays when data were compared by gestational age. Only two infants born prematurely showed delays on the IT-MAIS before and after correcting for age. These two infants were the same ones who showed delays in vocalization. They were both born at 24 weeks of gestation and had very low birth weights (500 and 862 grams, respectively). In addition, one of the infants born prematurely suffered from bronchopulmonary dysplasia (BPD). Preterm infants with very low birth weight and/or with BPD were found to be the infants at greatest risk for delays from the group of the infants born prematurely (Landry, Chapiesky, Fletcher, & Denson, 1988). This subgroup shows difficulties in many areas such as gross motor development (Singer, Yamashita, Lilien, Collin, & Baley, 1997), visual-motor integration, and performance IQ (Giacoia, Venkataraman, West-Wilson, & Faulkner, 1997; Hughes et al., 1999). Some studies found delay in the canonical babbling of this subgroup (Rvachew, Creighton, Feldman, & Sauve, 2005) as well as language delays (Foster-Cohen, Edgin, Champion, & Woodward, 2007). The third infant born prematurely

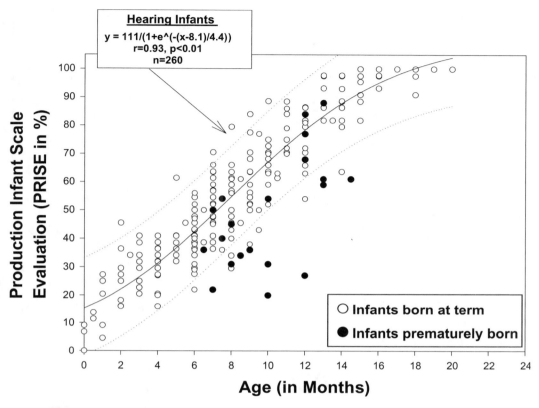

Figure 12–9. Individual PRISE scores of infants born prematurely (at less than 37 weeks) (*black circles*) and hearing infants born at full term (*open circles*) as a function of gestational age. Also shown is the best-fitting exponential function to the data of the full-term infants (*solid line*) and the ±2 SD (*dotted lines*).

that had a poor PRISE score achieved an IT-MAIS score within the normal range. The clinical recommendation for this infant was to participate in a follow-up program in order to monitor carefully his speech and language development.

Figure 12–11 shows the relationship between the PRISE and IT-MAIS scores of the infants born prematurely. It can be seen that the IT-MAIS can explain only 64% of the PRISE data. This is compared to a variance value of 87% in the full-term infants (see Figure 12–4). Figure 12–11 also shows

that the PRISE data lagged the IT-MAIS scores by approximately 10%. This is compared to similar absolute scores of IT-MAIS and PRISE in the full-term infants. One explanation for the differences in the results may be related to the difference in the sample sizes between the full term ($n = 143$) and the infants born prematurely ($n = 21$). It is also possible, however, that these differences resulted from factors not related to hearing (such as general maturation and motor development), particularly in infants born prematurely.

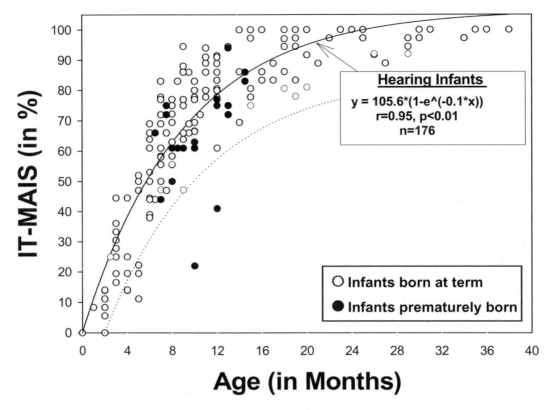

Figure 12–10. Individual IT-MAIS scores of infants born prematurely (at less than 37 weeks) (*black circles*) and hearing infants born at full term (*open circles*) as a function of gestational age. Also shown is the best-fitting exponential function to the data of the full-term infants (*solid line*) and the ±2 SD (*dotted lines*)

Question 7. Can the PRISE be validated with a direct behavioral measure?

As part of the process of validating the PRISE questionnaire, we correlated the PRISE data with a direct auditory behavioral measure of preference to child-directed speech (CDS) compared to reversed CDS (Segal & Kishon-Rabin, submitted). This was conducted in both normal-hearing and HI infants with cochlear implants. The underlying assumption of this work was that in order for infants

to acquire language they need to attend to the speech sounds of their ambient language and draw statistical conclusions (Saffran, Werker, & Werner, 2006). Thus, with obtaining auditory experience, infants begin to prefer and be more attentive to speech sounds than to nonspeech sounds (Colombo & Bundy, 1981; Cooper & Aslin, 1990; Fernald, 1985; Fernald & Kuhl, 1987). The use of reversed CDS allows for control of the temporal dynamics as well as for the spectral information of the nonspeech stimuli. Using the central fixation preference procedure

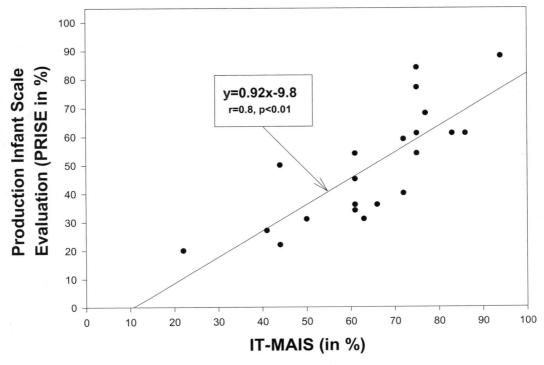

Figure 12–11. The relationship between PRISE and IT-MAIS scores of 21 infants born prematurely (before 37 weeks). Each circle represents data of one infant. The solid line shows the best-fitting function to the data.

(e.g., Cooper & Aslin, 1990; Houston et al., 2003; Shi & Werker, 2001), looking times were obtained from 9 infants with cochlear implants with a mean age of 24 months, 8 days (range: 19 months, 9 days to 33 months, 10 days, SD = 4.6 months, 7 days). Infants used their implants between 1 month and 14 months with an average of 5.7 months. Figure 12–12 displays the PRISE data of the implanted infants as a function of the preference they showed for the CDS compared to the reversed CDS. It can be seen that greater preference to CDS predicts higher PRISE scores. Although conclusions should be interpreted cautiously due to the small sample size, the data support the notion that

the relationship between emerging listening skills and preverbal vocalization is influenced by the child's accessibility to audible speech sounds. It should be noted that preference to CDS (compared to reversed CDS) was significantly correlated with listening experience but not with chronologic age. More specifically, the data of the three infants who were doing poorly on both tests could not be explained by age or maturation (because they are not the youngest), but rather by listening experience. Overall, these data contribute to the validation of the PRISE as an indirect measure of functional hearing.

Further support for the relationship between a direct auditory behavior test and

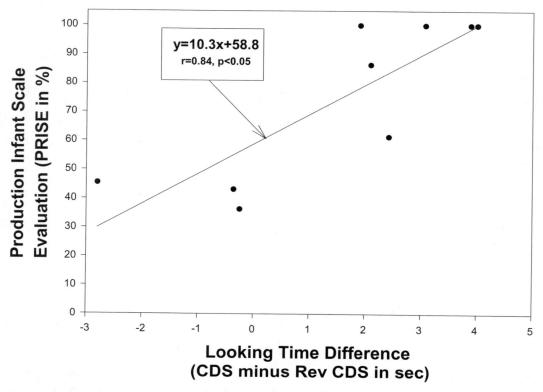

Figure 12–12. Preference to child-directed speech (CDS) over reversed CDS (Rev CDS) as a function of PRISE scores. Each circle represents data of one HI infant with a cochlear implant. Also shown is the best-fitting linear function to the data.

preverbal vocalizations is demonstrated in two individual HI infants after cochlear implantation. Figure 12–13A shows average PRISE scores at 1 and 4 months postimplantation of a HI infant who was implanted at 12.6 months. Also shown is the infant's preference to CDS compared to noise (looking time in seconds) and IT-MAIS scores. Similarly, Figure 12–13B shows average PRISE scores at 1, 2 and 4 months postimplantation of a HI infant who was implanted at 15.7 months. Also shown is the infant's preference to CDS compared to noise and the IT-MAIS scores. It can be seen that for both infants, the PRISE was sensitive to improvements in auditory skill development which resulted from auditory experience provided by the cochlear implant. The PRISE data also was in keeping with the infants' auditory preference to speech. Thus, the close relationship between a direct measure of functional hearing and preverbal vocal productions has been demonstrated in individual infants.

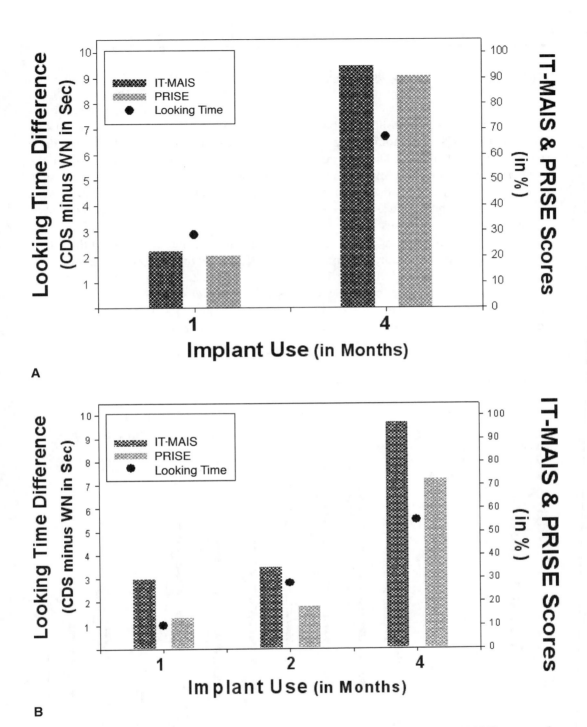

Figure 12–13. A. Changes in looking preference to CDS, PRISE and IT-MAIS scores for one HI infant with a cochlear implant at 1 and 4 months postimplantation, **B.** Changes in looking preference to CDS, PRISE, and IT-MAIS scores for a second HI infant with a cochlear implant at 1, 2, and 4 months of implant use.

Question 8. How reliable is parent report?

In order to test the reliability of parent report on the PRISE questionnaire, preverbal vocalizations of 30 normal-hearing infants between the ages of 5 and 18 months (mean = 11.8 months) were evaluated through two techniques. The first was by the standard parental interview as discussed above. The second was by an analysis of video-recordings conducted separately by two clinicians. The analysis of the preverbal vocalizations and subsequent scoring was conducted after viewing 20 minutes of video recording while the parents interacted with the infant. Note that when the clinicians interviewed the parents they did not see the infant. Similarly, the video recording focused on the infant so the clinician cannot recognize the infant. This was done to reduce any bias that may occur if the judging clinician associated the parent with the infant (Schauwers et al., 2004). Also, after each recording, the parent was asked whether the vocalizations on tape are typical (quality and quantity wise) of the infant. If not, new recordings were obtained.

Figure 12–14 displays the average scoring of each question of the PRISE as obtained by interviewing the parents in comparison to the results from video-analysis

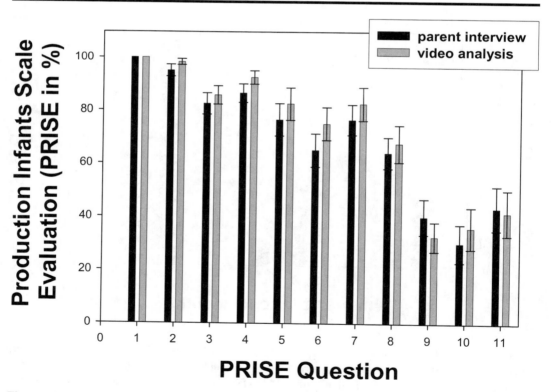

Figure 12–14. Mean score (in %) for each PRISE question as obtained by means of parent interview (*black bars*) and by video analysis (*gray bars*). Also shown are ±2 SD (from Kashkush, 2008).

scoring (Kashkush, 2008). It can be seen that the scoring using both techniques was similar for all questions ($p > 0.05$). These results support the use of parental interviewing as a reliable method for obtaining information regarding the preverbal vocalizations of their infant.

Question 9. How sensitive is the PRISE to abnormalities not related to hearing?

We suggest that unexpectedly low PRISE scores compared to normal IT-MAIS scores can be useful for alarming abnormalities not necessarily related to hearing. An example is the following case. KZ is a profoundly HI infant who was diagnosed at 3 months and fitted with a hearing aid at 4 months. Subsequently, this infant received a cochlear implant device at 12 months. Prior to implantation the IT-MAIS and PRISE scores were 2.5% and 31.8%, respectively. At 1 year post-implantation, the average IT-MAIS scores reached 85% whereas the mean PRISE score was 70%. A look at the individual PRISE questions showed an abnormal profile (Figure 12–15). Whereas questions 5, 6, 10 and 11 received maximum scores, questions 7, 8, and 9 showed lower scores. Considering the PRISE questions are in a hierarchical order of acquisition, the low scores of the intermediate questions were unexpected. These results suggested that the infant was

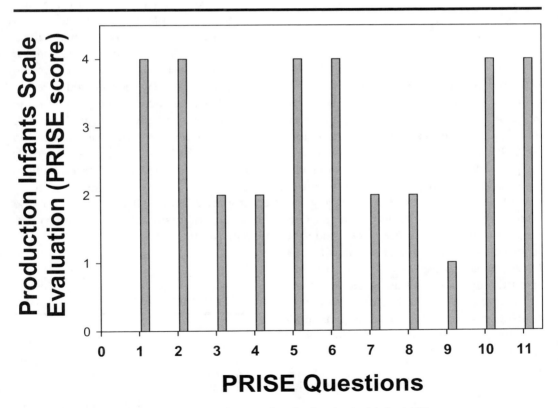

Figure 12–15. PRISE score for each question for implanted infant KZ.

at the one-word stage but with less than expected different consonant-vowel combinations. The IT-MAIS score suggested that this infant received sufficient auditory input. This infant was, therefore, directed to a clinician who specializes in speech disorders. A couple months later, KZ was diagnosed with dyspraxia which was not related to the hearing impairment. This is an example of a case that shows how use of the PRISE scores assisted in diagnosing a speech disorder at an early stage that otherwise may erroneously have been attributed to the hearing loss. Thus, integration of the PRISE and IT-MAIS data can alert one to problems not necessarily related to the hearing loss and that otherwise would not have been detected until much later.

Summary

In sum, we propose that the PRISE is an effective and sensitive tool for evaluating communicative skills of young infants. Because of the close relationship between auditory perception and speech production, we believe that the PRISE, although assessing preverbal vocalizations, provides valuable information regarding the development of the infant's auditory skills. Moreover, it has been shown to be sensitive to the various degrees of hearing loss from mild-moderate to profound hearing loss, as well as to unilateral hearing loss. These findings emphasize the importance of using the PRISE for evaluating very young infants at risk with hearing impairment, following their auditory and preverbal development, and assessing the effectiveness of the intervention. The fact that it is not influenced by language, easy and quick to administer and provides such valuable information suggests that the PRISE could be an essential tool in clinical settings. Moreover, its use in the clinic can be extended to infants at risk for developmental delays other than hearing, such as motoric (e.g., dyspraxia). It should be noted, however, that the efficacy of the PRISE is limited to the preverbal stage only. Also, the PRISE cannot replace auditory tests that can provide more analytical information regarding hearing. Its strength is to provide behavioral information that no other test can provide due to the infant's age and inability to cooperate. Finally, one should always bear in mind that because infants' productions are influenced by several factors, a low score on the PRISE can also be as a result of a deficit other than hearing.

Acknowledgments. We would like to thank Professor Minka Hildesheimer, head of the Speech and Hearing department and the Cochlear Implant team at the Sheba Medical Centre, and Dr. Drorit Ben-Itzhak, head of MICHA-Tel Aviv infants' program for the hearing impaired, for their cooperation and support for the work reported here. We would also like to acknowledge Dr. Daphne Ari-Even Roth and the undergraduate and graduate students at the Communication Disorders Dept, Tel-Aviv University for their valuable contribution and data collection. Finally, we would like to extend our deepest appreciation to all the parents of the numerous infants who were willing to participate in our studies.

References

Alexander, R., Boehme, R., & Cupps, B. (1993). *Normal development of functional motor skills: The first year of life*. Tucson, AZ: Therapy Skill Builders.

Apuzzo, M. L., & Yoshinaga-Itano, C. (1995). Early identification of infants with significant hearing loss and the Minnesota Child Development Inventory. *Seminars in Hearing, 16,* 124–139.

Bess, F. H. (1986). The unilaterally hearing-impaired child: A final comment. *Ear and Hearing, 7,* 52–54.

Bess, F. H., & Tharpe, A. M. (1986). Case history data on unilaterally hearing-impaired children. *Ear and Hearing, 7,* 14–19.

Best, C. T., McRoberts, G. W., & Sithole, N. M. (1988). Examination of perceptual reorganization for nonnative speech contrasts: Zulu click discrimination by English-speaking adults and infants. *Journal of Experimental Psychology: Human Perception and Performance, 14,* 345–360.

Bishop, D., Brown, B., & Robson, J. (1990). The relationship between phoneme discrimination, speech production and language comprehension in cerebral-palsied individuals. *Journal of Speech and Hearing Research, 33,* 210–219.

Bleile, K. M., Stark, R. E., & McGowan, S. J. (1993). Speech development in a child after decannulation: Further evidence that babbling facilitates later speech development. *Clinical Linguistics and Phonetics, 7,* 319–337.

Boothroyd, A. (1991). Assessment of speech perception capacity in profoundly deaf children. *American Journal of Otology, 12*(Suppl.), 67–72.

Brookhouser, P. E., Worthington, D. W., & Kelly, W. J. (1991). Unilateral hearing loss in children. *Laryngoscope, 101,* 1264–1272.

Cho Lieu, J. E. (2004). Speech-language and educational consequences of unilateral hearing loss in children. *Archives of Otolaryngology-Head and Neck Surgery, 130,* 524–530.

Cippone, P., Cuda, D., Benvenuti, M., Murri, A., & De Fillipis, A. (2006, March). *Prelexical language development: PRISE and IT-MAIS questionnaires normative data in the first year of life.* Paper presented at the 8th European symposium on pediatric cochlear implantation. Lido di Venezia, Italy.

Colombo, J., & Bundy, R. S. (1981). A method for the measurement of infant auditory selectivity. *Infant Behavior and Development, 4,* 219–223.

Conboy, B. T., Rivera-Gaxiola, M., Silva-Pereyra, J., & Kuhl, P. K. (2008). Event-related potential studies of early language processing at the phoneme, word, and sentence levels. In A. D. Friederici & G. Thierry (Eds.), *Early language development: Bridging brain and behavior* (pp. 23 –64). Philadelphia: John Benjamin.

Cone-Wesson, B. (2003). Electrophysiologic assessment of hearing infants: Compound nerve action potential, auditory brainstem response, and auditory steady state response. *Volta Review, 103*(4), 253–279.

Cooper, R. P., & Aslin, R. N. (1990). Preference for infant-directed speech in the first month after birth. *Child Development, 61,* 1584–1595.

Davis, J. M., Elfenbein, J., Schum, R., & Bentler, R. A. (1986). Effects of mild and moderate hearing impairments on language, educational, and psychosocial behavior of children. *Journal of Speech and Hearing Disorders, 51,* 53–62.

Davis, B. L., & MacNeilage, P. F. (2000). An embodiment perspective on the acquisition of speech perception. *Phonetica, 57,* 229–241.

Davis, B. L., MacNeilage, P. F., & Matyear, C. L. (2002). Acquisition of serial complexity in speech production: A comparison of phonetic and phonological approaches to first word production. *Phonetica, 59,* 75–107.

de Boysson-Bardies, B., Halle, P., Sagart, L., & Durand, C. (1989). A cross-linguistic investigation of vowel formants in babbling. *Journal of Child Language, 16,* 1–17.

de Boysson-Bardies, B., & Vihman, M. M. (1991). Adaptation to language: Evidence from babbling of infants according to target language. *Language: Journal of the Linguistic Society of America, 67,* 297–319.

Dore, J., Franklin, M. B., Miller, R. T., & Ramer, A. L. (1976). Transitional phenomena in early language acquisition. *Journal of Child Language, 3,* 13–29.

Dromi, E., & Ringwald-Frimerman, D. (1996). *Communication and language intervention with hearing-impaired children: The prelinguistic stage* [in Hebrew]. Tel Aviv, Israel: Tel Aviv University: Ramot.

Dyet, L. E., Kennea, N., Counsell, S. J., Maalouf, E. F., Ajayi-Obe, M., Duggan, P. J., et al. (2006).

Natural history of brain lesions in extremely preterm infants studied with serial magnetic resonance imaging from birth and neurodevelopmental assessment. *Pediatrics, 118*, 536–548.

Eilers, R. E., Wilson, W. R., & Moore, J. M. (1977). Developmental changes in speech discrimination in infants. *Journal of Speech and Hearing Research, 20*, 766–780.

Eimas, P. D., & Siqueland, E. R., Jusczyk, P., & Vigorito, J. (1971). Speech perception in infants. *Science, 171*, 303–306.

Eisenberg, L. S., Martinez, A. S., & Boothroyd, A. (2007). Assessing auditory capabilities in young children. *International Journal of Pediatric Otorhinolaryngology, 71*, 1339–1350.

Elbers, L. (1982). Operating principles in repetitive babbling: A cognitive approach. *Cognition, 12*, 45–63.

Fadiga, L., Craiqhero, L., Buccino, G., & Rizzolatti, G. (2002). Speech listening specifically modulates the excitability of tongue muscles: A TMS study. *European Journal of Neuroscience, 15*, 399–402.

Fennell, C. T., Byers-Heinlein, K., & Werker, J. F. (2007). Using speech sounds to guide word learning: The case of bilingual infants. *Child Development, 78*, 1510–1525.

Fenson, L., Dale, P. S., Reznick, J. S., Bates, E., Thal, D. J., & Pethick, S. J. (1994). Variability in early communicative development. *Monographs of the Society for Research in Child Development, 59*(5), 1–173.

Fernald, A. (1985). Four-month-old infants prefer to listen to motherese. *Infant Behavior and Development, 8*, 181–195.

Fernald, A., & Kuhl, P. K. (1987) Acoustic determinants of infant preference for motherese speech. *Infant Behavior and Development, 10*(3), 279–293.

Fletcher, S. J. (1992). *Articulation: A physiological approach.* San Diego, CA: Singular.

Foster-Cohen, S., Edgin, J. O., Champion, P. R., & Woodward, L. J. (2007). Early delayed language development in very preterm infants: Evidence from the MacArthur-Bates CDI. *Journal of Child Language, 34*, 655–675.

Fryauf-Bertschy, H., Tyler, R. S., Kelsay, D. M. R., & Gantz, B. J. (1997). Cochlear implant use by prelingually deafened children: The influences of age at implant and length of device use. *Journal of Speech, Language and Hearing Research, 40*, 183–199.

Galantucci, B., Fowler, C. A., & Turvey, M. T. (2006). The motor theory of speech perception reviewed. *Psychonomic Bulletin and Review, 13*, 361–377.

Giacoia, G. P., Venkataraman, P. S., West-Wilson, K. L., & Faulkner, M. J. (1997). Follow-up of school-age children with bronchopulmonary dysplasia. *Journal of Pediatrics, 130*, 400–408.

Hawkins, S. (1999). Looking for invariant correlates of linguistic units: Two classical theories of speech perception. In J. M. Pickett, (Ed.), *The acoustics of speech communication: Fundamentals, speech perception theory and technology* (pp. 198–231). Boston: Allyn & Bacon.

Hirschberg, J. (1999). Dysphonia in infants. *International Journal of Pediatric Otorhinolaryngology, 49*(Suppl. 1), S293–S296.

Horn, D. L., Houston, D. M., & Miyamoto, R. T. (2007). Speech discrimination skills in deaf infants before and after implantation. *Audiological Medicine, 5*, 232–241.

Houston, D. M., Horn, D. L., Qi, R., Ting, J. Y., & Gao, S. (2007). Assessing speech discrimination in individual infants. *Infancy, 12*, 119–145.

Houston, D. M., Pisoni, D. B., Kirk, K. I., Ying, E. A., & Miyamoto, R. T. (2003) Speech perception skills of deaf infants following cochlear implantation: A first report. *International Journal of Pediatric Otorhinolaryngology, 67*, 479–495.

Hughes, C. A., O'Gorman, L. A., Shyr, Y., Schork, M. A., Bozynski, M. E., & McCormick, M. C. (1999). Cognitive performance at school age of very low birth weight infants with bronchopulmonary dysplasia. *Journal of Development and Behavioral Pediatrics, 20*, 1–8.

Inder, T. E., Wells, S. J., Mogridge, N. B., Spencer, C., & Volpe, J. J. (2003). Defining the nature of the cerebral abnormalities in the premature infant: A qualitative magnetic resonance imaging study. *Journal of Pediatrics, 143*, 171–179.

Joint Committee on Infant Hearing. (2000). Year 2000 position statement: Principles and guidelines for early hearing detection and intervention programs. *American Journal of Audiology, 9*, 9–29.

Johnson, J. L., White, K. R., Widen, J. E., Gravel, J. S., James, M., Kennalley, T., et al. (2005). A multicenter evaluation of how many infants with permanent hearing loss pass a two-stage otoacoustic emissions/automated auditory brainstem response newborn hearing screening protocol. *Pediatrics, 116*, 663–672.

Kashkush, A. (2009). *Evaluating prelexical vocalization in Arab infants using video analysis and the PRISE.* Unpublished master's thesis, Communication Disorders Dept., Sackler Faculty of Medicine, Tel-Aviv University.

Katz, J. (Ed.) (1994). *Handbook of clinical audiology* (4th ed.). Baltimore: Williams & Wilkins.

Kemler-Nelson, D. G., Jusczyk, P. W., Mandel, D. R., Myers, J., Turk, A., & Gerken, L. (1995). The head-turn preference procedure for testing auditory perception. *Infant Behavior and Development, 18*, 111–116.

Kiese-Himmel, C. (2002). Unilateral sensorineural hearing impairment in childhood: Analysis of 31 consecutive cases. *International Journal of Audiology, 41*, 57–63.

Kirk, K. I., Miyamoto, R. T., Lento C. L., Ying, E., O'Neill T., & Fears B. (2002). Effects of age at implantation in young children. *Annals of Otology, Rhinology, and Laryngology, 111*(Suppl. 189), 69–73.

Kishon-Rabin, L., Rotshtein, S., & Taitelbaum, R. (2000). Identification of the relative onset time of a two-tone complex: Auditory sensitivity or language based? *Journal of Basic Clinical Physiology and Pharmacology, 11*, 259–271.

Kishon-Rabin, L., Taitelbaum, R., Muchnik, C., Gehtler, I., Kronenberg, J., & Hildesheimer, M. (2002). Development of speech perception and production in children with cochlear implants. *Annals of Otology, Rhinology, and Laryngology, 111*(Suppl. 189), 85–90.

Kishon-Rabin, L., Taitelbaum-Swead, R., Ezrati-Vinacour, R., & Hildesheimer, M. (2005). Prelexical vocalizations in normal hearing and hearing-impaired infants before and after cochlear implantation and its relation to early auditory skills. *Ear and Hearing, 26*(Suppl.), 17S–29S.

Koopmans-van Beinum, F. J., Clement, C. J., & van den Dikkenberg-Pot, I. (2001). Babbling and the lack of auditory speech perception: A matter of coordination? *Developmental Science, 4*, 61–70.

Kubo, T., Iwaki, T., & Sasaki, T. (2008). Auditory perception and speech production skills of children with cochlear implant assessed by means of questionnaire batteries. *Journal for Oto-Rhino-Laryngology and Its Related Specialties, 70*, 224–228.

Kuhl, P. K. (1985). Methods in the study of infant speech perception. In G. Gottlieb & N. A. Krasnegor, (Eds.), *Measurement of audition and vision in the first year of postnatal life: A methodological overview* (pp. 223–251). Norwood, NJ: Ablex.

Kuhl, P. K., & Meltzoff, A. N. (1996). Infant vocalizations in response to speech: Vocal imitation and developmental change. *Journal of the Acoustical Society of America, 100*, 2425–2438.

Kuhl, P. K., & Miller, J. D. (1978). Speech perception by the chinchilla: Identification function for synthetic VOT stimuli. *Journal of the Acoustical Society of America, 63*, 905–917.

Landry, S. H., Chapiesky, L., Fletcher, J. M., & Denson, S. (1988). Three-year outcomes for low birth weight infants: Differential effects of early medical complications. *Journal of Pediatric Psychology, 13*, 317–327.

Leshem, E., & Shuval, J. (Eds.). (1998). *Immigration to Israel: Sociological perspectives.* New Brunswick, NJ and London, England: Transaction.

Liberman, A. M., Cooper, F. S., Shankweiler, D. P., & Studdert-Kennedy, M. (1967). Perception of the speech code. *Psychological Review, 74*, 431–446.

Liberman, A. M., & Mattingly, I. G. (1985). The motor theory of speech perception revised. *Cognition, 21*, 1–36.

Locke, J. L. (1983). *Phonological acquisition and change.* New York: Academic Press.

Locke, J. L., & Pearson, D. M. (1990). Linguistic significance of babbling: Evidence from a tracheostomized infant. *Journal of Child Language, 17*, 1–16.

McKay, S., Gravel, J. S., & Tharpe, A. M. (2008). Amplification considerations for children with minimal or mild bilateral hearing loss and unilateral hearing loss. *Trends in Amplification, 12,* 43–54.

Mendel, L. L., & Danhauer, J. L. (1997). Test development and standardization. In L. L Mendel & J. L. Danhauer. (Eds.), *Audiologic evaluation and management and speech perception assessment* (pp. 7–14). San Diego, CA: Singular.

Menn, L. (1978). *Pattern, control and contrast in beginning speech: A case study in the development of word form and word function.* Bloomington: Indiana University Linguistic Club.

Miyamoto, R. T., Kirk, K. I., Svirsky, M. A., & Sehgal, S. T. (1999). Communication skills in pediatric cochlear implant recipients. *Acta Oto-Laryngologica, 119,* 219–224.

Moeller, M. P., Hoover, B., Putman, C., Arbataitis, K., Bohnenkamp, G., Peterson, B., et al. (2007). Vocalizations of infants with hearing loss compared with infants with normal hearing: Part I—Phonetic development. *Ear and Hearing, 28,* 605–627.

Mueller, H. A. (1997). Speech. In N.R. Finnie (Ed.), *Handling the young child with cerebral palsy at home* (2nd ed., pp. 112–117). Oxford: Butterworth-Heinemann.

Nittrouer, S. (2001). Challenging the notion of innate phonetic boundaries. *Journal of the Acoustical Society of America, 110,* 1598–1605.

Oller, D. K. (1980). The emergence of the sounds of speech in infancy. In G. Yeni-Komshian, J. F. Kavanagh, & C. A. Ferguson (Eds.), *Child phonology, Vol 1., Production* (pp. 93–112), New York: Academic Press.

Oller, D. K. (1986). Metaphonology and infant vocalization. In B. Lindblom, & R. Zetterstrom (Eds.), *Precursors of early speech* (pp. 21–36). New York: Stockton Press.

Oller, D. K., & Eilers, R. E. (1988). The role of audition in infant babbling. *Child Development, 2,* 441–449.

Oller, D. K., Eilers, R. E., Bull, D. H., & Carney, A. E. (1985). Prespeech vocalizations of a deaf infant: A comparison with normal methapho-nological development. *Journal of Speech and Hearing Research, 28,* 47–63.

Oller, D. K., Eilers, R. E., Neal, A. R., & Schwartz, H. K. (1999). Precursors to speech in infancy: The prediction of speech and language disorders. *Journal of Communication Disorders, 32,* 223–245.

Oller, D. K., Eilers, R. E., Urbano, R., & Cobo-Lewis, A. B. (1997). Development of precursors to speech in infants exposed to two languages. *Journal of Child Language, 24,* 407–425.

Paradis, J., & Genesee, F. (1996). Syntactic acquisition in bilingual children: Autonomous or interdependent? *Studies in Second Language Acquisition, 18,* 1–25.

Petito L. A., Katerelos M., Levy B. G., Gauna K., Tétreault K., & Ferraro, V. (2001). Bilingual signed and spoken language acquisition from birth: Implications for the mechanisms underlying early bilingual language acquisition. *Journal of Child Language, 28,* 453–496.

Pulvermüller, F., Huss, M., Kherif, F., Moscoso del Prado Martin, F., Hauk, O., & Shtyrov, Y. (2006). Motor cortex maps articulatory features of speech sounds. *Proceedings of the National Academy of Sciences, 103,* 7865–7870.

Raes, J., Michelsson, K., Dehaen, F., & Despontin, M. (1982). Cry analysis in infants with infectious and congenital disorders of the larynx. *International Journal of Pediatric Otorhinolaryngology, 4,* 157–169.

Robbins, A., Koch, D. B., Osberger, M. J., Zimmerman-Phillips, S., & Kishon-Rabin, L. (2004). Effect of age at cochlear implantation on auditory skill development in infants and toddlers. *Archives of Otolaryngology-Head and Neck Surgery, 130,* 570–574.

Robinshaw, H. M. (1995). Early intervention for hearing impairment: Differences in the timing of communicative and linguistic development. *British Journal of Audiology, 29,* 315–334.

Rvachew, S., Creighton, D., Feldman, N., & Sauve, R. (2005). Vocal development of infants with very low birth weight. *Clinical Linguistics and Phonetics, 19,* 275–294.

Saffran, J. R., Werker, J., & Werner, L. (2006). *The infant's auditory world: Hearing, speech, and the beginnings of language.* In W. Damon & R. M. Lerner (Series Eds.) & R. Siegler & D. Kuhn (Vol. Eds.), *Handbook of child psychology: Vol. 2. Cognition, perception and language* (6th ed., pp. 58–108). New York: Wiley.

Schauwers, K., Gillis, S., Daemers, K., De Beukelaer, C., & Govaerts, P. J. (2004). The onset of babbling and the audiological outcome in cochlear implantation between 5 and 20 months of age. *Otology and Neurotology, 25,* 263–270.

Segal, O., & Kishon-Rabin, L. (Manuscript submitted for publication). *Listening preference to child-directed speech compared to non-speech stimuli in hearing and hearing-impaired infants following cochlear implantation.*

Shi, R., & Werker, J. F. (2001). Six-month-old infants' preference for lexical words. *Psychological Science, 12,* 70–75.

Singer, L., Yamashita, T., Lilien, L., Collin, L., & Baley, J. (1997). A longitudinal study of developmental outcome of infants with bronchopulmonary dysplasia and very low birth weight. *Pediatrics, 100,* 987–993.

Sparrow, S. S., Balla, D. A., & Cicchetti, D. (1984). *Vineland Adaptive Behavior Scales.* Circle Pines, MN. American Guidance Service.

Stark, R. (1980). Stages of speech development in the first year of life. In G. H. Yeni-Komshian, J. F. Kavanagh, & C. A. Ferguson (Eds.), *Child Phonology, Vol. 1, Production* (pp. 73–92), New York: Academic Press.

Stark, R. (1986). Prespeech segmental feature development. In P. Fletcher & M. Garman (Eds.), *Language acquisition. Studies in first language development* (2nd ed., pp. 149–173). Cambridge: University Press.

Steinschneider, M., Schroeder, C. E., Arezzo, J. C., & Vaughan, H. G., Jr. (1995). Physiologic correlates of the voice onset time boundary in primary auditory cortex (A1) of the awake monkey: Temporal response patterns. *Brain and Language, 48,* 326–340.

Stoel-Gammon, C., & Cooper, J. A. (1984). Patterns of early lexical and phonological development. *Journal of Child Language, 11,* 247–271.

Svirsky, M. A., Teoh, S. W., & Neuburger, H. (2004). Development of language and speech perception in congenitally, profoundly deaf children as a function of age at cochlear implantation. *Audiology and Neuro-Otology, 9,* 223–233.

Taitelbaum-Swead, R., Kishon-Rabin, L., Kaplan-Neeman, R., Muchnik, C., Kronenberg, J., & Hildesheimer, M. (2005). Speech perception of children using Nucleus, Clarion or MED-EL cochlear implants. *International Journal of Pediatric Otorhinolaryngology, 69,* 1675–1683.

Tharpe, A. M. (2008). Unilateral and mild bilateral hearing loss in children: Past and current perspectives. *Trends in Amplification, 12,* 7–15.

Vihman, M. M. (1993). Variable paths to early word production. *Journal of Phonetics, 21,* 61–82.

Vihman, M. M. (2002). The role of mirror neurons in the ontogeny of speech. In M. Stamenov & V. Gallese (Eds.), *Mirror neurons and the evolution of brain and language* (pp. 305–314). Amsterdam: John Benjamin.

Waltzman, S. B., & Cohen, N. L. (1998). Cochlear implantation in children younger than 2 years old. *American Journal of Otology, 19,* 158–162.

Weber, C., Hahne, A., Friedrich, M., & Friederici, A. D. (2004). Discrimination of word stress in early infant perception: Electrophysiological evidence. *Brain Research. Cognitive Brain Research, 18,* 149–161.

Weber, C., Hahne, A., Friedrich, M., & Friederici, A. D. (2005). Reduced stress pattern discrimination in 5-month-olds as a marker of risk for later language impairment: Neurophysiological evidence. *Brain Research. Cognitive Brain Research, 25,* 180–187.

Werker, J. F., Shi, R., Desjardins, R., Pegg, J. E., Polka, L., & Patterson, M. (1998). Three methods for testing infant speech perception. In A. M. Slater (Ed.), *Perceptual development: Visual, auditory and speech perception in infancy* (pp. 389–420). East Sussex, UK: Psychology Press.

Westermann, G., & Reck Miranda, E. (2004). A new model of sensorimotor coupling in the development of speech. *Brain and Language, 89,* 393–400.

Wilson, S. M., Saygin, A. P., Sereno, M. I., & Iacoboni, M. (2004). Listening to speech activates motor areas involved in speech production. *Nature Neuroscience, 7,* 701–702.

Woodward, L. J., Anderson, P., Austin, N. C., Howard, K., & Inder, T. E. (2006). Neonatal MRI to predict neurodevelopmental outcomes in preterm infants. *New England Journal of Medicine, 355,* 685–694.

Yoshinaga-Itano, C. (2000). Development of audition and speech: Implications for early intervention with infants who are deaf or hard of hearing. In C. Yoshinaga-Itano & A. L. Sedey (Eds.), *Language, speech and social- emotional development of children who are deaf and hard of hearing: The early years* [Monograph]. *Volta Review, 100,* 213–234.

Yoshinaga-Itano, C., Sedey, A. L., Coulter, D. K., & Mehl, A. L. (1998). Language of early- and later-identified children with hearing loss. *Pediatrics, 102,* 1161–1171.

Zimmerman-Phillips, S., Robbins, A. M., & Osberger, M. J. (2000). Assessing cochlear implant benefit in very young children. *Annals of Otology, Rhinology, and Laryngology, 109* (Suppl. 185), 42–44.

APPENDIX 12–A
Issues Related to the Administration of the PRISE

The PRISE questionnaire is administrated by a speech-language pathologist or audiologist interviewing the parent(s). The parents are prompted by questions while provided with examples (Appendix 12–B) and are asked to describe the child's behavior. This interview is conducted in a similar manner to the IT-MAIS. The examiner scores the frequency of occurrence of the target behavior on the basis of parents' extensive reporting. Scores for each question range from 0 or never ("never demonstrate the behavior"); 1, rarely (25% of the time); 2, sometimes (50% of the time); 3, often (75% of the time); to 4, always (demonstrates the behavior 100% of the time). The PRISE contains 44 possible points (11 questions times maximum score of 4). Raw scores are transformed to percentages. It should be noted that the probes' scores are accumulated monotonically with age. That is, if a child for example, has vowel-like productions, it is clear that he or she shows vocal ability other than crying. Therefore, the child would receive the maximum score for questions 1 to 4. It should be noted, however, that if a child has a constant production for an object (e.g., "du" for a ball), but has only very little consonant repertoire and no variegated babbling, he should receive a 4 for questions 1 to 5, and for 7, but not for question 6.

The PRISE is easy to administer, and allows evaluating vocal behavior in a relatively short time. It is also based on information that is not limited to the testing room, and requires parents to be attentive to changes in their infants' communication behavior. In the last few years, we have urged parents to take the questionnaire home in order for them to observe their infant's vocalizations as described by the questionnaire. Usually, a week later they are interviewed.

APPENDIX 12–B
Example from the PRISE

The following are examples of two questions from the PRISE (6 and 11) with the additional prompts used by the interviewers to solicit information from the parents. Also shown are examples of parents' responses and subsequent scoring (Kishon-Rabin et al, 2005):

Example 1. *Question 6: Producing syllable-like, (consonant-vowel combination)—The vocalization stage*

Does the infant produce varied consonant and vowel combinations?

For example: when the infant plays with toys or addresses one of the family members, does he produce parts of words, such as: ba, du, pi, and so forth? Describe the sound variety which the infant produces in different situations during the day. Remember to ask the parents for the complete variety of sounds the infant produces.

Parents responses: ta, da, na, mu, ba

Scoring: The infant produces CV combinations with 5 to 6 different consonants. Therefore, a score of 3 is assigned for this question.

Key for scoring:

0—never produces consonant-vowel combination
1—produces combinations of vowel with 1 to 2 different consonants
2—produces combinations of vowel with 3 to 4 different consonants
3—produces combinations of vowel with 5 to 6 different consonants
4—produces combinations of vowel with 7 and more different consonants

Example 2. *Question 11: The One-Word Stage Does the child use a number of permanent sequences of sounds in relating to certain object (words)?*

For example: Does the child relate to his father regularly in a permanent name, such as: daddy or /dada/ or addresses men or people this way permanently. Does the child relate to a teddy bear such as: /tedi/ /edi/ or /dedi/ regularly? How many permanent sequences does the child use?

Write the words the child uses.

Parents response: /ama/ for mother ("ima" in Hebrew), /tata/ for grandma ("savta" in Hebrew), /fu/ for candle, /bai/ for hello, /ao/ for telephone (hello), /aba/ for daddy ("abba" in Hebrew).

Scoring: The infant uses 6 permanent sequences of sounds for 6 different objects. Therefore, a score of 2 is assigned for this question.

Key for scoring:

0—the child uses 2 or fewer words
1—the child uses 3 to 5 words
2—the child uses 6 to 7 words
3—the child uses 8 to 9 words
4—the child uses 10 words or more.

CHAPTER 13

Psychological Consideration in Pediatric Cochlear Implantation

JOHN F. KNUTSON
CARREN J. STIKA

Introduction

In the time since cochlear implants became available as an approved clinical prosthesis, considerable evidence has been accumulated that multichannel cochlear implants can result in significant audiologic and speech perception benefit in children with congenital or acquired deafness (Eisenberg et al., 2006; Flipsen & Colvard, 2006; Fryauf-Bertschy, Tyler, Kelsay, & Gantz, 1992; Gantz, Tyler, Tye-Murray, & Fryauf-Bertschy, 1994; Gantz, Tyler, Woodworth, Tye-Murray, & Fryauf-Bertschy, 1994; Houston, Pisoni, Kirk, Ying, & Miyamoto, 2003; Miyamoto, Osberger, Robbins, Myres, & Kessler, 1993; Nicholas & Geers, 2006; Pasanisi et al., 2002; Pulsifer, Salorio, & Niparko, 2003; Waltzman et al., 1997; Waltzman, Cohen, & Shapiro, 1995). Moreover, pediatric cochlear implants can result in other improvements in communicative capacity of profoundly deafened children, such as improved speech intelligibility (Chin, Tsai, & Gao, 2003; Miyamoto et al., 1997a; Seifert et al., 2002), enhanced expressive language skills (Geers, Nicholas, & Sedey, 2003a; Miyamoto, Svirsky, & Robbins, 1997b; Svirsky, Robbins, Kirk, Pisoni, & Miyamoto, 2000; Tomblin, Spencer, Flock, Tyler, & Gantz, 1999), and nonverbal communication skills such as turn-taking and attending (Lutman & Tait, 1995).

Although the research evidence occasions considerable optimism regarding the benefits that can be realized by a cochlear implant recipient, regardless of the index of benefit, the population of pediatric cochlear implant recipients continues to evidence great variability in outcome. Indeed, even within the context of contemporary state-of-the-art devices, the variability within devices is as great as the variability among devices. The variability in outcome not only raises important theoretical and practical questions about implant design for researchers and the implant industry, the variability in outcome can occasion challenging decisions for parents who elect to seek an implant for a child (Kluwin & Stewart, 2000; Vernon & Alles, 1995; Wever, 2002). Although the newer generation of implant designs, coupled with improved diagnosis of deafness and implantation at younger ages offers increased optimism, the articulation of a need for the identification of variables that can predict implant outcome by the NIH Consensus Development Conference (1995) continues to hold more than a decade after it was issued. The variance in outcome among cochlear implant recipients not only points to the need to develop strategies to predict and understand variability in outcome, it also points to the need to consider indices of outcome that go beyond the more common audiologic measures. In many respects, it is the variability in outcome that provides the justification for including a consideration of psychological assessments in cochlear implantation.

The use of psychological variables to predict implant benefit, or to assess implant outcomes, was proposed at the time clinical research with cochlear implants was just commencing and implants were purely investigational devices (e.g., Crary, Wexler, Berliner, & Miller, 1982; Miller, Duval, Berliner, Crary, & Wexler, 1978; Tiber, 1985). Although the putative utility of psychological variables has long been suggested, the investigation of psychological variables in implant outcomes has played a much less salient role than the investigations of other variables. In a technologically sophisticated biomedical field, it should not be surprising that psychological factors would be investigated less than the design and technology factors. However, in some respects the limited research can be attributed, in part, to the controversy as to how psychological variables should be assessed in deaf populations (Evans, 1989; McKenna, 1986, 1991; Pollard, 1996) and, in part, to the difficulties in applying standardized instruments to special populations, especially those who are very young and for whom reliable and valid measures are limited. Clearly, some standardized psychological instruments are not suitable for use with deaf populations due to their auditory and linguistic demands. It is also important to recognize that the use of non-standardized measures can compromise replicability across sites. Additionally, nonstandardized measures can reduce the likelihood of publication in archival journals and reduce the corpus of data that could be used to guide practice. Thus, although there are clear advantages to the use of standardized measures for assessing psychological child implant candidates and recipients, in some circumstances experimental procedures have been used that provided useful information. In short, although there is a general advantage to the use of standardized measures, less common and innovative measures may be required when evaluating young children who are deaf, and a consideration of such measures and assessment techniques are included in this chapter when they offer useful or potentially useful information.

One factor that complicates a review of psychological factors in pediatric cochlear implantation is the changing landscape with respect to who is a medically suitable candidate for implantation. When the U.S. Food and Drug Administration (FDA) first approved the use of cochlear implants in children, the recommended selection criteria for the pediatric population set a standard for children who were at least 2 years of age with profound bilateral sensorineural hearing loss. The child needed to have normal cochleae, and only those children who first demonstrated that little or no benefit from amplification or a vibrotactile device were considered. Although the primary goal of surgically implanting the child with the electronic device was to promote the development of audition and speech, at some cochlear implant centers a commitment to postoperative enrollment in intensive aural rehabilitation programs was thought to be essential. Children with other significant disabilities, such as developmental disabilities, autism, or visual impairments, were excluded because they were not considered capable of obtaining significant benefits from the surgically implanted device. Moreover, it was believed that children with some disabilities could not fully participate in the device-setting protocols; thus, they were excluded on practical grounds rather than because of evidence that they would not benefit from the device.

Over the years, the pediatric selection criteria have been broadened. Currently, children younger than 1 year of age, children with less severe degrees of hearing loss or with malformed cochleae, as well as children with additional disabilities, are receiving cochlear implants. Changes in the recommended selection criteria are largely due to significant improvements in cochlear implant technology and speech processing software, and a growing body of outcomes research that is documenting substantial benefits associated with cochlear implantation. Results of outcome research that shows impressive evidence regarding the critical importance of early intervention in minimizing detrimental effects of sensory deprivation on speech and language development have also played a persuasive role in lowering the age limit for cochlear implantation candidacy and coincidentally implanting some children who might later evidence significant disabilities. In less than 20 years, cochlear implantation has moved

from being an experimental procedure to an intervention that has widespread clinical acceptance. Indeed, today, cochlear implantation in young children has become almost ordinary in the pantheon of techniques for meeting the needs of profoundly deafened children.

Importantly, as the criteria for implanting a child have changed and the device has become less and less investigational, the context for considering psychological variables has changed as well. That is, the samples from which data were obtained even a decade ago might not be representative of the current population of implant candidates and recipients, complicating our ability to make use of some empirical findings. Additionally, as the population of implant recipients becomes younger, the availability of suitable assessment strategies becomes more limited. Consequently, many of the more pressing questions regarding the role of psychological assessments in cochlear implantation still do not have the empirical answers to unequivocally guide clinical services.

As the pediatric selection criteria have broadened, the scope of the preimplant assessment also has changed. During the early years of pediatric implantation, so as to ensure that implant candidates met the selection criteria and that parents fully understood the risks and benefits involved, many medical centers performing cochlear implant surgery required the child and parents to undergo a preoperative evaluation. This evaluation typically was conducted by a multidisciplinary team, often consisting of an otolaryngologist, audiologist, speech-language pathologist, educational specialist, and psychologist, with radiologic consultation available. Each discipline conducted a component of the preoperative evaluation designed to address relevant factors related to the child's candidacy. Together, the team decided whether the child and parents met the recommended criteria for cochlear implantation. Psychologists typically focused their efforts on evaluating a range of child attributes hypothesized to be related to implant benefit. They also considered parent attributes that could relate to the unique demands of parenting a pediatric implant recipient. More recently, as the clinical acceptability of implants has increased, as younger children are implanted, and as the procedure becomes more routine, a multidisciplinary team may not always be involved in the process (Berg, Ip, Hurst, & Herb, 2007). Moreover, psychologists are now less likely to participate in these multidisciplinary teams and in preoperative and postoperative counseling of the parents. However, some of the questions and management issues that psychologists might be best prepared to address continue to arise. Thus, we believe there is a continuing need to consider how psychological evaluations might provide useful information in the context of judging pediatric cochlear implant candidacy and in planning postoperative rehabilitative and educational services for those children who receive an implant.

Predicting Implant Outcome from Preimplant Psychological Variables

In an effort to better understand factors that may account for the variance in outcomes of cochlear implantation, a growing number of studies have focused attention on investigating the extent to which certain characteristics of the child may contribute to his or her ability to benefit from implantation, including intelligence, attention, age, psychosocial adjustment, and duration of implant use. Family characteristics that potentially play an influential role in deter-

mining postimplant benefit have also become the focus of increasing investigative interest. Although this body of research is still at its early stages of development, knowledge of current research findings is essential when judging a child's candidacy during the preoperative evaluation and when counseling parents regarding the potential benefit that their child may receive from a cochlear implant. Similarly, a consideration of relevant psychological variables and parental characteristics that may influence performance outcomes is imperative during the postoperative stages of pediatric cochlear implantation, so that follow-up care and rehabilitative services can be appropriately tailored to the unique needs of the individual child and family. Furthermore, with respect to investigative studies, because psychological variables may interact with other variables and affect outcomes, it is critical that studies of cochlear implant benefit take into account the potential influence of such variables so that inaccurate conclusions are not drawn from research results.

In the following section, we discuss some of the psychological variables that have been identified in the literature as potential sources of outcome variance. We also discuss the relevance of these research findings to clinical practice in contemporary pediatric cochlear implantation.

Child Factors

One psychological variable that has been postulated to predict implant benefit in children is intelligence. As noted previously, during the earlier years of pediatric cochlear implantation, children with cognitive developmental delays were precluded from receiving an implant. Although, intuitively, one might expect that intellectual ability would be a significant predictor of cochlear implantation success, research data do not always support this relation. Similar to research findings with adult cochlear implant recipients, outcome studies conducted with pediatric cochlear implants have yielded equivocal results regarding the association of measured intelligence with postimplant outcomes (e.g., Knutson, Ehlers, Ward, & Tyler, 2000a; Pyman, Blamey, Lacy, Clark, & Dowell, 2000; Tobey, Geers, Brenner, Altuna, & Gabbert, 2003). Lack of consistency in research findings may be due in part to methodological differences across a relatively small number of published studies. Studies investigating the relationship of intellectual ability and implant benefit have often employed different measures of cognitive ability and targeted different outcomes. Discrepancies in research findings also may be the result of inherent weaknesses in the reliability and validity of the instruments and assessment procedures with hearing-impaired samples. As noted previously, evaluating the cognitive skills in young children is challenging, and evaluating the intelligence of young deaf children with limited language skills using standardized assessment instruments is especially difficult. Consequently, efforts to capture a valid and reliable measure of cognitive skills in very young deaf children who are candidates for cochlear implants frankly may be too problematic.

With respect to existing published research that has investigated cognitive ability as a potential influence on outcome variance, although Knutson et al. (2000a) did not show a relation between presurgical nonverbal intelligence quotient (IQ) and speech perception measures, Geers, Brenner, and Davidson (2003b) reported that the Wechsler Intelligence Scale for Children—Third Edition (WISC-III) (Wechsler, 1991) Performance IQ score predicted speech perception in children implanted by age 5 with several years of implant experience.

Similarly, based on the same sample of subjects, Tobey et al. (2003) reported that the WISC-III Performance IQ score predicted the speech production of the children. There are, however, methodological limitations in that research that cast doubt on whether the WISC-III Performance IQ score can be used *presurgically* to predict implant benefit. First, the sample used in the Geers et al. (2003b) and Tobey et al. (2003) studies was not a prospective sample. Although the sample was very large, without establishing a prospective random sample, it is impossible to actually test a prediction model. Secondly, the WISC-III Performance score was obtained after years of implant use. In a study by Knutson, Wald, Ehlers, and Tyler (2000b), 46% of pediatric implant recipients evidenced a 0.5 standard deviation increase in Performance IQ after long-term implant use. Although Knutson et al. (2000b) did not report the correlations between the postimplant Performance IQ and the postimplant speech perception measures because they were not statistically significant, the absolute magnitude of the correlation that was provided to the authors of the present chapter closely approximated those reported in the Geers et al. (2003b) study, which had much greater statistical power. In short, recognizing the power difference between the two studies, it seems probable that the Geers et al. (2003b) and Tobey et al. (2003) correlations are more likely due to postimplant improvements in Performance IQ associated with the speech and language benefits following years of implant use rather than being due to the effective prediction of implant outcome with an IQ measure. At the very least, the Knutson et al. (2000b) data cast doubt on the utility of IQ alone in predicting implant outcome and would raise questions about limiting implantation to only those children who do not present with low IQ scores. Furthermore, as assessments of the intellectual status of very young children are quite unreliable, it would clearly be inappropriate to attempt to set IQ standards for implantation among the very young children who might be implant candidates in the current era.

Certainly, we do not mean to imply that the child's cognitive abilities should be simply ignored when judging candidacy and counseling parents regarding potential benefit from a cochlear implant. Knowledge regarding the child's cognitive development is valuable information relative to appreciating how a particular child functions in the world. In addition, a child's cognitive skills and learning potential can influence the child's progress following implantation, and the parents should be made aware of this. Furthermore, information regarding the child's intellectual ability and learning style are important factors that need to be considered when designing individualized postoperative services. Additionally, there are considerable adult data that suggest some special cognitive abilities involving working memory and signal detection are excellent predictors of both speech perception and music perception by adult implant users (Gfeller, Knutson, Woodworth, Witt, & De-Bus, 1998; Gfeller, Witt, Woodworth, Mehr, & Knutson, 2002; Gfeller, Woodworth, Robin, Witt, & Knutson, 1997; Knutson et al., 1991). Those methodologies have not been extended to children, but the adult data do suggest that some aspects of cognitive function beyond measured intelligence could play a role in pediatric implant benefit. In summary, although some cognitive abilities undoubtedly contribute to a child's experience with an implant, the current research evidence does not unequivocally support the notion that measured intelligence plays a direct or even primary role in predicting implant outcome. Consequently, earlier guidelines in pediatric cochlear implanta-

tion that recommended that children have at least average intelligence to be considered appropriate implant candidates may be overly conservative.

National annual surveys conducted by the Gallaudet Research Institute indicate that approximately 40 to 50% of children with hearing loss have additional disabilities of educational significance (Gallaudet Research Institute, 2007). Survey results indicated that among school-aged children with hearing loss, approximately 8% have mental retardation, another 3.8% have significant developmental delays, and at least 8% have specific learning disabilities. As the criteria for pediatric cochlear implantation continue to broaden, an increasing number of children with both hearing loss and other disabilities are being referred for cochlear implants. Understandably, parents of these children want to know about the potential benefits that may be realized by the child who receives a cochlear implant. Unfortunately, despite the large percentage of children with both hearing loss and other disabilities, there is a paucity of empirical research currently available that documents the outcomes of cochlear implantation for children with additional disabilities, including children with cognitive delays and learning difficulties. This is partly because children with multiple-handicaps were typically precluded from receiving implants during the earlier years of implantation. A review of the current literature on cochlear implant outcomes in children with multiple handicaps indicates a wide range of variability, with some reports suggesting limited benefit (e.g., Donaldson, Heavner, & Zwolan, 2004; Edwards, Frost, & Witham, 2006; Holt & Kirk, 2005; Pyman et al., 2000) and other reports proclaiming notable benefit (e.g., Fukuda et al., 2003; Waltzman, Scalchunes, & Cohen, 2000; Wiley, Jahnke, Meinzen-Deer, & Choo, 2005). The variability across reports may be due to different definitions of "benefit" and different criteria employed to measure it (Vlahovic & Sindigja, 2004). Additionally, there is considerable variability in the severity of the associated disabilities.

A recent study conducted by Holt and Kirk (2005) investigated the speech and language outcomes of children with cochlear implants who had cognitive delays in the borderline to mildly impaired range. Comparisons were made with a group of children with cochlear implants who had no additional developmental disabilities. Results indicated that although both groups of children showed significant gains in speech and language skills at 2 years after implantation, the children with the cognitive delays demonstrated significantly lower scores on two of the three measures of receptive and expressive language skills than did their normally developing implanted peers. Moreover, although the children with cognitive delays developed speech perception skills, they experienced considerably more difficulty with tasks involving higher level language skills. Based on the results of this study, the authors concluded that cochlear implantation in children with mild developmental delay can result in notable benefits. They added, however, that it remains unclear whether this would be the case for children with more significant cognitive delay or with additional disabilities. It also is important to note that children with borderline intelligence are expected to acquire language skills at a lower rate than children with average intelligence. Thus, the findings underscore the importance of establishing realistic parental expectations for outcomes as well as a consideration of managing the child following implantation.

In another recent study, Edwards et al. (2006) utilized retrospective case series analysis of young children, between the ages of 1.2 and 2.8 years, who were identified with cognitive delay prior to implantation. Progress in speech perception and speech intelligibility was assessed at 1 and 2 years post-implantation. Results indicated that the degree of developmental delay predicted speech intelligibility and speech perception outcomes, and that the children with greater delay demonstrated significantly less progress. Moreover, results indicated that developmental status was a better predictor of benefit than audiologic indices or the age at which their implant was activated. However, the authors concluded that evidence of cognitive delays should not be considered an automatic barrier to implantation, as mild delays were associated with progress in developing speech perception and speech production skills. They noted, though, that children who present with significant developmental delay may not be appropriate cochlear implant candidates, as the potential benefits are not sufficient to outweigh the risks. It also is worth noting, however, that children with significant developmental delays are more difficult to assess than children without such delays. Thus, some of the indices of poorer benefit from the implant might actually reflect difficulty in assessment rather than poor performance. Again, the findings raise questions about setting realistic expectations rather than setting exclusionary criteria.

Using retrospective review of data, Yang, Lin, Chen, and Wu (2004) compared auditory perception skills of prelingually deafened children with cochlear implants based on level of cognitive skills at preimplantation using the Bayley Scales of Infant Development (Bayley, 1993) for children younger than 3 years old, and either the Wechsler Preschool and Primary Scales of Intelligence-Revised (WPPSI-R) (Wechsler, 1989) or the Leiter International Performance Scale-Revised (Leiter-R) (Roid & Miller, 1997) for children who were older. Speech perception performance conducted at 1- and 2-years postimplantation was based on subjective ratings of the child's abilities according to a hierarchical 7-level scale of auditory perceptive ability, with the lowest level ("0") indicating no awareness of environmental sounds and the highest level ("7") representing the ability to use a telephone with a known speaker. Results of this study indicated that cognitive skills played a role in predicting the rate at which the children progressed through the speech perception. Children with cognitive delays tended to progress more slowly than the children without such delays. However, the authors concluded that although mental function may influence the child's rate of advancement in speech perception skills, all the children, despite their level of cognitive ability, did advance in the area of speech perception. The authors explained, however, that the children in their study who were identified as cognitively delayed were functioning mostly in the borderline range of cognitive ability. Consequently, they cautioned that it may not be possible to generalize their results to other groups of children with greater levels of cognitive impairment and more significant developmental delays.

Some investigators have challenged conclusions drawn from cochlear implantation outcomes research conducted with children with additional disabilities, emphasizing that a narrow focus on merely speech and language performance outcomes does not adequately capture the full range of benefits demonstrated by such children in daily situations (e.g., Edwards et al., 2006; Wiley et al., 2005). They assert that greater awareness of environmental sounds, improved attention, increased interest in the world, and overall enhancement of quality of life are valued benefits reported by parents, though these particular outcomes are frequently not addressed in cochlear implant research with children with multiple dis-

abilities (Wiley et al., 2005). With a broader view of potential benefit, the case against conservative psychological exclusionary criteria can be made.

Because some specialized cognitive measures have been useful in predicting implant benefit in adult users (e.g., Gfeller et al., 2000; Gfeller, Christ, Knutson, Witt, & Mehr, 2003; Knutson et al., 1991), there have been efforts to determine whether some cognitive measures might play a role in the outcome of pediatric implantation. However, testing young children who cannot use acoustic stimuli and who do not read or recognize standard characters occasions a great challenge for investigators attempting a downward extension of measures used successfully with adults. Of course, extending such measures to infants and toddlers would clearly be impossible. Because working memory is thought to be a component of the cognitive tasks that were successfully used to predict audiological outcomes with adult implant users, Cleary, Pisoni, and Kirk (2002) used a task that required children to reproduce sequential patterns of lighted signals as an index of working memory to predict implant outcome. Although this paradigm would seem to be an ideal test of working memory for the cochlear implant population, available data indicate it did not predict implant outcome when administered in a vision only modality. Thus, to date, investigators have not been successful in devising measures of specific cognitive function that are suitable for use *presurgically* with very young pediatric implant candidates. There are, however, other data based on older child implant users that strongly support the notion that working memory is an important factor in implant outcome.

David Pisoni and his colleagues (Cleary et al., 2002; Pisoni & Cleary, 2003; Pisoni & Geers, 2000) tested samples of children from different sites who used several different implant designs. In that work, the Digit Span subtest from the WISC-III was used to assess working memory in children and to predict performance on speech recognition scores. Digit Span involves the presentation of a series of numbers at the rate of one per second. The score is the length of the string that the subject can reproduce in correct order forward (as presented) or backward (reverse sequence of presentation). The test is usually presented aurally and is a part of such standardized IQ tests as the Wechsler Adult Intelligence Scale-Third Edition (WAIS-III) (Wechsler, 1997) and the WISC, as well as in laboratory tests of memory. Importantly, the Digit Span is easy to administer and is generally acknowledged to be a reliable and valid test of auditory working memory. Although researchers have obtained the Digit Span scores postimplantation, unlike the concerns raised earlier about "predicting" outcomes from postimplant intelligence tests, there is no reason to believe that a cochlear implant would affect the working memory that is assessed with that test. Thus, on the basis of the correlation between Digit Span performance and speech recognition tests, Pisoni and colleagues have concluded that working memory is critical for implant success because working memory is used to encode and manipulate the phonological representation of words by the child. In related findings that are consistent with the work of Pisoni and colleagues, Dawson, Busby, McKay, and Clark (2002), using subtests from the Kaufman Assessment Battery for Children (Kaufman & Kaufman, 1983), demonstrated that short-term memory is a significant predictor of receptive language in child implant users. Thus, like the data obtained from adult implant recipients, there is considerable evidence that working memory is important in achieving implant

benefit. Unfortunately, at the present time, there are no suitable measures of short-term working memory that can be administered to very young pediatric implant candidates to predict outcomes prospectively. Thus, although being able to assess working memory might be useful in predicting ultimate implant benefit and the trajectory of change, psychologists are not in a position to provide an assessment for very young congenitally deafened children. However, for older adventitiously deafened children who are implant candidates, efforts to assess working memory might be useful.

Research on the prediction of implant outcome with adult samples (e.g., Gfeller et al., 2003, 2000; Knutson et al., 1991) also implicates the role of attentional processes in implant benefit. Although such research has not been conducted to predict implant outcome with pediatric implant users, there are some data to suggest it might be possible to include assessments of attentional processes in pediatric implant assessments. For example, studies of attentional processes in deaf children and implant recipients have established the feasibility of assessing attention in young deaf children (e.g., Mitchell & Quittner, 1996; Quittner et al., 2007; Quittner, Smith, Osberger, Mitchell, & Katz, 1994; Tharpe, Ashmead, & Rothpletz, 2002). Thus, research on a combination of attentional processes and working memory as predictors in pediatric implant outcome might be a fertile area to explore. It will require an integration of basic developmental work together with clinical assessment strategies.

Duration of Implant Use

Although emerging evidence suggests that early implantation seems to result in more rapid gains in the ability to respond to acoustic stimuli, the data continue to indicate that ultimate implant benefit is achieved slowly over a relatively long period of time. Moreover, it is clear that functional experience with the implant contributes to the ultimate outcome—it is not just a matter of the "tincture of time." Whether reflected in speech perception, expressive language, or speech production, the trajectory of change follows a time course that may not reach an asymptote until 3 or more years postimplantation (Kiefer et al., 1996; Kirk, Miyamoto, Ying, Perdew, & Zuganelis, 2002; Miyamoto, Kirk, Robbins, Todd, & Riley, 1996; Miyamoto et al., 1997a; Mondain et al., 1997; Tye-Murray, Spencer, & Gilbert-Bedia, 1995; Tyler et al., 2000a, 2000b). Because the actual hours of implant use per day correlate with long-term implant benefit (Fryauf-Bertschy, Tyler, Kelsay, Gantz, & Woodworth, 1997; Wie, Falkenberg, Tvete, & Tomblin, 2007), it is reasonable to hypothesize a causal link between experience and benefit. Thus, there is good reason to consider psychological factors that are likely to influence hours of daily use of the implant in the assessment protocol. It should be noted that there has been some speculation that implant recipients who experience great initial benefit would be more likely to demonstrate more active use of the device, the time course for achieving benefit renders that hypothesis unlikely. That is, the time course of achieving benefit, even among those who get the greatest benefit, suggest that benefit-facilitated use would occur *after* a rather long period of use. Thus, for prelingually deafened children, available evidence on the time-course of benefit suggests that it is most probable that reliable use must precede benefit. Hence, identifying psychological factors that successfully predict reliable use of the implant may be critical for developing strategies to predict long-term or ultimate benefit.

When a young child receives a cochlear implant, the active use of the device is determined by the adult caregivers who manage the child's daily affairs. To the extent that parenting determines implant use during the initial period following hook-up and mapping, it is probable that family factors could play a critical role in implant outcome. Indeed, the important role of family factors in determining the use of implants and, ultimately, the audiologic outcome realized by children is supported by a number of different lines of evidence from several laboratories. In a recent study based on a large sample of children implanted by age 5 years who had 3 or more years of active implant use, Geers et al. (2003b) noted that children from smaller families, better educated families, and higher socioeconomic status (SES) families evidenced greater speech perception on standardized measures. Because the study was not based on a prospective sample, strong conclusions about factors that predict outcome cannot be made, but the study does identify several aspects of parenting that could contribute to implant outcome. For example, since family size per se is not likely to be an active variable determining implant outcome, it can be considered a proxy variable for family-based factors that could influence implant use. A simple probabilistic model would indicate that parents in smaller families can provide more direct attention, supervision, and resources to the implanted child relative to larger families. This is not inconsistent with other research on parenting in which family size plays an important role (Bassarath, 2001; Levine, Pollack, & Comfort, 2001).

Similarly, parental education and indices of SES can be viewed as proxy variables for those factors that result in greater educational and habilitative resources being made available to children. It should be noted, however, that it would clearly be unconscionable to restrict access to implants to children from small families from circumstances of advantage. Rather, these findings point to the need to make sure that all child implant recipients experience the levels of supervision, monitoring and habilitative resources that children from small advantaged families enjoy.

Because the use of the implant during the initial period following connection can play a critical role in ultimate implant outcomes (Te et al., 1996; Wie et al., 2007), for young children, the reliable early use of the implant is likely to be a direct consequence of the actions of parents. When initial use is not necessarily appreciated by the child, the parent will play a critical role in assuring that initial use. Unfortunately, there is evidence that some pediatric implant recipients cease implant use, and there are data suggesting that the rate of termination by child recipients is greater than among implanted adults (Rose, Vernon, & Pool, 1996; West & Stucky, 1995). Although those data were based on early work with implantation, the data provide a cautionary note to contemporary implant teams. While termination of implant use in the context of an absence of audiologic benefit should be neither surprising nor disturbing, data indicate that some termination of use by children occurs long before maximum benefit is likely to be achieved. Additionally, some children who use implants can be characterized as unreliable users, with parents of unreliable users failing to adequately maintain the speech processor, failing to provide fresh batteries for the device, or encouraging maximum hours of use. Termination of implant use prior to realizing benefit, or even unreliable implant use, occasions considerable concern because such unreliable

use is likely to result in reduced audiological benefit.

To determine whether psychological variables could predict unreliable use or premature termination of use, Knutson et al. (2000a) analyzed a constellation of preimplant psychological variables and implant use by 69 consecutively implanted children. Reliable and unreliable users were identified by the audiologists working with the children. The unreliable users were those children who had either completely ceased using the implant within 12 months of implant surgery, or who used the implant only at school. Notably, for unreliable users, implant use at school was often inconsistent, with teachers reporting poor speech processor maintenance. The unreliable users were significantly older than the reliable users ($t = 2.61$, $p < .05$). Although age of implantation is important in determining open-set and closed-set speech perception (e.g., Harrison et al. 2001), among unreliable users in the Knutson et al. (2000a) study, intermittent use occurred shortly after connection and well before substantial benefit would likely be achieved. Thus, it is probable that the lack of use would affect audiologic benefit rather than limited audiologic benefit associated with later implantation resulting in unreliable use.

To determine whether the reliable and unreliable users differed on psychological variables, the groups were compared on a set of variables selected a priori. Reliable users and non-reliable users did not differ on measured intelligence (mean IQ scores from the Leiter International Performance Scale (Arthur, 1949) and Hiskey-Nebraska Test of Learning Aptitude (Hiskey, 1955). Based on the mothers' preimplant completion of the Achenbach Child Behavior Checklist (CBCL) (Achenbach & Edelbrock, 1991), the group of reliable users exhibited significantly fewer externalizing behavior problems prior to implantation. Such evaluative instruments would not be suitable for implant candidates who are less than 18 months of age. However, observational strategies that would help to identify mothers who are having difficulty engaging their children and children who are evidencing precursors of externalizing behaviors, might identify those families who would be well served by providing parent management training to deal with early oppositional patterns that could compromise implant use.

Often clinicians and researchers need to gather information from parents about a range of child behaviors, including hours of daily implant use. The Parental Daily Report (PDR), a procedure pioneered by Chamberlain and Reid (1987), provides a means of gathering information that is not compromised by long-term recall. The PDR involves contacting a parent by telephone on five consecutive evenings to inquire as to whether the child displayed a range of target behaviors. Those behaviors can be general behavior problems as well as implant-related behaviors. To determine reliability of implant use, the PDR can be used to secure information from the parents as to the number of hours the child had worn the implant each day. Administered quarterly, a PDR assessment of hours of daily implant use can be used to monitor initial implant use and outcome as well as implant use during the developmental trajectory when implant benefit should be increasing. As an example, Knutson et al. (2000a) reported correlations between preimplant psychological measures and hours of implant use obtained with quarterly PDRs during the first three years following implantation. Results indicated no significant correlations between hours of use and age at implantation or intelligence. From the CBCL completed by the mothers, only the correlation between hours of use

and the Anxious/Depressed Scale was significant. Based on the mother's presurgical response to the Home Environment Questionnaire (HEQ) (Laing & Sines, 1982), hours of implant use was significantly and positively correlated with the Affiliation, Sociability, and Social Status Scales, accounting for 16 to 25% of the variance. Paralleling the HEQ scales, the mothers' rating of the child's sociability on the Missouri Children's Behavior Checklist (MCBC) (Sines, 1986, 1988), correlated significantly with hours of use. In short, mothers who described their children and their homes as more sociable and with more affiliation at preimplant had children who were more reliable users during the three years following implantation. Children who used the implant less were reported by their mothers to have more symptoms of anxiety and depression than those children who used the implant routinely. In general, these findings suggest that some preimplant child variables and characteristics of the home environment might be predictive of implant use. Moreover, these findings are not inconsistent with the Geers et al. (2003b) findings noted above, that more advantaged families with fewer children have better outcomes.

The Knutson et al. (2000a) study correlated presurgical psychological measures with standardized speech perception measures at 12, 24, and 36-month follow-up. Standardized nonverbal tests of intelligence administered presurgically did not predict implant benefit. Similarly, there was no consistent pattern of correlations between the speech perception measures and the CBCL Internalizing Scale (Achenbach & Edelbrock, 1991). Although correlations between the CBCL Externalizing Score and the 12-month audiological scores only approached statistical significance, all but two correlations were statistically significant at the 24- and 36-month follow-up sessions (all $r \geq 0.33$).

When considered in the context of the finding that the CBCL Externalizing Score was related to unreliable use, these correlations suggest children who present with externalizing behavior problems realize less benefit from implants, even when used for up to 36 months postimplant. Because nonusers and unreliable users were not represented in the sample upon which the correlations were based, the findings cannot be attributed to nonusers who would, of course, perform poorly. Thus, the Knutson et al. (2000a) study demonstrated that some maternal ratings of child behavior prior to implantation were predictive of both hours of implant use and speech perception scores after 36 months of implant use. Again, the findings point to the potential utility of assessing child behavior and parenting as pre-implant predictors and providing post-implant counseling and parent management training to those who might benefit.

Family Factors

Several studies identified additional family-based factors that could play an active role in the child's adaptation to the implant, its use, and the ultimate benefit that is obtained. Preisler, Tvingstedt, and Ahlstrom (2002) used analyses derived from video records of interactions in the home and in the preschool setting to document the complexity of predicting implant benefit from such observations. That study did, however, underscore the importance of the communicative interaction between the child and the parent(s) *prior* to implantation as a possible factor in implant outcome.

Preisler et al. (2002) also identified patterns of conflict that could arise between parents and children in the context of implant use. When the Preisler et al. (2002) findings are considered in the context of the Knutson et al. (2000a) study noted above, it seems probable that parents who have difficulty with supervising and effectively disciplining a child who is initially resistant to using the device might be at risk for having a child who achieves limited implant use and benefit. Similarly, Bat-Chava and Martin (2002) used qualitative methods to detail how parenting and child characteristics play a role in the sibling interactions in homes of children using implants or hearing aids, with data that could contribute to understanding how variables related to family size noted above operate in determining implant outcomes. Importantly, it is worth noting that family influences on implant outcome are not necessarily fixed at the time a child is implanted. For example, Paganga, Tucker, Harrigan, and Lutman (2001) described an intervention that facilitated the parent-child communication among pediatric implant users. Those findings provide a basis for optimism that home environments that occasion risk for implant recipients could be improved with effective parenting interventions.

Although communicative effectiveness and behavior management of the child has been implicated as a factor in determining implant benefit, it is also the case that the language environment of the child could play a role in determining implant outcome. For example, Stallings, Kirk, Chin, and Gao (2002) documented that greater word familiarity by parents was associated with improved child receptive vocabulary and their receptive and expressive language. Although such findings probably can be accounted for by the educational level and SES of the family (Geers et al., 2003b), when considered with the aforementioned studies, these findings provide another example how active parental involvement and parental communicative effectiveness could play an important role in determining implant outcome in children.

Psychological Consequences of Pediatric Cochlear Implantation

Parents seeking a cochlear implant for their child often raise questions about the broader consequences of implantation, beyond improved speech and language development and the ability to discern acoustic events. In short, questions arise as to what are the psychological consequences of implantation. The literature on the psychological status of hearing-impaired children can be used to focus a consideration of the putative psychological consequences of implantation. That literature tends to address two broad domains—psychosocial competence and cognitive development. The latter typically includes language development and academic progress. Increasingly, these research domains are placed in a developmental-interactive context, which takes into account the impact of the child's sensory status at various developmental stages while the child participates in a communicative environment that has social and educational consequences (see Marschark, 1993a; Schum, 2004). Such an approach is congruent with contemporary models of child development that place the child's behavior in a broad systems context (e.g., Cox & Paley, 1997). Such models argue for including age-appropriate, setting-specific, and interactive variables in the assessment of implant outcomes.

With respect to psychosocial competence, evidence exists that difficulties in communication are likely to compromise interactions with peers and the development of skillful interpersonal relationships (Rasing, 1993; Rasing & Duker, 1992). Thus, it is not surprising that hearing impairment, as a communicative difficulty, has been associated with compromised social competence. Indices of compromised psychological and social competence among hearing-impaired children have included impulsivity, distractibility, social immaturity, and tantrums (Greenberg & Kusché, 1989, 1993; Marschark, 1993b; Meadow, 1980; Mitchell & Quittner, 1996; Quittner et al., 1994; Watson, Henggeler, & Whelan, 1990). When that contemporary literature on the social competence of hearing-impaired children is considered, the importance of focusing on social competence and the presence or absence of behavioral problems as consequences of implantation is apparent. Moreover, because Levy-Schiff and Hoffman (1985) found that the degree of social competence was related to degree of hearing loss, it is reasonable to hypothesize that the degree of improvement in social competence following implantation should covary, albeit not perfectly, with degree of audiologic benefit.

Evidence also exists that family interaction can be influenced by the presence of a deaf child. Research has indicated that hearing parents of deaf children are more likely to use directing and controlling behaviors (Brinich, 1980; Greenberg, 1980) and to rely more on physical discipline (Schlesinger & Meadow, 1972) than parents of hearing children. This pattern of greater reliance on physical discipline also is thought to be reflected in the association between physical child abuse and communication impairments (Fox, Long, & Langlois, 1988; Knutson & Sullivan, 1993). Recently completed analog tests of disciplinary preferences indicate that mothers of child implant candidates and mothers of deaf children are more likely to endorse the use of physical discipline than mothers of normal-hearing children (Knutson, Johnson, & Sullivan, 2004). Moreover, because family stressors have been shown to magnify risk factors for poor adjustment (Abidin, Jenkins, & McGaughey, 1992; O'Grady & Metz, 1987) and because the presence of a deaf child can be identified as a chronic stressor (Burger et al., 2006; Pipp-Siegel, Sedey, & Yoshinaga, 2002; Quittner, Glueckauf, & Jackson, 1990), there is reason to hypothesize that family adjustment and family interaction could be adversely affected by the presence of a deaf child and that the implantation of that child could have an influence how the family functions (Quittner, Steck, & Rouiller, 1991). Importantly, there are data to suggest that cochlear implants affect communicative skills displayed with familiar adults (Lutman & Tait, 1995); as improved communication with familiar adults can include the child's parent, it is reasonable to expect that cochlear implants could positively influence family interactions. Such an expectation is often expressed by parents seeking an implant for a child when they are having difficulty parenting the child. It should be noted, however, that it would be appropriate to assist parents having difficulty managing their child rather than merely waiting and hoping that a cochlear implant will resolve such difficulties.

Questions have been raised regarding the degree to which child implant candidates and their parents are psychologically different than deaf children and parents who are not seeking an implant. Often such questions are posed by critics of implantation who argue that somehow seeking an implant for a child reflects an inability to adapt to the unique needs of the child. In responding to such questions, psychologists need to consider both the domains in which psychological outcomes of pediatric implantation could be established, as well as family-related variables. In one study relevant to that question, Knutson, Hinrichs, Gantz, and Tyler (1996) determined whether implant candidates presented with significant behavioral problems by comparing them to a sample of normal-hearing children who were presenting for psychological problems and behavioral difficulties and to a control sample obtained from other otolaryngological services unrelated to hearing loss. Parents of cochlear implant candidates were administered a number of standardized psychological tests, personality inventories, and child behavior rating scales. The instruments were selected because of their widespread use in research on child behavior and their established reliability and validity. Parents completed the Minnesota Multiphasic Personality Inventory (MMPI) (Hathaway & McKinley, 1943), the Home Environment Questionnaire (HEQ) (Laing & Sines, 1982; Sines, Clarke, & Lauer, 1984), the Child Behavior Checklist (CBCL) (Achenbach & Edelbrock, 1991), and the Missouri Child Behavior Checklist (Sines, 1986, 1988). In addition, these same instruments were administered to the two comparison groups. Most importantly, on most measures, the implant candidates and their parents were more similar to the otolaryngologic comparison group than the psychology clinic comparison group. In brief, the analyses generally supported the notion that child implant candidates and their families were *not* characterized by significant difficulty, and the study established the general absence of significant psychopathology among child implant candidates. This finding is important in the context of parents of deaf children continuing to be confronted by criticism from family and friends regarding the "controversy" of implantation. Although the implants are no longer investigational devices, and although evidence for benefit is far greater today than when that study was conducted, parents considering implantation for a deaf child continue to be confronted by family, neighbors, and others who question implantation on the basis of limited information or media depictions that continue to consider implantation controversial.

Although there was no evidence of severe psychopathology, several findings from the Knutson et al. (1996) paper did suggest that child implant candidates had significant *social* difficulties. On the HEQ, the mothers of the implant candidates indicated that their children experienced more rejection and inhospitable interactions outside the home than did children referred to the psychology clinic. Although it should be expected that children referred for behavioral problems would be rejected by members of their communities, it is not obvious that deaf children would experience even greater rejection. On the CBCL, maternal ratings of social participation and social competence of the implant candidates also were extremely low. Thus, although the implant candidates were not evidencing psychopathology, they were experiencing difficulties in social interactions with their peers. It should be emphasized that the preschool and early elementary-aged implant candidates in that research were older than most of the children receiving an implant today. Indeed, more recent studies are establishing a growing body of evidence indicating that children with early implantation show levels of self-esteem and social well-being that are comparable to those of their hearing peers (Bat-Chava, Martin, & Kosicw, 2005; Percy-Smith, Caye-Thomasen, Gudman, Jensen, & Thomsen, 2008; Sahli & Belgin, 2006). These findings point to improved social function as a possible psychological benefit of successful implant use.

Because interparent consistency is important in discipline and supervision, another potentially important finding reported by Knutson et al. (1996) related to the degree of agreement between mothers and fathers. When the responses of mothers and fathers were compared on the various scales, there were greater discrepancies between the reports of mothers and fathers from the implant group than between mothers and fathers in the other groups. Indeed, Knutson et al. (1996) reported that there was less concordance in parental reports within the implant group than would be expected on the basis of the available literature on mother-father agreement (Christensen, Margolin, & Sullaway, 1992; Greenbaum, Decrick, Prange, & Friedman, 1994; Hinshaw, Han, Erhardt, & Huber, 1992). Anecdotal evidence in clinical contexts often suggests that one parent assumes primary responsibility for meeting the needs of their hearing-impaired child. To the extent that shared parenting and consistency across parents may be important in facilitating implant usage and ultimate success, psychological evaluations focused on determining inter-parental congruence might be helpful in the context of working with parents who have difficulty assuring full use of the implant by the child.

Although the Knutson et al. (1996) study established the lack of psychopathology among families of child implant candidates, it did not contrast children and families who had sought an implant from those who had not sought an implant. Knutson, Boyd, Goldman, and Sullivan (1997a) contrasted implant candidates and their parents with a sample of deaf children and their parents who had elected not to seek a cochlear implant prior to the study or during the 3 years following data collection. Both groups of children and their parents completed the same protocol and the results were straightforward. There were no important differences between the children whose parents sought a cochlear implant and the children whose parents elected not to seek an implant on measures of intelligence, behavior, and the home environment. Although some statistically significant differences were detected, the absolute magnitude of those differences was clinically unimportant.

Although embracing a null hypothesis does not often advance science, Knutson et al. (1997a) concluded that it was quite appropriate in the comparison between implant-seeking families and those who did not seek an implant. With ample power, virtually identical means on most scales, and equal variance on each of the measures, the findings strongly supported the notion that children seeking an implant and their families are not behaviorally distinguishable from families who choose not to seek an implant for a congenitally deaf child. More importantly, the Knutson et al. (1996, 1997a) studies form a basis for arguing that assessment of the psychological outcomes of implants should focus on social competence and social interactions rather than indices of psychopathology.

The lack of concordance between mother and father descriptions of their children and the circumstances of their families in the Knutson et al. (1996) study, as well as in other areas of psychological research, can be used to cast doubt on the veridicality of parental report. As a result, direct observational methodologies have evolved as an important component for psychological assessment. Using micro- and macrolevel direct observational assessments of families of child implant candidates and those of deaf children who were not implant candidates, Knutson, Boyd, Reid, Mayne, and Fetrow (1997b) documented the methodological feasibility of laboratory tests of family interaction with implant candidates and recipients and provided substantive information about those families. Importantly, as the age at implantation has moved to include very young children, psychologists will be increasingly required to use systematic observations of the child rather than standardized psychological tests that can be administered to the child.

Knutson et al. (1997b) provided data that could have direct relevance to predicting implant outcome and assessing change following implantation. One important finding was that, like the Knutson et al. (1997a) study, there were no reliable differences between the sample of consecutively referred implant candidates and the comparison sample of families of deaf children who were not implant candidates. Thus, similar to the studies that used psychological tests and questionnaires, the implant-seeking families were not distinguishable from families who choose not to seek an implant for their child. Both sets of families did provide evidence of domains that can be examined in evaluating the psychological consequences of pediatric implantation.

When the observational data from the two samples of the Knutson et al. (1997b) study were contrasted with a large normative sample of families who did not have a hearing-impaired child, important differences were identified between families of deaf children and families without a deaf child. Although differences between the samples in the overall mean rate of some behaviors were interesting and somewhat counterintuitive (e.g., more frequent verbalizations by parents of deaf children), it was the lack of synchrony between the behavior of the parents and the behavior of the children that was most striking. Lack of synchrony refers to a circumstance where a child behavior (e.g., compliance) does not covary with the same parent behavior or a behavior (physical positive) that should be related to the child behavior. That is, on the basis of several theoretical models and existing empirical work with independent normative samples, it is possible to identify child and parent behaviors that evidence such child-parent synchrony. In the Knutson et al. (1997b) study, although the expected synchrony was readily apparent in the normative families, it was largely absent in the families of deaf children. As a result, Knutson et al. (1997b) suggested that patterns of increased synchrony in family interaction might be an outcome of implant use. Again, observational assessments of synchrony and reciprocity might be a useful domain for psychological assessments in the preimplant and postimplant period.

In addition to detailing patterns of family interactions, Knutson et al. (1997b) also described observations of implant candidates and recipients interacting with hearing peers in a standardized laboratory paradigm derived from the work of Gottman and Graziano (1983) and Dodge, Pettit, McClaskey, and Brown (1986). This peer interaction methodology is well established for assessing the social competence and friendships of children at least 6 years of age. In the paradigm used by Knutson et al. (1997b), two normal-hearing children engage in social play in a small room supplied with age-appropriate toys. After these two "host" children have played for 10 minutes, the implant candidate or recipient enters the room and is introduced to the host children. The experimenter departs and the three children are given an opportunity to play. Coded video-records of the play provides an assessment of the overtures the entering child makes to gain entry to the group and how they interact with age- and gender-matched peers. Moreover, it is a direct test of the challenges that deaf children and implant recipients confront when they are required to engage hearing children in a variety of contexts (e.g., Archbold, Nikolopoulos, Lutman, & O'Donoghue, 2002; Spencer, Koester, & Meadow-Orlans, 1994).

Approximately 40% of the children in the Knutson et al. (1997b) study failed to engage effectively in interaction with their peers. In general, social behaviors of the children who failed to enter and the children who entered less successfully were characterized by a pattern of social immaturity. Although efforts to identify variables that distinguished between the successful and unsuccessful entry was compromised by the lack of statistical power, age emerged as an important variable. That is, older children were more likely to enter than younger children. In a follow-up study, Boyd, Knutson, and Dahlstrom (2000) reported that short-term (less than 24 months) or long-term (more than 24 months) implant use was not associated with improved social competence on the peer entry task. Such findings are discouraging if enhanced social competence with hearing peers is a goal of implantation. However, Bat-Chava and Deignan (2001) provided qualitative and quantitative assessments indicating that peer relationships can evidence some improvement following implantation. Although these authors caution that peer communication difficulties persist post implantation, they also note the potential benefit in peer relationships that comes with implantation. Thus, there is some emerging objective evidence that improved social competence might be a benefit of pediatric implantation. Still, a psychologist working with an implant team might profitably work towards reducing social anxiety and increasing social skills much like successful programs for hearing children with social anxiety (e.g., Beidel, Turner, & Morris, 2000).

There are several other lines of evidence indicating that psychological benefit can be associated with pediatric implantation. For example, Knutson et al. (2000b) examined changes in Verbal and Performance IQ Scores from the WISC-III and changes in Internalizing and Externalizing behavior problems, as measured with the CBCL administered to the mothers. Standardized speech perception scores at 12, 24, and 36-month follow-up sessions were significantly correlated with mean Verbal IQ scores based on follow-up assessments that coincided with the audiological tests. Perhaps more importantly, 56% of the implanted sample evidenced a one-half standard deviation increase in Verbal IQ across the 3-year follow-up period. Additionally, 46% of the sample evidenced a one-half standard deviation increase in Performance IQ across the same follow-up period. Thus, although preimplant IQ scores were not correlated with audiologic benefit, improved audiologic performance was associated with improved measured intelligence at follow-up. To the extent that measured IQ predicts academic performance, these findings suggest it is reasonable to expect that implant benefit could also be realized in greater academic achievement as a long-term outcome. This is not to say that implants make children "brighter;" rather, their measured performance on some academically relevant tasks is enhanced.

Paralleling the findings with respect to measured intelligence, audiologic benefit was highly, but negatively, correlated with Externalizing and Total Problem scores at follow-up. That is, better audiologic performance was associated with few maternal reports of behavior problems. It was concluded by the authors that this pattern was probably an extension of the finding that parents who report externalizing problems with their children are likely to realize only modest benefit from implantation. Such findings are consistent with Robbins (2003) recent identification of compliance and behavioral management as an important consideration for clinicians working with young implant recipients. Thus, if psychological assessments were to identify behavior problems early in the postimplant period, effective parent management training might reduce behavior problems and increase the prospects for better audiologic benefit.

Although not based on a longitudinal assessment or a prospective sample, research by Geers et al. (2003a) and Nicholas and Geers (2003) provided data that are consistent with the conclusions of the Knutson et al (2000a) study. Geers et al. (2003a), using the WISC-III Similarities subtest as an index of verbal reasoning, provided evidence that speech perception benefit was associated with improved language skills. Additionally, based on a modified index of perceived competence and social acceptance, and parent ratings of emotional status, Nicholas and Geers (2003) were able to characterize their large sample of pediatric implant users as doing well psychologically.

Another factor that must be considered in psychological studies of implant outcome is the possibility that implants could have adverse psychological consequences. Although there are no systematic data to support the assertion that implants have pernicious effects on the lives of deaf children, that state of affairs has not prevented some critics of cochlear implants from asserting that adverse psychological sequelae will result when prelingually deafened children are implanted (Lane, 1996) or that failures and adverse consequences could be present among unstudied samples (Kluwin & Stewart, 2000). Although it is clearly true that some children and adolescents cease using the implant and their families might report dissatisfaction with the implant, such an outcome is not evidence that implants have *adverse* psychological effects. Additionally, some critics of implantation of prelingually deafened children have raised questions about the impact of implantation on the cultural identity of children and adolescents. However, a study by Wald and Knutson (2000) indicated that deaf adolescents with and without implants were comparable with respect to deaf and bicultural identities. Although the implanted adolescents had great hearing identity, that hearing identity was not associated with identifiable problems in either social adjustment or behavior problems.

It should be noted that the authors have received occasional reports and anecdotes of individual pediatric implant recipients who were described as evidencing significant behavior problems. Such anecdotes do not, however, provide evidence that the poor adjustment of an implanted child can be attributed to the implant itself. Some children, regardless of hearing status, will present with significant behavioral and emotional problems. Identifying a causal link between implantation and adverse outcomes requires the same standards of scholarship as establishing favorable outcomes. Thus, although it may be appropriate for clinicians and researchers to continue to include measures that can detect adverse effects of implantation, it is worth underscoring the fact that the present authors have not been able to locate any reports of adverse effects published in peer-reviewed archival journals. Sadly, the absence of evidence does not prevent popular media outlets and persons with fervently held beliefs to assert that implantation continues to be "controversial."

Implications Relative to the Preoperative Pediatric Evaluation

Although the selection criteria for children being considered for cochlear implants have broadened over the years, obviously not all children with hearing loss are suitable for cochlear implants, though the parents, or even occasionally the child or adolescent, might desire this form of intervention. Despite the substantial advances in the field of cochlear implants and the growing body of outcomes research demonstrating impressive benefits obtained by many children who receive cochlear implants at a young age, the decision to proceed with cochlear implantation as a form of intervention for a child with hearing loss is by no means a simple one. Careful consideration must be given to a number of factors before proceeding.

In the majority of cases, pediatric cochlear implantation is no longer viewed as a risky medical procedure; however, a review of the current literature indicates that it continues to be recommended that a multidisciplinary team be involved in the selection of appropriate pediatric candidates (Clark, 2003; Niparko & Blankenhorn, 2003; Zwolan, 2000). The advantage of a multidisciplinary team approach is that it allows for a variety of professional perspectives to be brought to the candidacy assessment, and ensures that multiple factors that may affect the outcome of cochlear implantation be considered. The multidisciplinary team not only gathers a broad base of information to use in the decision-making process regarding candidacy, but it also provides opportunity for the team to identify factors that may warrant further counseling and intervention.

The recommended implant team continues to include professionals from otolaryngology, audiology, speech-language pathology, psychology, and education (ASHA, 2004; Clark, 2003). Interestingly, whereas the roles of the surgeon, audiologist, and speech-language pathologist on the cochlear implant team are often well defined in the published literature, the role that the psychologist plays relative to the preoperative decision-making process is rarely discussed. In addition, although pediatric cochlear implant centers often indicate in their procedural descriptions that a psychological evaluation is conducted as part of the preoperative assessment, exactly what this presurgical psychological evaluation entails is not made clear. Guidelines that identify issues that should be addressed by the psychological evaluation are lacking. Evidence-based research that explains and supports these guidelines is rarely stipulated. Moreover, recommended methods for conducting a psychological evaluation that yield reliable and practical information relevant to the selection and management of children who are candidates for cochlear implants are nearly nonexistent. It could be, as the criteria for pediatric cochlear implantation broadens, that the value of the preoperative psychological evaluation may now be less relevant in terms of determining a child's eligibility and more critical in terms of identifying issues that merit attention and intervention postoperatively.

The field of cochlear implants in children is evolving rapidly. We now know so much more about outcomes for children with cochlear implants and variables that predict benefit. Consequently, guidelines established 15 years ago may be no longer appropriate. Given this dramatic change in the field, how do we now decide whether or not a child is an appropriate recipient of a cochlear implant? On what basis should this decision be made? What factors need to be considered and how should this information be obtained? Finally, what role does the psychologist play in pediatric cochlear implantation?

In the following section, we present recommendations and guidelines for conducting a preoperative psychological evaluation of pediatric CI candidates. These recommendations are based on the research evidence discussed earlier in this chapter coupled with over three decades of combined experience working with CI candidates and recipients. Because children ranging in age from infancy to adolescence are now being implanted, we have organized our recommendations according to broad age groups. Though some issues that require consideration during the preoperative psychological evaluation are critical regardless of the age of the child, there are also variables that are unique to children and adolescents at specific developmental stages.

Infants and Families

With the implementation of newborn hearing screening, parents are now being informed much earlier than they were in the past regarding the possibility that their child has a hearing loss. The vast majority of parents of hearing-impaired children—more than 90%—have had no experience with deafness prior to receiving the diagnosis of their child's hearing loss. Parents of newly diagnosed hearing-impaired children experience a range of emotions, including shock, anger, confusion, fear, and sadness (Kurtzer-White & Luterman, 2003). Understandably, parents of newly diagnosed hearing-impaired children are anxious parents (Feher-Prout, 1996; Luterman, 2001; Pipp-Siegel et al., 2002). They wonder how they will communicate with their child, how their child will learn to speak, and what the future entails. At the same time that parents are working to integrate the meaning of their child's diagnosis and trying to cope with a multitude of ensuing emotions, they are being placed in a position of having to make critical decisions regarding their child's long-term care.

It is common for parents of a child with a hearing loss, and particularly parents of a child with recently diagnosed hearing loss, to grapple with strong emotions regarding the meaning of the diagnosis and the wish to make the child's situation different. The kinds of emotions that parents frequently feel following the diagnosis of their child's hearing loss, as well as the process of coping with these feelings, have been conceptualized within the context of the grief cycle model (Clark & English, 2004; Kurtzer-White & Luterman, 2003). It has been postulated that many parents who are still in shock and feeling emotionally overwhelmed by their child's hearing loss may not have the psychological energy to respond to their child's communication and developmental needs (Calderon & Greenberg, 1999; Kurtzer-White & Luterman, 2003; Luterman, 1997; Meadow-Orlans, 1995). Moreover, parents who are still actively grieving and struggling to cope with the diagnosis of their child's hearing loss may be seeking an implant for their child based on inaccurate assumptions or "unrealistic expectations." Given the emotionally charged situation, parents of recently diagnosed children with hearing loss may have difficulty attending to and processing the information provided to them.

Hearing health care professionals who work with parents of children with recently diagnosed hearing loss need to be sensitive to issues related to the grieving process that may contribute to the parents' unrealistic expectations regarding cochlear implants and their motivation for seeking this treatment option (Kurtzer-White & Luterman, 2003). Some parents may believe that the cochlear implant will make their child "normal" and "function as a hearing person" (Kluwin & Stewart, 2000, p. 29). Certainly, the recent surge in media attention to the "miraculous benefits" of cochlear implants has done much to promote high expectations. Consequently, parents need to be educated regarding the fact that, although benefits from cochlear implantation can be significant and indeed remarkable at times, the device does not typically result in a child achieving fully normal hearing. Furthermore, as we have discussed throughout this chapter, parents need to appreciate that

outcome variability is considerable and our ability to make predictions regarding benefit for any one child is imprecise at this point. Although the modern device can result in substantial benefits, it is critical to place those benefits in the context of the time course of achieving those benefits, the importance of consistent use, and how the range of benefits can compare to results from amplification and other habilitative strategies.

Evaluating Expectations

It is often recommended that one of the goals of the preoperative evaluation is to determine whether the parents have "realistic expectations" regarding the benefits and limitations of a cochlear implant device. But how does one actually access the family's expectations and determine whether they are realistic? Frankly, we tend to agree with Zaidman-Zait and Most (2005), that the notion that we can reliably and accurately distinguish parents with "realistic expectations" from parents with "unrealistic expectations" may be a bit overoptimistic, especially given the lack of clear definition of this term and the wide variability in postimplantation outcomes. Moreover, as the benefits from implantation have advanced, the standards for what constitutes an "unrealistic" expectation also have changed. Expectations that were clearly unrealistic a decade or more ago are not necessarily unrealistic now. Finally, although there is a substantial body of research that provides evidence regarding a relationship between outcome expectations and satisfaction with benefits among new adult hearing aid users, little evidence-based research currently exists to guide clinical practice regarding the significance of evaluating the expectations of parents in pediatric cochlear implantation. On the other hand, intuitively it makes good clinical sense that professionals need to be sensitive to parents' hopes and expectations, and that the parents' motivations for pursuing a cochlear implant for their child need to be explored. Certainly, the wide variability in outcomes following pediatric cochlear implantation needs to be emphasized to parents. Importantly, attention needs to be given to parental expectations on an on-going basis, during both the preoperative evaluation process and the postimplantation rehabilitation stages.

Parents bring to the preoperative evaluation anticipation, expectations, questions, and fears. They hope that the cochlear implant will lead to successful results for their child and reduce the disabling effects of deafness. Although parents may be counseled by the cochlear implant team regarding the fact that a child with a cochlear implant does not function the same way as does a child with normal hearing, parents who are struggling with emotions related to their child's hearing loss may have difficulty accepting this information. Indeed, Zaidman-Zait and Most (2005) investigated maternal hopes and expectations regarding their child's outcomes following cochlear implantation and found that *all* the mothers participating in their study expressed relatively high expectations for improvement in their child's communication, social, and academic skills following cochlear implantation. Moreover, level of maternal expectation regarding the child's potential benefit from implantation did not vary much based on the child's individual characteristics (e.g., child's present age, duration and onset of hearing loss, length of time using the cochlear implant), all of which are known to be potential influences on outcomes. Hence, although professionals may counsel parents regarding the great variability in outcomes among children with cochlear implants, this knowledge does not seem to influence parents' level of expectations and hopes.

Despite the evidence presented, parents remain hopeful. Of course, this is understandable. All parents of deaf children who are seeking cochlear implants are hopeful and have high expectations for their child. Without such hopes it is improbable that they would seek an implant for their child. Professionals who counsel parents during the preoperative evaluation must keep in mind that parental hopes and expectations, as unrealistic as they may seem at times, can also play a positive role, as they can serve to inspire parents and motivate their involvement. Therefore, in this consideration of unrealistic expectations, we are not advocating efforts to dash those hopes. Professionals need to maintain a delicate balance between being supportive and encouraging, without inducing false and unrealistic expectations, while at the same time being realistic, but not squelching the sort of hopes that can motivate efforts and engender parental involvement. Recognizing the potentially significant relationship between parental hopes and expectations and subsequent parent involvement, coupled with the variability in children's outcomes following cochlear implantation, Zaidman-Zait and Most (2005) suggested that professionals involved in counseling parents during the preoperative evaluation not attempt to influence parents' expectations with regard to their child's potential outcomes. Instead, they recommended that the focus of counseling be on helping parents of cochlear implant candidates appreciate the demanding and intensive nature of the (re)habilitative process, as well as supporting and guiding their involvement in their child's education and development.

Evaluating Parental Commitment to Follow-Up Therapy

Because the rehabilitation process is demanding and requires intensive and dedicated long-term commitment on the part of the parents, another purpose of the preoperative evaluation is to assess the parents' commitment to these rehabilitation efforts. The importance of parental involvement in children's early intervention and school-based education programs is now well established, both for typically developing children and children with disabilities. Studies have consistently found that parents who are more involved in their children's education have children who are academically more successful (Epstein, 1990; Griffith, 1996; Grolnick & Slowiaczek, 1994). With respect to children with cochlear implants, though research is limited, studies indicate that parents' involvement in the child's rehabilitation and educational program is associated with positive effects on the child's speech and language development (DesJardin, 2005; Moeller, 2000; Spencer, 2004). In fact, given the crucial importance of parent involvement relative to the child's development, some multidisciplinary implant centers consider parent commitment to participation in the child's postoperative rehabilitation program as essential for cochlear implant candidacy (ASHA, 2004; Geers & Brenner, 2003).

Given the importance that parent involvement plays relative to beneficial outcomes for the young child with a cochlear implant, how should the parents' commitment to the postoperative efforts be evaluated? Although there has been some preliminary work conducted to develop questionnaires that can be used for this purpose, these assessment instruments have not been formally validated. Hence, similar to the process of evaluating the parents' expectations and motivation for seeking a cochlear implant for their child, a sensitive and supportive clinical interview will likely be the most effective means of gathering information regarding the parents' willingness and ability to participate in postoperative rehabilitation programs. A carefully designed discussion with parents can offer the opportunity to explore relevant issues as well as contribute to building a collaborative relationship between parent and professionals. Although this sort of evaluation technique may not yield definitive quantitative information that can be easily summed and the total score applied to judging a child's likeliness to benefit from a cochlear implant, it does provide a forum for exploring relevant issues and contributes to building a collaborative relationship between parents and professionals. Moreover, the information obtained from a clinically focused discussion with parents can be used to design follow-up intervention services and treatment programs that are directly relevant to the individual child and family.

Clinical Interview with Parents

The preoperative clinical interview with parents should be conducted with the purpose of eliciting information regarding:

1. the parents' emotional response relative to their child's hearing loss;
2. their hopes and expectations regarding the potential benefits of cochlear implantation for their child;
3. their understanding of the importance of follow through with postoperative therapy goals; and
4. their commitment to supporting the (re)habilitative process.

Although the goal of the clinical interview is to gather information regarding the child and family, it is important that the clinical interview be conducted with the clear intention of working collaboratively with the parents in effort to come to important decisions regarding the most likely adventitious way to manage the child's hearing loss. Parents will be less apt to be open and forthcoming with their thoughts, concerns, and feelings if they perceive the preoperative clinical interview as a qualifying examination which they and their child must both pass. The preoperative clinical interview should be viewed as an opportunity to build a collaborative relationship between parents and professionals—a partnership which ultimately increases the chances of obtaining successful outcomes for the hearing impaired child and family.

During the preoperative clinical interview, in effort to appreciate how the parents have adjusted to their child's hearing loss and to identify areas that might need further investigation and support, the following topics may be discussed:

1. How did the parents come to learn their child has a hearing loss?
2. How have the child and family (including the siblings) adjusted emotionally to the hearing loss?
3. Did the parents know other individuals who are deaf or hard of hearing prior to learning of their own child's hearing loss?
4. How supportive have family members and relatives been with respect to their child's hearing loss?
5. How supportive have their friends been regarding their child's hearing loss?

Parents' expectations and understanding of the benefits and limitations of a cochlear implant device also need to be carefully explored. For this purpose, the following topics may warrant discussion during the preoperative clinical interview:

1. How did the parents become interested in a cochlear implant for their child?
2. Do they know any other children with cochlear implants?
3. If they do, what are their impressions of how these children are doing?

4. What do they hope will be different if their child has a cochlear implant?
5. What would they most like to see improve?
6. What do they think might continue to be difficult for their child even after receiving a cochlear implant?

As discussed throughout this chapter, because parental involvement in the (re)habilitation process has been shown to be instrumental in postoperative services and enhancing the benefits of cochlear implantation and ultimately the child's progress, the clinical interview should address the parents' understanding of their responsibility to follow through with postoperative services. Some topic areas that may be appropriate for discussion during the preoperative clinical interview are the following:

1. Have the parents been involved in parent/infant educational services or programs?
2. If so, what aspects of these services or programs did they find to be most helpful?
3. Have they had any difficulty attending programs or services? If so, for what reasons?
4. Do they anticipate having difficulty attending educational programs in the future if their child receives a cochlear implant?
5. What issues might make attendance problematic?

Although parental involvement and engagement is important, it is also important to note that it would be inappropriate to hold pediatric implant candidates hostage to deficient or disengaged parents. Rather, in circumstances where parental involvement is likely to be limited or deficient, it would be desirable for implant teams to identify and facilitate alternative systems for providing the support and engagement that most typically comes from effective parents. Additionally, it is important for the implant team not to make decisions that regress on the socioeconomic status of the families. Poverty can certainly compromise effective parenting, but it is also the case that the circumstances of poverty can compromise the clinician's recognition of parental strengths and the prospects for full engagement in the implant process.

School-Aged Children

As cochlear implants are becoming an increasingly more common habilitation option for individuals who are deaf, it is not unusual for parents of school-aged children who are deaf, or even school-aged children themselves, to express an interest in obtaining an implant. A large body of research suggests that among congenitally and early deafened children, age of implantation correlates strongly with speech perception (Huang, Yang, Sher, Lin, & Wu, 2005; Kirk et al., 2002; Miyamoto et al., 1997a), with children implanted before the age of 3 years demonstrating better speech perception skills than do children implanted after the age of 3 years. However, some older children have been found to show benefit from cochlear implants (Osberger, Fisher, Zimmerman-Phillips, Geier, & Barker, 1998; Tomblin, Barker, & Hubbs, 2007). Given this variability in outcome, it is recommended that older children should not be automatically excluded as inappropriate cochlear implant candidates (Clark, 2003).

The purpose of the preoperative evaluation of school-aged children is essentially the same as that of the preoperative evaluation of very young children—that is, to explore reasons for seeking an implant and to determine whether the child can likely benefit from this form of intervention. Whereas the very young child is not able to express an opinion regarding the possibility of receiving a cochlear implant, the school-aged child certainly is. Therefore, it is important to actively include the older child in the preoperative evaluation process. Obviously, the motivation for receiving a cochlear implant and expectations regarding outcomes need to be explored from both the parents' and child's perspective, as suggested in the following questions:

1. Whose idea was it to seek a cochlear implant, the parents' or the child's?
2. What are the reasons that they are now seeking a cochlear implant?
3. What are they hoping will change?
4. Are there concerns or behaviors that the parents or child believe will change as a result of the cochlear implant?
5. How realistic are these expectations?
6. Does the child know any other individuals his or her age who have a cochlear implant?
7. How does the child currently communicate—sign language, speech, or a combination of sign language and speech?
8. Does the child have any other disabilities that may be impacting his or her communication abilities?

And finally, because a child's schedule of using his or her hearing aids is a strong predictor of the child's future willingness to use the cochlear implant, information relative to the child's attitude towards wearing his or her hearing aids should be explored.

Adolescents

As cochlear implantation is becoming more common and its related technology more advanced, hearing healthcare professionals and the implant team are encountering a greater number of older children seeking cochlear implants devices. The adolescent presents unique social and psychological issues that must be carefully addressed both during the preoperative evaluation and post-operatively. Topics addressed in the clinical interview with school-aged pediatric implant candidates are topics that should also be addressed with the adolescent implant candidate—for example, reasons for seeking a cochlear implant, expectations regarding benefits, and current use and attitude regarding amplification. However, adolescence introduces social and personal issues that are unique to that developmental period and warrant special consideration.

Adolescence frequently is characterized by a process of individuation from parents and a greater need for autonomy. Therefore, establishing separate yet integrated collaborative relationships with both the adolescent and his or her parents will be essential when working with this age group. The adolescent implant candidate should be encouraged to play an active role in the preoperative evaluation and the design and planning of postoperative rehabilitation goals. During the preoperative evaluation interview, careful attention should be given to exploring the extent to which the idea for obtaining a cochlear implant was the teenager's or the parents'. How motivated is the adolescent about having a cochlear implant device? Does he or she have conflicting feelings about obtaining a cochlear implant? Because teenagers are especially sensitive about appearing different from their peers and attention to self-image tends to take on greater significance during this stage of development, the teenager's concerns regarding the cosmetic aspects of the implant device should not be minimized. Indeed, it is important that these issues and concerns be carefully addressed. Peer pressure is also considerable during adolescence and may serve as a deterring or motivating factor. The teenage candidate may be reluctant to receive a cochlear implant, possibly due to pressure from his peers to remain "deaf." On a similar but alternative note, the teenager may want a cochlear implant because she is experiencing social and emotional difficulties with hearing peers and wishes to be "hearing." Whatever the case, clearly the motivation for seeking an implant needs to be explored carefully, both with the adolescent and the parents.

Regardless of whether the adolescent is emancipated, there are several reasons why the adult protocol might be more suitable for an adolescent than preadolescent children. They will increasingly need to use and maintain the device themselves. The decision process should not be one in which the use of the device can become a vehicle for challenging or debating their parents. Perhaps most importantly, the research literature that identifies psychological preimplant predictors for adult recipients might be applied to the adolescents. That is, the same protocol and the measures that cannot be used with young children could be applied to adolescent candidates (e.g., Knutson et al., 1991).

Utilizing Standardized Assessment Psychological Instruments

Use of standardized psychological assessment instruments may be warranted during the preoperative evaluation in order to gain specific information about the child's cognitive development and psychosocial functioning, as well as to identify certain behavioral characteristics that may compromise the child's ability to benefit from a cochlear implant (e.g., attention difficulties, impulsivity). Standardized assessment tools have the advantage of yielding scores that can be used to compare an individual child's performance on certain tasks with the performance of other children the same age. In addition, standardized assessment tools can help identify areas of strengths and weaknesses for a child, thereby enabling the rehabilitation treatment program to be tailored to the specific needs of the individual child and his or her family. Measures taken before and after implantation can be used to help track a child's progress and determine outcome benefits. And, certainly, the use of standardized measures is essential when conducting empirically based research so that research findings are readily interpretable and experimental procedures can be replicated by other investigators in the future.

Clearly there are many advantages of utilizing standardized psychological instruments to assess children with cochlear implants. However, as previously discussed, few standardized instruments may be appropriate for use with deaf children, and especially very young deaf children, due to the language and auditory processing demands of the measure. Noting these limitations, the following psychological standardized measures are suggested as potentially helpful for obtaining targeted information during the preoperative evaluation with young children with hearing loss, as well as for use in evidence-based outcome research on pediatric cochlear implantation. The list of assessment measures described below by no means should be considered exhaustive either in terms of the assessment instruments available or in terms of the domains that may warrant consideration.

Cognitive Functioning

The implant team may want to know information about the young child's cognitive skills. It is critically important when selecting assessment tools for use with deaf and hard-of-hearing children that the instrument's demands on audition and language be carefully considered. Unfortunately, intelligence testing of deaf and hard-of-hearing children has had a long history of inappropriate application of assessment instruments designed to evaluate the cognitive skills of typically hearing individuals, with limited regard to ways in which severe hearing loss may influence the child's performance on these measures (Marschack, 2006; Vernon, 2005). The following are popular standardized measures of cognitive ability that may be used to evaluate infants and toddlers with hearing loss.

Bayley Scales of Infant Development-Third Edition (BSID-III) (Bayley, 2005)

The BSID-III measures the cognitive and motor development of infants from 1 to 42 months of age. The test, which takes approximately 45 minutes, is administered individually by having the child respond to a series of stimuli and tasks. The Mental Scale yields a normalized standard score called the Mental Developmental Index. At the early developmental stages, the Mental Scale assesses a variety of skills and abilities, including sensory/perceptual, acquisition of object constancy, memory, learning, and problem solving. However, the test items designed for older infants often include tasks that require vocalization, beginning verbal communication skills, and complex language and concept formation. Hence, the hearing-impaired infant and toddler will likely fail these items, not because of issues related to cognitive weaknesses but because of the child's linguistic and auditory deficits.

Leiter International Performance Scale-Revised (Leiter-R) (Roid & Miller, 1997)

The Leiter-R is an individually administered test that examines conceptual ability, but does not require receptive or expressive communication skills. It is designed for individuals aged 2 years, 0 months through 20 years, 11 months. The Leiter-R has been regarded as particularly useful for evaluating the cognitive skills of children who are not easily assessed with more traditional and generally verbally based measures of intelligence. The test consists of game-like activities that require the examinee to apply spatial, visual, and conceptually mediated logical reasoning. The Leiter-R yields a general intelligence composite score and secondary cognitive ability scores in the following areas: Visualization (spatial), Reasoning, Attention, and Memory. It is relatively quick to administer (approximately 40 minutes for the six subtests on the Visualization and Reasoning Battery). However, the child must exhibit some sustained attention, which can be problematic for young children with hearing loss.

Mullen Scales of Early Learning (MSEL) (Mullen, 1995)

The Mullen Scales assess the cognitive functioning of young children from birth to 68 months. Based on the premise that a global measure of intellectual performance may mask uneven cognitive development, the MSEL assesses five skill areas, including gross motor (assessed from birth to 33 months) and four "cognitive" skills (assessed from birth to 68 months): fine motor, visual reception, receptive language, and expressive language. The MSEL accounts for differential development in distinct domains by structuring items to challenge

only the modality under test. Administration of the MSEL at age 1 year takes approximately 15 minutes; at age 3 years, test administration time increases to approximately 35 minutes.

Wechsler Preschool and Primary Scale of Intelligence-Third Edition (WPPSI-III) (Wechsler, 2002)

The WPPSI-III is an individually administered instrument that assesses the cognitive functions in children from 2 years, 6 months to 7 years, 3 months of age. For children younger than 4 years old, test administration takes approximately 30 to 45 minutes. For older children, test administration time increases to approximately one hour. The WPPSI-III provides standardized measures of a variety of abilities reflecting different aspects of intelligence. The test provides three IQ measures: Full Scale IQ, Verbal IQ, and Performance IQ. For young children with severe hearing loss and likely linguistic deficits, the Verbal Scale would not be an accurate measure of the child's cognitive aptitude as audition and expressive and receptive skills are required. However, the WPPSI-III Performance Scale has frequently been used to evaluate the cognitive skills of children with hearing loss as well as young children with speech and language difficulties.

Behavior Rating Inventory of Executive Function-Preschool Version (BRIEF-P) (Gioia, Espy, & Isquith, 2003)

Although the BRIEF-P is not a measure of intelligence per se, it does assess neuropsychological skills and behaviors that may interfere with a child's ability to make use of his or her cognitive potential (e.g., working memory, attention, inhibition). The BRIEF-P, which is designed for children between the ages of 2 years, 0 months and 5 years, 11 months, consists of a single Rating Form used by parents, teachers, and day care providers to rate a child's executive functions within the context of his or her everyday environments—home and preschool. The BRIEF-P consists of 63 items that measure various aspects of executive functioning: Inhibit, Shift, Emotional Control, Working Memory, and Plan/Organize. The clinical scales form three broad indexes (Inhibitory Self-Control, Flexibility, and Emergent Metacognition) and one composite score (Global Executive Composite). The BRIEF-P also provides two validity scales (Inconsistency and Negativity). It requires approximately 10 to 15 minutes to complete.

Social and Emotional Adjustment

The implant team may want to know something about the child's social and emotional adjustment. As discussed previously, the social-emotional adjustment of the child and compliance with daily use-time of the implant device has been found to have a significant effect on outcome.

Behavior Assessment System for Children, Second Edition (BASC-2) (Reynolds & Kamphaus, 2004)

The BASC-2 is a comprehensive set of rating scales for children between the ages of 2 years, 0 months and 21 years, 11 months that measure both problem behaviors and competencies in the home, community, and school setting. Parents or caregivers and teachers can complete forms at three age levels: preschool (ages 2 to 5), child (ages 6 to 11),

and adolescent (ages 12 to 21). Completion of forms takes about 10 to 20 minutes. The parent-report BASC-2 for preschoolers includes nine problem-behavior scales: Aggression, Anxiety, Attention, Atypicality, Depression, Hyperactivity, Somatization, and Withdrawal; and four adaptive (or competency) scales: Activities of Daily Living, Adaptability, Functional Communication, and Social Skills. The teacher-report addresses the same areas except for Activities of Daily Living.

Child Behavior Checklist for 1.5–5 (CBCL/1.5–5) (Achenbach & Rescorla, 2000)

The CBCL/1.5–5 is a measure of behavioral and emotional problems for use with children between the ages of 1.5 and 5 years. The CBCL/1.5–5 is composed of 99 items rated by parents about the child which yield three domains and related subscales: (a) Internalizing domain, which includes Emotional Reactive, Anxious/Depressed, Somatic Complaints, and Withdrawn subscales; (b) Externalizing domain, which is comprised of Attention Problems and Aggressive Behavior; and Total Problems Score, which is composed of the Internalizing domain, Externalizing domain, Sleep Problems and Other Problems. Several DSM-Oriented scales have been created to address Affective Problems, Anxiety Problems, Pervasive Developmental Problems, Attention Deficit/Hyperactivity Problems, and Oppositional Defiant Problems.

Caretaker-Teacher Report Form 1.5–5 (C-TRF 1.5–5) (Achenbach & Rescorla, 2001)

The C-TRF 1.5–5 is similar to the CBCL, but is designed to be completed by service providers, daycare providers, and teachers regarding behavioral problems, disabilities, what concerns the respondent most about the child, and the best things about the child.

Infant Toddler Social and Emotional Assessment (ITSEA) (Carter & Briggs-Gowan, 2005; Carter & Briggs-Gowan, 2006)

The ITSEA is a parent-report questionnaire, comprised of 161 items, that assesses social-emotional/behavioral problems and competencies in 12- to 36-month-old children. The ITSEA includes three problem domains: Externalizing (i.e., Activity/Impulsivity, Aggression/Defiance, and Peer Aggression scales); Internalizing (i.e., Depression/Withdrawal, General Anxiety, Separation Distress, and Inhibition to Novelty scales), and Dysregulation (i.e., Sleep, Negative Emotionality, Eating, and Sensory Sensitivity scales). Parents rate how well each statement describes their child's behavior in the past month on a 3-point scale: (0) Not true/rarely, (1) Somewhat true/sometimes, and (2) Very true/often. A "no opportunity" code and an outgrown code are provided for some items. Higher scores on the Externalizing and Dysregulation scales reflect greater levels of problem behaviors; higher scores on the Competence scales indicate greater competence. In addition to measuring problem behaviors in early childhood, the ITSEA assesses social emotional competencies, or adaptive behaviors. The Competence Domain of the ITSEA is composed of 37 items measuring behaviors that develop in early childhood in the areas of empathy, compliance, prosocial peer, attention skills, mastery motivation, and imitation/play. Higher scores indicate greater competence.

Adaptive Behavior

Vineland Adaptive Behavior Scales-Second Edition (Vineland-II) (Sparrow, Balla, & Cicchetti, 2005)

The Vineland-II is an individually administered measure of personal and social sufficiency for ages birth to 90 years. The Vineland-II assesses adaptive functioning in four domains: Communication, Daily Living Skills, Socialization, and Motor Skills domains. The Vineland-II is a revision of the Vineland Adaptive Behavior Scales (VABS) (Sparrow, Ballow, & Cicchetti, 1984). The new edition has added items in each of the four domains, and especially in the birth through 3-year range. The increased item density during the early developmental years allows for a more complete picture of the very young child's strengths and weaknesses and growth in adaptive functioning (Sparrow et al., 2005). The Vineland-II gathers data using a semistructure interview, in which the parent (or caregiver) is asked to identify the skills and behaviors the child demonstrates on a regular basis. Communication skills include such things as understanding the meaning of yes and no and naming (using speech or sign language) at least 10 objects; daily living skills include feeding self with fork and letting someone know when diapers are wet or soiled; socialization skills include smiling or making sounds when approached by a familiar person and choosing to play with other children; and motor skills include sitting supported for one minute. Administration of the Vineland-11 for infants and toddlers takes approximately 20 minutes. For older children and adolescents, test administration time increases to approximately 45 to 60 minutes. A Parent/ Caregiver Rating Form also is available and covers the same content as the Survey Interview, but uses a rating scale format. This alternative method is suggested when time or access is limited.

Vineland Adaptive Behavior Scales–Second Edition, Teacher Rating Form (Sparrow et al., 2005)

The Vineland-II Teacher Rating Form assesses adaptive behavior for children in school, preschool, or a structured daycare setting (ages 36 months and older). The Teacher Rating Form contains the same Domains as the Survey Forms but covers content that a teacher would observe in a classroom or preschool setting. For example, the Communications Domain measures how a child listens, pays attention, and uses words to speak and write. The Daily Living Skills Domain evaluates a child's daily habits and hygiene; understanding about time, money, and math; and ability to follow rules and routines. The Socialization Domain measures how a child interacts with others, uses play and leisure time, and demonstrates responsibility and sensitivity to others. The Motor Skills Domain assesses both gross and fine motor skills.

Parental Stress

Parenting Stress Index, 3rd Edition (PSI) (Abidin, 1995)

The PSI is a 101-item questionnaire that identifies the magnitude of stress in the parent-child system. It is designed to target dysfunctional parenting and predicts the potential for parental behavior problems and child adjustment difficulties within the family system. The PSI yields a Total Stress Score as well as scale scores related to child and parent characteristics. It takes the parent

around 20-25 minutes to complete. A Short Form of the PSI is also available, which is composed of 36 items from the full-length PSI. It can be completed in approximately 10 to 15 minutes. Similar to the full-length PSI, the Short Form PSI yields a Total Stress Score.

Parental Sensitivity and Emotionally Availability

Emotional Availability Scales-3rd Edition (EA Scale); (Biringen, Robinson, & Emde, 1993)

The EA Scales is a measure that assesses six dimensions of the emotional availability of the parent toward the child and of the child toward the parent. Using a 10-minute videotaped play interaction between mother and child, the EA Scales is designed to systematically assess the parental dimensions of sensitivity, structuring, non-intrusiveness, and non-hostility. The child dimensions include the child's responsiveness to the parent and the child's involvement of the parent. The Maternal Sensitivity Scale assesses mother's responsiveness to her child in terms of timing, flexibility, the quality and appropriateness of her affect, and her negotiation of conflictual situations. This scale is rated on a 9-point scale, with a score of 1 indicating lack of sensitivity and a score of 9 indicating high sensitivity. The Maternal Structuring/Intrusiveness Scale assesses the extent that the mother scaffolds her child's play and sets limits without being intrusive or controlling. It is evaluated on a 5-point scale, with a score of 1 indicating an absence of structuring and a score of 5 indicating optimal structuring. The Non-intrusiveness scale measures the parent's ability to be available to the child without being intrusive or overly directive. This scale is rated on a 5-point scale, with a score of 1 indicating intrusive and a score of 5 indicating nonintrusive. The Parental Non-Hostility scale judges the degree of the parent's overt and covert maternal hostility using a 5-point scale, with a score of 1 indicating overt and blatant hostility and 5 indicating no observed hostility.

The Child's Responsiveness Scale assesses the child's display of pleasure and eagerness to engage the mother in interaction using a 7-point scale. A score of 1 indicates lack of responsiveness and a score of 7 indicates an optimal balance between responsiveness to the parent and autonomous activities. The Child Involvement with Parent Scale assesses the degree to which the child attends to the parent and engages the parent in play. A score of 1 indicates absence of involvement and a score of 7 indicates optimal involvement in which the child shows a balance between autonomous play and drawing the parent into interaction.

Parental Involvement and Self-Efficacy

Scale of Parental Involvement and Self-Efficacy (SPISE) (DesJardin, 2003)

The SPISE was designed to measure parents' perspectives about specific skills necessary to work with their young child with hearing loss and the extent to which parents perceive themselves as involved in skills related to their child's sensory device use and strategies to develop their child's speech-language acquisition. The SPISE consists of three sections: Demographic Information, Maternal Self-Efficacy, and Parental Involvement. The Maternal Self-Efficacy section consists of ten questions that are rated on a 7-point Likert-type scale ranging from 1 ("not at all") to 7 ("very much"). Items in this section represent mothers' perceptions of their degree of influence on the child's auditory development. Issues tapped include her role in early intervention; degree to which the mother feels competent in care and follow-through with the child's daily amplification; degree to which the mother feels she can make a difference in her child's language development; and the extent to which she believes that she has the knowledge and competence to follow-through with speech/language activities. The section on Parental Involvement consists of twelve questions that represent parent involvement in the use of their child's amplification and early intervention program. For a more comprehensive discussion of this measure, the reader is referred to DesJardin's chapter (Chapter 17) in this book.

Maternal Efficacy Scale (Teti & Gelfand, 1991)

The Maternal Efficacy Scale is a 10-item parent questionnaire designed to assess maternal perceptions of effectiveness in several domains of childcare, such as soothing the child, knowing what the child wants, getting the child to understand what the mother wants). Items are rated on a 4-point scale, with higher scores indicating higher feelings of effectiveness.

Conclusion

The field of pediatric cochlear implantation has advanced considerably over the past 20 years. Despite the accumulating evidence of positive benefits resulting from pediatric cochlear implantation, large variation in outcomes for children implanted continues to exist for reasons which we are not yet fully able to explain. Moreover, predictions of outcome in the individual case are not nearly as advanced as clinicians and parents might hope. We now know so much more about the variables that may lead to improved auditory speech recognition and speech production ability in hearing-impaired children after cochlear implantation. However, we are just beginning to scratch the surface with research in the efficacy of pediatric cochlear implantation on psychological and social-emotional domains, and research on putative predictors of implant outcome has not advanced with the implantation of younger and younger children and some changes in the devices. Although cochlear implantation may no longer be viewed as a high-risk medical procedure, the choice whether or not to pursue implantation is not a simple one. Parents of hearing-impaired children and the professionals who serve these children and their families want to know what the potential benefits will be.

In this chapter we have reviewed the existing research and clinical information as to how psychological variables might play a role in predicting and understanding implant benefit and how psychological change can follow implant use. Based on that review, we have addressed the ways in which psychologists on an implant team contribute to the preoperative evaluation and continue to serve as a vital part of the organization and system for helping to determine children who are appropriate pediatric implant candidates. We also have emphasized, however, as the criteria for pediatric cochlear implantation shifts and evolves over time, so too does the focus and purpose of the psychologist in the preoperative evaluation. We believe that the true value of the preoperative psychological evaluation rests not so much in its function to determine who is or who is not eligible for implantation. Rather, the preoperative psychological evaluation,

in concert with other activities of the implant team, offers the opportunity to partner with parents of hearing-impaired children and identify those issues that potentially promote or possibly interfere with optimal developmental outcomes for the child. Moreover, the information obtained from the psychological preoperative evaluation can be used to help design and advocate for follow-up intervention services and treatment programs that are directly relevant to the needs of the individual child and family. The authors continue to believe that psychological variables in pediatric cochlear implantation retain their currency and that psychological research with pediatric cochlear implant candidates and recipients continues to be an important area of inquiry and that such research should guide improved clinical practice.

Acknowledgments. Preparation of this chapter was supported, in part, by grant 2 P50 DC00242 from the National Institute on Deafness and Other Communication Disorders, NIH; grant M01-RR-59 from the General Clinical Research Centers Program, National Center for Research Resources, NIH; the Lions Clubs International Foundation; and Iowa Lions Foundation.

References

Abidin, R. R. (1995). *Parenting Stress Index* (3rd ed.). Lutz, FL: Psychological Assessment Resources.

Abidin, R. R., Jenkins, C. L., & McGaughey, M. C. (1992). The relationship of early family variables to children's subsequent behavioral adjustment. *Journal of Clinical Child Psychology, 21*, 60–69.

Achenbach, T. M., & Edelbrock, C. (1991). *Manual for child behavior checklist*. Burlington, VT: University of Vermont, Department of Psychiatry.

Achenbach, T. M., & Rescorla, L. A. (2000). *Manual for the ASEBA Preschool Forms and Profiles (1.5-5)*. Burlington, VT: University of Vermont, Research Center for Children, Youth and Families.

Achenbach, T. M., & Rescorla, L. A. (2001). *Manual for the ASEBA Caretaker-Teacher Report Forms and Profiles (1.5-5)*. Burlington, VT: University of Vermont, Research Center for Children, Youth and Families.

American Speech-Language-Hearing Association. (2004). *Cochlear implants* [Technical report]. Available from http://www.asha.org/policy

Archbold, S. M., Nikolopoulos, T. P., Lutman, M. E., & O'Donoghue, G. M. (2002). The educational settings of profoundly deaf children with cochlear implants compared with age-matched peers with hearing aids: Implications for management. *International Journal of Audiology, 41*, 157-161.

Arthur, G. (1949). The Arthur adaptation of the Leiter International Performance Scale. *Journal of Clinical Psychology, 5*, 345-349.

Bassarath, L. (2001). Conduct Disorder: A biopsychosocial review. *Canadian Journal of Psychiatry/La Revue Canadienne de Psychiatrie, 46*, 609-616.

Bat-Chava, Y., & Deignan, E. (2001). Peer relationships of children with cochlear implants, *Journal of Deaf Studies and Deaf Education, 6*, 186-199.

Bat-Chava, Y., & Martin, D. (2002). Sibling relationships for deaf children: The impact of child and family characteristics, *Rehabilitation Psychology, 47*, 73-91.

Bat-Chava, Y., Martin, D., & Kosciw, J. G. (2005). Longitudinal improvements in communication and socialization of deaf children with cochlear implants and hearing aids: Evidence from parental reports. *Journal of Child Psychology and Psychiatry, 46*, 1287-1296.

Bayley, N. (2005). *Bayley Scales of Infant Development, Third Edition*. San Antonio, TX: Pearson Education.

Beidel, D. C., Turner, S. M., & Morris, T. L. (2000). Behavioral treatment of childhood social phobia. *Journal of Consulting and Clinical Psychology, 68*, 1072-1080.

Berg, A. L., Ip, S. C., Hurst, M., & Herb, A. (2007). Cochlear implants in young children: Informed consent as a process and current practices. *American Journal of Audiology, 16*, 13-28.

Biringen, Z., Robinson, J., & Emde, R. (1993). *Emotional Availability Scale*. Denver: University of Colorado Health Sciences Center, Department of Human Development and Family Studies.

Biringen, Z., Robinson, J., & Emde, R. (1998). *Emotional Availability Scales (3rd ed.), Infancy/Early Childhood Version*. Denver: University of Colorado Health Sciences Center, Department of Human Development and Family Studies.

Boyd, R. C., Knutson, J. F., & Dahlstrom, A. J. (2000). Social interaction of pediatric cochlear implant recipients with age-matched peers. *Annals of Otology, Rhinology, and Laryngology, 109*(Suppl. 185), 105-109.

Brinich, P. M. (1980). Childhood deafness and maternal control. *Journal of Communication Disorders, 13*, 75-81.

Burger, T., Spahn, C., Richter, B., Eissele, S., Lohle, E., & Bengel, J. (2006). Psychic stress and quality of life in parents during decisive phases in the therapy of their hearing-impaired children. *Ear and Hearing, 27*, 313-320.

Calderon, R., & Greenberg, M. (1999). Stress and coping in hearing mothers of deaf and hard of hearing children: Factors affecting mother and child adjustment. *American Annals of the Deaf, 144*, 7-18.

Carter, A. S., & Briggs-Gowan, M. (2005). *ITSEA/BITSEA Infant Toddler and Brief Infant Toddler Social Emotional Assessment Examiner's manual*. San Antonio, TX: Harcourt Assessment.

Carter, A. S., & Briggs-Gowan, M. (2006). *ITSEA Infant-Toddler and Brief Infant Toddler Social Emotional Assessment Examiner's manual*. San Antonio, TX: Harcourt Assessment.

Chamberlain, P., & Reid, J. B. (1987). Parent observation and report of child symptoms, *Behavioral Assessment, 9*, 97-109.

Chin, S. B., Tsai, P. L., & Gao, S. (2003). Connected speech intelligibility of children with cochlear implants and children with normal hearing.

American Journal of Speech-Language Pathology, 12, 440–451.

Christensen, A., Margolin, G., & Sullaway, M. (1992). Interparental agreement on child behavior problems. *Psychological Assessment, 4*, 419–425.

Clark, G. (2003). *Cochlear implants: Fundamentals and applications.* New York: Springer-Verlag.

Clark, J. G., & English, K. M. (2004). *Counseling in audiologic practice: Helping patients and families adjust to hearing loss.* Boston: Pearson Education.

Cleary, M., Pisoni, D. B., & Kirk, K. I. (2002). Working memory spans as predictors of spoken word recognition and receptive vocabulary in children with cochlear implants, *Volta Review, 102*, 259–280.

Cox, M. J., & Paley, B. (1997). Families as systems, *Annual Review of Psychology, 48*, 243–267.

Crary, W. G., Wexler, M., Berliner, K. I., & Miller, L. W. (1982). Psychometric studies and clinical interviews with cochlear implant patients. *Annals of Otology, Rhinology, and Laryngology, 91*(Suppl. 91), 55–81.

Dawson, P. W., Busby, P. A., McKay, C. M., & Clark, G. M. (2002). Short-term auditory memory in children using cochlear implants and its relevance to receptive language. *Journal of Speech, Language, and Hearing Research, 45*, 789–801.

DesJardin, J. L. (2003). Assessing parental perceptions of self-efficacy and involvement in families of young children with hearing loss. *Volta Review, 103*, 391–409.

DesJardin, J. L. (2005). Maternal perceptions of self-efficacy and involvement in the auditory development of young children with prelingual deafness. *Journal of Early Intervention, 27*, 193–209.

Dodge, K. A., Pettit, G. S., McClaskey, C. L., & Brown, M. M. (1986). Social competence in children. *Monographs of the Society for Research in Child Development, 51*(2, Serial No. 213).

Donaldson, A. I., Heavner, K. S., & Zwolan, T. A. (2004). Measuring progress in children with autism spectrum disorder who have cochlear implants. *Archives of Otolaryngology-Head and Neck Surgery, 130*, 666–671.

Edwards, L. C., Frost, R., & Witham, F. (2006). Developmental delay and outcomes in paediatric cochlear implantation: Implications for candidacy. *International Journal of Pediatric Otorhinolaryngology, 70*, 1593–1600.

Eisenberg, L. S., Johnson, K. C., Martinez, A. S., Cokely, C. G., Tobey, E. A., Quittner, A. L., Fink, N. E., Wang, N. Y., Niparko, J. K., & CDaCI Investigative Team. (2006). Speech recognition at 1-year follow-up in the Childhood Development after Cochlear Implantation Study: Methods and preliminary findings. *Audiology and Neurotology, 11*, 259–268.

Epstein, J. I. (1990). School and family connections: Theory, research, and implications for integrating sociologies of education and family. *Marriage and Family Review, 15*, 99–126.

Evans, J. W. (1989). Thoughts on the psychosocial implications of cochlear implantation in children. In E. Owens & D. K. Kessler (Eds.), *Cochlear implants in young deaf children* (pp. 307–314). Boston: College-Hill Press.

Feher-Prout, T. (1996). Stress and coping in families with deaf children. *Journal of Deaf Studies and Deaf Education, 1*, 155–166.

Flipsen, P., Jr., & Colvard, L. G. (2006). Intelligibility of conversational speech produced by children with cochlear implants. *Journal of Communication Disorders, 39*, 93–108.

Fox, L., Long, S. H., & Langlois, A. (1988). Patterns of language comprehension deficit in abused and neglected children. *Journal of Speech and Hearing Disorders, 53*, 239–244.

Fryauf-Bertschy, H., Tyler, R. S., Kelsay, D. M., & Gantz, B. J. (1992). Performance over time of congenitally deaf and postlingually deafened children using a multichannel cochlear implant. *Journal of Speech and Hearing Research, 35*, 913–920.

Fryauf-Bertschy, H., Tyler, R. S., Kelsay, D. M., Gantz, B. J., & Woodworth, G. G. (1997). Cochlear implant use by prelingually deafened children: The influences of age at implant and length of device use. *Journal of Speech, Language, and Hearing Research, 40*, 183–199.

Fukuda, S., Fukushima, K., Maeda, Y., Tsukamura, K., Nagayasu, R., Toida, N., et al. (2003). Language development of a multiply handicapped child after cochlear implantation. *Interna-*

tional Journal of Pediatric Otorhinolaryngology, 67, 627-633.

Gallaudet Research Institute. (December 2006). *Regional and national summary report of data from the 2006-2007 annual survey of deaf and hard of hearing children and youth.* Washington, DC: GRI, Gallaudet University.

Gantz, B. J., Tyler, R. S., Tye-Murray, N., & Fryauf-Bertschy, H. (1994). Long term results of multichannel cochlear implants in congenitally deaf children. In I. J. Hochmair-Desoyer & E. S. Hochmair (Eds.), *Advances in cochlear implants* (pp. 528-533). Vienna: Manz.

Gantz, B. J., Tyler, R. S., Woodworth, G. G., Tye-Murray, N., & Fryauf-Bertschy, H. (1994). Results of multichannel cochlear implants in congenital and acquired prelingual deafness in children: Five-year followup. *American Journal of Otology, 15*(Suppl. 2), 1-7.

Geers, A., & Brenner, C. (2003). Background and educational characteristics of prelingually deaf children implanted before 5 years of age. *Ear and Hearing, 24*(Suppl.), 2S-14S.

Geers, A. E., Brenner, C., & Davidson, L. (2003b). Factors associated with development of speech perception skills in children implanted by age five. *Ear and Hearing, 24*(Suppl.), 24S-35S.

Geers, A. E., Nicholas, J. G., & Sedey, A. L. (2003a). Language skills of children with early cochlear implantation. *Ear and Hearing, 24*(Suppl.), 46S-58S.

Gfeller, K., Christ, A., Knutson, J. F., Witt, S., & Mehr, M. (2003). The effects of familiarity and complexity on appraisal of complex songs by cochlear implant recipients and normal hearing adults. *Journal of Music Therapy, 40,* 78-112.

Gfeller, K., Christ, A., Knutson, J. F., Witt, S., Murray, K. T., & Tyler, R. S. (2000). Musical backgrounds, listening habits, and aesthetic enjoyment of adult cochlear implant recipients. *Journal of American Academic Audiology, 11,* 390-406.

Gfeller, K., Knutson, J. F., Woodworth, G., Witt, S., & DeBus, B. (1998). Timbral recognition and appraisal by adult cochlear implant users and normally hearing adults. *Journal of the American Academy of Audiology, 9,* 1-19.

Gfeller, K., Witt, S. A., Spencer, L. J., & Tomblin, B. (1998). Musical involvement and enjoyment

of children who use cochlear implants. *Volta Review, 100,* 213-233.

Gfeller, K., Witt, S., Woodworth, G., Mehr, M. A., & Knutson, J. F. (2002). Effects of frequency, instrumental family and cochlear implant type of timbre recognition and appraisal. *Annals of Otology, Rhinology, and Laryngology, 111,* 349-356.

Gfeller, K., Woodworth, G., Robin, D. A., Witt, S., & Knutson, J. F. (1997). Perception of rhythmic and sequential pitch patterns by normally hearing adults and adult cochlear implant users. *Ear and Hearing, 18,* 252-260.

Gioia, G. A., Espy, K. A., & Isquith, P. K. (2003). *Behavior Rating Inventory of Executive Function—Preschool Version™ (BRIEF-P™).* Lutz, FL: Psychological Assessment Resources.

Gottman, J. M., & Graziano, W. G. (1983). How children become friends. *Monographs of the Society for Research in Child Development, 48*(3, Serial No. 201).

Greenbaum, P. E., Decrick, R. F., Prange, M. E., & Friedman, R. M. (1994). Parent, teacher, and child ratings of problem behaviors of youngsters with serious emotional disturbances. *Psychological Assessment, 6,* 141-148.

Greenberg, M. T. (1980). Social interactions between deaf preschoolers and their mothers: The effects of communication method and communication competence. *Developmental Psychology, 16,* 465-474.

Greenberg, M. T., & Kusche, C. A. (1989). Cognitive, personal, and social development of deaf children and adolescents. In M. C. Wang, M. C. Reynolds, & H. J. Walberg. (Eds.), *The handbook of special education: Research and practice* (Vols. 1-3, pp. 95-129). Oxford, England: Pergamon Press.

Greenberg, M. T., & Kusche, C. A. (1993). *Promoting social and emotional development in deaf children.* Seattle: University of Washington Press.

Griffith, J. (1996). Relation of parental involvement, empowerment, and school traits to student academic performance. *Journal of Educational Research, 90,* 33-41.

Grolnick, W. S., & Slowiaczek, M. L. (1994). Parents' involvement in children's schooling: A multidimensional conceptualization and motivational model. *Child Development, 65,* 237-252.

Harrison, R. V., Panesar, J., El-Hakim, H., Abdolell, M., Mount, R. J., & Papsin, B. (2001). The effects of age of cochlear implantation on speech perception outcomes in prelingually deaf children. *Scandinavian Audiology Supplement, 53,* 73-78.

Hathaway, S. R., & McKinley, J. C. (1943). *Minnesota Multiphasic Personality Inventory.* Minneapolis: University of Minnesota.

Hinshaw, S. P., Han, S. S., Erhardt, D., & Huber, A. (1992). Internalizing and externalizing behavior problems in preschool children: Correspondence among parent and teacher ratings and behavior observations. *Journal of Clinical Child Psychology, 21,* 143-150.

Hiskey M. S. (1955). *Hiskey-Nebraska Test of Learning Aptitude.* Lincoln, NE: College View Printers.

Holt, R. F., & Kirk, K. I. (2005). Speech and language development in cognitively delayed children with cochlear implants. *Ear and Hearing, 26,* 132-148.

Houston, D. M., Pisoni, D. B., Kirk, K. I., Ying, E. A., & Miyamoto, R. T. (2003). Speech perception skills of deaf infants following cochlear implantation: A first report. *International Journal of Pediatric Otorhinolaryngology, 67,* 479-495.

Huang, C. Y., Yang, H. M., Sher, Y. J., Lin, Y. H., & Wu, J. L. (2005). Speech intelligibility of Mandarian-speaking deaf childeren with cochlear implants. *International Journal of Pediatric Otorhinolaryngology, 69,* 505-511.

Kaufman, A. S., & Kaufman, N. L. (1983). *Kaufman Assessment Battery for Children (K-ABC).* Circle Pine, MN: American Guidance Service.

Kiefer, J., Gall, V., Desloovere, C., Knecht, R., Mikowski, A., & von Ilberg, C. (1996). A follow-up study of long-term results after cochlear implantation in children and adolescents. *European Archives of Oto-Rhino-Laryngology, 253,* 158-166.

Kirk, K. I., Miyamoto, R. T., Ying, E. A., Perdew, A. E., & Zuganelis, H. (2002). Cochlear implantation in young children: Effects of age at implantation and communication mode. *Volta Review, 102,* 127-144.

Kluwin, T. N., & Stewart, D. A. (2000). Cochlear implants for younger children: A preliminary description of the parental decision process and outcomes. *American Annals of the Deaf, 145,* 26-32.

Knutson, J. F., Boyd, R. C., Goldman, M., & Sullivan, P. M. (1997a). Psychological characteristics of child cochlear implant candidates and children with hearing impairments. *Ear and Hearing, 18,* 355-363.

Knutson, J. F., Boyd, R. C., Reid, J. B., Mayne, T., & Fetrow, R. (1997b). Observational assessments of the interaction of implant recipients with family and peers: Preliminary findings. *Otolaryngology-Head and Neck Surgery, 117,* 196-207.

Knutson, J. F., Ehlers, S. L., Wald, R. L., & Tyler, R. S. (2000a). Psychological predictors of pediatric cochlear implant use and benefit. *Annals of Otology, Rhinology, and Laryngology, 109*(Suppl. 185), 100-103.

Knutson, J. F., Hinrichs, J. V., Gantz, B. J., & Tyler, R. S. (1996). Psychological variables and cochlear implant success: Implications for adolescent recipients. In P. M. Sullivan & P. E. Brookhouser (Eds.), *Deaf adolescents: Puzzles, problems, and promises. Proceedings of the Fourth National Conference on the Habilitation and Rehabilitation of Hearing Impaired Adolescents* (pp. 47-67). Omaha, NE: Boys Town Press.

Knutson, J. F., Hinrichs, J. V., Tyler, R. S, Gantz, B. J., Schartz, H. A., & Woodworth, G. (1991). Psychological predictors of audiological outcomes of multichannel cochlear implants: Preliminary findings. *Annals of Otology, Rhinology, and Laryngology, 100,* 817-822.

Knutson, J. F., Johnson, C., & Sullivan, P. M. (2004). Disciplinary choices of mothers of deaf children and mothers of normally hearing children. *Child Abuse and Neglect, 28,* 925-937.

Knutson, J. F., & Sullivan, P. M. (1993). Communicative disorders as a risk factor in abuse. *Topics in Language Disorders, 13,* 1-14.

Knutson, J. F., Wald, R. L., Ehlers, S. L., & Tyler, R. S. (2000b). Psychological consequences of pediatric cochlear implant use. *Annuals of Otology, Rhinology, and Laryngology, 109*(Suppl. 185), 109-111.

Kurtzer-White, E., & Luterman, D. (2003). Families and children with hearing loss: Grief and counseling. *Mental Retardation and Developmental Disabilities Research Reviews*, 9, 232–245.

Laing, J. A., & Sines, J. O. (1982). The Home Environment Questionnaire: An instrument for assessing several behaviorally relevant dimensions of children's environments. *Journal of Pediatric Psychology*, 7, 425–449.

Lane, H. (1996, February). *Ethical consideration of pediatric cochlear implantation*. Paper presented at the Sixth Symposium on Cochlear Implants in Children, Miami, FL.

Levine, J. A., Pollack, H., & Comfort, M. E. (2001). Academic and behavioral outcomes among the children of young mothers. *Journal of Marriage and the Family*, 63, 355–369.

Levy-Schiff, R., & Hoffman, M. A. (1985). Social behaviour of hearing-impaired and normally-hearing preschoolers, *British Journal of Educational Psychology*, 55, 111–118.

Luterman, D. (1997). Emotional aspects of deafness. *Volta Review*, 99, 78–83.

Luterman, D. (2001). *Counseling persons with communication disorders and their families* (4th ed.). Austin, TX: Pro-Ed.

Lutman, M. E., & Tait, D. M. (1995). Early communicative behavior in young children receiving cochlear implants: Factor analysis of turn-taking and gaze orientation. *Annals of Otology, Rhinology, and Laryngology*, *104*(Suppl. 166), 397–399.

Marschark, M. (1993a). Origins and interactions in the social, cognitive, and language development of deaf children. In M. Marschark & M. D. Clark (Eds.), *Psychological perspectives on deafness* (pp. 7–26). Hillsdale, NJ: Lawrence Erlbaum Associates.

Marschark, M. (1993b). *Psychological development of deaf children*. New York: Oxford University Press.

Marschark, M. (2006). Intellectual functioning of deaf adults and children: Answers and questions. *European Journal of Cognitive Psychology*, 18, 70–89.

McKenna, L. (1986). The psychological assessment of cochlear implant patients. *British Journal of Audiology*, 20, 29–34.

McKenna, L. (1991). The assessment of psychological variables in cochlear implant patients. In H. Cooper (Ed.), *Cochlear implants: A practical guide* (pp. 125–145). San Diego, CA: Singular.

Meadow, K. P. (1980). *Deafness and child development*. Berkeley: University of California Press.

Meadow-Orlans, K. P. (1995). Sources of stress for mothers and fathers of deaf and hard of hearing infants. *American Annals of the Deaf*, *140*, 352–357.

Miller, L., Duvall, S., Berliner, K., Crary, W. G., & Wexler, M. (1978). Cochlear implants: A psychological perspective. *Journal of the Oto-Laryngological Society of Australia*, 4, 201–203.

Mitchell, T. V., & Quittner, A. L. (1996). Multimethod study of attention and behavior problems in hearing-impaired children. *Journal of Clinical Child Psychology*, 25, 83–96.

Miyamoto, R. T., Kirk, K. I., Robbins, A. M., Todd, S., & Riley, A. (1996). Speech perception and speech production skills of children with multichannel cochlear implants. *Acta Oto-Laryngologica*, 116, 240–243.

Miyamoto, R. T., Osberger, M. J., Robbins, A. M., Myres, W. A., & Kessler, K. (1993). Prelingually deafened children's performance with the Nucleus multichannel cochlear implant. *American Journal of Otology*, 14, 437–445.

Miyamoto, R. T., Svirsky, M., Kirk, K. I., Robbins, A. M., Todd, S., & Riley, A. (1997a). Speech intelligibility of children with multichannel cochlear implants. *Annals of Otology, Rhinology, and Laryngology*, *106*(Suppl. 168), 35–36.

Miyamato, R. T., Svirsky, M. A., & Robbins, A. M. (1997b). Enhancement of expressive language in prelingually deaf children with cochlear implants. *Acta Oto-Laryngologica*, *117*(2), 154–157.

Moeller, M. P. (2000). Early intervention and language development in children who are deaf and hard of hearing. *Pediatrics*, *106*, e43, 1–9.

Mondain, M., Sillon, M., Vieu, A., Lanvin, M., Reuillard-Artieres, F., Tobey, E., et al. (1997). Speech perception skills and speech production intelligibility in French children with prelingual deafness and cochlear implants.

Archives of Otolaryonology-Head and Neck Surgery, 123, 181–184.

Mullen, E. M. (1995). *Mullen Scales of Early Learning* (AGS ed.). Circle Pines, MN: American Guidance Service.

National Institute on Deafness and Other Communication Disorders. (1995). Cochlear implants in adults and children. *NIH Consensus Statement, 13*(2), 1–30.

Nicholas, J. G., & Geers, A. E. (2003). Personal, social, and family adjustment in school-aged children with a cochlear implant. *Ear and Hearing, 24*(Suppl.), 69S–81S.

Nicholas, J. G., & Geers, A. E. (2006). The process and early outcomes of cochlear implantation by three years of age. In P. E. Spencer & M. Marschark (Eds.), *Advances in the spoken language development of deaf and hard of hearing children* (pp. 271–297). New York: Oxford University Press.

Niparko, J. K., & Blankenhorn, R. (2003). Cochlear implants in young children. *Mental Retardation and Developmental Disabilities Research Review, 9*, 267–273.

O'Grady, D., & Metz, J. R. (1987). Resilience in children at high risk for psychological disorder. *Journal of Pediatric Psychology, 12*, 3–23.

Osberger, M. J., Fisher, L., Zimmerman-Phillips, S., Geier, L., & Barker, M. (1998). Speech recognition performance of older children with cochlear implants. *American Journal of Otology, 19*, 152–175.

Paganga, S., Tucker, E., Harrigan, S., & Lutman, M. (2001). Evaluating training courses for parents of children with cochlear implants. *International Journal of Language and Communication Disorders, 36*, 517–522.

Pasanisi, E., Bacciu, A., Vincenti, V., Guida, M., Berghenti, M. T., Barbot, A., Panu, F., & Bacciu, S. (2002). Comparison of speech perception benefits with SPEAK and ACE coding strategies in pediatric Nucleus C124M cochlear implant recipients. *International Journal of Pediatric Otorhinolaryngology, 64*, 159–163.

Percy-Smith, L., Caye-Thomasen, P., Gudman, M., Jensen, J. H., & Thomsen, J. (2008). Self-esteem and social well-being of children with cochlear implant compared to normal-hearing children. *International Journal of Pediatric Otorhinolaryngology, 72*, 1113–1120.

Pipp-Siegel, S., Sedey, A. L., & Yoshinaga-Itano, C. (2002). Predictors of parental stress in mothers of young children with hearing loss. *Journal of Deaf Studies and Deaf Education, 7*, 1–17.

Pisoni, D. B., & Cleary, M. (2003). Measures of working memory span and verbal rehearsal speed in deaf children after cochlear implantation. *Ear and Hearing, 24*(Suppl.), 106–120.

Pisoni, D. B., & Geers, A. (2000). Working memory in deaf children with cochlear implants: Correlations between digit span and measures of spoken language processing. *Annals of Otology, Rhinology, and Laryngology, 109* (Suppl. 185), 92–93.

Pollard, R. Q., Jr. (1996). Conceptualizing and conducting preoperative psychological assessments of cochlear implant candidates, *Journal of Deaf Studies and Deaf Education, 1*, 16–28.

Preisler, G., Tvingstedt, A. L., & Ahlstrom, M. (2002). A psychosocial follow-up study of deaf preschool children using cochlear implants. *Child: Care, Health and Development, 28*, 403–418.

Pulsifer, M. B., Salorio, C. F., & Niparko, J. K. (2003). Developmental, audiological, and speech perception functioning in children after cochlear implant surgery. *Archives of Pediatrics and Adolescent Medicine, 157*, 552–558.

Pyman, B., Blamey, P., Lacy, P., Clark, G., & Dowell, R. (2000). The development of speech perception in children using cochlear implants: Effects of etiologic and delayed milestones. *American Journal of Otology, 21*, 57–61.

Quittner, A. L., Barker, D. H., Snell, C., Cruz, I., McDonald, L-G., Grimley, M. E., Botteri, M., Marciel, K., & CDaCI Investigative Team. (2007). Improvements in visual attention in deaf infants and toddlers after cochlear implantation. *Audiological Medicine, 5*, 242–249.

Quittner, A. L., Glueckauf, R. L., & Jackson, D. N. (1990). Chronic parenting stress: Moderating versus mediating effects of social support. *Journal of Personality and Social Psychology, 59*, 1266-1278.

Quittner, A. L., Smith, L. B., Osberger, M. J., Mitchell, T. V., & Katz, D. B. (1994). The impact of audition on the development of visual attention. *Psychological Science, 5*, 347-353.

Quittner, A. L., Steck, J. T., & Rouiller, R. L. (1991). Cochlear implants in children: A study of parental stress and adjustment. *American Journal of Otology, 12*(Suppl.), 95-104.

Rasing, E. J. (1993). Effects of a multifaceted training procedure on the social behaviors of hearing-impaired children with severe language disabilities: A replication. *Journal of Applied Behavior Analysis, 26*, 405-406.

Rasing, E. J., & Duker, P. C. (1992). Effects of a multifaceted training procedure on the acquisition and generalization of social behaviors in language-disabled deaf children. *Journal of Applied Behavior Analysis, 25*, 723-734.

Reynolds, C. R., & Kamphaus, R. W. (2004). *Behavior Assessment System for Children-Second Edition.* Circle Pines, MN: American Guidance Service.

Robbins, A. M. (2003). Communication intervention for infants and toddlers with cochlear implants. *Topics in Language Disorders, 23*, 16-28.

Roid, G. H., & Miller, L. J. (1997). *Leiter International Performance Scale-Revised.* Wood Dale, IL: Stoelting.

Rose, D. E., Vernon, M., & Pool, A. F. (1996). Cochlear implants in prelingually deaf children. *American Annals of the Deaf, 141*, 258-262.

Sahli, S., & Belgin, E. (2006). Comparison of self-esteem level of adolescent with cochlear implant and normal hearing. *International Journal of Pediatric Otorhinolaryngology, 70*, 1601-1608.

Schlesinger, H., & Meadow, K. (1972). *Sound and sign: Child deafness and mental health.* Berkeley: University of California Press.

Schum, R. (2004). Psychological assessment of children with multiple handicaps who have hearing loss [Monograph]. *Volta Review, 104*, 237-255.

Seifert, E., Oswald, M., Bruns, U., Vischer, M., Kompis, M., & Haeusler, R. (2002). Changes of voice and articulation in children with cochlear implants. *International Journal of Pediatric Otorhinolaryngology, 66*, 115-123.

Sines, J. O. (1986). Normative data for the revised Missouri Children's Behavior Checklist-Parent Form (MCBC-P). *Journal of Abnormal Child Psychology, 14*, 89-94.

Sines, J. O. (1988). Teachers' norms and teacher-parent agreement on the Missouri Children's Behavior Checklist. *Journal of School Psychology, 26*, 413-416.

Sines, J. O., Clarke, W. M., & Lauer, R. M. (1984). Home Environment Questionnaire. *Journal of Abnormal Child Psychology, 12*, 519-529.

Sparrow, S., Balla, D., & Cicchetti, D. (1984). *Vineland Adaptive Behavior Scales: Survey Form manual.* Circle Pines, MN: American Guidance Service.

Sparrow, S. S., Balla, D. A., & Cicchetti, D. V. (2005). *Vineland Adaptive Behavior Scales, Second Edition: Survey Forms manual.* Circle Pines, MN: American Guidance Service.

Spencer, P. E. (2004). Language at 12 and 18 months: Characteristics and accessibility of linguistic models. In K. Meadow-Orlans, P. Spencer, & L. Koester (Eds.). *The world of deaf infants* (pp. 147-167). New York: Oxford University Press.

Spencer, P., Koester, L. S., & Meadow-Orlans, K. (1994). Communicative interactions of deaf and hearing children in a day care center. An exploratory study. *American Annals of the Deaf, 139*, 512-518.

Stallings, L. M., Kirk, K. I., Chin, S. B., & Gao, S. (2002). Parent word familiarity and the language development of pediatric cochlear implant users. *Volta Review, 102*, 237-258.

Svirsky, M. A., Robbins, A. M., Kirk, K. I., Pisoni, D. B., & Miyamoto, R. T. (2000). Language development in profoundly deaf children with cochlear implants. *Psychological Science, 11*, 153-158.

Te, G. O., Hamilton, M. J., Rizer, F. M., Schatz, K. A., Arkis, P. N., & Rose, H. C. (1996). Early speech changes in children with multichannel cochlear implants, *Otolaryngology-Head and Neck Surgery, 115*, 508-512.

Teti, D. M., & Gelfand, D. M. (1991). Behavioral competence among mothers of infants in the first year: The mediational role of maternal self-efficacy. *Child Development*, *62*, 918–929.

Tharpe, A. M., Ashmead, D. H., & Rothpletz, A. M. (2002). Visual attention in children with normal hearing, children with hearing aids, and children with cochlear implants. *Journal of Speech, Language, and Hearing Research*, *45*, 403–413.

Tiber, N. (1985). A psychological evaluation of cochlear implants in children. *Ear and Hearing*, *6*(Suppl.), 48–51.

Tobey, E. A., Geers, A. E., Brenner, C., Altuna, D., & Gabbert, G. (2003). Factors associated with development of speech production skills in children implanted by age five. *Ear and Hearing*, *24*(Suppl.), 36S–46S.

Tomblin, J. B., Barker, B. A., & Hubbs, S. (2007). Developmental constraints on language development in children with cochlear implants. *International Journal of Audiology*, *46*, 512–523.

Tomblin, J. B., Spencer, L., Flock, S., Tyler, R., & Gantz, B. (1999). A comparison of language achievement in children with cochlear implants and children using hearing aids. *Journal of Speech, Language, and Hearing Research*, *42*, 497–511.

Tye-Murray, N., Spencer, L., & Gilbert-Bedia, E. (1995). Relationships between speech production and speech perception skills in young cochlear-implant users. *Journal of the Acoustical Society of America*, *98*, 2454–2460.

Tyler, R. S., Kelsay, D. M., Teagle, H. F., Rubinstein, J. T., Gantz, B. J., & Christ, A. M. (2000a). Seven-year speech perception results and the effects of age, residual hearing and preimplant speech perception in prelingually deaf children using the Nucleus and Clarion cochlear implants. *Advances in Oto-Rhino-Laryngology*, *57*, 305–310.

Tyler, R. S., Teagle, H. F., Kelsay, D. M., Gantz, B. J., Woodworth, G. G., & Parkinson, A. J. (2000b). Speech perception by prelingually deaf children after six years of cochlear implant use: Effects of age at implantation. *Annals of Otology, Rhinology, and Laryngology*, *109* (Suppl.185), 82–84.

Vernon, M. (2005). Fifty years of research on the intelligence of deaf and hard-of-hearing children: A review of literature and discussion of implications. *Journal of Deaf Studies and Deaf Education*, *10*, 225–231.

Vernon, M., & Alles, C. D. (1995). Issues in the use of cochlear implants with prelingually deaf children. *American Annals of the Deaf*, *139*(5), 485–492.

Vlahovic, S., & Sindija, B. (2004). The influence of potentially limiting factors on paediatric outcomes following cochlear implantation. *International Journal of Pediatric Otorhinolaryngology*, *68*, 1167–1174.

Wald, R., & Knutson, J. F. (2000). Deaf culture identity of adolescents with and without cochlear implants. *Annals of Otology, Rhinology, and Laryngology*, *109*(Suppl. 185), 87–89.

Waltzman, S. B., Cohen, N. L., Gomolin, R. H., Green, J. E., Shapiro, W. H., Hoffman, R. A., et al. (1997). Open-set speech perception in congenitally deaf children using cochlear implants. *American Journal of Otology*, *18*, 342–349.

Waltzman, S., Cohen, N., & Shapiro W. (1995). Effects of cochlear implantation on the young deaf child. *Advances in Oto-Rhino-Laryngology*, *50*, 125–128.

Waltzman, S. B., Scalchunes, V., & Cohen, N. L. (2000). Performance of multiply handicapped children using cochlear implants. *American Journal of Otology*, *21*, 329–335.

Watson, S. M., Henggeler, S. W., & Whelan, J. P. (1990). Family functioning and the social adaptation of hearing impaired youths. *Journal of Abnormal Psychology*, *18*, 143–163.

Wechsler, D. (1989). *Wechsler Preschool and Primary Scales of Intelligence*. San Antonio, TX: The Psychological Corporation.

Wechsler, D. (1991). *Wechsler Intelligence Scale for Children-Third Edition*. San Antonio, TX: The Psychological Corporation.

Wechsler, D. (1997). *Wechsler Adult Intelligence Scale-Third Edition*. San Antonio, TX: The Psychological Corporation.

Wechsler, D. (2002). *Wechsler Preschool and Primary Scales of Intelligence-Third Edition*. San Antonio, TX: The Psychological Corporation.

West, R. E., & Stucky, J. (1995) Cochlear implantation outcomes: Experience with the Nucleus 22 implant. *Annals of Otology, Rhinology, and Laryngology, 104*(Suppl. 166), 447–449.

Wever, C. C. (2002). *Parenting deaf children in the era of cochlear implantation: A narrative-ethical analysis.* Master's thesis, University of Nijmegen, The Netherlands.

Wie, O. B., Falkenberg, E. S., Tvete, O., & Tomblin, B. (2007). Children with a cochlear implant: Characteristics and determinants of speech recognition, speech-recognition growth rate, and speech production. *International Journal of Audiology, 46,* 232–243.

Wiley, S., Jahnke, M., Meinzen-Deer, J., & Choo, D. (2005). Perceived qualitative benefits of cochlear implants in children with multi-handicaps. *International Journal of Pediatric Otorhinolaryngology, 69,* 791–798.

Yang, H-M., Lin, C-Y., Chen, Y-J., & Wu, J-L. (2004). The auditory performance of children using cochlear implants: Effects of mental function. *International Journal of Pediatric Otorhinolaryngology, 68,* 1185–1188.

Zaidman-Zait, A., & Most, T. (2005). Cochlear implants in children with hearing loss: Maternal expectations and impact on the family. *Volta Review, 105,* 129–150.

Zwolan, T. A. (2000). Selection criteria and evaluation. In S. B. Waltzman & N. L. Cohen (Eds.), *Cochlear implants* (pp. 63–76). New York: Thieme Medical.

CHAPTER 14

Outcomes in Cochlear Implantation: Assessment of Quality of Life Impact and Economic Evaluation of the Cochlear Implant

FRANK R. LIN
JOHN K. NIPARKO
HOWARD W. FRANCIS

Introduction

Trends in clinical research increasingly emphasize the importance of assessing the impact of a medical treatment on an individual's day-to-day life (Drummond & Maynard, 1993). Methods in outcomes research survey an intervention's performance in real life when implemented on populations of individuals who not only vary in their patterns of utilizing an intervention, but also vary in their candidacy characteristics, demographic backgrounds, and clinical resources surrounding the intervention.

There are myriad perspectives regarding "outcome" that might be considered and then compared to a baseline. Historically health-related outcomes in children have been conceptualized clinically in terms of morbidity and mortality (American Medical Association, 1990). In both children and adults, however, health is best defined multidimensionally. Stated otherwise, physical, mental, and social well-being should be assessed not simply by the presence or absence of disease (World Health Organization, 1948). Assessment of multidimensional health in terms of quality of life impact is emerging as an important outcome measure in clinical studies.

A conceptual model for understanding how various measures could be used to evaluate patient outcomes has been developed by Wilson and Cleary (1995) (Figure 14–1).

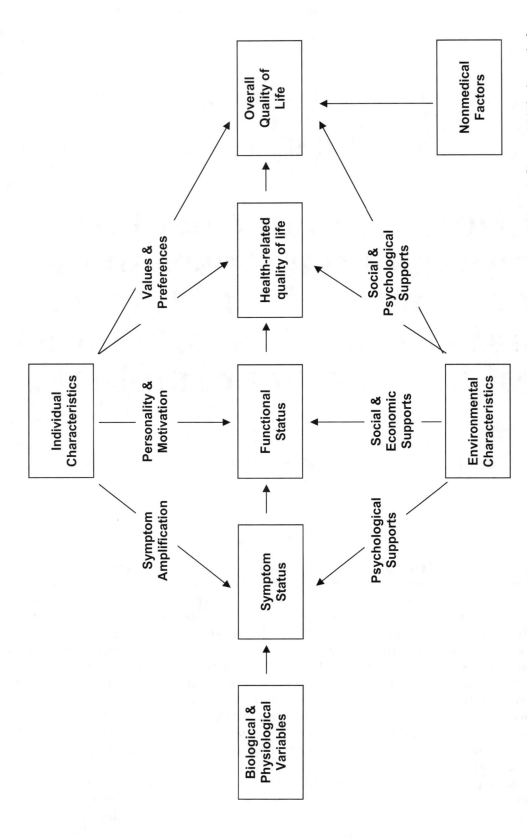

Figure 14–1. Conceptual model of relationships among measures of patient outcome (adapted from Wilson & Cleary, 1995). *Journal of the American Medical Association, 273,* 59–65. Copyright © (1995) American Medical Association. All rights reserved.

Biological and physiological variables (e.g., connexin 26 mutation leading to impaired cochlear function) serve as the basis for an individual's symptom status (e.g., degree of hearing loss). These domains then underlie an individual's functional status and subsequent health-related and overall quality of life. Relationships between any two domains can additionally be mediated by individual characteristics (personality, values, motivation), and environmental characteristics (social and economic supports).

In the Wilson and Cleary (1995) model, quality of life (QoL) reflects an individual's contentment or satisfaction with life. Numerous factors contribute to this perception: health status, non-medical factors, and individual and environmental characteristics. Nonmedical factors are perhaps the most understated element of this model as these would include such items as financial status and living environment. From a clinical perspective, however, rather than focusing on an individual's overall QoL, we generally choose to focus on only those domains that are affected by one's health and comprise health-related quality of life (HRQL) (Spilker & Revicki, 1996). HRQL is broadly understood to incorporate aspects of physical, social, and mental well-being in accordance with the World Health Organization's definition of health (WHO, 1948).

Applying Outcomes Research to Cost-Effectiveness

Market forces have induced medical care providers, from sole practitioner to large health maintenance organizations, to justify interventions based not only on safety and efficacy, but also on cost-effectiveness. This is particularly true when new technologies are considered, as health care costs have grown with the expense associated with modern medical technologies (Samuel, 1988).

Methods of assessing cost-effectiveness evaluate health interventions based on the relationship between the resources consumed (costs) and the resultant health outcomes (effects). Such analyses provide a quantified assessment of the value provided and seek to describe the impact of an intervention in terms of benefit and cost. Thus, an outcome can be practically assessed with respect to the costs for the care, rehabilitation, and maintenance associated with a particular treatment. Such research provides the basis for solving problems of medical economics, rating the effectiveness of interventions, and optimizing use of health care dollars.

Financial constraints on health care and special education services at the federal, state, and local levels increasingly mandate assessments of outcomes in preschool and school-aged children. Such assessments are likely to be important in shaping policy toward childhood hearing impairment. For example, outcomes analysis in childhood cochlear implantation will further inform discussions of universal screening of hearing in newborns. Early identification likely impacts the subsequent evaluation and management of candidates for cochlear implantation. Evaluating the impact of age of identification on cochlear implant results thus provides key outcomes data in the appraisal of different options for screening hearing in young children. An on-going analysis of a variety of outcomes will also contribute constructively to the social discourse on the appropriateness of cochlear implantation in children.

The effectiveness of an intervention may be evaluated in the context of its cost in several ways. These methods differ in the manner in which outcomes are valued. In **cost-benefit** analysis, outcomes are valued in financial terms, usually with respect to future health care expenditures saved.

Cost-benefit ratio =
Net costs (cumulative evaluation, treatment, maintenance in $s) /
Net monetary effects (in $s)

In **cost-effectiveness** analysis, outcomes are measured in natural units of clinical effects. Clinical effects are often expressed in life years saved but, depending on the study, effects may be expressed in any unit of measure deemed clinically significant. For example, in comparing different anti-hypertensive intervention strategies, mm Hg of blood pressure reduction may be an appropriate unit of measure. The key feature of cost-effectiveness analysis is that one does not need to assign a dollar value to the outcome.

Cost-effectiveness ratio =
Net costs (cumulative evaluation, treatment, maintenance in $s) /
Net effects (measured in units of clinical effects)

A form of cost-effectiveness analysis that rates outcome in terms of changes in life expectancy *and* health-related quality of life is **cost-utility** analysis. The unit of outcome measure is not just life years, but **quality-adjusted life years** (QALYs). In this approach, life years (life expectancy) are converted into QALYs by a quality-of-life conversion factor termed "health utility." Health utility represents one particular method of quantifying HRQL where health utility scores represent a valuation of one's health status expressed on a scale from 0.00 (death) to 1.00 (perfect health). This valuation can be directly elicited from individuals using one of three commonly used utility metrics, the visual analogue scale (VAS), time tradeoff (TTO), and standard gamble (SG) (Froberg & Kane, 1989). Alternatively, health utility valuations can also be obtained by using scores that are imputed from population-based valuations of functional ability and health attributes (e.g., Health Utilities Index [Feeny, Torrance, & Furlong, 1996] or Euro-QoL [Rabin & de Charro, 2001] instruments). QALYs are then calculated as the product of an individual's life expectancy and health utility. Therefore, for an individual with a life expectancy of 30 years but who has a health utility of 0.5, the calculated QALYs would be 15. QALYs are subsequently used as the denominator in cost-utility calculations:

Cost-utility ratio =
Net costs (cumulative evaluation, treatment, maintenance in $s) /
Net effects (measured in QALYs)

For example, although treatments for hearing rehabilitation have little impact on longevity, they commonly result in improved awareness and, possibly, enhanced communication. These factors change quality of life. For this reason, cost-utility provides an appropriate measurement tool for rating effects relative to associated costs.

Because QALYs incorporate generic changes in life expectancy and quality of life resulting from an intervention, cost per QALY of diverse interventions can be compared. Substantial improvement in the quality of life resulting from an intervention decreases the cost incurred per QALY. The lower the cost per QALY, or the greater the number of QALYs obtained at a given cost, the greater the cost-effectiveness of an intervention.

Cost-Utility of Cochlear Implantation in Adults

As hearing rehabilitation presumably improves audition and communication, and has little impact on longevity, cost-utility analysis provides an appropriate measure of hearing rehabilitation. A number of cost-utility studies have been performed to assess cochlear implantation in adults (Evans, Seeger, & Lehnhardt, 1995; Fugain, Severns, Braspenning, Brokx, & van den Broek, 1998; Harris, Anderson, & Novak, 1995; Lea, 1991; Lea & Hailey, 1995; Palmer, Niparko, Wyatt, Rothman, & de Lissovoy, 1999; Summerfield, Marshall, & Davis, 1995; six studies in Summerfield & Marshall, 1995; U.K. Cochlear Implant Study Group, 2004; Wyatt & Niparko, 1995; Wyatt, Niparko, Rothman, & de Lissovoy, 1995a; Wyatt, Niparko, Rothman, & de Lissovoy, 1995b; Wyatt, Niparko, Rothman, & de Lissovoy, 1996). Ten of these studies used models of cost and benefit, though four report duplicate results. Seven of the studies have tracked actual costs and performed outcome measurements in cohorts of patients. Costs per QALY for the cochlear implant (CI) in adult users were determined using clinical cost data accumulated through pre-, post-, and operative phases of implantation. Benefits were determined by measuring health utility before and after implantation; the difference in health utility values was then translated into an increased number of QALYs associated with cochlear implantation.

Generally, these studies have reported:

1. patient data on adults (age >18 years) with bilateral, postlingual, profound deafness,
2. a decrement in health utility associated with profound deafness on a scale from 0.00 (death) to 1.00 (perfect health),
3. a subsequent gain in health utility following cochlear implantation,
4. a cost-utility value in terms of $/QALY.

These studies provide information that not only sheds light on the impact of cochlear implantation, but also may help to further understanding of the impact of acquired profound hearing impairment on quality of life.

Pooled results from adults with profound deafness ($n = 497$) yielded a decrement in health utility of −0.46 (95% confidence interval: −0.44 to −0.48) from a "perfect health" score of 1.00 (i.e., 1.00 − 0.46 = health utility of 0.54). The majority of these studies have concluded that the CI compares favorably to other accepted health interventions, but the reported range of results is considerable. Health utility gains varied from +0.07 to +0.30, yielding cost-utility values of $9,000 to $31,177/QALY. Pooled results from seven studies ($n = 520$) indicated a health utility gain from cochlear implantation of +0.26 (95% confidence interval: +0.24 to +0.28) yielding an improvement from the above "profoundly deaf" health utility of 0.54 to 0.80. This resulted in a weighted average cost-utility figure from cochlear implantation of $12,847/QALY.

A recent study performed by the U.K. CI study group also established the effect of the relaxation of candidacy criteria on cost-utility ratios among postlingually deafened adults (U.K. CI Study Group, 2004). In this prospective cohort study, the cost-utility of cochlear implantation in traditional candidates (adults with no open-set speech recognition under aided conditions without visual cues) and candidates who were able to achieve up to 50% open-set speech recognition under aided conditions was compared. Although utility scores increased for both groups after CI, greater gains and hence improved cost-utility were seen in traditional candidates rather than those with some aidable hearing. Interestingly, for both groups of patients, little utility gain and unfavorable cost-utility ratios were seen in individuals who had been profoundly deaf for greater than 30 to 40 years.

One limitation of the above studies relates to the difficulty in comparing the health utility gain from those who receive a cochlear implant to controls who do not. Controls are defined as adults with bilateral, postlingual, profound deafness who have not received a cochlear implant. They may be on the waiting list to receive an implant, or rejected as an implant candidate for medical or insurance reasons, or may not wish to receive an implant. Palmer et al. (1999) followed 16 control patients prospectively for 1 year along with 46 implanted patients. Whereas there was a +0.20 increase in health utility (0.58 to 0.78) in the implanted group, the control group reported the same baseline health utility with no change after 1 year (0.58 and 0.58, respectively).

Taken together, the above observations suggest that severe to profound hearing loss has an impact on quality of life that is both substantial and measurable, and that cochlear implantation is associated with marked improvement in self-rated measures of quality of life. The CI produces effects that favorably influence cost-effectiveness ratios, and cochlear implantation appears to represent an effective use of health care dollars.

Outcomes After Pediatric Cochlear Implantation

As an intervention that uniquely bridges the medical and educational aspects of rehabilitation in childhood deafness, cochlear implantation should be assessed for its costs and communication-related outcomes

as well as level of audiologic benefit. That is, the benefits of pediatric cochlear implantation can be assessed with broad measures that are likely interrelated:

1. Traditional measures of functional outcomes, including tests of speech perception, language, and communication skills;
2. Impact on educational performance, utilization of special education resources, and cost-benefit considerations;
3. Perceived changes in HRQL and cost-effectiveness studies.

Until the long-term effects of the cochlear implant on educational achievement and vocational outcome are known, the assessment of educational independence, verbal language skills and literacy can serve as preliminary outcome measures. Measures that reflect the development of these skills have been shown to predict educational and vocational outcome in hearing impaired children without cochlear implants (Holt, 1994; Kasen,Ouellette, & Cohen, 1990; Saur, Coggiola, Long, & Simonson, 1986; Trybus & Karchmer, 1977).

Auditory perception appears to be critical to a number of cognitive processes. Tests of attention reveal that hearing-impaired children have deficits in their selective visual attention, suggesting that auditory input affects the development of attention skills (Quittner, Steck, & Rouiller, 1991). Profoundly hearing-impaired children who receive a CI demonstrate improved visual attention skills that eventually match those of age-matched peers with less severe hearing impairments who are able to use hearing aids. Fundamental cognitive domains such as attention reasonably can be expected to exert a broad impact on quality of life. However, measurement of such effects represents a considerable challenge in clinical research.

Measurement of Functional Outcomes

While the evaluation of functional outcomes can be straightforward and routine in adults, the evaluation of outcomes in the prelingually deafened child during an early period (≤5 years old) of cognitive immaturity is much more difficult. In the former case, the patient can simply be asked "How is your hearing with the implant?" or alternatively, a standardized auditory perceptual or speech test can be applied. In contrast, with the prelingually deaf 3-year-old, cognitive immaturity limits the application of many tests, and scores on other tests can often be grossly confounded by the child's level of cooperation with the examiner (Thoutenhoofd et al., 2005). Consequently, current approaches to functional assessment of the young CI child focus on the *comprehensive* assessment of the breadth of a child's skills since each test reveals only a limited picture of a child's abilities. This approach of comprehensive assessment coupled with treatment strategies/decisions based on this framework most likely offers the best chance of ensuring future success given that long-term scholastic, social, and behavioral development will derive from early functional abilities.

Conceptual Model of Measuring Functional Outcomes

A conceptual framework provided by the World Health Organization's International Classification of Functioning (ICF) is useful to understand the role of current outcome instruments (World Health Organization, 2001). The ICF provides a systematic taxonomy for understanding human functioning where functioning is composed of two components (body functions/structures and activities/participation), and each component is subsequently hierarchically coded and classified with progressively greater detail (Table 14–1) (World Health Organization, 2001).

TABLE 14–1. Overview of the International Classification of Functioning

	Functioning & Disability	
Components	Body Functions and Structures	Activities and Participation
Domains	Body functions and structures	Life areas (tasks, actions)
Constructs	Change in body function (physiologic)	Capacity: Executing tasks in a standard environment
	Change in body structures (anatomic)	Performance: Executing tasks in the current environment
Positive aspect	Functional and structural integrity	Activities Participation
	Functioning	
Negative aspect	Impairment	Activity limitation Participation restriction
	Disability	

Source: From *International Classification of Functioning, Disability, and Health.* Copyright (2001). World Health Organization. Reprinted with permission.

Body functions/structures refer to the physiological functions of body systems and anatomical parts of the body. Aspects of body functions/structure salient to prelingual childhood deafness are detailed in Table 14–2 and broadly encompass hearing, voice, and speech functions. In contrast, the activities/participation component of the ICF refers to the execution of a task and involvement in life situations. Examples include communicating with receiving and producing spoken messages and initiating spoken conversations (see Table 14–2).

Most importantly, domains of the activities/participation component of the ICF can be further qualified by *capacity* versus

TABLE 14–2. Salient Domains of the International Classification of Functioning (ICF) and Current Measures Used in Pediatric Cochlear Implantation

Components	Functioning	
	Body Functions & Structures	*Activities & Participation*
Relevant domains*	Sensory functions b230 Hearing functions Voice & speech functions b310 Voice functions b320 Articulation functions b330 Fluency and rhythm of speech functions b340 Alternative vocalization functions	Learning & applying knowledge d115 Listening Communication d310 Receiving spoken messages d315 Receiving nonverbal messages d320 Receiving formal sign language messages d330 Speaking d340 Producing messages in formal sign language d350 Conversation d360 Using communication devices
Examples of commonly used instruments	1. Meaningful Auditory Integration Scale 2. Early Speech Perception Test 3. Pediatric Speech Intelligibility Test 4. Lexical Neighborhood Test 5. Multisyallabic Lexical Neighborhood Test 6. Audiometry	*Capacity* 1. Reynell Developmental Language Scales 2. MacArthur Communicative Development Inventory *Performance* 1. Functioning after Pediatric Cochlear Implantation (FAPCI) instrument

*The specified domains and ICF codes are a small sample of the complete ICF taxonomy and represent the domains felt to be the most relevant for studying functioning in young children with CI's. Many items are further subclassified with greater detail in the ICF taxonomy (e.g., Hearing functions [b230] has subclassifications of Sound detection [b2300], Sound discrimination [b2301], Localization of sound source [b2303], Lateralization of sound [b2303], and Speech discrimination [b2304]).

performance. Capacity refers to an individual's abilities in a standardized environment whereas performance indicates an individual's abilities in a real-world environment. For example, a child's ability to communicate by understanding a spoken message (d310, see Table 14–2) could be measured in a clinic setting where there are no distracting noises and the child is one-on-one with the examiner (capacity). Alternatively, this same functional domain could also be measured in the child's home environment where multiple other environmental factors are present (performance).

The ICF model is particularly apt for understanding functioning in CI children because it brings together two competing models of disability that are analogous to models of deafness (Munoz-Baell & Ruiz, 2000; Simeonsson, 2003; Ustun, Chatterji, Bickenbach, Kostanjsek, & Schneider, 2003). Medical models view functioning and disability as a result of pathology and as being

best addressed through clinical interventions (Figure 14–2, impact of health condition on components of functioning). Sociocultural models, on the other hand, conceptualize disability as a socially created problem and deafness as a cultural identity that is best addressed by reducing the barriers that deaf individuals face in interacting with the hearing mainstream (see Figure 14–2, functioning impacted by environmental and personal factors) (Munoz-Baell & Ruiz, 2000).

The ICF synthesizes these two approaches toward disability into a *biopsychosocial* model that integrates useful components of each approach (Ustun et al., 2003). Using this conceptual model, we can better understand how two children with cochlear implants could have vastly different levels of functioning. For example, both children could be affected by the same underlying health condition (e.g., connexin 26 mutation that leads to congenital deafness), but the functioning of both children would also

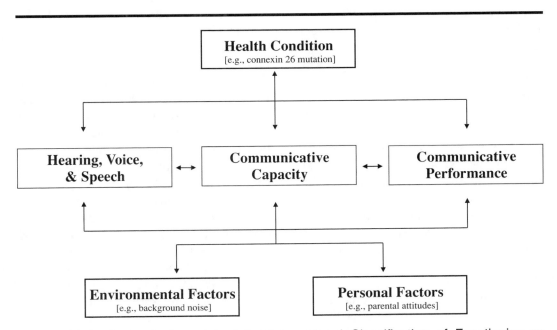

Figure 14–2. Conceptual model of the International Classification of Functioning as applied to deafness and cochlear implantation.

be impacted by environmental factors such as family relationships and attitudes and personal factors such as the child's innate intelligence and personality.

Current Instruments for Comprehensive Functional Assessment

Comprehensive assessment of a child's functioning, therefore, necessarily incorporates instruments that probe: (1) hearing, voice, and speech (body functions); (2) communicative capacity; and (3) communicative performance. Based on historical models of aural rehabilitation, efforts at assessing functioning in CI children have primarily focused on open- and closed-set speech perception, given that this was often the highest functional level that a deaf child using bilateral hearing aids could achieve (Carney & Moeller, 1998). Consequently, there is a wide range of outcome measures available for probing this domain (see Table 14–2). With early intervention and cochlear implantation, however, many CI children have far surpassed just basic speech recognition. Prospective studies of early cochlear implantation have now incorporated normal hearing children as controls, signifying the expected gains that deaf children with CIs can be expected to make with respect to language (Fink et al., 2007).

Measures of communicative capacity reflect a child's ability to use language in ideal (clinic) conditions. Such measures evaluate a child's progress after CI (see Table 14–2). In a longitudinal, multisite study of CI outcomes after early implantation, measures of communicative capacity using either the Reynell Developmental Language Scales (Reynell & Gruber, 1990) or MacArthur-Bates Communicative Development Inventories (Fenson et al., 2007) better reflected parental perceptions of a child's abilities at home than a closed-set measure of speech

perception (Lin et al., 2008). Other authors have also suggested that measures of speech perception administered in a structured setting may be poor indicators of a child's true performance in home settings (Thoutenhoofd et al., 2005; Vidas, Hassan, & Parnes, 1992).

A direct measure of a child's ability to use language and communicate in real-world settings (communicative performance) has only recently been developed (see Table 14–2). Previously, the ability to assess a child's ability to communicate relied mainly on a clinician's subjective observations of a child's abilities in clinic and from eliciting the feedback of parents. The recently developed Functioning after Pediatric Cochlear Implantation (FAPCI) instrument is a 23-item psychometrically validated metric that objectively quantifies a cochlear-implanted child's communicative performance (i.e., ability to communicate in real-world settings) (Lin et al., 2007). This instrument was designed for CI children <6 years-old and 4 years of CI experience were needed before maximal FAPCI scores were obtained.

The critical importance of measuring communicative performance in addition to other functional domains (speech and language) is highlighted by several factors. Previous models of childhood development have established the absolute importance of effective early parent-child communication for optimal cognitive, behavioral, and social development (Marschark, 1993). Early acquisition of *synchrony* and *reciprocity* in parent-child communicative interactions sets the foundation for parent-child bonding and establishes the child's subsequent ability for exploration, learning, and social interactions (Vaccari & Marschark, 1997). In contrast to measures of speech and language, only a measure of communicative performance would directly probe the quality of these parent-child communicative interactions.

From the perspective of parents and health care decision makers, there also is a strong indication that measures of communicative performance may be paramount. The diagnosis of deafness is almost universally a surprise to parents given that it is rarely diagnosed prenatally. Faced with this unanticipated event, parents are confronted with a stunning array of therapeutic and rehabilitative options and the need to be an informed decision maker on behalf of their child (Schwartz, 2007). Should cochlear implantation be pursued or is Deaf culture and sign language a better option? If cochlear implantation is indeed chosen, when should surgery be performed and what kind of auditory rehabilitation should be pursued? Evaluation measures reflecting the expected evolution of a child's real-world abilities may represent the most intuitive and relevant outcome that parents would need to consider in their decision-making process. From the perspective of health care decision makers, there has also been an increasing emphasis placed on measuring effectiveness rather than efficacy. Recent nonbinding recommendations from the Food and Drug Administration (FDA) emphasizing that some treatment effects are known only to the patient, have called for the use of patient-reported measures that directly reflect outcomes pertinent to the patient and family (U.S. Department of Health and Human Services, 2006).

Educational Outcomes After Early Cochlear Implantation and Cost-Benefit Analysis

In the United States "special education" is defined as unconventional instruction for children who do not benefit optimally from conventional educational practices or have impaired access to conventional instruction due to disability (Lloyd, Singh, & Repp, 1991; Mastropieri & Scruggs, 1987; Smith & Luckasson, 1992; Snell, 1993). These services are delivered to those with physical and communication handicaps, sensory disabilities (blindness and deafness), differences in intellectual capacity (gifted and mentally retarded), emotional or behavioral disturbances, and learning disabilities. Education of the hearing-impaired student often draws on all aspects of special education in order to foster both receptive and expressive communication skills, particularly when verbal communication is the objective. Special instructional services typically include individualized teaching techniques, materials, equipment, facilities, and related support services.

Mandates regarding services and environments for deaf education derive from laws of compulsory education. Legislative action in the United States, particularly the Education for All Handicapped Children Act of 1974, defined specific requirements for schooling students with disabilities, including the hearing impaired. These mandates compel systems of education to avail students with disabilities, at no cost, a public education in the least-restrictive environment—one that approximates, as closely as possible, that experienced by nondisabled students. To address the specific needs of disabled children, this legislation stipulates that:

1. individualized education plans (IEPs) reflect faithfully a student's educational needs;
2. the educational options that are provided to disabled students cannot be constrained by their handicap.

Given the substantial costs associated with special education, an analysis of patterns of usage of educational resources is a logical first step in analysis of the cost-effectiveness of technologies such as the cochlear implant that may impact educational placement.

Placement and Speech and Language Rehabilitative Services

Consideration of a hearing-impaired child's educational needs is multifaceted. For example, a self-contained classroom may provide more focused remediation of educational deficits, but also provides limited access to models of spoken language. Such language models can enhance language acquisition for hearing impaired children (McCormick & Schiefelbusch, 1990). Although children with disabilities can benefit from participation with other children, they are often enrolled in a program offered by a neighborhood school (Lloyd et al., 1991). "Mainstreaming," "inclusion" or "integration" is conceptually consistent with the legal mandate for education in a minimally restrictive environment. Indeed, in the United States two-thirds of students with disabilities receive the majority of their instruction in regular education classes.

The appropriateness of mainstreaming hearing-impaired children is highly debatable (Northern & Downs, 1991). For the hearing-impaired child, placement in a mainstream setting often introduces demands for related support services to enhance speech understanding.

In addition to placement alternatives, specialized support services are an intervention mainstay in most special education settings. Interpreters, speech-language pathologists, itinerant teachers of the deaf, instructional assistants, and academic tutors provide services to augment classroom

instruction in our region. Provision of these services is determined based not only on the educational needs of the child, but also on logistical issues such as availability of appropriate professionals, budgetary limitations, and legislative requirements. These factors often will affect a child's placement more than educational needs. Moreover, the family's psychosocial status and support play a critical role in the child's (re)habilitation and likely affect placement (Quittner et al., 1991).

Clinical investigators have analyzed preliminarily the impact of cochlear implantation on school placement (Francis, Koch, Wyatt, & Niparko 1999; Koch, Wyatt, Francis, & Niparko, 1997; Nottingham Paediatric Cochlear Implant Programme, 1997). These investigations found mainstreaming rates of 58% after two years of implant experience (Nottingham Paediatric Cochlear Implant Programme, 1997) and 75% after four years of implant experience (Francis et al., 1999). These rates exceed the (control) rates of mainstreaming of unimplanted children with similar levels of baseline hearing by five-(Nottingham Paediatric Cochlear Implant Programme, 1997) to two-fold (Francis et al., 1999). However, such figures ignore the large numbers of variables affecting placement, and greater detail of analysis is required as described below. Moreover, given the variability in educational placement and services, models that track the use of educational resources by hearing-impaired children are likely to be regionally specific.

The Educational Resource Matrix

The Educational Resource Matrix (ERM) (Figure 14-3) has been developed to map educational placement and the use of rehabilitation resources by hearing-impaired children (Koch et al., 1997). The ERM serves

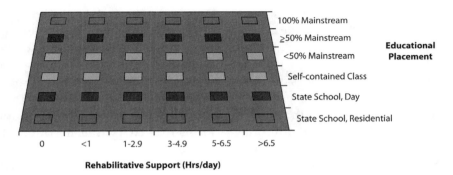

Figure 14–3. Educational resource matrix (ERM) model.

as a model recognizing that programs, services, and policies related to the education of hearing-impaired children vary markedly across the United States, but offers a basis on which to begin appraisal of the cost benefit of cochlear implants in children in the United States.

The ERM stratifies qualitative aspects of school setting and levels of rehabilitative support based on the experience of the rehabilitation team at the Johns Hopkins University Cochlear Implant Program (The Listening Center at Johns Hopkins). The school environment is monitored by the CI rehabilitation team, affording the observation of classroom placement and use of special educational services over years. Because of variability in the resources and policies of school districts, changes in classroom placement by an implanted child are not a sufficient indication of progress in educational independence. Most noticeable was the observation that a change in classroom placement was often accompanied by changes in the need for support services. The ERM makes it possible to follow both placement and resource usage over time to provide a first approximation of educational independence. Through school visits, teacher and parent interviews, and review of individual education plans, trends

in educational independence in implanted children are compared with those of unimplanted severely to profoundly hearing-impaired students. Assigning real costs to coordinates on the ERM enables estimates of cost-benefit ratios associated with levels of educational independence (Francis et al., 1999; Koch et al., 1997).

Stratification of educational placement reflects a continuum from full mainstream placement (within the child's local school) to residential placement at a state school for the deaf. Typically, public school districts often incorporate partial mainstreaming into programs of deaf education. Educational setting is indexed according to the degree of student independence according to six categories:

1. Full mainstream in regular classroom and school;
2. Greater than 50% of the school day spent in a regular classroom and school; less than 50% of the school day spent in a special education classroom;
3. Less than 50% of the school day spent in a regular classroom and school; greater than 50% of the school day spent in a special education classroom;
4. Full-time placement in a special education classroom in a regular school;

5. State school for the deaf: Day student;
6. State school for the deaf: Residential student.

Specialized support includes the use of related services designed to enhance communication. The ERM reflects the range of specialty services often required by hearing-impaired students. Teachers of the hearing-impaired, itinerant special educators, speech-language pathologists, educational audiologists, interpreters (sign language, cued speech, oral), occupational therapists, and/or instructional assistants may be required. Use of these services is based on a 6.5-hour school day and are averaged over a 5 day week. In cases where the child attends a half-day program, divisions are based on percentage of total time spent in school. Support services vary along a continuum of:

1. No support services
2. Less than 1 hour per day
3. 1 to 2.9 hours per day
4. 3 to 4.9 hours per day
5. 5 to 6.5 hours per day
6. More than 6.5 hours per day

Observed Trends in Educational Placement and Resource Use

In a study of 35 implanted school-aged children from the Johns Hopkins Cochlear Implant Program, a positive correlation between the length of implant experience and the incidence of placement in mainstream classrooms was observed. Whereas classroom placement remained static in the first 2 years of implantation, the rate of mainstream placement increased to 30% in the second 2 years of implant experience, and 75% among children with over 4 years of experience. In an age-matched group of nonimplanted children there was also a positive trend toward increased mainstream placement, but at older ages and at lower rates compared to the implanted group. There was also a decline in the use of support services by fully mainstreamed implanted children with increasing implant experience. When compared to an age-matched group of nonimplanted fully mainstreamed hearing-impaired children, implanted children used a quarter of the number of support hours. More so than the trend toward mainstream placement itself, this decline in the use of special education services suggests a substantial evolution in language skills and educational independence by implanted children within the first 4 years of their implant experience.

In the third and fourth years of implant experience, as children began their transition toward mainstream placement, 4 out of 10 children demonstrated an increase in the use of support services whereas others showed a decline. The variable use of special support services by implanted children in transition speaks to a complex array of factors that may influence the path of educational migration by a cochlear implanted child, including the presence of concomitant learning disabilities, the effectiveness of preimplant intervention, the age at implantation, and the resources and policies of the school.

Cost-Benefit Considerations in Children

Because cost data can be assigned to location points within the ERM, the ERM can be used to generate longitudinal data on relative costs of education. This is critical in calculating cost-benefit ratios concerning multichannel cochlear implants (Wyatt et al., 1995a). Educational costs can be assigned to variables in the ERM based on actual budgetary data. For example, costs used to assess the impact of observed educational trends on the cost-benefit of multiple CIs was derived from the 1995 State of Maryland Department of Education Budget (Francis et al., 1999). The lower right corner represents one extreme of the matrix, the cost of full-time education in a state school for the deaf at $42,000/year (see Figure 14–3). The upper left corner represents the other extreme, the cost of the education of a fully mainstreamed child who does not require support, at $6,106/year. Hourly costs associated with speech and language support were derived from salary figures for public school speech pathologists and interpreters for school year 1995 to 1996, and was estimated at $23/hr for the state of Maryland. Cost figures for cochlear implantation should include the cost of evaluation, placement of the implant, rehabilitation, device maintenance, and allowances for potential complications as previously described (Wyatt et al., 1995a). This was estimated to be $43,000 based on 1997 cost data from the Listening Center at Johns Hopkins.

A cost-benefit analysis was performed with financial projections covering the 13-year period of education for children implanted at 3 and 5 years of age (Francis et al., 1999). The analysis was performed for four different educational scenarios that reflect observed trends in the use of educational resources by implanted children. Due to the lack of data on the use of educational resources by implanted children in high school, an assumption was made that patterns of placement and use of support services remained static from middle into high school. The cost of implantation and kindergarten to 12th grade education was compared to the educational costs associated with observed trends in the use of educational resources by a nonimplanted age-matched cohort. Future costs and savings were discounted at 5% per annum to reflect

accurately the time value of money. Educational costs for a 3-year-old child who receives a CI may be compared to that of non-implanted children in a regular public school or a residential state school for the deaf. Cost savings associated with cochlear implantation from this perspective range from $30,000 to $200,000. There is a similar cost-savings associated with cochlear implantation at 5 years of age, even in the scenario where progression to full-time mainstream placement is the most delayed ($27,000 to $192,000 cost savings).

Cost-benefit projections based on observed advancement toward educational independence and very conservative cost figures indicate an extremely favorable net present value of the implant. The ERM illustrates that small increases in educational independence can result in annual savings in educational expenses that, when generalized to populations of implanted children, likely results in an overall cost savings associated with increased educational independence. However, these cost-benefit projections must be supplemented with measures of the impact on quality of life in order to determine the overall cost-effectiveness of cochlear implants in children.

Cost-Effectiveness Considerations in Children

Cost-effectiveness ratios of CIs in children must incorporate a range of considerations that extend beyond cost-benefit analyses (Hutton, Politi, & Seeger, 1995; Wyatt et al., 1995a). Broad measures of benefit in pediatric cochlear implantation may be measured in terms of communication outcomes, educational benefit, and perceived quality of life as reflected by social adjustment and physical, mental, and emotional health states.

Determining the quality of life associated with CIs in children presents substantial challenges. There are difficulties in assessing quality of life changes in children across developmental phases, as methods for assessing quality of life in children are not as well established as in the adult population. Most measures rely on parental opinion or reporting, which reflect the change in quality of life as perceived by the parent. In a systematic review of HRQL after pediatric cochlear implantation, the authors found substantial heterogeneity in the instruments that had been used to assess HRQL (Lin & Niparko, 2006). Most studies either used ad hoc instruments designed specifically for the purposes of the study and/or instruments that had no prior psychometric validation. The use of an unvalidated instrument without a framework for interpreting scores (i.e., normative values) only allows for broad qualitative conclusions. In the systematic review, no validated, deafness-specific HRQL instruments were found to be available. Well-validated, generic HRQL instruments that included health utility metrics, however, were found to be sensitive to deafness and feasible for studying HRQL in CI children.

Quality of life impact greatly affects perceived benefit as indicated by self-ratings, and it is not valid to assume that this impact will match that seen in postlingual adults with cochlear implants (see section "Cost-Utility of Cochlear Implantation in Adults"). Because many of the costs of an intervention such as the multichannel CI are "upfront," and are tied to surgical treatment and initial audiologic and rehabilitative services, the device would appear to be more cost-effective in children than in adults given longer periods of use in children. That is, cost-effectiveness of an intervention

is greatly enhanced by durability as sustained benefits effectively diminish the cost per QALY. However, predictions of long-term cost-effectiveness cannot be made based on expected period of use alone. For example, it may be that the perceived decrement in quality of life for prelingual childhood deafness is considered less than that for postlingual adult deafness.

Cost-Utility in Childhood Cochlear Implantation

The cost-utility of pediatric cochlear implantation remains a concern because of high costs, difficulty assessing benefit in very young subjects who cannot self-report, and lack of data to compare with the diversity of accepted medical interventions in other populations. With lifetime pediatric cochlear implantation costs estimated between $50,000 and $100,000 per case (Francis et al., 1999), the aggregate cost for the estimated 200,000 American children who meet criteria for implantation could be as great as $20 billion (Blanchfield, Feldman, & Dunbar, 1999). Rising health care costs, due in part to medical advances such as the cochlear implant, have led to pressures that discourage the implementation of new technologies. Cost-effectiveness and cost-utility studies are now recognized as the approach of choice in guiding decisions of health care rationing under conditions of budget constraints (Russell, Gold, Siegel, Daniels, & Weinstein, 1996).

Earlier published cost-utility analyses of the cochlear implant in children were limited by using health utilities obtained from adult patients (O'Neill, O'Donoghue, Archbold, & Normand, 2000; Summerfield & Marshall, 1995) or hypothetically estimated utilities of a deaf child (Carter & Hailey, 1999; Hutton et al., 1995; Lea, 1991; Lea &

Hailey, 1995). These studies yielded cost-utility ratios that fell out over a wide range ($3,141 to $25,450/QALY). These studies used a repeated measures of utility approach. This is a standard method of deriving benefit effects when implementing the Health Resource Allocation Strategy in evaluating an intervention relative to treatments for different disorders (Patrick & Erickson, 1993). Untreated controls were not included in these studies and conclusions about different interventions in deafness are not possible.

More recent studies have overcome these methodologic hurdles by directly quantifying health utility changes in children (Barton, Stacey, Fortnum, & Summerfield, 2006; Cheng et al., 2000) and including comparisons with nonimplanted children (Barton et al., 2006). Cheng et al. (2000) surveyed parents of a cohort of 78 children (average age 7.4 years, with 1.9 years of cochlear implant use) who received multichannel implants at Johns Hopkins University to determine direct and total cost to society per QALY. Parents of profoundly deaf children (n = 48) awaiting cochlear implantation served as a comparison group to assess validity of recall. Parents rated their child's health state "now," "immediately before," and "one year before" the cochlear implant using the Time Trade-Off (TTO), Visual Analogue Scale (VAS), and Health Utilities Index—Mark III (HUI). Mean VAS scores increased 0.27 on a scale from 0 to 1 (from 0.59 "immediately before" to 0.86 "now"), TTO scores increased 0.22 (from 0.75 to 0.97), and HUI scores increased 0.39 (from 0.25 to 0.64). Discounted direct medical costs were $60,228, yielding cost-utility ratios of $9,029/QALY using the TTO, $7,500/QALY using the VAS, and $5,197/QALY using the HUI. Including indirect costs, such as reduced educational expenses, the cochlear implant yielded a net savings of $53,198 per child. Based on assessments from a single center, childhood cochlear implantation produces a positive impact on quality of life at reasonable direct costs and results in societal savings.

Barton et al. (2006) built on this earlier work by expanding cost-utility calculations to estimate how various child and family-centered factors (e.g., preoperative hearing level, age at implantation, family socioeconomic status) would impact health utility scores in the United Kingdom. In addition, they also estimated the incremental additional costs associated with cochlear implantation versus providing hearing aids. Using a cross-sectional cohort of 403 implanted children, and 1863 nonimplanted children and the HUI Mark 3 instrument, the authors utilized linear regression models to estimate health utility gains associated with cochlear implantation and corresponding QALY's. Cost-effectiveness was found to be more favorable for children with a greater degree of preoperative hearing loss and for children who were implanted at an earlier age. Cost-utility estimates ranged from €40,660/QALY for children implanted at age 6 with an average preoperative hearing level of 105 dB to €10,798/QALY for children implanted at age 3 and with a preoperative hearing level of 125 dB.

Summary

Studies of real-world outcomes after cochlear implantation are now available. These studies have assessed multiple attributes of quality of life and health status to determine utility gained from the multichannel cochlear implant. The precise cost-utility results varied between studies, likely owing to differences in methods used to value benefit, the level of benefit actually obtained, and differences in costs associated with the intervention.

Nonetheless, these appraisals consistently indicate that the multichannel cochlear implant occupies a highly favorable position in terms of its cost-effectiveness relative to other medical and surgical interventions employed within the United States. Such studies are also important in analyzing the needed components of programs of rehabilitation and future directions for clinical intervention. Furthermore, third-party payers, consumers, and health care providers now need to make decisions based on economic and health outcomes data. These studies shed new light on the importance of access to hearing care.

Current research in pediatric cochlear implantation is focused on measuring benefit in ways that will complement traditional audiologic outcomes, namely, educational benefit, communicative performance in real-world settings, and perceived quality of life, particularly as such outcomes unfold in recipients' adult lives. This will allow the expression of cost-benefit, cost-effectiveness, and cost-utility ratios that assess the larger personal and societal impact of the cochlear implant on childhood deafness.

References

Barton, G. R., Stacey, P. C., Fortnum, H. M., & Summerfield, A. Q. (2006). Hearing-impaired children in the United Kingdom, IV: Cost-effectiveness of pediatric cochlear implantation. *Ear and Hearing, 27*, 575–588.

Blanchfield, B. B., Feldman, J. J., & Dunbar, J. (1999). The severely to profoundly hearing impaired population in the United States: prevalence and demographics. *Policy Analysis Brief. H Series, 1*, 1–4.

Carney, A. E., & Moeller, M. P. (1998). Treatment efficacy: Hearing loss in children. *Journal of Speech, Language, and Hearing Research, 41*, 61–84.

Carter, R., & Hailey, D. (1999). Economic evaluation of the cochlear implant. *International Journal of Technology Assessment in Health Care, 15*, 520–530.

Cheng, A. K., Rubin, H. R., Powe, N. R., Mellon, N. K., Francis, H. W., & Niparko, J. K. (2000). Cost-utility analysis of the cochlear implant in children. *Journal of the American Medical Association, 284*, 850–856.

Drummond, M., & Maynard, F. (Eds.). (1993). *Purchasing and providing cost-effective health care.* Edinburgh: Churchill-Livingstone.

Evans, A. R., Seeger, T., & Lehnhardt, M. (1995). Cost-utility analysis of cochlear implants. *Annals of Otology, Rhinology, and Laryngology, 104*(Suppl. 166), 239–240.

Feeny, D., Torrance, G. W., & Furlong, W. (1996). Health utilities index. In B. Spilker (Ed.), *Quality of life and pharmacoeconomics in clinical trials* (2nd ed., pp. 239–252). Philadelphia: Lippincott-Raven.

Fenson, L., Marchman, V. A., Thal, D., Dale, P. S., Reznick, J. S., & Bates, E. (2007). *MacArthur-Bates Communicative Development Inventories: User guide and technical manual* (2nd ed.). Baltimore: Paul H. Brookes.

Fink, N. E., Wang, N. Y., Visaya, J., Niparko, J. K., Quittner, A., Eisenberg, L. S., Tobey, E.A., & CDaCI Investigative Team. (2007). Childhood Development after Cochlear Implantation (CDaCI) study: Design and baseline characteristics. *Cochlear Implants International, 8*, 92–116.

Francis, H. W., Koch, M. E., Wyatt, J. R., & Niparko, J. K. (1999). Trends in educational placement and cost-benefit consideration in children with cochlear implants. *Archives of Otolaryngology-Head and Neck Surgery, 125*, 499–505.

Froberg, D. G., & Kane, R. L. (1989). Methodology for measuring health-state preferences—II: Scaling methods. *Journal of Clinical Epidemiology, 42*, 459–471.

Fugain, C., Severns, J. L., Braspenning, J. C., Brokx, J. P., & van den Broek, P. (1998). Economic evaluation of cochlear implants in children. In *Abstracts from the 4th European*

Symposium on Pediatric Cochlear Implantation, June 14-17, 1998: Hertogenbosch, the Netherlands.

Gans, J. E., Blyth, D. A., Elster, A. B., & Gaveras, L. L. (1990). *American adolescents: How healthy are they?* (Profiles of Adolescent Health Series, Vol. I). Chicago: American Medical Association.

Harris, J. P., Anderson, J. P., & Novak, R. (1995). An outcomes study of cochlear implants in deaf patients: Audiologic, economic and quality of life changes. *Archives of Otolaryngology-Head and Neck Surgery, 121,* 398-404.

Holt, J. (1994). Classroom attributes and achievement scores for deaf and hard of hearing students. *American Annals of the Deaf, 139,* 430-437.

Hutton, J., Politi, C., & Seeger, T. (1995). Cost-effectiveness of cochlear implantation of children. A preliminary model for the UK. *Advances in Oto-Rhino-Laryngology, 50,* 201-206.

Kasen, S., Ouellette, R., & Cohen, P. (1990). Mainstreaming and postsecondary educational and employment status of a rubella cohort. *American Annals of the Deaf, 135,* 22-26.

Koch, M. E., Wyatt, J. R., Francis, H. W., & Niparko, J. K. (1997). A model of educational resource use by children with cochlear implants. *Otolaryngology-Head and Neck Surgery, 117,* 174-179.

Lea, A. R. (1991). *Cochlear implants.* Canberra, Australia: Australian Government Publication Service.

Lea, A. R., & Hailey, D. M. (1995). The cochlear implant. A technology for the profoundly deaf. *Medical Progress Through Technology, 21,* 47-52.

Lin, F. R., Ceh, K., Bervinchak, D., Riley, A., Miech, R., & Niparko J. K. (2007). Development of a communicative performance scale for pediatric cochlear implantation. *Ear and Hearing, 28,* 703-712.

Lin, F. R., & Niparko, J. K. (2006). Measuring health-related quality of life after pediatric cochlear implantation: A systematic review. *International Journal of Pediatric Otorhinolaryngology, 70,* 1695-1706.

Lin, F. R., Wang, N. Y., Fink, N. E., Quittner, A. L., Eisenberg, L. S., Tobey, E. A., Niparko, J. K., & CDaCI Investigative Team. (2008). Assessing the use of speech and language measures in relation to parental perceptions of development after early cochlear implantation. *Otology and Neurotology, 29,* 208-213.

Lloyd, J. W., Singh, N. N., & Repp, A. C. (1991). *The regular education initiative: Alternative perspectives on concepts, issues, and models.* Sycamore, IL: Sycamore Publishing.

Marschark, M. (1993). *Psychological development of deaf children.* New York: Oxford University Press.

Mastropieri, M. A., & Scruggs, T. E. (1987). *Effective instruction for special education.* Austin, TX: Pro-Ed.

McCormick, L., & Schiefelbusch, R. L. (1990). *Early language intervention.* Princeton, NJ: Merrill.

Munoz-Baell, I. M., & Ruiz, M. T. (2000). Empowering the deaf. Let the deaf be deaf. *Journal of Epidemiology and Community Health, 54,* 40-44.

Northern, J. L., & Downs, M. P. (Eds.). (1991). Education of hearing-impaired children. In *Hearing in children* (pp. 323-354). Baltimore: Williams and Wilkins.

Nottingham Paediatric Cochlear Implant Programme. (1997). *Outcomes for paediatric cochlear implantation in Nottingham: Safe, effective, efficient.* Progress Report. Nottingham, UK.

O'Neill, C., O'Donoghue, G. M., Archbold, S. M., & Normand, C. (2000). A cost-utility analysis of pediatric cochlear implantation. *Laryngoscope, 110,* 156-160.

Palmer, C. S., Niparko, J. K., Wyatt, J. R., Rothman, M., & de Lissovoy, G. (1999). A prospective study of the cost-utility of the multichannel cochlear implant. *Archives of Otolaryngology-Head and Neck Surgery, 125,* 1221-1228.

Patrick, D., & Erickson, P. (1993). *Health status and health policy: Quality of life in health care evaluation and resource allocation* (pp. 27-57). New York: Oxford University Press.

Quittner, A. L., Steck, J. T., & Rouiller, R. L. (1991). Cochlear implants in children: A study of parental stress and adjustment. *American Journal of Otology, 12*(Suppl.), 95–104.

Rabin, R., & de Charro, F. (2001). EQ-5D: A measure of health status from the EuroQol Group. *Annals of Medicine, 33,* 337–343.

Reynell, J. K., & Gruber, C. P. (1990). *Reynell Developmental Language Scales* (US ed.). Los Angeles: Western Psychological Services.

Russell, L. B., Gold, M. R., Siegel, J. E., Daniels, N., & Weinstein, M. C. (1996). The role of cost-effectiveness analysis in health and medicine. Panel on cost-effectiveness in health and medicine. *Journal of the American Medical Association, 276,* 1172–1177.

Samuel, F. E., Jr. (1988). Technology and costs: Complex relationship. *Hospitals, 62,* 72.

Saur, R., Coggiola, D., Long, G., & Simonson, J. (1986). Educational mainstreaming and the career development of hearing-impaired students: A longitudinal analysis. *Volta Review, 88,* 79–88.

Schwartz, S. (2007). *Choices in deafness: A parents' guide to communication options.* Bethesda, MD: Woodbine House.

Simeonsson, R. J. (2003). Classification of communication disabilities in children: Contribution of the International Classification on Functioning, Disability and Health. *International Journal of Audiology, 42*(Suppl 1), 2–8.

Smith, D., & Luckasson, R. (1992). Introduction to special education: Teaching in an age of challenge. *Teacher Magazine Reader.* Boston: Allyn & Bacon.

Snell, M. E. (Ed.) (1993). *Systematic instruction of people with severe disabilities* (4th ed.). New York: MacMillan/Merrill.

Spilker, B., & Revicki, D. (1996). Taxonomy of Quality of Life. In B. Spilker (Ed.), *Quality of life and pharmacoeconomics in clinical trials* (2nd ed., pp. 25–31). Philadelphia: Lippincott-Raven.

Summerfield, A. Q., & Marshall, D. H., (1995). *Cochlear implantation in the UK 1990–1994: Report by the MCR Institute of the hearing research on the evaluation of the National Cochlear Implant Programme.* London: HMSO.

Summerfield, A. Q., Marshall, D. H., & Davis, A. C. (1995). Cochlear implantation: Demands, costs, and utility. *Annals of Otology, Rhinology, and Laryngology, 104*(Suppl. 166), 245–248.

Thoutenhoofd, E. D., Archbold, S. M., Gregory, S., Lutman, M. E., Nikolopoulos, T. P., & Sach, T. H. (2005). *Paediatric cochlear implantation: Evaluating outcomes.* London: Whurr.

Trybus, R. J., & Karchmer, M. A. (1977). School achievement scores of hearing impaired children: National data on achievement status and growth patterns. *American Annals of the Deaf, 122,* 62–69.

U.S. Department of Health and Human Services, Food and Drug Administration. (2006). *Guidance for industry: Patient-reported outcome measures: Use in medical product development to support labeling claims.* Rockville, MD: Center for Biologics Evaluation and Research.

Ustun, T. B., Chatterji, S., Bickenbach, J., Kostanjsek, N., & Schneider, M. (2003). The International Classification of Functioning, Disability and Health: A new tool for understanding disability and health. *Disability and Rehabilitation, 25,* 565–571.

U.K. Cochlear Implant Study Group. (2004). Criteria of candidacy for unilateral cochlear implantation in postlingually deafened adults II: Cost-effectiveness analysis. *Ear and Hearing, 25,* 336–360.

Vaccari, C., & Marschark, M. (1997). Communication between parents and deaf children: Implications for social-emotional development. *Journal of Child Psychology and Psychiatry and Allied Disciplines, 38,* 793–801.

Vidas, S., Hassan, R., & Parnes, L. S. (1992). Real-life performance considerations of four pediatric multi-channel cochlear implant recipients. *Journal of Otolaryngology, 21,* 387–393.

Wilson, I. B., & Cleary, P. D. (1995). Linking clinical variables with health-related quality of life. A conceptual model of patient outcomes. *Journal of the American Medical Association, 273,* 59–65.

World Health Organization. (1948). *World Health Organization Constitution.* Basic Documents, Official Publications. Geneva: WHO Press.

World Health Organization. (2001). *International Classification Of Functioning, Disability, And Health.* Geneva: WHO Press.

Wyatt, J. R., & Niparko, J. K. (1995). Evaluating the cost effectiveness of hearing rehabilitation. In: C. Cummings, J. M. Frederickson, L. A. Harker, C. J. Krause, & D. E. Schuller (Eds.), *Otolaryngology: Head and neck surgery update* (2nd ed., pp. 112–125). St. Louis, MO: Mosby Year Book.

Wyatt, J. R., Niparko, J. K., Rothman, M. L., & de Lissovoy, G. V. (1995a). Cost-effectiveness of the multi-channel cochlear implant. *American Journal of Otology, 16*, 52–62.

Wyatt, J. R., Niparko, J. K., Rothman, M. L., & de Lissovoy, G. V. (1995b). Cost-effectiveness of the multichannel cochlear implant. *Annals of Otology, Rhinology, and Laryngology, 104*(Suppl. 166), 248–250.

Wyatt, J. R., Niparko, J. K., Rothman, M., & de Lissovoy, G. (1996). Cost utility of the multi-channel cochlear implant in 258 profoundly deaf individuals. *Laryngoscope, 106*, 816–821.

CHAPTER 15

Auditory-Verbal Therapy and Babies

SYLVIA F. ROTFLEISCH

Introduction

Today most newborns are screened for hearing loss before they leave the hospital. They are referred to an audiologist if they fail the screening and undergo diagnostic assessment within a few weeks of their birth. Upon confirmation of hearing loss, hearing aids are fitted and aided audiograms eventually are obtained. Thus, infants with hearing loss gain at least some access to sound very early in their lives.

The field has changed dramatically. Newborn infant screening, employing auditory brainstem response (ABR) and otoacoustic emissions (OAEs), has significantly lowered the age of the population we service. Early identification of hearing loss necessitates a change in intervention. Auditory-Verbal (AV) therapy is one habilitative approach that is advocated for the infants identified with hearing loss. This approach provides an auditory-focused intervention in which the caregiver is given training as part of the therapy. The caregiver learns from auditory experts how to teach their young baby how to listen and to develop spoken language competence.

The success of AV therapy is evident from select research findings. Goldberg and Flexer (2001) completed a survey of AV therapy graduates who were 18 years or older and had participated in an AV program for at least 3 years. Their survey reported that more than 98% of the AV graduates obtained a university education. In comparison, Blanchfield, Feldman, and Dunbar (2001) reported that 46% of the general deaf and hard-of-hearing population had some attendance at a college level. These numbers also are comparable to 60% of the general U.S. population of students. Another set of statistics indicates that 53% of the deaf and hard-of-hearing population had a family income of less than $25,000 as compared to 35% of the general U.S. population (Blanchfield et al., 2001). Individual income of 60% of AV graduates was over $25,000 (Goldberg & Flexer, 2001). Robertson and Flexer (1993) reported data on 37 children with hearing loss who used listening as their primary mode of communication. For 30 of these children, scores on reading tests were higher than the 50th percentile. Individuals included in studies who followed the AV approach appear to be functioning at a higher level on a number of important variables in comparison to the overall deaf and hard-of-hearing population.

In this chapter a strong auditory approach is advocated. A brief overview is presented, describing normal development in the areas of auditory processes, language development, communication, and speech acquisition. The acoustics of speech are briefly reviewed, which are relevant to any auditory sensory device being utilized. Also discussed are those aspects critical to the AV therapy intervention model, such as parent education and counseling. The normal sequence of skills in typical development provides a foundation for what should be achieved by the young child. This information helps in determining appropriate goals, ongoing progress, and efficacy of the sensory devices. Recommended initial goals are outlined and the implementation of these goals illustrated through examples of play and everyday parent/adult child interactions and therapy. Progression of goals beyond initial skills are included in illustrative cases and discussions.

Intervention

With the implementation of objective screening instrumentation, such as ABR and OAE, along with the option of cochlear implantation at increasingly younger ages, there is a need for conventional therapy models to be re-examined. Traditional remedial models, both individual and school-based programs, do not meet the needs of the infant with hearing loss. In the past, professionals conducting well-baby visits would refer the child who was not responding to sounds or not acquir-

ing speech and language to an audiologist or speech-language pathologist (SLP). For example, the toddler and parent would arrive at the SLP's office presenting with a language delay. Assessments would be administered to confirm the delay and establish standardized scores with the deficits identified. Then rehabilitation could begin. The child would be scheduled for therapy appointments one or more times per week, or would be placed in a setting with peers demonstrating similar deficits. The parent would bring the toddler to therapy and sit in the waiting room or the parent would walk the child into the classroom and hope there would be no tears when they turn to leave. Traditional remedial therapy models are not applicable or appropriate to the infant. A more current scenario has the parent entering the audiology clinic, a 4-week-old infant in arms, newly diagnosed with hearing loss after having failed the hearing screening. Earmold impressions are taken and sent off to the lab while the family waits for the earmolds to arrive and hearing aids to be dispensed.

This scenario does not fit well with the older remedial model. First, one cannot separate the baby from the caregiver. Second, the infant may or may not demonstrate delays in the skill areas of auditory, speech, and language with the existing standardized tests. The baby is best served by progressing through the same developmental sequence of skills as a typically developing hearing child in order to acquire the foundation for becoming a competent spoken language communicator. An AV therapy approach fits such a scenario more readily than the traditional model, as the parent or primary caregiver is an integral player in the intervention model. A parent-infant model is an effective approach for promoting auditory, speech, and language development of babies using hearing aids and/or cochlear implants. AV therapy, as defined by its principles (Table 15–1), incorporates the parent/caregiver as a crit-

TABLE 15–1. Principles of LSLS Auditory-Verbal Therapy*

1. Promote early diagnosis of hearing loss in newborns, infants, toddlers, and young children, followed by immediate audiologic management and Auditory-Verbal therapy.

2. Recommend immediate assessment and use of appropriate, state-of-the-art hearing technology to obtain maximum benefits of auditory stimulation.

3. Guide and coach parents[1] to help their child use hearing as the primary sensory modality in developing spoken language without the use of sign language or emphasis on lipreading.

4. Guide and coach parents[1] to become the primary facilitators of their child's listening and spoken language development through active consistent participation in individualized Auditory-Verbal therapy.

5. Guide and coach parents[1] to create environments that support listening for the acquisition of spoken language throughout the child's daily activities.

6. Guide and coach parents[1] to help their child integrate listening and spoken language into all aspects of the child's life.

7. Guide and coach parents[1] to use natural developmental patterns of audition, speech, language, cognition, and communication.

8. Guide and coach parents help their child self-monitor spoken language through listening.

9. Administer ongoing formal and informal diagnostic assessments to develop individualized Auditory-Verbal treatment plans, to monitor progress and to evaluate the effectiveness of the plans for the child and family.

10. Promote education in regular schools with peers who have typical hearing and with appropriate services from early childhood onward.

*An Auditory-Verbal Practice requires all 10 principles.

[1]The term "parents" also includes grandparents, relatives, guardians, and any caregivers who interact with the child.

Source: (Adapted from the Principles originally developed by Doreen Pollack, 1970.) Adopted by the AG Bell Academy for Listening and Spoken Language®, July 26, 2007. Permission to adapt by Alexander Graham Bell Association for the Deaf and Hard of Hearing, Washington, D.C.

ical team member. The principles define parent/caregiver and use this terminology to imply the primary caregiver. These terms are used interchangeably in this chapter. Intervention is removed from the clinical setting as it becomes an ongoing part of the child's daily interactions. Essentially, the caregiver is taught to interact with the baby in a manner which facilitates the natural development of audition, speech, and language on a daily basis. The logic behind this model assumes that the parent has the most to gain and is highly motivated to have his or her baby succeed. Therapists who see the baby and caregiver on a regular basis primarily focus on the parent during the session. Counseling is a critical component of work with parents of children with hearing loss whether newly diagnosed or several months into the intervention process.

Speech and language competence is the goal of auditory-based therapy approaches. These approaches, currently and in the past, have been referred to as Auditory-Visual, Auditory-Oral, Auditory-Verbal, Acoupedic, Unisensory, and Aural. A critical difference in approaches relates to the use of audition as it integrates with other sensory modalities, such as vision and touch. Audition is the primary sensory modality used in an AV therapy approach, and though other senses are introduced to supplement the auditory input, the practice advocates "putting it back into hearing." The delivery models for auditory-based approaches vary from the parent-infant to small groups and classes in similar settings with peers who have hearing loss of varying degrees. An AV therapy approach recommends education in regular schools with peers who have typical hearing.

Communication Development

In the following sections the sequence of normal development are outlined in several areas, which are most pertinent to the baby who is deaf or hard-of-hearing. Infants' skills do not develop in isolation; many areas are dependent on each other and are integrally tied. Speech production ability is dependent on motor development as well as audition. Speech is typically a reflection of hearing abilities. Though not discussed in this chapter, cognitive and other areas of development for babies and young children must be taken into consideration when planning appropriate activities for the child. The child's gross motor, fine motor, cognitive levels of functioning must be understood to set up the activity for success in therapy.

Using Sound Meaningfully: Auditory Comprehension of Language

Typically developing infants follow a normal sequence of development in all areas of development. One expects infants from birth to 3 months, with usual access to sound, to be responsive to their auditory environment. New parents of typically developing infants watch this development with expectation and amazement. They don't agonize over every skill unless they do not see expected changes, or the pediatrician expresses concerns or feels there are delays. Babies' detection and localization responses develop in a well-documented manner over their first years of life.

Auditory Development

Auditory detection and discrimination is developmental (Weir, 1979; Werner & Gillenwater, 1990; Werner & Mancl, 1993; Yoshinaga-Itano & Sedey, 2000). From an early stage, babies with hearing loss show deficits most closely related to and dependent upon their hearing abilities. When babies are initially fitted with their sensory devices —hearing aids or cochlear implants—they must begin the process of learning to listen. They will be tested by the audiologist, possibly resulting in an audiogram with aided thresholds, and the parents might be under the impression that now the child hears— perhaps even believe that they hear normally as does a typically developing child (Table 15–2). Babies who are just beginning to listen will not react consistently in an everyday environment. Parent education must incorporate the typical developmental stages with an explanation of the child's need for experienced listening in order to develop early auditory skills. Hearing-impaired babies, after gaining access to auditory information, must begin to progress through the stages. Monitoring responses to sounds is one of the first goals. The parents must understand that skills require time to develop and, in monitoring these skills, progress can be determined in terms of the baby's functional use of audition. Professionals educate parents about the normal developmental stages so that they understand the sequence and time frame. It is common for parents to think that as soon the sensory device is appropriately adjusted, the child will begin to behave as other children of the same chronologic age, such as immediately beginning to babble, respond to their name, or produce words.

Providing a sensory device does not immediately propel a child into the auditory skill level of a hearing child of the same chronologic age. Upon receiving sound, the child with hearing loss typically exhibits the auditory skills of a newborn. Regardless of the child's chronologic age, the child's hearing age is referenced to the time he or she begins to use their sensory device. The skills of a baby with a hearing age of 4 months should be compared to a typically developing child of 4 months. The use of hearing age allows for a more appropriate monitoring and comparison of skill levels. It also helps to determine if skills are emerging in an appropriate sequence and time frame. Babies have the ability to respond to differences in speech sounds soon after birth (for a review see Jusczyk & Luce, 2002). This is a critical piece of information for us to understand, explain to parents, and be aware that those babies had exposure to sounds in utero for several months (Birnholtz & Benacceraf, 1983). Monitoring these responses in therapy sessions as well as from parental input, provides important information about the development of specific auditory attention and localization skills. It is important to watch the baby's responses to voices, a critical auditory cue for the development of spoken language. The situations in which infants learn to listen and understand sounds should be in a natural setting and not in controlled, clinical situations, such as those in an audio booth. The actual signal reaching the infant's ears will depend on the acoustics of their various surroundings, intensity of the sounds, and the functioning of their sensory device to consider just a few.

TABLE 15–2. Infants' Responses and Localization

Infant Responses and Localization: Newborns to 24 Months	
0–4 months Normal infant is aroused from sleep by sound signals of 90 dB (SPL) in a noisy environment, 50–70 dB (SPL) in quiet.	**9–13 months** Baby directly locates a sound source of 25–35 dB (SPL) to the side and below.
3–4 months Normal infant begins to make a rudimentary head-turn toward a sound signal 50–60 dB (SPL).	**13–16 months** Toddler localizes directly sound signals of 25–30 dB (SPL) to the side and below; indirectly above.
4–7 months Baby turns head directly toward the side of a signal 40–50 dB (SPL) but cannot find it above or below.	**16–21 months** Toddler localizes directly sound signals of 25–30 dB (SPL) on the side, below and above.
7–9 months Baby directly locates a sound source of 30–40 dB (SPL) to the side and indirectly below.	**21–24 months** Child locates directly a sound signal of 25 dB (SPL) at all angles.

Source: Adapted from Northern and Downs (1991).

As we watch for initial reactions and evidence that the infant is responding to sound, we must look for clear unambiguous behaviors. Parents also must learn that babies have subtle ways of responding. Widening of eyes, turning head or looking around, change in sucking rate, change in movement of the body, and change of vocalization patterns (starting or stopping) are all normal reactions for a baby to have when hearing a sound. These behaviors may be manifested when the auditory event begins or possibly at the cessation of the signal.

Auditory abilities are noted when babies demonstrate an understanding of the non-segmental aspects of speech, such as inflection and syllabification. Babies will not respond or show interest to conversation that is not intended for them, but when the voice changes and has increased inflection and other nonsegmental cues, the baby will respond and attend to the voice. Once babies are consistently responding and attending to voices, the infant then responds to changes in tone of voice, to music, to friendly or angry tones, intonation patterns and to their own name—features that are related to the nonsegmental aspects of speech. Specific intonation patterns will become associated with routines in the child's life and are recognized by the infant as they anticipate what will happen based on the adult vocalizations. From this stage, monitoring of auditory development is integrally tied to the development of auditory comprehension of language—also referred to as receptive language (Table 15–3). Additionally, as babies begin to vocalize more consistently, their auditory abilities are reflected by various aspects of auditory feedback—also referred to as speech production, in which they begin to demonstrate vocal control over the new sounds they produce in their emerging vocal play (see the section on speech production below).

Babies begin to understand simple instructions or requests, especially when context is available. With more auditory experience, infants learn to determine word boundaries and listen when spoken to as they become aware of the interaction during spoken communication. By 1 year of age, babies typically will recognize a few initial words, such as "no," their name, "mommy," "daddy," and a few common objects of significance. This is an indication of an increased ability to differentiate a variety of segmental aspects of speech within the vowels and consonants. By 18 months babies are typically able to point to named objects and recognize many names of familiar people, objects, and body parts. They demonstrate an understanding of simple commands, requests and questions. The young child's expressive vocabulary is beginning to grow and they usually have more than five words—primarily nouns and names, which they use consistently. They tend to still use jargon at this age and will manipulate the nonsegmental aspects to convey emotional aspects as they communicate. Initially, comprehension of the first 10 to 50 words progresses more rapidly than retrieval (or expression) of these words. Children will have acquired these words receptively by about 1 year, 1 month (Benedict, 1979). By the time the child has reached 2 years of age, he or she is demonstrating more advanced auditory discrimination and recognition abilities. Auditory memory has improved, which is demonstrated by the child's abilities to attend to simple songs, stories, and rhymes.

Communication

Communication begins with a deliberate attempt by the baby to convey meaning. The attempt to communicate cannot be determined by one behavior. Young children demonstrate communicative intent prior to their use of linguistic units. Linguists define

TABLE 15–3. Normal Developmental Milestones

Audition and Auditory Comprehension of Language	Expressive Language/Preverbal Vocalization and Communication
0–3 months	**0–3 months**
• Turns head toward direction of sound	• Begins to imitate sounds
• increases or decreases sucking behavior in response to sound	• Laughs
• Startles to loud sounds	• Makes pleasure sounds (cooing, gooing)
• Quiets or smiles when spoken to	• Cries differently for different needs
• Seems to recognize your voice and quiets if crying	
• Looks at speaker and smiles	
4–6 months	**4–6 months**
• Responds to changes in tone of your voice	• Vocalizes excitement and displeasure
• Notices toys that make sounds	• Babbling sounds more speechlike with many different sounds, including p, b, and m
• Localizes sound	• Vocalization with intonation
• Pays attention to music	
• Responds to human voices without visual cues by turning his head and eyes	
• Responds appropriately to friendly and angry tones	
• Responds to name	
7–12 months	**7–12 months**
• Emergence of naming insight	• Enjoys games like peek-o-boo and pat-a-cake
• Understands simple instructions/requests, especially if vocal or physical cues are given ("Come here," "Want more?")	• Emergence of gestures—reaching, waves bye-bye, rejects objects, "pick me up"
• Responds to "no"	• Babbles with inflection
• Recognizes name	• Babbling has both long and short groups of sounds such as "tata upup bibibibi"
• Listens when spoken to	• Uses speech or non-crying sounds to get and keep attention
• Is aware of the social value of speech	• Imitates different speech sounds/ familiar words
• Recognizes words for common items like "cup," "shoe," "juice"	• Says "dada" and "mama," which correlates with the person
	• Says 2–3 words besides "mama" and "dada" although they may not be clear
	• Uses exclamations, such as "oh-oh!"

continues

TABLE 15–3. *continued*

Audition and Auditory Comprehension of Language	Expressive Language/Preverbal Vocalization and Communication
18 months	**18 months**
• Points to object or picture when it's named	• Waves good-bye and plays pat-a-cake
• Recognizes names of familiar people, objects and body parts	• Makes the "sounds" of familiar animals
• Understands about 50 words	• Uses words such as "more" to make wants known
• Follows simple commands and understands simple questions (gives a toy, "Roll the ball," "Kiss the baby," "Where's your shoe?")	• Has vocabulary of 5 to 20 words, including names
	• Begins to have dramatic increase in vocabulary
• Brings object from another room when asked	• Vocabulary made up chiefly of nouns
	• Names a number of objects common to his surroundings
	• Some echolalia (repeating a word or phrase over and over)
	• Much jargon with emotional content
24 months	**24 months**
• Listens to simple stories, songs, and rhymes	• Says more words every month
• Follows 2–3 simple, related commands	• Uses some 1-2 word questions ("Where kitty?" "Go bye-bye?" "What's that?")
• Understands several action words	• Uses many different consonant sounds at the beginning of words
• Points to smaller body parts	• Is able to use at least two prepositions, usually chosen from the following: in, on, under
• Understands complex sentences	• Vocabulary of approximately 150–300 words
	• Knows and says about 50 words with two to three syllables
	• Can use two pronouns correctly: I, me, mine, you, although me and I are often confused
	• Begins using simple prepositions, such as "with" and "for"
	• Mean length of utterance is given as 1.2 words
	• Combines two words such as "daddy bye-bye"

Source: Compiled from American Speech-Language Hearing Association; Brown, (1973); Bzoch, League, and Brown, (2003); Child Development Institute; Foster, (1990); Gleason, (1997); Learning Disabilities Association of America (1999); Mayo Clinic; Zimmerman, Steiner, and Pond, (2002).

true communication as demonstrating the existence of two simultaneous attention components: (1) attention to the object of the communication, and (2) attention to the person with whom one is communicating. However, even prior to these behaviors, adults will typically respond to the infants' actions or vocalizations in a manner that assumes the baby is intentionally communicating. The parent learns early that the child has different vocalizations for various needs. As infants begin to use their voices, caregivers can differentiate a contented sound from one of hunger, or from a voice indicating distress. In such circumstances, the infant typically will elicit a response from the adults due to their interpretations of these vocalizations. There are several specific behaviors, both vocal and nonvocal, that suggest communicative intent by the baby. These are: (1) continuing with a behavior (such as a reach or a vocalization) until it is responded to; (2) showing distress at an object or a person, but ceasing when the person responds; (3) reaching toward something that is clearly out of reach; (4) using consistent or 'ritualized' facial expressions, gestures, or vocalizations, such as "ga" when indicating things; and (5) combining gaze at a person with some other behavior such as a facial expression, a vocalization, or a hand gesture (Foster, 1990). The emergence of communicative intention is not known, but the most common practice is to look for evidence of several different behaviors as discussed earlier, and at that point make the determination that the child is probably attempting to communicate. It is our response to the child that treats the vocalizations 'as if' they were communicative. This response reinforces the child's behavior. Early pragmatic functions, as listed by Dore (1975), include labeling, repeating, answering, requesting action, requesting, calling, greeting, protesting, and practicing. These functions are evidenced in prelinguistic conversations and at the one-word stage of linguistic communication.

A very basic premise in spoken language communication that enables one to participate in conversation is "turn-taking." Communication requires that one communicative partner speaks while the other one listens. Then the roles reverse—essentially, you talk, I listen, then I talk and you listen. One must provide adequate information so that the listener can determine the topic and relationship between the referents through semantic construction. From early infancy vocalizations can be reinforced and fostered into this critical turn-taking behavior. Along with the different turn-taking behaviors, mutual eye contact is determined to be critical for success in communication. These basic skills begin to develop from early infancy and develop into complex spoken interactions. In addition to the vocal behaviors involved in communication, there are many elements which are nonverbal and develop prior to, or in tandem with, other foundation behaviors of communication. The combination of vocal and nonvocal components allows for communicative competence. Most common nonvocal gestures of communicative intent and their approximate age at emergence include: reaching (extending a hand to reach an object out of reach) at 6 months; waving bye-bye (waving or flapping of hands) at 9 months; rejection (pushing away an object or person or turning away from what is not desired) at 9 months; "pick me up" (raising arms when he/she wants to be picked up) at 10 months; pointing (extending arm and finger in the direction of an object) at 11 months; offering (combination of reaching and grasping along with offering and releasing) and shaking head "no" at about 1 year, 2 months (Foster, 1990). As the different pragmatic functions emerge, even prior to real words, children are capable of advanced prelinguistic stages, revolving around the here and now, and use these stages to initiate and engage in multiple turns which are indicative of complex conversational structures.

Auditory Retrieval

Babies vocalize both excitement and displeasure. Parents soon learn to interpret and predict their child's needs, based on the sounds of these initial vocalizations and the progression through babbling stages. Once again consider that the different elements of audition, speech, and language cannot be isolated from one another, and the development of these abilities is interconnected (see Table 15–3). At a given time, babies develop insight into the symbolic nature of an arbitrary sequence of speech phonemes. At about the time when first words are about to emerge, babies have three primary types of speech acts: speech play, modulated canonical babbling, and protowords. Speech play is the child playing and practicing specific phonemes and is not considered to be communicative. Canonical babbling and jargoning, implied by the intonation contour, is superimposed on the string of syllables being produced. Protowords, also referred to as word approximations, are articulated utterances that hold meaning. At about 1 year of age, these utterances are typically recognized by parents as the baby's first words. These often include "dada" and "mama," which correlate with the person, or as reduplicative or one-syllable word approximations (e.g., "baba" for bottle or "da" for dog). These word approximations are a reflection of the child's limits with regard to his or her phoneme repertoire and the ability to combine sounds.

There is a slow progression of the baby's vocabulary over the next several months, followed by a dramatic increase at about the age of 16 to18 months. Growth of vocabulary differs for comprehension and retrieval as the first 50 words are attained. Expressive vocabulary acquisition is slower and follows receptive vocabulary acquisition. Children will have acquired 50 words receptively before they are able to produce 10 words expressively. Typically developing, hearing babies acquire receptive vocabulary at a rate of approximately 22 words per month during the time span while they expand their comprehension from 10 to 50 words. Expressive vocabulary is acquired at a rate of about nine words per month during the period while they are at the 10- to 50-word stage. They will acquire the 50-word level of expressive vocabulary by about 1 year, 6 months (Benedict, 1979). Children will use a single word with an intonation curve to modify the meaning of the communication. The two-word stage follows soon thereafter, as the child's expressive vocabulary continues to develop. It appears that the form and functions used by children are similar even across different languages. The toddler combining three words or more is considered to be at the stage of telegraphic speech. Some define this as the stage when no function words are being used but when syntax, word order and phrasing emerge. However others point out that some telegraphic phrases are syntactically complete (Foster, 1990). Generally speaking we expect 1-year-old infants to speak in one-word utterances, and 2-year-olds to be combining words and speaking in two-word utterances (Brown, 1973).

Speech Production

Stages of children's preverbal vocalizations are not random. There are predictable, specific stages that children move through which deserve inspection. The understanding of normal speech development allows for the prediction and appropriate facilitation of phonemes to be acquired. Classifying misarticulations and omissions assists in determining whether these errors are developmental in nature or are a result of poor auditory access to the speech signal. Oller and his colleagues have extensively documented infant preverbal vocalization patterns during the first year of life (Oller, 1980; Oller & Eilers, 1988; Oller, Eilers, Neal, & Schwartz, 1999), as shown in Table 15–4. The types of sounds produced are ordered sequentially and occur regardless of language in the home or socioeconomic level. It is known that parents' responses help in the development of speech production. Social and vocal reinforcement increases the quantity of the babbling but not the consonants used. The vocalization stages have some overlap. Development of speech begins with the birth cry, but not all sounds are treated as precursors to speech. Sounds that are not related to speech production are referred to as reflexive vocalizations and include a variety of sounds: fixed vocal sounds (crying, laughing, and moaning), vegetative sounds (coughing, sneezing, and burping), squealing, growling, raspberries, and grunts (Foster, 1990).

Babies develop control of their non-segmentals and vowels in vocal play. Consonant production develops through babbling. The late onset of canonical babbling is a predictor of later speech and language disabilities (Oller et al., 1999) and infants with severe hearing impairment are at risk of not developing canonical babbling (Eilers & Oller, 1994). Syllabic and word production consists of rapid consonant-to-vowel transitions which are essential for typical speech development. Babies appear to produce words using phonemes mastered through babbling (Oller, Wieman, Doyle, & Ross,

1976). Professionals who provide intervention for infants who are deaf and hard-of-hearing must encourage and promote canonical babbling to promote mastery of sounds.

There is a developmental progression of articulation in that certain phoneme classes are mastered before we can expect other phoneme classes to be mastered. It is generally accepted that the pattern of articulatory development won't be completed until at least 7 to 8 years of age and even later. Occurring at about 3 years of age, the consonants mastered first are p, b, m, n, w, h. These phonemes include different speech features, such as manner of production (plosives, nasals, one fricative [h] and one semivowel [w]). In addition, there is a voicing feature within the plosive feature ([b] versus [p]) and a place cue difference within the nasal feature ([m] versus [n]). Later developing consonants include: k, g, d, t, and "ng." These consonants show voicing contrasts ([d] versus [t]; [g] versus [k]) and place cue contrasts ([d] versus [g]; [k] versus [t]) within the plosive manner. The nasal feature for the English language is completed with the addition of the "ng," another place contrast within this manner. The complete sequence of mastery (Sander, 1972) is provided in Figure 15–1.

Parental Education

One challenging aspect for professionals who are new to the principles of AV therapy is often in teaching and empowering parents to be their baby's primary teacher. Teaching children to listen and speak may initially seem very complicated to parents as they embark on AV therapy. Therefore, parent education becomes a focal point in intervention in the model whereby the caregiver is a critical partner in their child's development. This style of intervention

TABLE 15–4. Stages of Infant Vocal Development

Stage/Age	Features
Quasi-resonant sounds, Reflexive vocalizations 0–2 months	• Quasi-resonant sounds are normal phonation but typically not full use of resonating in the vocal cavity • Small quantity of vowels or coos (fully resonant sounds) • Reflexive vocalizations and vegetative sounds • Infant has mouth partially open and produces an utterance
"Gooing" "Cooing" 2–3 months	• Control over quasi-resonant sounds—most frequent sounds • Increase in controlled repetitive utterances with a preference for velar sounds • Back articulations which may be due to gravity • Beginning of laughter • Crying is very tense and usually nonspeechy at this age
Fully resonant sounds 4–6 months	• Using full resonant sounds with mouths wide open • Controlled number of vocalization types—vocal play with pitch, intensity • Increased use of vowel-like productions • Practice and play with the nonsegmentals • Sounds like singing when happy • Limited production of consonant-like productions • Raspberries, squealing, growling • Occasional marginal babbling—closure of the vocal tract combined with a vowel-like production
Reduplicated babbling 7–10 months	• Canonical babbling—syllabification characteristics similar to mature productions • Reduplicative syllables (mamama, bababa) utterance with little variation • Nonreduplicated utterances—single consonant common (ba, ada, imi)
Variegated babbling 11–12 months	• Characteristics of language • Longer utterances with variety of consonant and vowel productions • Variety of syllabic stress within utterances • Referred to as gibberish, modulated babble or jargoning

Source: Compiled from Oller (1980); Oller and Eilers, 1988; Oller, Eilers, Neal, and Schwartz (1999).

aligns with Luterman's proposed humanistic approach, in which the clinician and the client are equal partners (Luterman, 1984). Parents learn the theoretical basis and practical skills necessary for effective facilitation of their child's development. By teaching parents to be the primary facilitators of the child's skills, they will subsequently be pre-

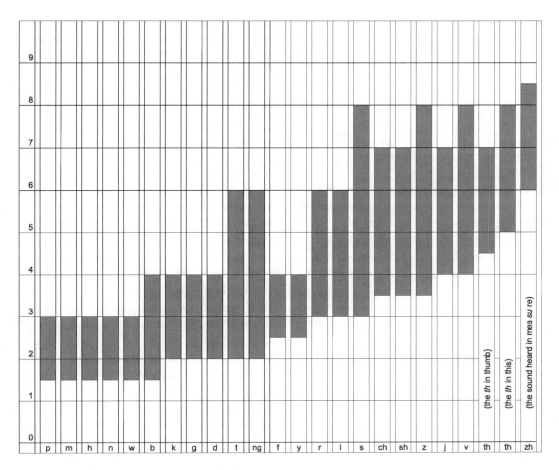

Figure 15–1. Vowel formant and speech sound development chart according to age range (years) at emergence. Adapted from Sander (1972). Permission to adapt by the American Speech-Language-Hearing Association.

pared to advocate for their child through the different stages of their development. Parents also assist by observing and reporting back to the AV therapist about their child's progress. They are taught to understand: (1) their child's current level of functioning; (2) what skills and stages will follow; and (3) what behaviors they should be monitoring. Therapy sessions must have clearly defined goals, which are explained to the parent. The sessions focus on designated goals; the AV therapist demonstrates the prerequisite skills that the child has acquired and the targeted skills being devel-

oped. Parents must learn the sequence of normal development as it relates to their child's development, and must learn to incorporate the therapeutic strategies and techniques into everyday interactions with their youngster. During therapy sessions, the therapist must monitor the parents' interaction style and assist in reinforcing those aspects of communication that will facilitate their child's development. Therapists watch for and teach the typical elements of parents' communication interactions, which include such various elements as voice pitch and intensity, turn-taking skills, and audition-maximizing strategies. Facilitating optimum use of these strategies through modeling and reinforcement can ensure a good interaction style.

Acoustics of Speech

A natural starting point is to teach parents about the audiogram and speech acoustics. This is considered to be one of the first and essential aspects of parent education. Parents have so many questions about their child's hearing that they often don't know where to begin. Parents do not typically understand the fundamentals of an audiogram; the explanation provided at initial diagnosis is often not comprehended due to the shock of the diagnosis. It is wise to assume that anything after the "your child is deaf" statement was not completely absorbed. Technical terms must be explained in language that is understandable. The technical terms and acronyms: OAEs—otoacoustic emissions; ABRs—auditory brainstem responses; SAT—speech awareness thresholds; VRA—visual reinforcement audiometry; CPA—conditioned play audiometry; and so forth, are often very confusing. Parents must have an understanding of critical information to allow them to comprehend their infant's hearing loss and to make appropriate decisions.

Information relating to the audiologic tests and the audiogram can easily be presented during the initial therapy session. As this explanation begins, so too will the questions and the start of your relationship with the parents. Aspects to present include the basics of an audiogram—the representation of the frequencies in hertz (Hz) from low to high. Understanding the relationship of these frequencies to speech and language is critical for parents. However, it can be explained that music has frequencies that we do not test—both higher and lower pitch sounds that allow for the ability to hear and

appreciate music. This is an important concept to keep in mind as we encourage singing with babies. Intensity, or decibel (dB) level (referenced to Hearing Level or HL), is represented on the vertical axis of the audiogram—progressing from quiet to louder levels. Parents must comprehend that the threshold of a tone, noise, or speech is defined as sound that is detected 50% of the time.

When assessing the speech of a hearing-impaired child, professionals often follow the remedial model proposed by Daniel Ling (1976, 2002), which organizes speech assessment and teaching by features that are intended to be taught in a systematic approach. The rationale underlying the sequence of teaching encompasses normal development, speech acoustics, and speech intelligibility. Ling's Phonetic Level Evaluation (PLE) (Ling, 2002) and proposed intervention order is as follows: nonsegmentals (also referred to as suprasegmentals); vowels and diphthongs; consonants by manner of production; consonants by place of production; voice/voiceless consonants; and consonant blends.

The nonsegmentals include those features of duration, intensity, and pitch. Ling explains that the nonsegmentals are the underlying foundations of speech intelligibility and they convey meaning. For example, through variations in stress and pitch, a phrase is interpreted to be either a question or a statement. Important to parents is the understanding that development and control of the nonsegmental aspects of speech is more critical than development of some individual phonemes.

Segmentals refer to the phonemes, or vowels and consonants. Explaining the acoustic structure of vowels will assist the parents in understanding the ways in which these properties are perceived, which subsequently will impact the development of a child's vowel productions. The vowels are represented as vocal tract resonances, which can be visually displayed in terms of their frequency/intensity components as a function of time. The visual representation, known as the spectrogram, displays the characteristic acoustic features known as formants, or harmonics of the fundamental frequency (i.e., the frequency of the vocal folds as they vibrate). Formant structure determines which vowel is being produced and consists of a set of resonances that contains energy in specific frequency regions. The first two formants characterize the vowel being produced and convey the acoustic information required for identifying vowels. The first or the lower frequency energy cluster is referred to as the first formant (F_1) and the second, being the higher frequency energy, is referred to as the second formant (F_2). Anatomically, as air is exhaled from the lungs and moves through the vocal tract, the different positions of the articulators (i.e., lips and tongue) determine the resonant characteristics (formants) that define specific vowels. Examining the vowel formant chart displayed in Figure 15–2, one realizes that there are vowels that share the

same first formant. Therefore, it is the second formant that is particularly important for differentiating one vowel from another. The problem arises for hearing-impaired children who might not detect F_2 due to the nature of their hearing loss and/or the limited frequency bandwidth of their sensory device. Inability to detect F_2 will result in an inability to differentiate vowels with the same first formant but different second formant, for example, [oo] versus [ee]. A diphthong is the technical term for two vowels that merge, such as [ou] or [oi]. Vowels and diphthongs are important because they also convey nonsegmental (or prosodic) information, including speech rhythm, rate, and stress, as well as some acoustic cues for accents and dialects.

The basic linguistic unit is the syllable, composed of consonants (C) and vowels (V). Syllables are characterized by combinations of Vs and Cs, such as CV, VC, CVC, and VCV. In addition to the vowels and consonants, an important acoustic cue is the frequency transition between the phonemes.

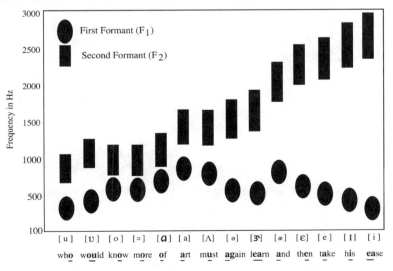

Figure 15–2. Vowel formant chart. *Source*: (Adapted from Aural habilitation—The foundations of verbal learning in hearing-impaired children by Ling, D. & Ling, A., 1978.) Permission to adapt by Alexander Graham Bell Association for the Deaf and Hard of Hearing, Washington, D.C.

Consonants typically are classified according to the features of manner, place, and voicing. These basic features are important to describe to parents. The "manner" feature refers to the manner in which the consonant is produced. These are categorized as plosives, nasals, fricatives, liquids, affricates, and semivowels (Table 15–5). It is important to note that plosives are also referred to as stops; however, in this chapter, a stop is used to indicate an unreleased plosive such as [t] in *bat* or [b] in *cab*. Consonant manner is reliant on frequency, timing, and intensity acoustic cues.

Consonant place of production refers to the location in the oral cavity where the articulators (i.e., lips, alveolar ridge, and palate) are positioned for producing the consonant. Acoustically, consonant place is reliant on high-frequency cues and, therefore, is most susceptible to the effects of hearing loss. The anatomic terms that define consonant place are detailed in Table 15–6.

Consonant voicing denotes whether the vocal folds are vibrating or not vibrating when the consonant is produced. Voicing cues rely heavily on duration of the phoneme (e.g., [b] versus [p]). Parents typically assume that if you are using your voice that the vocal folds are vibrating. Having the parents place their hand on the front of their throat while producing "ah" allows them to feel the vibrations of the vocal folds. With their hand still on their throat, they produce an "sss" and instantly understand that, even though it is counter intuitive, one can speak without "voicing." Whispering an entire sentence clearly illustrates this point. We complete a blank consonant chart in a session that shows the different consonants together thinking of the three features that define a consonant and integrating some of the principles which we have discussed thus far. It is advisable to go slowly through this theoretical information over the course of several sessions. Incorporating this new terminology in therapy sessions by redefining the terms or having the parents explain them allows for practical and applicable reinforcement of the new concepts.

TABLE 15–5. Consonant Manner of Production

Plosives	an exploding sound where we build up the pressure and then get a sudden burst of air coming out almost like an explosion.
Nasals	a resonating of the air in the nasal passage where the mouth is typically closed and the structure (velopharyngeal port) which opens and closes the nasal cavity is open to allow the air into the nasal cavity where it resonates.
Fricatives	blowing sounds with friction between the articulators and the produced airstream which must go through the oral (mouth) cavity.
Liquids (Approximants)	two articulators are close to each other preventing a strong breath stream or turbulence causing the sound energy to be blocked or obstructed.
Affricates	a combination of a fricative and a stop plosive.
Semivowels (Approximants, glides)	the sound made by the movement between two vowels.

Source: Compiled from Ladefoged (2006).

TABLE 15–6. Anatomical Terms for Place of Production

Anatomic Terms	Location
Bilabial	both lips
Labiodental	lips and teeth—(lower lip and upper front teeth)
Linguadental	tongue tip and teeth
Alveolar	tongue tip and alveolar ridge (behind the teeth)
Palatal	front of tongue (tongue blade) and hard palate
Velar	back of tongue (tongue dorsum) and hard palate
Glottal	originating at the vocal folds

In addition to educating the parents, summarizing this information in a methodical way assists the therapist in establishing therapy goals. It is particularly helpful to consider "essential principles" and portray the acoustic properties of nonsegmentals and segmentals. It is important for parents to understand that nonsegmental and low-frequency segmental cues are more accessible to hearing-impaired children. It is an appropriate expectation that the development of auditory detection and discrimination abilities will progress from easier skills, using acoustic cues that are the most accessible, to the more difficult skills incorporating less accessible acoustic cues. Nonsegmental information is carried by the vowels and, therefore, hearing up to 1000 Hz provides access to at least the first formants F_1 of all vowels and provides information that enables detection and some discrimination of these features. Because discrimination of the vowels is dependent upon access to the second formant of the vowels, audibility to 3000 Hz is required to discriminate all the vowels. Access to acoustic cues for speech features, particularly the consonant features, is included in much more detail in Table 15-7.

The acoustic information conveyed by low frequencies includes nonsegmentals, F_1 and some F_2 vowel information, most consonant manner information, nasal murmur, and consonant voicing cues. In contrast, high frequencies, which are typically more difficult and less accessible, include F_2 of many vowels; consonant place cues; and the fricatives classified under consonant manner (Table 15-8) (Rotfleisch, 2000).

With a grasp of speech acoustics, as related to the audiogram, we can overlay a child's detection abilities on the audiogram and then have much more information about their potential for auditory development. This provides an opportunity to look at an audiogram as more than merely detection, but as containing potential information about discrimination to postulate a "functional audiogram" (Rotfleisch, 2000). Sometimes this can be done using a detection audiogram or sometimes the reverse process allows part of the audiogram to be predicted based on skills. Given some particular abilities and/or difficulties that are observed in a child's performance, though not necessarily a comprehensive picture, reasonable assumptions can be made about an audiogram. However as discussed previously, an audiogram primarily reflects detection thresholds as a function of frequency and does not ensure discrimination abilities. The predictions that can be made from the detection audiogram are impacted by other factors, such as neural survival and the use of the sensory device. Results from more formal tests that measure speech perception and spoken word recognition (detailed in other chapters) provide a more complete profile regarding the child's auditory abilities, difficulties, and emerging skills. On the basis of all obtainable data, appropriate goals can be established.

TABLE 15–7. Acoustic Cues for Speech Features

Vocalization	Consonants: Manner of Production
• minimum of up to 750 Hz to hear all • 125 Hz—male fundamental frequency • 250 Hz low harmonics • 250 Hz fundamental frequency of female and child voices • 500 Hz harmonics of most voices	• 500 Hz—primary cues, for most consonants • 2000 Hz—additional cues • 750 Hz—allows for ability to discriminate nasals from plosives • 300 Hz nasal murmur—m n "ng" • 1500 Hz—laterals liquids r, l • 2000 Hz unvoiced plosives—p, k, t • 2000 Hz—turbulent noise of fricatives sh, f, th (unvoiced) • 4000 Hz—turbulent noise of voiced and unvoiced fricatives • 4000 Hz fricatives and affricates
Nonsegmentals	**Consonants: Place of Production**
• mainly low-frequency information • information is carried by the vowels • can learn to discriminate if have hearing up to 1000 Hz	• F_2 transition and burst frequency at 1500–4000 Hz • 2000 Hz primary cues • 4000 Hz secondary cues
Vowels & Diphthongs	**Consonants: Voicing**
• 1000 Hz to detect all vowels • 3000 Hz to discriminate • 250 Hz F_1 of high back and front vowels • 500 Hz F_1 of most vowels • 1000 Hz F_2 of back and central vowels • 2000 Hz F_2 of front vowels	• 250 Hz • 500 Hz and below, and duration and intensity differences • 750 Hz for vocal fold vibration • 3000 Hz for unvoiced • voiced at least one formant present at or below 700 Hz, • voiceless no energy below 1000 Hz

Source: Compiled from Ling (1976, 1989).

TABLE 15–8. Accessible Speech Cues as a Function of Frequency

Low-frequency information *Easier, more accessible*	High-frequency information *More difficult, less accessible*
Nonsegmentals—duration, intensity, pitch	Vowels—remaining F_2
Vowels—F_1 and some F_2	Consonant place cues
Consonant manner information	Consonant manner cues (fricatives)
Voicing cues	
Nasal murmur	

Parental Counseling

Counseling is a critical component of work with parents of children with hearing loss whether newly diagnosed or several months into their intervention. Expectant parents have an image of their perfect newborn with ten tiny perfect fingers and toes, everything brand new and a miracle. The diagnosis of a disability or impairment of any nature, therefore, contradicts their vision, hopes and dreams for their perfect baby. Parents of newly diagnosed babies with hearing loss must go through stages of grieving and must cope with the diagnosis of hearing loss. Luterman (1984) acknowledges the loss of the dream of a normal child, is indeed a loss which must be grieved. The stages that people will go through in accepting a hearing loss are the same as those noted in the acceptance of other serious loss in one's life cycle. Kubler-Ross (1969) first wrote about these stages regarding terminally ill patients learning to cope with their own imminent death. Since her initial work with the grief process, many applications have emerged from her groundbreaking research. Her outlined stages of the grief process include denial, anger, bargaining, depression, and acceptance. Luterman believes that these stages are instrumental in understanding parental reactions to the diagnosis of hearing loss and their inevitable grieving. As professionals we should neither attempt to escape nor avoid this crisis. Luterman feels this is a beginning framework but that we must not oversimplify the process. He explores Erikson's life cycle and stages of development (Erikson, 1950) and presumes how they would be impacted by a communicative disorder. Most relevant are Erikson's early stages of childhood involving the development of the child's ego with regard to the following conflicts: trust versus mistrust, autonomy versus shame or doubt, and initiative versus guilt. Because of parental grief, Luterman suggests that the child may be denied the consistency and the responsiveness that will foster the development of trust. With diminished language abilities, the parents may not have the ability to explain clearly the rules to their young child, which may limit most of the child's experiences—particularly those that may be potentially harmful. These parental issues may restrict the young hearing-impaired child's development of both autonomy and initiative. As professionals working with young infants and toddlers, an understanding of the normal developmental stages of ego and self-esteem throughout the life cycle, as outlined by Erikson (1950), provides a more global understanding of child development.

Habilitation

Early intervention with a hearing-impaired infant requires habilitation, rather than rehabilitation, as the infant will be developing new skills, which have never been acquired. An auditory training model and hierarchy proposed by Erber (1982) progresses from detection and discrimination to identification and comprehension. More recently, auditory learning has become a more common way to think of the role of audition in habilitation. Mischook and Cole (1986) proposed a model for auditory learning in which Erber's levels overlapped in such a way that comprehension became the center of the learning process. The American Speech-Language-Hearing Association (ASHA) Task Force on Central Auditory Processing Consensus Development (1996) proposed a model of defined auditory processes more closely focused on the child's specific abilities or deficits.

In this chapter, a habilitative approach is taken that combines the ASHA-identified processes with the Mischook and Cole (1986) model. In addition, because the interdependence of the different skills is not clearly addressed in these models, the "Chocolate Chip Cookie Theory" advocated by the author (Rotfleisch, 2001), is incorporated. This theory uses the example of baking cookies to illustrate the important points and principles in the habilitation of the deaf and hard-of-hearing child in the process of learning spoken language. In this analogy, one considers the cookie "ingredients" along with the skills needed to become a competent communicator through an AV approach. The process of mixing the cookie dough and implementing therapy goals demonstrates that all components need to be combined. Consider the different ingredients in the recipe for a chocolate chip cookie and the possible variations in recipes, including the use of different ingredients such as nuts, semisweet versus milk chocolate chips, butter, versus shortening or margarine, and even using different cooking equipment or utensils. Though the resulting cookies are different, they still are chocolate chip cookies. However, we can tell from the flavor if the cookie has the perfect quantity of butter, not enough sugar or an inadequate amount of chocolate chips. Once baked, it is not possible to separate the sugar from the flour from the eggs. When looking at the "recipes" of the required skills for a child who is deaf or hard-of-hearing, "bakers" may have different variations or components. Typically the obvious "ingredients" include auditory processes, receptive and expressive language, pragmatics, speech, and then those skills that are a reflection of the child's unique "equipment" or experiences, such as behavior, preschool experiences, or sibling interactions. Just like the variability in cookie recipes, the "ingredi-ents" may vary, but we are still "baking" or working toward a competent spoken language communicator.

Consider again the "baked cookies"; the "ingredients" or skills cannot really be separated from each other, as in the cookie. It does not matter how clear the articulation is if you do not have the language and pragmatic skills for communication. It does not matter if the language is age appropriate if the child does not listen or participate in a conversation, respond appropriately and use language for "real" communication. It does not matter how age appropriate the language is if the speech is unintelligible. Accordingly, when working with the young child, interaction necessitates an overlapping of skills. When the child is presented with a simple command or stereotypic phrase within their comprehension, such as "time for lunch," they must attend to the auditory signal and determine that the speech sounds are different and meaningful at the level of their abilities. The child typically will demonstrate auditory comprehension by responding appropriately to the adult's conversational contribution by moving toward the table or saying "mmm" to indicate that they are planning to eat. At a more complex level it is critical to analyze all the elements during the interaction. Plurals emerge expressively in hearing children with a language level between 2 and 3 years of age. By that age, they have learned to listen and comprehend plural forms. Babies with hearing loss often have poorer access to high-frequency sounds and their sensory device must provide sufficient audibility to these sounds to enable development of this skill. Looking at the auditory processes involved in acquiring the [s] or [z] plural forms is an excellent example to illustrate the overlap and interdependence on the different skills. The child must have consistent access through their sensory device to the [s] or [z] to learn to attend to high frequency, relatively low energy speech sounds. As the child learns to attend to the sounds, discrimination and auditory recognition must be facilitated. If the word is embedded within a phrase or a sentence, the child must be able to attend to, discriminate and recognize the [s] or [z] sounds and show memory for the sequencing of the phonemes. Furthermore, he or she must develop the concept of the plural form and then associate the form with the appropriate phonemes [s] and [z] in word final position. Auditory memory and sequencing come into play as the child develops this skill. Lastly, the child must be able to produce the phoneme to be able to produce the plural form. Similar processes are implemented for other aspects of language. As in the chocolate chip cookie analogy, audition is not isolated from speech and language when interacting with the child. All these components are interrelated in a successful communicative act and all "ingredients" need to be integrated. This is particularly critical when interacting with the child in a natural everyday situation.

Established goals should reflect the normal sequence of development, although it must be acknowledged that even with the most advanced sensory aid technology, acquisition of some skills will be difficult. The therapist working with babies and their families, therefore, must have knowledge in many areas, particularly in the areas of normal and deviant development in audition, speech and language. The therapist's understanding of speech and the effects of hearing loss will be important for informal information gathering and in designing individualized diagnostic therapy. Knowledge in these areas will allow the therapist to determine if the child's progress is appropriate regarding the specific sequence of skill development as well as the time frame

to develop the ability. The therapist must be able to determine if slow progress is a result of poor access to auditory information or to possible developmental delays. Thus, the therapist must be able to monitor the child's overall performance to determine whether he or she is accessing the acoustic signal and is able to use the information in a meaningful way, or whether he or she is a candidate for other sensory device technology, such as a different hearing aid or a cochlear implant. It is imperative that the therapist work closely with the child's audiologist and provide relevant information regarding programming of the hearing aid and/or cochlear implant.

Some important premises in habilitation are recommended regardless of specific goals:

1. Audiograms are an indication of detection but not a guarantee of accessibility of the complete auditory stimulus required for various discrimination abilities or higher auditory skills.
2. The therapist works in collaboration with the primary caregiver to determine the developing skills of the baby.
3. The therapist must make a determination regarding the developing behaviors if they are normal development or deviant behaviors related to the hearing loss that might require prevention or remediation.
4. The therapist must be able to monitor skill development to determine the appropriateness and sequence of the task and the time frame for which the skill is expected to emerge.

The typical sequence of skills shown below is based on the assumption that the baby has a typical sensorineural hearing loss with more hearing in the low frequencies relative to the higher frequencies. Under this assumption, the recommended sequence for auditory learning is as follows:

- Nonsegmentals
- Vowels which vary by first formant information
- Consonants—manner of production
- Consonants—voicing feature
- Vowels which vary by second formant information
- Consonants with high frequencies elements such as the fricative manner
- Consonants—place cues.

It is important to note that children progress at different rates for different skills. If a child's skills develop outside of the expected sequence, the therapist should still attempt to reinforce and expand the new behavior. Experience with cochlear implants has shown that children with implants often have greater access to many of the high-frequency sounds than they had with hearing aids. Thus, we might predict that some fricatives are particularly salient for these children. However, consonant place information remains difficult even with current sensory devices. Auditory access through newer sensory devices will need to be considered as they become available to determine if the recommended sequence of skills needs to be revised.

Initial auditory development progresses as the baby begins to associate meaning with the auditory signal. Babies listening to music, voices, and intonation contours, take advantage of the low-frequency range. As mentioned earlier, the nonsegmental aspects of speech are typically more accessible than the segmentals. As babies begin to understand a few basic phrases or commands and some typical first words, discrimination of the vowels and a few consonants will typically allow for this level of language com-

prehension. As vocabulary grows, words containing low-frequency phonemes will be easier to learn than words containing high-frequency phonemes. In essence, babies typically access and attend to simples songs and rhymes within their lower-frequency range and eventually extract known words within these familiar patterns. As listening skills emerge, young children with hearing loss begin to use their voice to communicate. The access of low-frequency acoustic cues enables vocalization of the nonsegmental aspects of speech and vowels. The first consonants that typically emerge are [p, b, m, w, h].

The early emergence of pragmatic functions in prelinguistic conversations and at the one-word level are easily fostered in babies who are deaf and hard-of-hearing, partly due to their dependence on the intonation contour and other nonsegmental aspects of speech. Spoken language, first evidenced with word approximations, requires access to basic vowels and some initial consonants. As the word approximations evolve from one to two syllable words along with intonation contours, babies with usable low-frequency hearing have access to much of the auditory cues that promote continued emergence of new vocabulary. It is important to note that those babies who become candidates for cochlear implants, their previously learned skills will transition readily with continued habilitation.

Therapy Goals, Techniques, and Examples

Three babies, all at early but slightly different stages of listening, are presented. The set of initial habilitation goals, treatment plans, and definitions (Tables 15–9A and 15–9B) are indicated for a period of 6 months and are appropriate for each of these

TABLE 15–9A. Initial Habilitation Goals

	Jessica	Lucy	Billy
1. Auditory Processes for Using Sound Meaningfully			
1.1. Auditory Attention			
1.1.a. Monitor, facilitate and reinforce awareness of voices including parents' and a variety of speech sounds.	X		X
1.1.b. Monitor responses to a variety of sounds including loud, sudden noises, voices of different quality, tones, music, and singing.	X	X	X
1.1.c. Condition to consistently respond, discriminate and imitate the 6 sounds [m, oo, ah, ee, sh, s].		X	
1.1.d. Monitor and reinforce awareness of environmental sounds.	X		X
1.1.e. Monitor and facilitate localization responses to speech and environmental sounds.	X		
1.1.f. Monitor, facilitate and reinforce awareness of nonsegmental aspects of speech—duration, intensity, and pitch.	X	X	X
1.2. Auditory Memory			
1.2.a. Develop, reinforce and expand auditory memory to one to two items.	X	X	X
1.3. Auditory Discrimination and Identification			
1.3.a. Monitor, facilitate and expand auditory discrimination ability for the nonsegmental aspects of speech—duration, intensity, and pitch.	X	X	X
1.3.b. Monitor, facilitate and expand auditory discrimination ability for a variety of vowels and diphthongs to include a variety of mid-neutral and low-frequency vowels.	X	X	X
1.3.c. Monitor, facilitate and expand auditory discrimination ability for frontal and bilabial consonants (b, p, w, m) with vowel variety by manner of production and voicing cues.		X	X
1.3.d. Monitor, facilitate and expand auditory discrimination ability for phrases on the basis of rhythmic structure and known words.		X	X
1.3.e. Monitor, facilitate and expand auditory discrimination ability for words consisting of varying syllabification—1, 2, or 3 syllables in a limited set.			X

continues

TABLE 15–9A. *continued*

	Jessica	Lucy	Billy
1.3.f. Monitor, facilitate and expand auditory discrimination ability for emerging phonemes and those produced by varying manners of production, place, and voice cues.		X	X

1.4. Auditory Integration

	Jessica	Lucy	Billy
1.4.a. Facilitate ability to attend to auditory signal while engaged in a motor task or when visually engaged in an activity.	X	X	X

2. Auditory Processes for Learning to Talk

2.1. Auditory Feedback

	Jessica	Lucy	Billy
2.1.a. Facilitate, monitor, reinforce, and expand variety of vocalizations and phrase babbling.	X	X	X
2.1.b. Facilitate, monitor, reinforce, and expand imitations, turn-taking and vocalizations spontaneously, in prompted situations and with modeling.	X	X	X
2.1.c. Facilitate, monitor, reinforce, and expand use of vocalizations as communicative intent.	X	X	X
2.1.d. Facilitate, monitor, reinforce, and expand control of nonsegmental aspects of speech (duration, intensity, pitch) at phonetic level.	X	X	X
2.1.e. Facilitate, monitor, reinforce, and expand productions to include a variety of low, mid, and high-frequency vowels and diphthongs.	X	X	X
2.1.f. Facilitate, monitor, reinforce stages of babbling in appropriate sequence and quality of productions from cooing to reduplicative to canonical.	X	X	
2.1.g. Facilitate, monitor, reinforce, and expand babbling of frontal and bilabial consonants [b, p, w, m] with emerging vowel variety at phonetic level.		X	X
2.1.h. Facilitate, monitor, reinforce, and expand fricative breath stream of (h, sh) at phonetic level.		X	X
2.1.i. Facilitate, monitor, reinforce, and expand phoneme productions at phonetic level and emerging phonologic level.		X	X

TABLE 15–9A. *continued*

	Jessica	Lucy	Billy
3. Auditory Processes for Learning to Language			
3.1. Auditory Recognition			
3.1.a. Facilitate, monitor, reinforce, and expand the ability to recognize objects by associated sounds, which vary in nonsegmental qualities and vowel content.	X	X	X
3.1.b. Facilitate, monitor, reinforce, and expand the ability to recognize words by nonsegmental qualities (duration, syllables) and vowel content.	X	X	X
3.1.c. Facilitate, monitor, reinforce, and expand the ability to recognize phrases on the basis of rhythmic structure, known words and contextual cues.		X	X
3.2. Auditory Sequencing			
3.2.a. Facilitate and expand imitations of one to two-syllable functional words.		X	X
3.3. Auditory Comprehension			
3.3.a. Facilitate, monitor, reinforce, and expand auditory comprehension of words and phrases without contextual cues.		X	X
3.3.b. Facilitate, monitor, reinforce, and expand the ability to identify objects for animals and vehicles by associated sounds, which vary in nonsegmental qualities and vowel content.	X	X	X
3.3.c. Facilitate, monitor, reinforce, and expand the ability to comprehend words by nonsegmental qualities (duration, syllables) and vowel content.	X		X
3.3.d. Facilitate, monitor, reinforce, and expand auditory comprehension of phrases based on one to two known words (directives and statements) or rhythmic pattern.		X	X
3.3.e. Facilitate, monitor, reinforce, and expand auditory comprehension of language in the areas of functional words, phrases (up, down, bye-bye, all gone, more), nouns, verbs, and adjectives.		X	X
3.3.f. Monitor and record auditory comprehension of vocabulary every 2 months.	X	X	X

continues

TABLE 15–9A. *continued*

	Jessica	Lucy	Billy
3.4. Auditory Retrieval			
3.4.a. Stimulate spontaneous expressive language in the areas of functional words, phrases, nouns, verbs, and adjectives.		X	X
3.4.b. Facilitate imitation and spontaneous productions of phrases using correct nonsegmental aspects, phoneme content, and syllabification.		X	X
3.4.c. Facilitate and expand consistent use of speech and word approximations to communicate a variety of pragmatic functions (requesting, protesting, responding, turn-taking, attention-getting).		X	X
3.4.d. Elicit a variety of pragmatic functions with vocalizations and nonvocal gestures.	X	X	X
3.4.e. Monitor and record expressive vocabulary every 2 months.		X	X

babies. Three scripts presenting scenes from sample therapy sessions and a scene at home follow to illustrate some effective activities and interactions. The discussions clarify which recommended initial goals have been implemented. These scenarios then illustrate how a variety of targeted goals can be integrated and ways in which the different goals interact and overlap. In addition, some of the therapist's contribution or the techniques used by the parent will be discussed. The next level of habilitation goals is included along with a discussion about the progression to these skills.

Therapy sessions focus on an open interchange between the parent and therapist as they discuss the parental observations noted since the previous session. The discussions revolve around implementation of goals, addressing prevalent issues, and monitoring the child's and parent's behaviors or reactions. The therapist always asks if the parent has any specific questions or concerns. These questions or concerns are best dealt with at the beginning of the session in order to meet the needs of the parent. The principle of habilitation is to facilitate the normal sequence of auditory development within the child's capabilities. Initial intervention with young infants should focus on the interaction of the parent and child. The underlying premise of communication begins from a very young age and should demonstrate a natural interaction style between parent and child. If this natural behavior has been disrupted due to the psychological impact of the diagnosis of hearing loss, it is critical to re-establish the interaction. This may start with the parent making eye contact with their baby and then talking to, cooing and singing to the baby. The next step would be to facilitate consistent turn-taking between the parent and baby through observation of this interaction. Activities at this point would be to determine the baby's attention to sounds, control of his or her

TABLE 15–9B. Operational Definitions of 10 Auditory Processes Taught for Verbal Communication and Environmental Monitoring

---

Auditory Processes for Using Sound Meaningfully

Auditory Attention

Focusing one's selective attention on sound. Hearing becomes an active listening sense and a passive source of information. Advanced stages of attention include hearing at a distance, listening in the presence of background noise, and understanding over the telephone.

Auditory Memory

Remembering what one heard to perform cognitive functions in the working memory. Both short-term and long-term memory are needed to attach meaning to sound. Auditory memory span must also be developed in order to remember sequences of sounds for understanding words, phrases, sentences, and stories.

Auditory Discrimination

Judging two sounds as different: this is necessary so meaning can be assigned to each sound. It leads to the recognition of environmental sounds and the use of speech.

Auditory Integration

Experiencing sound in all activities; for sound to be useful, it must be associated, or integrated, with other sensory experiences.

Auditory Processes for Learning to Talk

Auditory Feedback

Hearing the sounds produced by ones own speech muscles when talking. Hearing is the sense through which normal hearing infants learn to speak. It also is used to monitor and correct the pitch, loudness, vocal rhythm, and articulation as one speaks.

Auditory Processes for Learning Language

Auditory Recognition

Associating a sound with its referent; that is, the symbolic function of sound.

Auditory Sequencing

Remembering the order of sounds heard. We must learn to retain sounds in their correct order for understanding the word, phrase, or sentence spoken.

Auditory Comprehension

Understanding the linguistic structures of the language; these include the semantic, syntactic, morphologic, and pragmatic aspects of the language.

Auditory Retrieval

Using words that are stored in our memory. With this skill, we can use spoken language to express our thoughts and use spontaneous, expressive communication.

Auditory Application

Applying all of the above auditory functions when using arbitrary symbols, such as letters for reading and writing, and numbers for mathematics. This allows for learning in school, at work, and in daily life.

Source: Adapted from Daniel (1990). Permission to adapt by Linda Daniel.

vocalizations, and development of initial auditory, speech and language skills. The parent learns to vocalize to the child by playing with the nonsegmental aspects of speech as carried by the vowels. A pause is important to allow the child an opportunity to vocalize. Any vocalization by the infant is treated as a turn within the communicative interchange and the parent learns to react to it and respond back to reinforce this behavior. Infants' vocalizations should go through the babbling stages. However, depending on the severity of the hearing loss or with some older babies who have stopped babbling or vocalizing, they may not return to and progress through the babbling stages. Early responses to a variety of sounds from the home environment, everyday experiences, and therapy sessions must be monitored and noted. As responses become more consistent, the therapist facilitates listening to a variety of sounds and speech while encouraging vocal play and reacting to the infant's vocalizations. The caregiver must understand what the therapist is doing and the reasons why they are doing it. Thus, it is the therapist's role to model and/or explain what is occurring throughout the session so that the parent can implement the same goals and strategies at home. Parents become creative and will let the clinician know what they are doing at home after they have been provided with some understanding of what the baby needs to learn next.

AV Therapy Techniques

Enhancing Perception

The young child's ability to attend, discriminate, remember, and comprehend different words will depend on a variety of acoustic cues. For example, a child with early skills may be able to discriminate between the words "hot" versus "hot dog" versus "happy" because he or she extracts the nonsegmental cues, specifically number of syllables and stress pattern. Words such as "hat" and "hot" differ acoustically by vowel content. Words with consonants that vary by manner of production ("hat" versus "mat") or voicing ("bat" versus "pat") may be discriminated more easily than words that contrast place cues ("cake" versus "take" or "mat" versus "gnat"). However, this child may or may not discriminate words that they are not yet able to produce. The child with emerging abilities requires ongoing reinforcement. Providing many speech pattern contrasts in meaningful contexts will reinforce current skills and expand upon them. New and more difficult contrasts should be introduced and facilitated in the areas of the attention, discrimination, memory, production, and comprehension by contrasting those phonemes that are being misperceived and confused. Often isolating the phoneme out of the word, and appropriately acoustic highlighting the contrast enhances the correct perception, discrimination and production. Correcting and enhancing the child's perception allows for better perception and production.

The Expectant Pause

The expectant pause is an effective tool in that it helps the parent find the right balance between speaking and pausing. This balance gives the message that it is time for the baby to take a turn.

Acoustic Highlighting

Acoustic highlighting is a technique which makes a particular sound or word salient. There are a variety of ways to accomplish this. Acoustic highlighting can be accomplished by manipulating the nonsegmentals, for example by making the word louder, longer in duration or varying the pitch. An unvoiced consonant is more salient when it is whispered either in isolation or with the word or phrase.

Auditory Closure

Auditory closure requires the child to "fill in the blank." Parents often do this naturally by allowing the child to complete the phrase or sentence. This technique can be used effectively by pausing and letting the child fill in the key word in the phrase or song.

Expansion

Expansion is an effective strategy to facilitate many skills and goals. When the child says a word or word approximation, the caregiver responds by using that word plus a few others to expand upon the communicative contribution. Words can be combined to produce a phrase or short sentence. This strategy reinforces the child's communication by repeating their word to make it clear that the child's language was understood. Expansion also increases the child's attention, discrimination and auditory memory.

Listen

The primary sense modality used in AV therapy is audition. There are many strategies that can be used to assist in providing an auditory-only input when appropriate. The child focuses on hearing by having the talker strategically positioning themselves behind or at the side. Joint attention has the child and therapist or parent attending to an object or toy as it is being discussed. This facilitates the normal progression of communication development, provides auditory input with some reinforcement. A hand cue (i.e., a hand held in front of the mouth) is a technique used by some clinicians to prevent lipreading. Using a hand

cue is a technique that has been long associated with AV therapy for obstructing the view of the mouth or to prompt a response. However, this strategy blocks a portion of the auditory information and makes it more difficult for the child to access the auditory event. To prevent this, some clinicians use a "listening" hoop with an acoustically transparent fabric. Neither of these approaches fosters natural interaction and would not be recommended with a parent infant interaction. The AV philosophy does not advocate complete absence of visual input. When visual input becomes necessary, the situation can be manipulated to meet that need.

Case Studies: Initial Habilitation Goals

Three cases are presented: Jessica, Lucy, and Billy. All are at different stages in their AV therapy. The commentary following each script is accompanied by Table 15–9A, which provides the goals and skill sets for each child.

Jessica

Jessica was diagnosed at 4 months with a profound bilateral sensorineural hearing loss and was fitted bilaterally with hearing aids. She was implanted at 1 year of age, following the hearing aid trial. Her hearing aids provided some access to low-frequency sounds, evident in her use of the nonsegmentals and low-frequency neutral vowels. Initial stimulation of the cochlear implant (CI) occurred at the age of 1 year, 1 month. Jessica tolerated the CI from the initial fitting and now wears it all waking hours. She has been listening with her CI for 1 month. She plays appropriately with toys, interacts with adults, and has age-appropriate developmental milestones.

Auditory Processes for Using Sound Meaningfully

Auditory Detection and Attention. Jessica responds well to a variety of sounds using her implant. She enjoys listening to music and voices. She frequently points to or touches her ear when she hears a sound. She does not yet respond to all of the six Ling sounds [m, oo, ah, ee, sh, s] (Ling, 2002/2003). Awareness to "sh," plosives and nasals are inconsistent. No consistent response has been noted for [s].

Auditory Discrimination. Jessica has begun to discriminate some of the nonsegmental aspects of speech; duration, intensity and pitch as noted in her imitative and spontaneous productions. In therapy sessions it was noted that she has changed from a vowel to an [m] when provided with auditory-only input.

Auditory Processes for Learning to Talk

Auditory Feedback. Jessica has increased her spontaneous vocalizations and is using her voice to turn-take with adults. She has begun to modulate the nonsegmental aspects of speech—duration, intensity, and pitch in her spontaneous productions. Her vocalizations tend to be of an appropriate intensity and she varies her pitch. She is producing a few vowels including but not limited to: "u" as in "but," "e" as in "bed," and "oo" as in "boot." She produces the consonants [m], [p], and [b] and will combine them with a vowel. At this time she is not producing any other consonants consistently.

Auditory Processes for Learning Language

Auditory Comprehension and Auditory Retrieval. Standardized language testing indicated an age-equivalent score of 9 months for receptive language and 7 months for expressive language. Jessica has become aware that using her voice is an effective means of gaining attention and eliciting a response to her needs. She understands a few words. Jessica demonstrates excellent eye contact and has used her voice to turn-take with her mother and the therapist on many occasions. She has begun to imitate some words which she hears and has spontaneous word approximations for "push," "bye bye," "poop," "up," and "hot."

Guiding the Parent. Jessica's mother interacts the way most caregivers do, using caregiver's speech. She uses more inflection, exclamations, slower speech, whispering, simple language, baby talk words, many questions, names rather than pronouns, and elaborations of what the child says. Jessica and her mother worked on a variety of skills and initial goals while interacting in a very natural way. The therapist has guided the mother in ways to be talking to the baby and reinforcing the skills that are effective in achieving the targeted goals. The therapist has instructed the mother to respond to the child's vocalizations and provides reinforcement when the mother naturally uses her interactions to work towards specific therapy goals.

Sound object associations (Vaughan, 1981) have long been a tool used by AV therapists (Table 15–10). Animal and vehicle sounds should be selected to have specific nonsegmental patterns and vowel content that infants respond to at the beginning stages of auditory attention, discrimination and feedback. Different durational patterns can be imitated by babies. Approximations for animal or vehicle sounds may be considered the infant's first attempts at producing words, reinforcing the child's understanding that an arbitrary sequence and combination of sounds has meaning. There tends

TABLE 15–10. Preliminary Word List

SOUND–OBJECT ASSOCIATIONS		PEOPLE AND OBJECTS	
Vehicles		Mommy	eye
boat—bababab		Daddy	nose
car (truck, bus)—brrr beep, beep		baby	mouth
airplane—aaaa		shoe	watch—tictoc
train—ch, ch, ch ooo		**VERBS**	
Animals		Sh, go to sleep	wash, wash, wash
cat—meow		sit down	walk, walk, walk
dog—woof woof		pull	shake, shake
cow—moo		up, up, up	round and round
horse—neigh		down	have a drink
pig—oink oink		push	bounce the ball
lamb—ba-a-a-a		pop	Oh-o, it fell down
duck—quack, quack		blow	
fish—(no sound)		**ADJECTIVES**	
rabbit, frog—hop, hop, hop		hot	more
bird—peep peep		cold	all gone
chicken—cluck		soft	dirty
rooster—cock-a-doodle-doo		broken	wet
goat—ma-a-a-a		mmm, that's good	

to be a limited vocabulary which is at the core of what is said to babies and what is repeated. These key words may show some variation from one family to another, but key words such as mommy, daddy, bottle, up, down, more, eat, to list a few, are part of the baby's listening experience. Reinforcing sound-object associations and limited, but repeated, vocabulary helps to set up successful interactions. Beginning therapy with auditory attention and discrimination, as well as focusing on vocal patterns most likely to emerge following the normal sequence of communication development, promotes suc-

cess. Monitoring the infant's emerging abilities also helps to determine if the sensory device is providing adequate audibility.

Scenario: Jessica

Mother
Hi Jessica
Says in an excited sing-songy voice, as she walks to the baby sitting on the blanket pulling rings from a stacking toy. She pauses and waits for a response.

Mother
Hi Jessica

She repeats exactly the same way, from closer and talking slightly louder. Baby stops what she is doing and looks at mother who is now sitting in front of her and leaning down towards her.

Jessica
Ah

Baby vocalizes a very short sound, as she looks up at her mother's face, mouth and then eyes.

Mother
Hiiii Jessica. You heard mommy.
I heard Jessica.

With lots of intonation and excitement in her voice.

Jessica
Ah

Mother
I know Jessica. Let's play.

Says immediately and smiles again still maintaining eye contact.

Jessica
Aaaah

Coos the baby, smiling back at her mother continuing to make eye contact.

Mother
OK Jessica. Let's play!

Turning around to get a toy from behind her.

Therapist
Perfect—this is just what we want. You are using your voice in a very fun way for her to listen to—all that "motherese" we have been talking about. You spoke to her and paused for her to take a turn and she did—I think three times. Then as soon as she responded with her voice you answered her. We are establishing foundations for basic communication—turn-taking, pausing and listening. We want to encourage this as much as possible. I talk, you listen, then you talk and I listen. Let's

see if you can get several more turns, be sure to remember to pause long enough to give Jessica the opportunity to vocalize.

Commentary

In reference to specific goals shown in Table 15–9A, the mother had the baby attend to her voice (1.1.a.) and used lots of inflection to get her attention and have her listen to the nonsegmental aspects of speech (1.1.f.). She is establishing turn-taking by immediately responding to her vocalizations (2.1.b.). Mother is encouraging Jessica to use her voice to babble or coo and to communicate. This provides reinforcement and encourages more vocalization (2.1.a., 2.1.c.). The therapist reinforces the mother's behaviors and explains how to proceed to the next stage. The therapist is being very positive and telling mother all the good things she is doing, which encourages the mother to repeat those behaviors.

Mother
Yaah Jessica! What should mommy
and Jessica play?

Using with a question intonation contour, holding the toy behind her but turning to look at the baby.

Jessica
Ah

Mother
Does Jessica want to play with
the choo choo?

Holding a toy train behind her back but making eye contact with the baby.

Jessica
Aah

Mother
Yes?

She pauses.

Mother
Ok! Here's the choo choo

Holding up the toy train in front of the baby and between them as they had been in mutual gaze.

Jessica
Aah
Baby reaches toward the toy.

Therapist
OK, let's see if we can get her to change the duration. Remember the nonsegmental aspects of duration/intensity/pitch. Let's see if we can get her vocalization to sound more like yours . . . maybe—but maybe not—she will use the duration information. Duration is usually the first nonsegmental feature. As we know she will sometimes produce a longer vowel sound—she may continue to do that or she may try to imitate the pitch change. Alternatively, she may change the vowel if she listens and realizes what you are saying isn't the same as the "ah." We know she has been cooing different vowels. So try acoustically highlighting the "oooo" so it is THE most interesting thing you are saying and see if she will pay attention to the difference in the sounds. But she may not change anything. Go ahead and try.

Mother
The train goes Ch ch oooooo
Making her voice sound like the whistle on a train with an up and down intonation contour and holding the toy between them.

Jessica
Aah
Reaching for the toy.

Mother
Ch ch ooooooooo
Moving the train to hold the baby's interest.

Jessica
Aaaaah

Therapist
OK! Did you catch that?

Mother
What?

Therapist
I think she might have produced a longer duration attempt and that's great! All the other times when she talked to you, she made a short sound—but this last one was really longer. Also great is that she is using her hearing first, you told her what you were going to do before you showed her the toy. You first had her listen and then you reinforced the auditory message by showing her the toy. This is a great strategy to use regularly. Now you are both going to look at the train and talk about it. She knows you are talking about the train. You are both paying attention to the train. We call that joint attention. She doesn't have to look at you when you are talking. Let's see if she will do it again—but she may not. Remember to pause to let her know it is her turn.

Commentary
In these turns the baby is listening to the durational information which the mother is making to characterize the train. She uses her voice with a different quality almost like singing (1.1.b.). Jessica is repeatedly provided with the auditory signal, which has very specific nonsegmental patterns and vowel content. She is learning to pay attention to the sound, hear it as different and approximate the sound (1.1.f, 1.3.a, 2.1.b., 2.1.d.). Jessica will learn to associate the sounds with the given object, and other objects will be associated with different nonsegmental patterns and speech patterns (3.1.a, 3.3.b).

The therapist is reinforcing concepts about nonsegmentals and reminding the mother about the order of acquisition, including commenting about what the baby has done before so trying to elicit it again. She explains the concept of joint attention and the auditory strategy of "talking" to establish auditory integration. The baby doesn't need to be looking at the mother when she speaks. The therapist reinforces the need to pause, and gives positive feedback to the mother by bringing up all the great things that she has done.

Mother
Ch ch oooooo

Jessica
Ah Aaaaaah

Therapist
Yah Jessica, Ch ch oooooo
says the train
With enthusiasm looking at the baby who looks toward the therapist.

Therapist
FABULOUS job mom! She did a short sound and a longer sound! We want Jessica to know how excited we are about that. She is trying to imitate the durational cues she is hearing by using her voice. Do it some more so she can keep listening to the different vowel. Then we will try to change it to a different duration and different vowel for the rabbit.

Mother
ch ch oooooo
Says the mother making the "ooo" sound louder, longer and with the same sing-songy pitch as previously.

Jessica
ah Aaaaaah

Mother
Ch ch oooooo
Replies the mother with the same intonation pattern used previously.

Mother
Ch ch oooo that's the choo choo

Jessica
Ooo

Mother
Oooooo

Jessica
Oooo
Says Jessica reaching for the toy

Mother
Ch ch ooooo
That's the train. Does Jessica want to hold the train?
Smiling and talking enthusiastically as she holds the train in front of the baby within her reach, giving the toy train to the baby as she reaches the train, mom keeps her hands on the train as well.

Therapist
Ch ch oooooo says the train.
FABULOUS job mom! So did you catch what happened?

Mother
Yes! She actually listened to the sound and changed it.

Therapist
You are right, mom! You are teaching her to hear different vowels and different durations of speech sounds and then to tell her what she is hearing. That is fantastic. She is learning to listen and to change the sound because she is engaged with you and you are conversing with her so she wants to talk to you . . . and grab the train.
Mother and therapist both laugh!

Mother
Ch ch oooooo that's the train.
It says choo choo
Baby is busily playing and looking at the toy

Mother
Jessica! Listen.

Points to her ear, pushes on the train to make the whistle "toot" as the baby looks at her

Jessica's eyes widen and she looks toward the toy.

Mother
Jessica! Good listening.
I know you heard that didn't you?
Mommy hears that!
She points at her ear and then Jessica's, shaking her head up and down and smiling.

Mother
Listen again. Mommy hears that!
Tooting the train whistle as the baby is playing with the toy train. Again she points at her ear and then Jessica's ear, shaking her head up and down and smiling.

Therapist
Ok, now let's take out the rabbit and you say "hop hop hop." Remember to say it first before you show it to her—the same as you did with the train.

Mother
Jessica! What should Jessica and mommy play?
Calling the baby by her name and using with a question intonation contour, holding the toy rabbit behind her but turning to look at the baby and making eye contact.

Jessica
Uh

Mother
Hop hop hop. Should Jessica play with the bunny rabbit?
Holding up the toy rabbit in front of the baby and between them as they both gaze.

Mother
That's the bunny. The bunny goes hop hop hop.

Jessica
Ah

Therapist
That was nice, you called her and she turned to you. You told her about the rabbit before you took it out. Try to do just the hop hop and make it important so maybe she will try to imitate that.

Mother
Hop hop hop

Jessica
Aah aah aah

Mother
Hop hop hop

Therapist
That is great. She changed the duration to a short repeated sound. Let's go for the vowel. I remember that you told me she has done this vowel in her babbling.
I'm going to make the vowel the most important thing for her to listen to by acoustically highlighting it. We can do this with a vowel by making it a bit longer, or a bit louder. Let's see if we can get her to change it. hOp hOp hOp hOp.

Jessica
Aah aah aah
Baby reaches for toy and as mom moves the rabbit as if it is hopping through the air.

Mother
hOp hOp hOp hOp
Mother moves the bunny in a hopping motion in front of the baby as she moves forward grabbing the toy.

Jessica
Aah aah aah

Mother
hOp hOp hOp hOp
Still waving the bunny in the air.

Jessica
Aaw

Mother
hOp hOp hOp hOp

Therapist

That's it! She changed the vowel and is trying to say the right one, but we lost the duration. Ok!! Don't give her the toy yet. Let her listen and play with the sound and her voice and match what she hears—her perception, with what she says, her production.

Mother

hOp hOp hOp hOp

Holding the bunny in the air in front of the baby but high up out of her reach as they both look at the toy.

Jessica

Aaw

Mother

hOp hOp hOp hOp

Moving the bunny down and looking at the baby, who continues to look at the toy.

Jessica

Aaw aaw

Reaching again for the toy and moving towards it and grabbing it.

Mother

Hop hop hop! That's the rabbit.
Hop hop hop!!!
She really hears that doesn't she?
She says with excitement looking at the baby and then the therapist.

Therapist

She sure does and even more than that you are teaching her to hear sounds as different—long, short, repeated, different vowels. And you are teaching her to use her hearing for auditory feedback to start with a good foundation for her speech intelligibility!
Jessica! Hop hop hop

Jessica

Aw aw

Mother

hop hop hop hop Yah, I heard that!

Jessica

Aw aw

Commentary

Mother is continuing to incorporate the goals as mentioned above with turn-taking, attending to voice, listening to variety of nonsegmental patterns, encouraging communicative intent, and reinforcing the sound-object association. She uses a variety of strategies, such as joint attention, caregiver speech, expansion, acoustic highlighting, and pausing. At this time we are focusing on her approximation of duration and change in vowels. The next step is to get both features correct. As the baby is not able to produce the "ch," sound a reasonable approximation would be the correct duration and vowel—"oo oo ooooo." While playing with the train, Jessica listens to the train whistle (1.1.d.) and localization responses are facilitated (1.1.e). She continues to listen to the three parts of the sounds associated with the train and the noun, thereby working on her auditory memory (1.2.a.). Through acoustic highlighting and repetition, the baby showed auditory discrimination ability for the vowel she was producing and the vowel which she was hearing from her mother and the therapist (1.3.b). The auditory input allowed Jessica to discriminate duration and the vowel. The use of this vocalization was encouraged as were the pragmatic functions of turn-taking and requesting with communicative intent (2.1.a, 2.1.b, 2.1.c., 2.1.d., 2.1.e., 2.1.f.). This type of activity leads to development of sound recognition as well as associating objects with sounds and words (3.1.a, 3.1.b, 3.3.b, 3.3.c). In addition, the baby is learning to listen while actively engaged in holding, manipulating, and looking at an object (1.4.a.).

The therapist is positively reinforcing the child and the mother in this scenario. The child vocalizes during the interaction. The mother is instructed to continue this activity to determine if several more productions are elicited. This activity also reinforces the auditory feedback loop; the child hears the sound and produces the same sound using her emerging ability to match her perception and production. The therapist encourages auditory integration while she and Jessica are engaged in play to allow the child to integrate listening with other activities. The child is learning to listen while doing other things. The therapist then directs the mother to use a toy that will have a different durational pattern and a different vowel.

Jessica is demonstrating consistent and basic responses to a variety of sounds, learning to listen to the durational information in speech and to some vowels. These skills need to be expanded before progressing to the next level of skills, that is, learning to attend to and discriminate intensity, pitch, additional vowels as well as producing these aspects of speech. Through everyday interactions and sound object associations, other skills such as labeling, comprehension, auditory retrieval, and protowords are reinforced.

Lucy

Lucy was diagnosed at birth with a severe-to-profound bilateral sensorineural hearing loss. She was aided at 2 months and wore hearing aids for most of her waking hours. She currently uses a cochlear implant, which was activated at 1 year, 1 month. She has been listening with her cochlear implant for 3 months. Lucy has been seen for AV therapy since diagnosed with hearing loss. She is cooperative, easily engaged in sessions and plays appropriately with the variety of toys and materials presented to her. She is very social and interactive. All of her developmental milestones have been age appropriate.

Auditory Processes for Using Sound Meaningfully

Auditory Detection and Attention. Lucy showed detection of sounds soon after her latest mapping appointment. At the present time, Lucy is responding to all six of the Ling sounds [m, oo, ah, ee, sh, s]. This is a good prognostic indication for the development of the different speech sounds. Lucy shows consistent responses to sounds. Furthermore, she imitates "bababa" and produces this string of phonemes spontaneously.

Auditory Memory. Lucy is demonstrating some short-term auditory memory for a few speech patterns, which she will imitate from an auditory-only model, such as "round and round and round" or "dot dot dot."

Auditory Discrimination. Lucy is beginning to attend to and discriminate between differing nonsegmental patterns, particularly durational cues. She will imitate some patterns, such as "shake shake shake", "round and round and round," "dot dot dot," and "no" based on durational information, intonation patterns and some vowel productions. She has produced a few different vowels with auditory-only input. She imitates the number of syllables and articulates two [p] phonemes for the word "purple" when requesting a purple marker. This indicates that she has acquired voicing cues. Lucy approximated "dot dot dot" using the [d] phoneme. Mother reports that she will frequently babble with the [d].

Auditory Processes for Learning to Talk

Auditory Feedback. Mother reports that Lucy "found her voice" last week. She reported babbling at home with [b] and [m] sounds and attempts to say "bye-bye" and "no." She is producing a variety of vowels at this time including primarily: "o" as in "boat," "e" as in "bed," "ow" as in "bowwow," "oo" as in "book," "ay" as in "bay," "ee" as in "beep," and "oo" as in "boot."

She uses a variety of consonants and babbling in therapy sessions. Mother reports that she most frequently produces the following consonants: [b, p, d, m, w].

She produces high-pitch sounds in an attempt to imitate the "sh." It is not yet accurate nor does it have any fricative quality.

Auditory Processes for Learning Language

Auditory Comprehension and Auditory Retrieval. Lucy vocalizes with good oral production, makes eye contact, responds consistently and has communicative intent. She is showing comprehension of a few words mostly with visual information cue or with contextual information in addition to the auditory model. Lucy is using a few word approximations at this time, mostly prompted or imitated. Her most common productions to date include: "No," "Lucy," "bye-bye," "up up up," "ow," "dot dot dot," and "round and round and round."

Lucy's language abilities were assessed with a standardized evaluation, with results indicating an age equivalent of 12 months for both receptive and expressive language.

Everyday activities such as diaper changing, meal times, dressing, and getting in and out of the car are routine, repetitive, and necessary. This mother has been learning to take advantage of some of these rituals from during the day in such a way that she is able incorporate some targeted goals. Lucy's mother incorporates modifications in those routines which reinforce many of the goals. She also has strategically placed specific items and toys so that she might easily incorporate them in songs and sound-object play during the day. This strategy ensures that she is using every day situations to maximize her daughter's potential. Activities of daily living naturally incorporate the meaningful everyday language along with repetitions needed to facilitate the development of competent young communicators.

Scenario: Lucy

Lucy
Aaaah ah bababa
Vocalizing to get mom's attention.

Mother
Yes Lucy-Lu! Mommy's here!
What do you want?
Mother walks toward the baby walking around the kitchen.

Lucy
Aaaah ah bababa
Looking at mother and making eye contact.

Mother
Peeyoo!
Mother wrinkles up her nose as she gets closer to Lucy and makes funny face.

Lucy
Aah ooo
Looking up at her mother but walking away.

Mother
PEEEEYoooo
Acoustically highlighting the "ee" vowel.

Lucy
Eeee yooooo
Still walking away from her mother.

Mother
Peeyoo! What a stinky diaper!

Lucy
Eee yooo

Mother
Peeyoo! Let's change that stinky diaper.

Lucy
Eeeeyooo Eeeeyooo Eeeeyooo
She says approximating mother's intonation curve more closely every repetition.

Mother
Peeeyooo! Peeyooo! Peeyoo!
Let's change that stinky diaper.
Continuing to use the intonation pattern and chasing after Lucy.

Lucy
Eeeyooo!

Mother
I'm going to GET YOU Lucy-Lu!
Mom says in a playful sing-songy manner but doesn't provide any contextual cue as to what she is about to do.

Lucy
Oooo Ooo
As she tries to run away from her mother anticipating that she is going to come and catch her.

Mother
I GOT YOU Lucy-Lu!
Mother reaches out her hands and quickly steps over to get Lucy. Lucy holds her moms' hands and looks up at her mother.

Mother
Let's do our walking walking song.
Holding her hands so she is standing in front of her facing forward so they can walk with Lucy's hands stretched up.

Lucy
Waw Waw Waw Waw

Mother
Yah—walking walking Let's go!
We're walking to the changing table
Mother stands behind Lucy and holds Lucy's hands out at the sides as they begin to walk.

Mother
Walking, walking, walking, walking

Mom sings as they take deliberate steps with each word.

Lucy
Aw aw aw
Lucy vocalizes at the same time as her mother is singing "walking."

Mother
Hop hop hop

Lucy
Aw aw aw
Lucy vocalizes at the same time as her mother is singing "hop hop hop" and is beginning to giggle.

Mother
Hop hop hop
Singing and making little hops pulling Lucy up by the arms to have her hopping with the words to the song.

Lucy
Aw aw aw
Lucy vocalizes along with her mother, looks up at her mother and giggles in anticipation of what is going to happen as she mother reaches down and holds her under the arms.

Mother
Now we are running
Now we are running
Singing as she moves quickly across the floor holding and moving Lucy across the floor.

Lucy
She giggles and looks from her mother and then in front of her as they approach her room.

Mother
Now let's STOP!
Now let's STOP!
Mom's singing stops abruptly at "stop"and she suddenly stops moving and holds Lucy still as she continues to giggle and laugh looking at her mother.

Commentary

Lucy is learning to listen all the time to a variety of sounds, voice qualities and singing throughout her everyday activities (1.1.b.) and has learned that they have meaning. Mother incorporates a variety of different stereotypic phrases during the course of their interaction (Peeyoo let's change a stinky diaper, I'm going to get you Lucy-Lu!, Let's do our song) and Lucy is paying attention to what is being said, learning to understand the meaning based on the nonsegmental pattern, intonation, and contextual cues. She is being encouraged to imitate some of the key words (1.1.f., 1.2.a., 1.3.a., 1.3.d., 3.1.b., 3.1.c., 3.2.a.). When Lucy is attempting to approximate some expressions or words based on the duration, pitch, vowel content or some consonants, mother acoustically highlights the missing or incorrect sound(s) to help with her attention, discrimination and feedback through matching her perception with her production (1.3.b. 1.3.c, 2.1.d., 2.1.e.). Mother has primarily focused on the vowels and nonsegmentals in this portion of their interaction (1.3.f.). Throughout the interchange, mother makes it apparent through her interaction style, language, turn-taking, and body language that she expects Lucy to take part in the conversations and interactions (2.1.a., 2.1.b., 2.1.c., 2.1.f., 2.1.i., 3.1.a.). Lucy is learning to attend to and discriminate words and phrases. She has been learning that sounds have meaning and now she is attending to the variety of auditory information with and without contextual cues as she anticipates what is going to happen (1.2.a., 3.3.a, 3.3.c. 3.3.d, 3.3.e.). As she attempts to imitate and spontaneously produce some of the words, Lucy's feedback loop is being reinforced within the limits of her phonologic repertoire (3.4.a., 3.4.b., 3.4.c., 3.4.d.). The interaction to this point is very natural; mother incorporates the auditory signal and expects Lucy to be listening

while she is responding to the song with mother standing behind her (1.4.a.). It is obvious from the interchange between mother and daughter that listening is expected all the time. Mother naturally uses hearing, acoustically highlights and pauses.

Mother
Here we are!
As she bends down to pick her up she pauses and looks at Lucy with anticipation and waits.

Lucy
Uh uh uh

Mother
Up up up up up you go Lucy-Lu
She whispers "up up up" to acoustically highlight the [p].

Lucy
Uh uh uh
Repeats as her mother is picking her up onto the changing table.

Mother
Puh Puh Puh
Whispers as she looks at Lucy playfully.

Lucy
Puh puh

Mother
Up up up up
She says again.

Lucy
Pup up

Mother
Ma ma ma ma
With a pronounced intonation contour emphasizing different pitches. Mom playfully babbles with Lucy as she seems to be interested in practicing and making sounds at this time.

Lucy
Mamamamamama

She babbles back playfully smiling at her mother and wiggling on the changing table.

Mother
Bababa
She says playful with intonation looking at Lucy and leaning over her as she lies her down on the changing table.

Lucy
Bababababababababababababa
Does a very long string with variations in pitch and intensity.

Mother
Bababababa hahahahahahahaha
Repeats back some of what Lucy produced and then changes and whispers the string of "ha"s.

Lucy
Hhhhhaaaaa
Whispers back to her mom and smiles. Takes a board book that her mother gives her and looks at it, turning the pages and holding it above her face, thereby blocking her view of her mother.

Mother
Ah
Lucy stops looking at the book and pauses, looking at mother who looks at her with an expectant pause.

Lucy
Ah

Mother
Good listening Lucy, you heard "ah."
The airplane goes ahhh.
Lucy puts down the book as mother gives her a toy airplane. Mother begins to unsnap the baby's clothes.

Mother
Mmmm
Speaks when Lucy is quiet and is looking at the toy airplane.

Lucy
Mmm
Lucy stops looking at the book, pauses, and imitates.

Mother
Good listening Lucy, you heard mmmmm. Yummy!
She rubs Lucy's tummy when she says "mm" and then she waits until Lucy is engaged and not looking at her to say the next sound.

Mother
Sssshhhh
When Lucy is looking at her book. Mother is careful not to blow too much when she is making this sound to be certain that Lucy is listening and not just feeling the breath stream.

Lucy
Eeeeeeeeeeeee
She produces a high pitch vowel sound. She looks at her mom and smiles, she holds her finger up to her mouth in a "sh be quiet" gesture.

Mother
Good listening Lucy, that's right.
Shhhh the baby is sleeping.
Mother whispers the end of the sentence to indicate quiet.

Lucy
Aaaa
She talks in a whisper imitating the intensity her mother modeled. Mother continues taking off the baby's clothes.

Mother
Shhhhh
Holding her finger to her mouth as Lucy looks at her. She waits until Lucy begins to look at the airplane toy and manipulate it.

Mother
Oooo

Lucy

Oooo

Imitates almost immediately.

Mother

I heard you Lucy, you said "ooo."

Here's the police car. It goes oooo.
Mother adds an intonation contour to imitate a siren and lets Lucy play with the toy car. Mother is careful to wait for it to be quiet and for Lucy not to be watching her.

Mother

Eeee

Lucy

Eeee

Mother

Good listening Lucy, you heard eeeee
Again, Mother is careful to wait for it to be quiet and for Lucy not to be watching her.

Mother

Sssss

Lucy turns and looks at her mother as hears the sound.

Mother

Good listening! You heard me! sssssssss
She smiles and continues with the diapering business at hand.

Commentary

Mother continues with the expectation that Lucy is listening to, will attend to, discriminate, comprehend, and produce a variety of sounds that include singing, stereotypic phrases, different nonsegmental patterns, and consonant and vowel combinations. In addition mother does some more structured tasks to assess her detection, attention, and discrimination abilities for the six Ling sounds, nonsegmentals, speech phonemes, and productions that reinforce feedback of nonsegmentals, vowels, bilabial consonants, and the fricative breath stream (1.1.c., 1.3.a., 1.3.b., 1.3.c., 1.3.f., 2.1.a., 2.1.d., 2.1.e., 2.1.f.). Mother did her best to produce the sounds while Lucy was not looking directly

at her or while she was engaged with a book or toy, or by using joint attention (1.4.a.). Eliciting productions from Lucy allows her to incorporate the goals relating to auditory feedback and reinforce the correct perception at Lucy's appropriate skill level (2.1.b., 2.1.c., 2.1.g., 2.1.h., 2.1.i.). Though she was not "correcting" Lucy's speech per se, the correct perception was being facilitated and reinforced, thereby enhancing and developing her perception. As Mother knows that Lucy is able to produce a better approximation for "up up up" than "Uh uh uh," her approximation for this little phrase is accurate in terms of nonsegmental pattern (duration and pitch contour) and vowel production even though it does not include the [p]. When Mother whispers "puh, puh, puh" to acoustically highlight the unvoiced plosive, she helps her child attend to the missing phoneme in her production (2.1.g., 3.4.b.). In addition, mother is incorporating the elements of comprehension and language retrieval by having different sounds represent items, providing some meaning associated with them, and using the sounds in short sentences or phrases so that Lucy attends to the auditory information (3.1.a., 3.1.b., 3.1.c., 3.3.a., 3.3.b., 3.3.c., 3.3.e., 3.4.a.). Moreover, Lucy is listening to sounds as well as some key words (1.2.a., 3.2.a., 3.3.d.). Throughout the interaction, mother continues to reinforce principles of communication and various pragmatic functions (3.4.c, 3.4.d.).

Mother

Yah, now should we make your mobile
go ROUND'n' ROUND'n' ROUND?
She uses an intonation contour and stresses "round," she looks at Lucy and then looks up at the mobile.

Mother

Round 'n' round 'n'round 'n'round?
She asks again with a rising intonation pattern and waits, and waits a bit longer than

one might usually expect in a conversation. Looks at Lucy with anticipation, raised eyebrows, and shrugs her shoulders.

Lucy
Ow ow

Mother
OK—Mommy will make it go
round 'n' round 'n' round.

Lucy
Ow ow ow

Mother
Mommy will WIND it up.
Turning the knob on the mobile as Lucy watches and smiles in anticipation.

Mother
Turn turn turn.
Holds the mobile with one hand as she begins to wind it with the other.

Mother
Ready? Listen!
Pointing to her ear.

Lucy
Aaaaahhhh
Lucy watches as the cows go around and the music begins to play and vocalizes as if she is trying to sing with the music.

Mother
I know Lucy hears the music. La la la
Mom hums and sings along with the music.

Mother
Mommy hears the music!

Mother
Round and round and round the cows
are going round.
Round and round and round.

Lucy
Aaaaah
Baby looking at mobile and through her control of the nonsegmentals in her vocal play, she sounds as if she is trying to sing with the music.

Mother
Round and round
She says in a sing song way almost like the music from the mobile.

Lucy
Mmmm
The baby reaches for the cow.

Mother
Moooo. That's the cow. Moooo.
Mother reaches for a toy cow on the side of the changing table. She looks at the cow and then at Lucy.

Lucy
Oooooo

Mother
Just like the cows going round and
round. MMMMMoooooo
Mom accepts Lucy's communication and shows her that she understands it. She acoustically highlights the "m" which is missing from Lucy's production.

Lucy
Mm ooo
Looking at her mom and then at the cow and back at mom.

Mother
Old McDonald had a farm
E-I-E-I-O

Mother
And on that farm he had aaaaaaa
Holds the syllable and note for "aaa," she looks at the cow and touches it to wiggle it and looks at Lucy waiting for her to talk.

Lucy
Looks at mother and cow.

Mother
Cow!
E-I-E-I-O
With a mmmmmoooo mmooo
here and a . . .
Again, she holds the syllable and note for "aaa," she looks at the cow and touches it to

wiggle it and looks at Lucy waiting for her to talk.

Lucy
Mmmmm
Vocalizes and smiles.

Mother
Moo moo there
Here a moo
There a moo
Everywhere a mooooo mooooo
She smiles and nods as Lucy vocalizes. She changes to "moo" as she hears Lucy begin her vocalization and slows down and elongates the vowel in "moo" each time to allow Lucy to join in with her all the time trying to change her diaper!

Lucy
Mmmmm mmmmm
Lucy joins in and keeps vocalizing all the time mother is singing.

Mother
Old McDonald had a farm
E-I-E-I-O
And on that farm he had aaaaaa
She looks to the other farm animal toys and looks at Lucy raising her eyebrows and smiling in a way of inviting her to pick the next animal.

Commentary
In this part of the scenario, Lucy again is listening to a variety of sounds and voice features as she listens to her mother talking and singing, as well as to the music from the mobile (1.1.b., 1.1.f, 1.3.a.). Mother is acoustically highlighting one to two items throughout her interaction and while she is singing "Old McDonald" (1.2.a., 1.3.d.). Lucy listens to the salient intonation patterns in stereotypic phrases (Table 15–11) and songs, highlighted by vowels and consonant features (1.3.b., 1.3.c., 1.3.f.). Mother elongates the

TABLE 15–11. Common Stereotypic and Functional Phrases

Bye-bye	Push it down	Where is it?	What do you say?
Sit down	Push hard	Wave bye bye to . . .	Put it there
Stand up	Open it	Time for bed	Hurry up
Help me	Be careful	Comb your hair	Wait a minute
Turn it off	May I have . . .	Eat your . . .	Fell down/fall down
Take it off	I do	Blow your nose	I forget
Put it on	No more	Pick you up	No thank you
Put it down	All gone	Good job	Yes thank you
Push me	Time for . . . breakfast/snack/ lunch/bath	Give me five	You're welcome
That's enough		Turn around	I don't know
Happy Birthday	Let's go . . .	Stand on your toes	Wink your eye
Close your eyes	Brush your teeth	Read a book	Blow a kiss
Clean up	Daddy's home	Yuck, what a stinky diaper	Knock on the door

[m] to help Lucy attend to the sound and to discriminate the nasal murmur in contrast to the long "ooo" vowel. Lucy must attend, discriminate, and produce the contrast, and she must attend to both elements within "moo." Mother interacts with her naturally and expects her to be listening while she is manipulating a toy and not looking at her (1.4.a.). Mother pauses and makes eye contact in a way which conveys the message that Lucy is to vocalize and participate (2.1.a., 2.1.b., 2.1.c.). She has many contrasts within the stereotypic phrases (round 'n' round 'n' round, Ready Listen, I hear. . .), the familiar and repetitive song she sings, and the key words which she stresses such as "mooo," "turn turn turn." These provide ample opportunities to reinforce her discrimination abilities for phonemes and for the language comprehension and retrieval that mother is establishing (3.1.a, 3.1.b., 3.1.c., 3.3.a., 3.3.b., 3.3.c). Mother reinforces the perception-production model and encourages Lucy to improve her control of the nonsegmentals, vowels, and emerging consonants (2.1.d., 2.1.e., 2.1.f., 2.1.g., 2.1.i., 3.2.a.).

Mother has implemented a variety of strategies and techniques. She uses auditory closure within the song by encouraging Lucy to participate and complete the phrase. She is very strategic in using her activities of daily living—the mobile and specific toys at the changing table. These activities involve the repetition of sounds for the farm animals, vehicles, and a Ling six-sound check. She incorporates singing into many of the daily routines.

Billy

Billy was diagnosed at 10 months with a severe-to-profound sensorineural hearing loss in his right ear and a profound sensorineural hearing loss in his left ear. He was diagnosed with questionable enlarged vestibular aque-ducts and he may have had normal hearing up until 8 months, when he sustained a bump to his head. His parents noted several months later that he had stopped babbling and he was no longer frightened by the loud noises that he had reacted to when he was younger. He was aided at 11 months and wore his hearing aids for most of his waking hours. No consistent responses were noted with his hearing aids. At the age of 1 year, 4 months he underwent surgery for a cochlear implant in his right ear; the implant was activated at 1 year, 6 months. He now uses his implant consistently and appears to be benefiting from the auditory information provided. He requests his implant as soon as he wakes up in the morning and often will not let his parents take off the device when he goes to sleep. His parents are pursuing a second implant for him at this time. Billy is cooperative, interacts well with adults during the therapy sessions, and plays appropriately with toys presented to him. He has been using his CI for 6 months. All developmental milestones are age-appropriate to date.

Auditory Processes for Using Sound Meaningfully

Auditory Attention. Billy is able to attend to a variety of auditory signals including speech and environmental sounds. He is able to attend to a key word embedded within a short phrase or sentence when acoustically highlighted. He attends to a variety of stereotypic phrases many of which are specific to his family and experience.

Auditory Memory. Billy displays consistent auditory memory for one key word and is able to remember and repeat a series of three to five consonant-vowel combinations. He will repeat familiar key words embedded within phrases when they are acoustically highlighted.

Auditory Discrimination and Integration. Billy is consistently responding to and discriminating between all of the Ling six sounds, indicating that he is able to detect all aspects of speech with his CI. He demonstrates awareness to environmental sounds and responds to his name when called from a distance. He also is attending to different intensities of sounds, music, and quiet voices or whispers. He is able to attend to nonsegmental and segmental information through audition only. He attends to and discriminates familiar, context-related language when he is occupied in a play activity. He is able to attend to sentences auditory-only containing one to two familiar words. He understands multiple stereotypic phrases, which are used at home, and he is comprehending phrases containing one to two key words (see Table 15–11. Billy's spoken approximations tend to be accurate by syllable and vowel content, as are his productions in response to a word that has been modeled for him.

Auditory Processes for Learning to Talk

Auditory Feedback. At the present time Billy uses a variety of vowel sounds consistently in his spontaneous babbling and word approximations. These include but are not limited to:

"o" as in "bomb,"

"ow" as in "bow wow,"

"o" as in "bomb,"

"u" as in "but,"

"ee" as in "beep,"

"ai" as in "bye bye,"

"i" as in "big,"

"oo" as in "boot,"

"oo" as in "book,"

"a" as in "bad."

He has an increased his spontaneous use of consonants. His phonemes are emerging in an appropriate sequence, which indicates good access to the auditory information.

He most typically produces the following phonemes: plosives (b, p, t. d); nasals (m, n); fricatives (h, sh); and, semivowels (w, y).

Auditory Processes for Learning Language

Auditory Recognition. Billy has acquired many new word approximations in the past months, which are indicative of his developing recognition of auditory patterns.

Auditory Comprehension and Auditory Retrieval. Billy's language abilities were assessed with a standardized evaluation. Test results indicated an age equivalent of 20 months in receptive language and 18 months in expressive language.

Billy has a growing expressive vocabulary of basic words, which he uses spontaneously but the words are not yet clearly articulated. He produces sounds for many vehicles and animals. Billy approximates about 30 words. These words include but are not limited to: more, mommy, roll roll, shoes, uh oh, up, hot, ouch, pull, shake, Billy, moo, help, ball, bounce, teddy bear, shake, milk, daddy, ch ch ooo, airplane, go, train, no, night night, thank you, open, push, bang bang, bye bye, and aaah (airplane). Billy understands many more words than he produces. He still uses some jargon when communicating.

Scenario: Billy

Mother
What should we play with next?
Looking at several toys on the shelf beside the table and then at Billy.

Billy
Puh

Looks at mom, who then looks at the toys while he finishes scribbling on a paper with markers.

Therapist

Billy—draw more. I'm going to talk to mommy. Round and round.
Alright, he is happy with the markers for right now. So, let's talk about what goals we are going to be able to incorporate with the toys.
Putting her hand gently on mother's hand to get her attention and initiating the discussion while letting Billy continue drawing.

Mother

We can certainly get him to use lots of his words with any of these toys. I know he wants the play-doh.

Therapist

OK, perfect. Try to hold back and let him come out with the language first without you giving it to him. But if you want him using words he knows, then use short sentences and put one to two familiar words in the phrases. This also is a good exercise to develop memory for these two words. He knows "open" and "help," and those are words you are about to use. You can say something like "I'll help you open the play-doh." Try to acoustically highlight the words only if you think he really didn't pull out the word from the phrase. Remember, if he is using these words spontaneously, he should recognize them and should be able to attend to them within short sentences. What else can we work on?

Mother

Listening to me while he is busy playing with the play-doh.

Therapist

Absolutely. He was busy drawing, and he looked up at you when you asked what he wanted to play with. That was great that he was paying attention. You can reinforce his listening to you. What else can you think of?

Mother

Making his speech clearer.

Therapist

Perfect. And also improving upon his listening skills. Better attention and matching what he hears with what he says will reinforce his understanding. So, right off the bat, we can get him to listen and better approximate the words for play-doh or puzzle or whatever toy he wants. If it was the play-doh, is "puh" the best approximation you think he can do?

Mother

No, he can do a [d]

Therapist

Good place to start. You can get him to listen and do better approximations.

Mother

Ok, what should I do?

Therapist

Ask him again and he will probably tell you "puh" again. So, he may mean puzzle, but we both know he likes play-doh much more than puzzles. So I think you need to let him know you aren't sure what he means or that you think he means puzzle. I bet he will protest if you try to give him the puzzle or just say "no" if you let him know you think he said puzzle.

Mother

Doesn't that mean not giving him what he wants even if we know what he wants?

Therapist

Wait wait wait, Do you REALLY know what he wants by what he communicated? He was drawing so he didn't point to anything and it wasn't close enough for him to grab it.

Mother

Weeeellll, maybe not. So how do I tell him that I don't know what he means? He doesn't understand those words.

Therapist

He will understand by the way you phrase it, body language and intonation. You can tell him that. You are letting him know that you want to know what he means, but you aren't sure. Then you can help him listen to the words again, so he can improve his approximation and then have more successful communication interactions with you. You really want to understand, so convey that to him in your response. You aren't questioning him to be mean. You are attempting to improve the communication by having him attend to the words, discriminate how the words are different, and then match his perception and production for nonsegmentals, vowels and consonants. THEN, you can give him what he REALLY wants, because you will know! This is a great way to work on a number of targeted goals!

Mother

So I ask for the [d] in Doh?

Therapist

Yes, try to do that. But, what about the number of syllables and the vowels he used? I know has acquired the concept of duration, so I think he should be able to produce both vowels with the [d]. The [p] in "play" isn't really a [p] in isolation because it blends with the [l]. So he may substitute the blend with a [p] or just omit it entirely. But he should produce two syllables with the correct vowels and a [d] in the second syllable. Right?

Mother

For sure. So if he doesn't produce the [p], I shouldn't whisper or acoustically highlight it, is that right?

Therapist

Right—might be too much unless he tries to produce it. Have him attempt the other sounds that you know he can produce. Also, remember once he has all the toys, he has the control. You have the most control while you have the object or while he needs your help. So give him the toys slowly and not all the parts at the same time. That way he needs to interact with you in order to obtain all the parts. OK go for it!

Mother

Billy, what should we play with next? Pointing at several toys on the shelf beside the table and then looking at Billy.

Billy

Puh

Looks at mom, who then looks at the toys as he puts down his marker, now finished scribbling on a paper and ready to move on to another toy.

Mother

I don't know what you mean. What should we play with? Cars? The puzzle? PLAY-DOH? Making eye contact with Billy and pointing with a finger to each choice.

Billy

Puh

Mother

Puzzle? You want to play with the puzzle? Pointing at the puzzle and reaching with her hand as if she is going to pick it up.

Billy

NO! Shaking his head 'no" and pointing at the play-doh.

Mother

NO, not the puzzle. Billy wants the

PLAY-Doh! Billy wants to play with
play-doh?
Shaking her head and then reaching toward
the play-doh and grabbing several canisters
with different colors of play-doh.

Billy
Puh

Mother
Puh—it sounds like Puzzle, but you want
PLAY-Doh! You want to play with
PLAY-DOH. Listen. PLAY-DOH.

Billy
Ay oh

Mother
Good try! Listen again, play-DOH.

Billy
Ay Doh

Mother
Alright, I understand We'll play with
play-doh. What color do you want? We
have so many! Which one?
Mom has several containers of play-doh and
is holding them close to her body.

Billy
Ah be de wa de mah to wa
Jargoning with an excited voice.

Mother
I know—we have so many!
Which one do you want?
With lots of excitement and vocal play.

Billy
Ah be de wa de mah to wa
Babbles excitedly with a similar intonation
contour to the one mother just used, rapidly looking at his mom and then the play-
doh and back at his mother.

Mother
We have different colors—purple,
blue, green, yellow
Shows each one as she names them.

Billy
Wah ba dauh

Mother
Yah I know you WANT play-doh.
Which one?

Billy
Grabs at the purple.

Mother
Oh—I think you want purple. It's not
OK to grab. Use your voice. Just tell me
that you want purple. Purple.
Holding up the purple but not too close in
front of him and making eye contact.

Billy
Puhpuh

Mother
Purple! You want purple! I thought so.
Here is the purple play-doh.
Hands him the play-doh container, sealed
shut and puts the other play-doh away on
the shelf.

Billy
Puh puh

Mother
Yes—I gave you the purple!
You have purple play-doh.

Therapist
FABULOUS! Nice getting him to listen
while he was busy and then improving his
production. You really let him know you
wanted to understand what he was
saying. Your expansions were great. When
he said one word, you used the same
word and let him know you understood
what he communicated. Then you used
the expansion technique and put the
words into little phrases. That facilitates
his auditory memory, his attention, and
recognition of words within phrases.
This way you are improving and
reinforcing his communication.

Mother
What should we do?
Pauses for a long time, raises her eyebrows, leans forward, shrugs her shoulders in a quizzical, questioning manner.

Billy
Open

Mother
Pull it open! OK, you pull it open.

Billy
Open
He holds out the play-doh and asks by raising his pitch to produce a question.

Mother
You need help to open the play-doh?

Billy
Hep

Mother
I'll help open the play-doh.

Billy
Open

Mother
Wow! It's stuck. We need to pull it open. I need to PULL . . . Pull, pull, pull!

Billy
Puh, puh, puh

Mother
There! I pulled it open!

Billy
Open

Mother
I pulled the play-doh open!
What do you say?

Billy
An you!

Mother
Yes—Thank you is right. You're welcome!

Billy
(babble string)
Showing he can't get the play doh out of the container and sounding frustrated.

Mother
Uh O! The play-doh is stuck!

Billy
Uh O!

Mother
What should we do?

Billy
Hep
Holding out the play-doh for his mother to take it.

Mother
I'll help you. Let's shake, shake shake!
Puts her hand on the play-doh and turns it over.

Billy
Shay shay shay

Mother
Hmmmm, That's not working.

Billy
Shay shay

Mother
Yes I did shake it, but it didn't work. I can bang on the table. Bang, bang, bang.

Billy
Ba ba ba

Mother
Bang bang bang on the table.
Listen it's going to be loud.

Billy
Ba ba ba

Mother
I heard that! Bang bang bang.
Mother smashes the container on the table repeatedly.

Billy
Ba ba ba

Mother
I think we got it! Yeah.
Gives the play-doh to Billy and he plays
with it.

Therapist
FABULOUS! Great expansions and
working on getting him to listen to two
key items. See if you can do that when
you give him choices with the cookie
cutters. Also, remember we were trying to
get him to listen to words that have
different numbers of syllables. You can
find different molds for words with different syllables—dog, airplane, teddy bear—
gives you one, two and three syllables.
There lots of different things in there.

Billy
Oh oh oh
Moving and gesturing with his hands as if
he is rolling the play-doh.

Mother
Roll roll roll the play-doh.
We need a rolling pin.
She rummages in the basket of play-doh
related toys.

Billy
Oh oh oh
Watching his mother as she looks for the
rolling pin.

Mother
There you go.
Roll, roll roll the play-doh
Finds the rolling pin and holds it out for
Billy to take.

Billy
Oh oh oh
He says as he attempts to roll the play-doh.

Mother
Great! You are rolling the play-doh.
My turn.

Billy
Oh oh oh
Continuing to roll and seeming to not be lis-
tening.

Mother
Mommy's turn please!
Reaching out for the rolling pin.

Billy
(Babble string)
Keeps rolling and seems to be saying that
he is not going to share.

Mother
I know you want to roll the play-doh.
Mommy's turn and then you can
roll more.

Billy
More
Shaking his head as he rolls out the play-
doh.

Mother
You want to roll more.
Mommy's turn now.
Taking the rolling pin as Billy passes it to her,
not too certain that he wants to give it up.

Billy
(Babble string)
As if he is reluctantly giving it to her but
reminding her she has to give it back.

Mother
Thank you! I'll give it back. Roll roll roll.
I'm rolling the play-doh.

Therapist
Lovely turn-taking mom! He is mostly very
engaged in what he is doing but still really
listening to you whether or not he is
looking at you. And you keep talking to
him and pausing until he takes his turn.
That is great. It is interesting that
sometimes he takes a longer time—which
means he may be thinking about what he
wants to say, and then if it has a key word

that you used, he is pulling it out of the phrase, remembering it, and using it spontaneously. I also like the way he tells you with his jargon that he isn't happy about giving it to you. It's adorable!

Billy
More?

Mother
Ok, you want to roll more?

Billy
More!
Smiling and reaching for the rolling pin.

Mother
Here you go.
Holding it out, raising her eyebrows, leaning toward him, and waiting for his response as she gets ready to let go of the rolling pin.

Billy
An you

Mother
You're welcome!

Commentary
Billy listens throughout this play activity (1.4.a.). Mother appropriately lets him listen to the noise that is relevant to their activity, such as when they bang the play-doh container on the table (1.1.d.). He attends to and discriminates between a variety of nonsegmental features, vowels and consonants (1.3.a., 1.3.b., 1.3.c., 1.3.f.), and demonstrates auditory feedback through his many spontaneous productions. There is clearly an established conversational interaction in which he participates; he uses his voice to produce specific phonemes (2.1.a., 2.1.c., 2.1.d., 2.1.e., 2.1.g., 2.1.i.). In addition, he shows an expanded use of one to two syllable words (3.2.a.). Mother and Billy demonstrate very good turn-taking and communication skills (3.4.d.). Billy is tuned into Mother's voice (1.1.a.). He is aware of the nonsegmental

aspects of her vocalizations and understands when she asks a question (1.1.f., 1.3.a., 2.1.b.). As they continue to play, Billy demonstrates auditory comprehension and retrieval abilities. He associates a variety of objects with their sounds, which suggests that these words had emerged when he was younger (1.3.a., 3.3.b.). He understands words, phrases, and questions (with and without context) based on one to two known words (directives and statements) or rhythmic pattern. Furthermore, he uses a variety of functional words, phrases, nouns, and verbs for a variety of pragmatic functions (3.1.b., 3.3.a., 3.3.c., 3.3.d., 3.3.e., 3.4.a., 3.4.b., 3.4.c.).

Mother
Let's see—we could make an airplane that goes "aaaah."

Billy
Aaaah

Mother
Yes, the airplane goes "aaah." Or we could make a train, that goes . . .
Mother holds the airplane as she talks about it and hides the train in her hand waiting for him to respond to her prompt before she completes the phrase.

Billy
Sh sh ooooo

Mother
CH CH ooooo says the train.
Billy wants the train?
She shows the train cookie cutter.

Billy
Ayn

Mother
The train goes . . .
She pauses and looks with expectation.

Billy
Sh sh ooooo

Reaching for the train mold, taking it from his mother, and putting it on the play-doh.

Mother
The train—CH Ch ooooooo.
Push down and make the train.

Billy
Ayn

Mother
PUSH on the TRAIN.

Billy
Push

Mother
Push down on the play-doh.

Billy
Push

Mother
Push down. Push down on the train.

Billy
Dow

Mother
Let's push it out of the mold. Wow.
Here's the choo choo train.

Billy
Ayn

Therapist
Lovely turn-taking. You used some auditory closure very effectively. If he says "down" again—we should see if he will say the [n]. Let's see if we can get him to listen to the different words with different syllables.

Mother
I don't know how to do that.

Therapist
Ok. Let me show you. I'm going to use different words—one syllable, two syllables, and three syllables.

Turning to Billy, the therapist takes three molds in her hand and shows them to Billy, but doesn't give them to him yet.

Therapist
That's the car.

Billy
Aw

Therapist
I have the car. This is the airplane.

Billy
Upane

Therapist
This is the Teddy bear.

Billy
Teddy beh

Therapist
Good listening Billy, I have a car, an airplane and a Teddy bear.
Shows each one again as she says their name.

Therapist
So I had him listening to the number of syllables and he actually produced lovely approximations of them by syllable, vowel and some consonants. Are there any sounds you think he can produce better?

Mother
I don't think so, I thought they sounded great and was surprised he didn't need to repeat them.

Therapist
That's probably because we are giving him tasks in which we are setting him up for success. He CAN do syllables; he has great vowel variety and some nice emerging consonants, which he is mastering in word imitations. He has a great auditory feedback loop going for him. He is really listening! Ok, now have him pick two of the three items, but always do it in the

same order. If he gets one correct, continue to repeat the two objects because we are working on two-item auditory memory. This is a bit harder for him but he knows these items, loves play-doh, so this is a great activity to practice.

Mother
Billy, let's get the car and the teddy bear. Billy is reaching for the car, because he wants it, but mom who now has the molds is keeping her hands cupped so he can't have them yet.

Mother
You can make the car. I want to make the teddy bear. Will you get the car and the teddy bear?

Billy
Teddy beh?
With a clear rising intonation pattern that denotes a question.

Therapist
So that is very typical. He remembered the last item he heard, even though he really wants the car. So now he can retain "teddy bear" in his short-term auditory memory and concentrate on the other item. Be sure to acoustically highlight the car as he didn't get that one, and repeat both items.

Mother
Yes but we need the car and the teddy bear.

Billy
Teddy beh . . . ah

Mother
Yes—get the car for you and the teddy bear for me

Billy
Teddy beh

Mother
Car and the teddy bear.

Billy
Teddy beh

Mother
Car and the teddy bear.

Billy
Ah

Mother
YES! The car and the Teddy bear.
Billy reaches for both molds. She lets him take them and but then takes the teddy bear as he begins playing with the car.

Mother
Thank you for the teddy bear and now you have the car. Let's put them in the play-doh.

Therapist
So what just happened there?

Mother
He picked two items but I needed to repeat and repeat and repeat.

Therapist
Good for both of you. You persisted with the two items and he was able to do it. Yes, it did take some repetition. You didn't need to repeat it quite that many times, but this is probably one of the first times he has successfully completed this task. So this represented a structured activity for a two-item auditory memory task. You accomplished it with two key words, spoken in short phrases, while expanding language for him.

Commentary
Mother continues with many goals as discussed above with regard to attending, discriminating, and feedback. She makes certain that Billy is listening to her by being very

involved in the activity and expecting his consistent participation in the communication regardless of how exciting the activity is for him (1.1.a., 1.1.b.). She contrasts words and short phrases, with different syllables and nonsegmental patterns (1.1.f., 1.3.a., 1.3.b). Mother makes good use of acoustic highlighting, auditory closure, joint attention, and expansions in this segment.

The emergence of new skills is evident for both Billy and his mother. Mother is learning to have a greater expectation in terms of consistency in Billy's productions. Furthermore, she is learning to balance several goals in one activity. This includes enhancing his listening, facilitating his production, and maintaining the balance of conversation so that the most important elements remain—interaction and communication (2.1.a., 2.1.b., 2.1.c., 2.1.d., 2.1.e., 2.1.g., 2.1.h., 2.1.i.). This activity also requires her to monitor his discrimination of nonsegmentals, vowels, and consonants (1.3.a., 1.3.b., 1.3.c., 1.3.d., 1.3.f.). The natural evolution of these features is to develop auditory discrimination and comprehension ability for words and phrases based on those features, including ones that vary in numbers of syllables, known words, and phrases (1.3.e., 3.1.a., 3.1.b., 3.1.c., 3.3.a., 3.3.c., 3.3.d., 3.3.e.). Mother is learning to facilitate Billy's two item auditory memory by having him listen to two familiar key words in phrases when she expands his language or models it by having him select two known items from a small set (1.2.a.). These auditory processes of discrimination, recognition, and comprehension facilitate retrieval. With consistent use of the speech phonemes within his repertoire (2.1.i., 3.4.c.), his spontaneous expressive language is expanding by one- to two-syllable functional words and by functional words, phrases, nouns, verbs, and adjectives (3.2.a., 3.4.a, 3.4.b., 3.4.d.).

Billy has accomplished most of the goals that were initially targeted. From this point, all of his current skills must be reinforced. More advanced goals for the beginning listener are targeted, as described under "Advanced Beginner Habilitation Goals" found in Table 15–12. The new goals reinforce current abilities but add more advanced skills. Billy's capabilities are referenced to normal development. In most areas, foundation skills are introduced at the beginner listening level, ensuring that the auditory skills of detection, attention, discrimination, feedback, identification, comprehension, and retrieval are progressing.

Conclusion

Early diagnosis of hearing loss in newborns is now a reality. Current and emerging technology is providing auditory access to babies with hearing loss. A strong auditory-focused intervention facilitates parent-infant interaction and communication development. This approach takes into consideration the normal sequence of development in the areas of auditory processing, language development, communication, and speech acquisition. Auditory-Verbal therapy, in particular, provides an intervention model designed to maximize the baby's potential to develop spoken language competence.

TABLE 15–12. Advanced Beginner Habilitation Goals

1. Auditory Processes for Using Sound Meaningfully

Auditory Attention

- Reinforce and expand ability to consistently respond, discriminate and imitate the 6 sounds [m, oo, ah, ee, sh, s].
- Reinforce discrimination of phonemes by manner, place, and voicing cues when presented at normal intensity, with decreased voice intensity and increased distance.
- Reinforce consistent attention to word final consonants.
- Indicate when cochlear implant is off or not working.
- Reinforce and facilitate responses to name and other auditory signals from increasing distances using the cochlear implant.
- Facilitate ability to attend through audition only to sentences of 3 to 6 words.
- Facilitate attention for auditory only recognition and comprehension tasks.

Auditory Memory

- Expand and reinforce an auditory memory for 2 to 4 items.

Auditory Discrimination

- Condition to consistently respond, discriminate and imitate the 6 sounds [m, oo, ah, ee, sh, s].
- Expand awareness of environmental sounds.
- Reinforce and expand ability to attend to auditory information for discrimination of nonsegmentals information.
- Reinforce and expand ability to attend to auditory information for discrimination of vowels.
- Facilitate and reinforce ability to attend to auditory information for discrimination of various manners of production.
- Facilitate and reinforce ability to attend to auditory information for discrimination of voicing cues within a variety of manners of production.
- Facilitate ability to attend to auditory information for discrimination of place cues within a variety of manners of production.
- Facilitate auditory discrimination of phrases on the basis of rhythmic structure and known words.
- Discriminate words consisting of varying syllabification—1, 2, or 3 syllables in a limited set.
- Reinforce attending to voices when motorically or visually occupied in play.

Auditory Integration

- Facilitate and reinforce use of audition only for closed-set discrimination.
- Facilitate and reinforce use of audition when actively engaged in activities.

2. Auditory Processes for Learning to Talk

Auditory Feedback

- Continue to monitor, reinforce, and expand variety of vocalizations and phrase babbling.
- Develop and expand control of nonsegmental aspects of speech (duration, intensity, pitch) at phonetic and phonologic levels.

TABLE 15–12. *continued*

- Expand productions to include a variety of low, mid, and high-frequency vowels and diphthongs.
- Practice syllabic babble and alternating with consonants varying in manner and voice.
- Expand and reinforce consistent productions of consonants of varying in manner and voice.
- Expand and reinforce consistent productions of consonants of the fricative and affricate manners including initially, but not limited to, [s, sh, h, f, ch] with vowel variety at a phonologic level.
- Expand and reinforce consistent productions of consonants of differing place cues within a variety of manners of production.
- Facilitate and correct speech productions through imitations, turn-taking, and spontaneous vocalizations in prompted situations and with modeling of language stimulus varying by nonsegmental aspects, vowels, and consonant content at phonologic level.
- Facilitate and reinforce consistent production of word final consonants.

3. Auditory Processes for Learning Language

Auditory Recognition
- Identify objects by associated sounds, which vary in nonsegmental qualities and vowel content.
- Develop and reinforce auditory recognition of phrases on the basis of rhythmic structure, known words, and contextual cues.

Auditory Sequencing
- Facilitate and expand imitations of one to four-syllable functional words and phrases.

Auditory Comprehension
- Stimulate and expand auditory comprehension of language in the areas of functional words, phrases (up, down, bye-bye, all gone, more), nouns, verbs, and adjectives.
- Develop and reinforce auditory comprehension of phrases without contextual cues.
- Develop and reinforce auditory comprehension of phrases based on one to two known words (directives and statements) or rhythmic pattern.
- Monitor and record auditory comprehension of vocabulary every 2 months.

Auditory Retrieval
- Stimulate expressive language in the areas of functional words, phrases, nouns, verbs, and adjectives.
- Monitor and record expressive vocabulary every 2 months.
- Facilitate imitation on demand of phrases using correct nonsegmental aspects, phoneme content, and syllabification.
- Facilitate and expand consistent use of speech and word approximations to communicate a variety of pragmatic functions (e.g., requesting, protesting, responding, turn-taking, attention-getting).
- Elicit a variety of pragmatic functions.

References

American Speech-Language-Hearing Association. (2005a). *(Central) auditory processing disorders*. Available at http://www.asha.org/members/deskref-journals/deskref/default .

American Speech-Language-Hearing Association Task Force on Central Auditory Processing Consensus Development. (1996).

Benedict, H. (1979). Early lexical development: Comprehension and production. *Journal of Child Language, 6*, 183–200.

Birnholtz, J. C., & Benacerraf, B. R. (1983). The development of human fetal hearing. *Science, 222*, 516–518.

Blanchfield, B., Feldman, J., & Dunbar, J. (2001). The severely to profoundly hearing impaired population in the United States: Prevalence estimates and demographics. *Journal of the American Academy of Audiology, 12*, 183–189.

Boothroyd, A. (1982). *Hearing impairments in young children*. Englewood Cliffs, NJ: Prentice-Hall.

Brown, R. W. (1973). *A first language: The early stages*. Cambridge, MA: Harvard University Press.

Bzoch, K. R., League, R., & Brown, V. (2003). *Receptive-Expressive Emergent Language Test (3rd ed.) Examiner's manual*. Austin, TX: Pro-Ed.

Daniel, L. (1990). HEAR In Dallas log notes form.

Daniel, L., Daniloff, R., & Schuckers, G. (1999). ALPS: A language rehabilitation program for children with cochlear implants. *Journal of Louisiana Allied Health Professionals, 2*.

Does Your Child Hear and Talk? (n.d.). Retrieved October 8, 2008, from http://www.asha.org/public/speech/development/chart.htm

Dore, J. (1975). Holophrases, speech acts and language universals. *Journal of Child Language, 2*, 21–40.

Downs, M. P. (1995). Universal newborn hearing screening—The Colorado study. *International Journal of Pediatric Otorhinolaryngology, 32*, 257–259.

Eilers, R., & Oller, D. K. (1994). Infant vocalizations and the early diagnosis of severe hearing impairment. *Journal of Pediatrics, 124*(2), 199–203.

Erber, N. P. (1982). *Auditory training*. Washington, DC: Alexander Graham Bell Association for the Deaf.

Erikson, E. H. (1950). *Childhood and society* (2nd ed.). New York: Norton.

Foster, S. H. (1990). *The communicative competence of young children*. New York: Wesley Longman Limited.

Geers, A. (2003). Predictors of reading skill development in children with early cochlear implantation. *Ear and Hearing, 24*(Suppl.), 59S–68S.

Gleason, J. B. (1997). *The development of language* (4th ed.). Boston: Allyn and Bacon.

Goldberg, D. M., & Flexer, C. (2001). Auditory-verbal graduates: An updated outcome survey of clinical efficacy. *Journal of the American Academy of Audiology, 12*, 406–414.

Kubler-Ross, E. (1969). *On death and dying*. New York: Macmillan.

Ladefoged, P. (2006). *A course in phonetics* (5th ed.). Boston: Thomson Wadsworth.

Language Development in Children (n.d.). Retrieved October 8, 2008, from http://www.childdevelopmentinfo.com/development/language_development.shtml

Ling, D. (1976, 2002). *Speech and the hearing-impaired child: Theory and practice* (2nd ed., 2002). Washington, DC: Alexander Graham Bell Association for the Deaf.

Ling, D. (1989). *Foundations of spoken language for hearing-impaired children*. Washington, DC: Alexander Graham Bell Association for the Deaf.

Ling, D. (2002/03). The six-sound test. *The Listener, Winter*, pp. 52–53.

Ling, D., & Ling, A. (1978). *Aural habilitation—The foundations of verbal learning in hearing-impaired children*. Washington, DC: Alexander Graham Bell Association for the Deaf.

Luterman, D. (1984). *Counseling the communicatively disordered and their families*. Boston: Little Brown and Company.

Luterman, D. (1987). *Deafness in the family*. Boston: Little, Brown and Company.

Mayo Clinic. (n.d.). Retrieved October 8, 2008, from http://www.mayoclinic.com/health/infant-development/AN01026

Mischook, M., & Cole, E. (1986). Auditory learning and teaching of hearing-impaired children. In E. Cole & H. Gregory (Eds.), Auditory learning, *Volta Review, 88*(5), 67–81.

Northern, J. L., & Downs, M. P. (1991). Behavioral hearing testing of children. In *Hearing in children.* (4th ed., pp. 139–187). Baltimore: Williams & Wilkins.

Oller, D. K. (1980). The emergence of the sounds of speech in infancy. In G. Yeni-Komishian, J. Kavanagh, & C. Ferguson (Eds.), *Child phonology Vol. 1: Production* (pp. 93–112). New York: Academic Press.

Oller, D. K., & Eilers, R. E. (1988). The role of audition in infant babbling. *Child Development, 59,* 441–449.

Oller, D. K., Eilers, R., Bull, D., & Carney, A. (1985). Prespeech vocalizations of a deaf infant: A comparison with normal metaphonological development. *Journal of Speech and Hearing Research, 28,* 47–63.

Oller, D. K., Eilers, R. E., Neal, A. R., & Schwartz, H. K. (1999). Precursors to speech in infancy: The prediction of speech and language disorders. *Journal of Communication Disorders, 32,* 223–245.

Oller, D. K., Wieman L. A., Doyle W. J., & Ross, C. (1976). Infant babbling and speech. *Journal of Child Language, 3,* 1–12.

Pollack, D. (1970). *Educational audiology for the limited hearing infant.* Springfield, IL: Charles C. Thomas.

Robertson, L., & Flexer, C. (1993). Reading development: A parent survey of children with hearing impairment who developed speech and language through the auditory-verbal method. *Volta Review, 95*(3), 253–261.

Rotfleisch, S. (2000). Soda bottles and submarines: Essential speech acoustics. *The Listener, Summer,* pp. 51–56.

Rotfleisch, S. (2001). E = mc² (English equals milk and cookies too!). *The Listener, Fall,* pp. 39–42.

Sander, E. K. (1972). When are speech sounds learned? *Journal of Speech and Hearing Disorders, 37,* 55–63.

Speech Language Milestone Chart. (n.d.). Retrieved October 8, 2008, from http://www.ldonline.org/article/6313

Vaughan, P. (1981). *Learning to listen.* Ontario, Canada: General Publishing.

Weir, C. (1979). Auditory frequency sensitivity of human newborns: Some data with improved acoustic and behavioral controls. *Perception and Psychophysics, 26,* 287–294.

Werner, L. A., & Gillenwater, J. M. (1990). Pure-tone sensitivity of 2- to 5-week old infants. *Infant Behavior and Development, 13,* 355–375.

Werner, L. A., & Mancl, L. R. (1993). Pure-tone thresholds of 1-month-old human infants. *Journal of the Acoustical Society of America, 93,* 23–67.

Yoshinaga-Itano, C., & Sedey, A. L. (2000) Language, speech, and social-emotional development of children who are deaf or hard-of-hearing: The early years, *Volta Review, 100,* 181–211.

Zimmerman, I. L., Steiner, V. G., & Pond, R. E. (2002). *Preschool Language Scale* (4th ed.), Examiner's manual. San Antonio, TX: The Psychological Corporation.

CHAPTER 16

Educational Considerations: From Listening to Literacy

MARY ELLEN NEVINS
PATRICIA M. CHUTE

Introduction

The educational system is a conduit that children enter in childhood and emerge into adulthood. This system is charged with providing the academic and social skills to become productive members of society. Every child has an opportunity to reach his or her personal best in an educational system whose variability supports (or constrains) the child's individual potential. Despite the fact that legislation has mandated that all children have the right to a quality educational experience, there are many challenges in the system that create barriers to success. This is particularly true for children with special needs. Children using cochlear implants can take advantage of the best the system has to offer but may still be susceptible to the limitations of individual educational programs.

Educational Outcomes of Children with Cochlear Implants

With more than 20 years of pediatric cochlear implant data available, the educational implications of implantation are becoming apparent. Children whose only challenge is severe to profound sensorineural hearing loss receive maximal benefit from the potential of the device. This allows them the opportunity to achieve academic parity with their typically developing age mates (Nicholas & Geers, 2006). Unfortunately, this outcome is not representative of the population of children with cochlear implants presenting with "special circumstances" which override what the device can offer. That being said, however, research has demonstrated that deaf children with cochlear implants will receive auditory benefit from the device that is superior to that afforded by traditional hearing aids (Geers, 1997; Stacey, Fortnum, Barton, & Summerfield, 2006). With this as a backdrop, educational considerations for children with implants need to be viewed within the context of the academic system, the child with the implant and the interaction between the two.

Categorical Nomenclature

A number of researchers and interventionists have written on the topic of implant performance outcomes and have categorized them into different user groups. When comparing implant users to hearing aid users, categories have been labeled "gold," "silver," or "bronze" (Robbins, Kirk, Osberger, & Ertmer, 1995). The Spoken Language Predictor introduced by Geers and Moog (1987) used a 4-point numerical scale of speech perception ability to forecast the potential of any child to develop oral communication skills. Speech perception was ranked from "1" no pattern perception, "2" pattern perception, "3" some word recognition, and "4" consistent word recognition. This was later adapted to include levels "5" and "6" to account for the open set speech recognition made possible by the cochlear implant.

In a recent publication describing "auditory inclination" for children who use sign communication prior to implantation, Chute and Nevins (2006) have used terms such as "excellent, good, and limited" auditory skill development. In this chapter, a novel conceptualization linked to a child's ability to use auditory skills to achieve language and academic parity is offered for the purpose of driving subsequent discussions regarding an individual child's performance in the classroom. The first group of children to be identified is one in which auditory skill development allows students to achieve at levels within a *commensurate range* when compared to their typically developing peers. A second group includes children who make good use of their auditory access and are within the *capable range* in the classroom with supports, but will not likely achieve the language and academic success enjoyed by the *commensurate* group. A final group presents with other physiologic or learning issues that places their achievement in the *challenged range* when compared to their chronological peers. The reader is reminded that children with or without hearing loss will demonstrate a span of performance that can vary from subject to subject and skill to skill. Within the heterogeneous organization of grouping that is common in schools, children who are classified as "A" or excellent students sit alongside children who are considered "C" or average students. This scope of performance is typical throughout the educational system and reminds professionals of the fact that children in any of the categories noted above will also reflect this range. However, if a particular child's "personal best" is to be an "A" student and he or she is unable to achieve that potential, then an analysis of placement and services is warranted.

Commensurate Performers

Children who ultimately perform within the range of their typically developing peers are likely to be those who have been identified and implanted early, have a short duration of deafness and have had timely access to excellent early intervention services. A family-centered approach in which parents take an active role in providing language input at home is the cornerstone of habilitation services for this young age group (Harrigan & Nikolopoulos, 2002; Simser, 1999). Skill development that takes place in the natural environment in a top down fashion more similar to that of hearing children is generally believed to be effective in the acquisition of listening and spoken language for youngsters with hearing loss. Children whose performance places them within the **commensurate range** show evidence of a learning trajectory that parallels typically developing children. In other words, a year's growth (or more) is expected in a year's time across all domains, especially linguistics.

Capable Performers

Children who are considered *capable* performers develop auditory skills that support their spoken language and academic learning. Their auditory perceptual abilities are improved over their hearing aid capabilities but they do not catch up to their typically developing peers linguistically and academically. There are delays that preclude them from achieving at a level that is the same as their hearing peers but not as pronounced as the group in the *challenged* range. Generally, this group has accessed implantation at older ages and/or presents with a mild language or auditory processing issue. Research suggests that this group may constitute a substantial number of cochlear implant recipients (Nicholas & Geers, 2007) and, therefore, presents with diverse habilitation needs.

Challenged Performers

Children who are *challenged* to take advantage of the auditory potential of the implant generally present with some cognitive involvement or have specific auditory processing issues. The cochlear implant cannot overcome the physiologic factors that are present in these children. Auditory access for children with cognitive involvement may provide quality of life enhancement and basic functional skills. Habilitation for the *challenged* child should be undertaken using a whole child perspective with realistic expectations and the knowledge that reaching the point of personal best may be a slow and laborious process.

These categorical ranges are postulated with the understanding that there can be movement between categories for some children as a result of quality and quantity of services. Speech and hearing professionals can assist a child in moving in an upward manner thus ensuring the child reaches his/ her personal best. Conversely, limitations in service provision and lack of knowledge and skills on the part of personnel may result in a child's downward movement within the range or to another lower category. For example, a child who receives a cochlear implant and is enrolled in a school environment in which few opportunities for listening and spoken language are provided will have limited outcomes. Properly selected habilitation strategies aimed specifically at the child's performance range will allow the implant user to maintain status within the current performance range or provide the impetus to move in an upward direction.

Broad Educational Principles

The temptation to view children with cochlear implants outside of the larger context of general educational principles results in a narrow view of how and where the child can achieve academically. It may be considered that at the root of all learning is Vygotsky's "Zone of Proximal Development

(ZPD)" (Vygotsky, 1962). Briefly stated, the Zone of Proximal Development is conceptualized as an area just beyond the point at which a child can perform a task independently. Mediation or assistance provided by an adult (parent, teacher, or even a more accomplished peer) can assist in accomplishing a skill too difficult for the child on his or her own but within reach when the proper guidance is provided. This basic concept may then be regarded as an underlying premise to the Individualized Educational Plan (IEP). IEPs identify present level of functioning; when the next or "proximal" skill is targeted for intervention, the student is far more likely to accomplish it than one further along on a skill development continuum.

Children placed in classrooms in which the instruction is either too easy or too difficult may be "engaged" in an activity, but will not be learning if they already know the concept or it is beyond their ZPD. For any child in any classroom, then, the implicit goal is to maximize academic learning time. It may be prudent to revisit the concept of academic learning time (ALT) as an educational principle for consideration of planning instruction for the child with a cochlear implant. ALT is representative of the amount of time a student spends attending to challenging academic activities while performing those tasks with a high degree of success (Berliner, 1978; Vockell, 2008). It is maximized when a child's placement allows him/her to function within the ZPD and where true learning takes place.

Classroom Settings, ZPD and ALT

Although a large number of children with cochlear implants are in the mainstream, this educational setting is not the only place

(nor is it always the best place) for them. Inclusive classrooms (regular education classrooms that are co-taught by a general education teacher and a teacher of children with hearing loss), self-contained classrooms and schools for the deaf may also be appropriate placements for children with cochlear implants. Unfortunately, in many locations, there is not a continuum of choices available to a child due to lack of population density or limited availability of qualified professionals. This is particularly problematic when children in the mid-*capable range* are placed in a mainstream classroom. It is possible that most, if not all, instruction will be beyond a child's ZPD and, as a result, true academic learning time is limited. Similarly, a child in the *commensurate range* in a classroom for children with hearing loss may be exposed to instruction that is geared to children with lesser abilities. In this case, instruction is not challenging enough and the mandate for instruction within the Zone is left unheeded. Success in the classroom for each of these children will be diminished if instruction is not planned with the "laserlike focus" required to meet the individual educational needs of the child.

Specific Auditory Skill Development

With a presumption of application of the concepts discussed above, there are two additional notions that may help frame auditory habilitation recommendations for an individual child. These include *auditory inclination* (Chute & Nevins, 2006) and *learning trajectory.* Auditory inclination is defined as the "child's own responsiveness to spoken language input" (Chute & Nevins, 2006 p. 132) once auditory access has been provided. Until and unless the child with a severe to profound hearing loss receives a cochlear implant, it is impossible to assess any child's auditory inclination. This, in turn, suggests that it is possible for a child to receive a cochlear implant at a later age and subsequently take advantage of a "native" auditory inclination. Auditory inclination, in effect, drives the pace of movement through an auditory skills hierarchy. Children with excellent auditory inclination are expected to move more rapidly toward auditory comprehension than children with good or limited auditory inclination. The latter group may likely never reach this highest level of auditory skill. This rate of movement through the auditory skills curriculum may be conceptualized as a line called a learning trajectory. Learning trajectories represent the slope of achievement in any skill area that can be defined as either steep (indicating rapid progress), shallow (signaling slow progress) or medial (representing a constant and steady rate of progress over time). Recipients who show a negative trajectory should be evaluated by a team to determine the cause for this unusual outcome. It should be noted that the learning trajectory is a fluid, dynamic parameter that changes over time and should not be determined by smaller day to day performance variations. Learning trajectory will be influenced by a number of confounding factors. For a complete discussion of factors that affect the slope of learning, the reader is referred to a discussion of the Zone of Cochlear Implant Performance in Chute and Nevins (2006).

Creating a profile of the child with a cochlear implant is the first step in planning appropriate auditory habilitation. A number of questions need to be answered to determine the quality and quantity of service delivery. Information to be gathered includes:

- What was the age of the child at implantation?
- What was the duration of severe to profound deafness?

- What is the duration of implant use?
- What is the current level of auditory skill development?
- How would the auditory learning trajectory be categorized?
- What is the categorization of auditory inclination?

A number of possible scenarios may emerge from this profile review that will drive the nature of the auditory habilitation plan. One subset of students is represented by those who are long term users with established auditory skills. These students demonstrate medial to steep learning trajectories and excellent auditory inclination. This places them in the *commensurate range* of performance and dictates a particular habilitative plan. This plan may include listening in noise, making inferences from connected discourse materials presented auditorily, or fine tuning discrimination by practicing minimal pair contrasts embedded in sentence contexts. Another subset is that of newly implanted recipients who are at the early levels of skill development. Because they have a short duration of implant use, assessment of learning trajectory and auditory inclination must be reserved until after a period of aggressive auditory management. This would suggest a very different habilitative plan. Depending on the age of the child habilitation may be more top-down than bottom-up. Generally speaking, the younger the child, the more the intervention focuses on comprehension and identification of words, sentences and simple connected discourse in a naturalistic setting. The older the child, the more likely it is that skill development will take place in a structured setting and follow a stepwise hierarchy emphasizing pattern recognition with subsequent building to word identification in closed sets. A third subset comprises the long term user with good inclination and a medial to shallow trajectory and performing in the *capable* range. The habilitation plan appropriate for these children outlines continued auditory skill development that systematically moves from increasingly larger closed sets to bridge sets to open sets to support their continued capable functioning. Still another subset of implant recipients is the mid- to long-term user presenting with a shallow trajectory and limited auditory inclination for which a cause may or may not be evident. Their performance in the *challenged range* requires a habilitative plan that emphasizes audition as a support to speechreading. Listening-only skills are limited to basic functional abilities and incorporate more detection than discrimination tasks.

Principles That Drive Effective Auditory Skill Development

It is apparent, then, that there is no single habilitation plan that will be appropriate for all children with cochlear implants. However, there are a number of guiding principles that are universal to the development and implementation of effective habilitation. When working on the development of auditory skills with school-aged children, it is imperative to promote collaboration between and among teachers and speech and hearing professionals, and to recommend the use of the classroom curriculum whenever possible. By adhering to these principles, the ability to formulate authentic auditory learning lessons both within and outside of the classroom will be facilitated. Although published auditory curricula such as the Speech Perception Instructional Curriculum Evaluation, SPICE (Moog, Biedenstein, & Davidson, 1995); Development

Approach to Successful Listening II, DASL II (Stout & Windle, 1992); and Classroom G O A L S (Firzst & Reeder, 1996) are available for the novice professional and serve as a guide through the hierarchy of auditory skills, they tend to utilize content that is decontextualized. Furthermore, each auditory skill often has a designated activity which precludes group work for children at various auditory skill levels. In contrast, when a curricular activity is overlaid with auditory skill development, the resultant lesson can be customized to challenge each child at his or her own auditory level. This may be observed in the classroom teacher's plan for a unit on the post office. Vocabulary such as *stamp*, *letter*, and *mail carrier* may be presented in a closed set for a child with pattern perception ability, whereas children with segmental ability may listen for *envelope*, *magazine*, or *circular* within the same broad activity. Children with auditory comprehension ability may be asked to "Put the magazine in Mrs. Jackson's mailbox and the letter in Ms. Addison's mailbox." Whether the speech-language pathologist reviews, extends or complements the post office unit in the individual therapy setting, it is vital that a two way communication mechanism is in place to support the use of classroom content in building skills. The reader is directed to Chute and Nevins (2006) for a comprehensive discussion of auditory work infused into classroom content.

Regardless of the nature of the auditory activities, in order to truly develop the auditory system, there must be an opportunity for the child to listen without visual cues. Depending on the philosophical orientation of the individual practitioner and/or the range within which the child functions, the speech and hearing professional might initially set up the listening activity using sign plus audition, vision (as in speechreading) plus audition, or go directly to audition alone. Whether the auditory input is the initial stimulus of the activity or the final, carefully developed plans that maximize academic learning time provide the child with more opportunities for listening and spoken language growth.

Spoken Language Competence

The auditory access provided by the cochlear implant has created a listening environment in which many deaf children are able to learn language in a manner similar to their typically developing peers. In the early years of listening and language development, severely and profoundly deaf children with cochlear implants often make substantive growth in their spoken language abilities (Nicholas & Geers, 2006). Children who have excellent auditory inclination may also demonstrate a medial to steep learning trajectory in spoken language development. They may keep pace with their typically developing peers such that, in a group, it may be hard to identify the child with hearing loss. Their top-down learning of language occurs in a naturalistic auditory environment that allows the child to induce syntactic rules through exposure to mature language models. When children learn language in this fashion, their performance can be considered to be representative of the commensurate range. Despite this noteworthy accomplishment, children with hearing loss using cochlear implants will still require continued services from language experts such as a teacher of deaf children and a speech and language pathologist. As a collaborative team, these professionals will offer the language vigilance needed by implant recipients as they enter the educational system faced with the dual task of content

learning and continued language development. General education classroom teachers do not have the explicit linguistic expertise to "drive the language bus"; in fact, language is but a transparent vehicle for teaching the content of science, social studies, and even math. This is not unlike the issues facing students who come to school as second language learners. In fact, Gibbons (2002) has written eloquently on integrating language and subject learning in the mainstream classroom for students for whom English is not a first language. In her practical text, *Scaffolding Language Scaffolding Learning* she outlines explicit ways "to look at language not through it." Gibbons maintains that efforts to include explicit language instruction will benefit more the second language learner; the monolingual English user will likely benefit from a language-focused curriculum (as will children with hearing loss).

Similarly, teachers of literacy and the language arts in general education classrooms assume an intact spoken language system, from which decoding and comprehension tasks and mature grammar usage emerges. The child with an implant demonstrating commensurate spoken language skills at age 5 years is charged with the task of developing the complex syntactic structures that will support later reading with comprehension from the rapid paced discourse of the mainstream classroom. This places the student at a distinct disadvantage when compared to his or her typically developing peers, especially in noisy classrooms. Unless there is a language expert to monitor the development of such sophisticated language devices as indirect discourse, the perfect tenses, relativization of clauses and the use of figurative language, to name just a few of the complexities of complex language, the child with an implant runs the risk of losing commensurate status.

Teachers and speech language pathologists may implement tools such as the Cottage Acquisition Scales of Listening Language and Speech, CASLLS-Complex Level (Wilkes, 1999) and the Teacher Assessment of Spoken Language, TASL, (Moog & Biedenstein, 2003) as a roadmap for systematic complex syntactic development.

In the same way that auditory skill development can be paired with content, so too can language structures be considered simultaneously with the subject matter concepts. The best of all possible worlds is an integrated habilitation plan that encourages listening, language and speech skill development in the context of curricular material that reinforces content. The reader is directed to Appendix 16–A where sample content excerpts present vocabulary and language for the child in a mainstream classroom with an emphasis on expanding sophisticated language structures for the *commensurate* student. A second paragraph (see Appendix 16–A) is written for the child performing within the *capable* range in either an itinerant-supported mainstream classroom or in a small instruction, self-contained program for students with hearing loss. The final paragraph (see Appendix 16–A) is representative of the functional nature of the Food Pyramid content for the student *challenged* to use listening and spoken language skills.

Beginning the Reading Process

Spoken language is the cornerstone from which literacy is launched. Therefore, all efforts to develop competence in the various components of spoken language contribute to the acquisition of subsequent literacy skills. When thinking about literacy instruction, it is tempting to view code-breaking as the start of real reading. However, attention to the concept of precursors to literacy (van Kleeck & Schuele, 1987) or the emergence of literacy (van Kleeck, 2006) has catapulted literacy into the domain of parents and early interventionists. Recognizing the fact that so much of children's success in later reading is built on a rich knowledge base, the early and constant accrual of world knowledge either through direct or indirect experiences is highly encouraged. Children with implants now have the capacity to participate in an experience with real time auditory access to the language of that experience (as opposed to the tedious preteaching or reteaching of the event and its language). This enhances the child's ability to store and retrieve the actors, sequential elements and the labels of any particular experience to be referenced in later reading activities. For example, a young child may watch dad fill a flat bicycle tire with air from a pump. Dad explains what he is doing and the child learns the vocabulary and action of this task. Perhaps dad may even let his son pump some air into the tire himself. The child will see that the tire inflates and the bike can be ridden once again. That same little boy may later find himself reading a story about a boy on a bike ride who gets a flat tire. He will know what is needed because of his own personal experience with the "pump." He will form a hypothesis and read ahead to see if the boy does indeed find someone with a pump. It is not just his decoding skills that allow him to read *p-u-m-p* as pump; his own world knowledge contributes to his effective reading as well.

Despite the fact that it may appear simplistic to say that building a child's world experiences is a worthy activity in preparation for reading, parents and professionals working with young children are strongly encouraged to do so. Sharing books is one way to broaden world experiences without even leaving the house. These indirect experience builders will also serve to support later reading with comprehension and it is NEVER too early to introduce books at home. The reader is referred to Jim Trelease's *Read Aloud Handbook* (2001), a book that can be recommended to parents and professionals alike.

A second activity that contributes to later literacy is the development of a rich spoken language vocabulary. As one of the first tasks in reading instruction is to learn to read known words (Gunning, 1996) the greater the store of spoken vocabulary words a child brings to the reading task the more he or she can focus on the decoding task. While the word "mop" is easy to decode from a phonic standpoint, if a child does not know that word or concept in the spoken vocabulary (perhaps the brand name *Swiffer* has replaced this lexical item for today's youngsters), decoding will simply result in word calling and not real comprehension. This is not unlike adults sounding out a foreign word for which they do not know the meaning. But this example paints too rudimentary a picture. The greater challenge is to keep the momentum of early vocabulary accrual well into the elementary and high school years. The task of vocabulary learning is monumental; it has been suggested that in order to keep pace, children need to learn a minimum of eight new words a day throughout their school-aged years. It is well documented that children with good vocabularies tend to be good readers and vice versa (Stanovich, 1986). Unfortunately, children with limited vocabularies are frustrated by their reading and tend to disengage from the reading task. With this as a vicious cycle of defeat, reading skills fail to improve and reading achievement languishes. Once again, there are a number of excellent books written expressly for the purpose of stimulating vocabulary growth for all students and the reader is referred to Beck, McKeown, and Kucan (2002) and Johnson (2001).

Breaking the Code

Although there are numerous ways to learn to read, utilizing a phonics approach to teaching reading is, once again, the approach of choice in many educational programs today. Regardless of the particular phonics program that is implemented, the basic premise of phonics is matching alphabetic letters to the sounds of our spoken language. Despite the fact that there are a number of irregularities in the sound symbol match-up in English, learning to read via a phonic approach appears to be an efficient way to break the code for many fledgling readers. The good news for cochlear implant recipients is that the auditory access provided by the device should allow a child to hear the low intensity, high frequency consonants that are necessary for comprehensive sound-symbol recognition. The obvious connection between phoneme perception, speech production and phonics, suggests that all previous auditory and speech work to which a child has been exposed, contributes to the task of learning to read. In fact, in her book "Growing a Reader from Birth," written for parents of typically developing children, author Dianne McGuinness (2004) states, "The skills needed to become an expert listener are the same skills needed to become an expert reader (p. 9)." This is indeed heartening for those speech and hearing and educational professionals who have provided intervention to develop spoken language comprehension. Having worked with our youngest children to assist them in acquiring language competence, the professionals involved in early intervention and preschool education are charged with this task and have actually been setting the stage for later reading achievement. Citing McGuinness (2004) yet again, measures of language comprehension predict reading comprehension with 50% accuracy; measures of decoding predict later reading comprehension with 10% accuracy. It would appear, then, that decoding is a necessary, but insufficient skill to account for all the effort that is required for reading with comprehension. Thus, code breaking ability, in tandem with a plentiful store of vocabulary, abundant world knowledge, and a rich language base prepares the child for reading development in subsequent literacy activities in school.

Later Reading and Academic Achievement

It is at approximately the third or fourth grade level that a child's reading passes from the phase considered "learning to read" to that considered "reading to learn." According to Fountas and Pinnell (2001) this level is representative of a mature reading ability which indicates that a child can independently interact with text and build meaning from it. Instruction continues in the language arts to support reading more mature themes. Developing control and understanding of sophisticated literacy devices such as humor, irony, and satire, foreshadowing and flashback, and the figurative and metaphorical use of language also are important aspects of advanced reading instruction. If a student's ability to read at increasingly sophisticated levels fails to keep pace with his or her peers, there may be a need to seek support to provide more individualized reading and discussion in advance of classroom activities. Another consideration is to identify alternative reading selections which offer a more simplistic version of the text or to substitute easier content that mirrors the theme of the originally assigned book. At the same time as reading literature demands grow, the requirement to read independently in the content areas of science and social studies increases almost exponentially. The teacher/speech-language pathologist may also wish to monitor a student's comprehension of complex concepts presented in content texts. A student may require concepts to be reframed into more accessible language depending on the skills and abilities with which they present. Despite the well-meaning intentions of the No Child Left Behind legislation (2001), students who are required to read materials at the frustration level of reading will be disheartened by the futility of their attempt and may disengage from any effort to continue their literacy learning. The good news is that more deaf children have been able to break through the fourth grade reading ceiling that limited them for so many years (Spencer, Barker, & Tomblin, 2003). Despite this achievement, the majority of children educated in mainstream environments still face many educational challenges (Archbold & O'Donoghue, 2007; Chute & Nevins, 2003).

Educational Challenges for Children with Cochlear Implants

Chute and Nevins (2003) identified five areas of educational challenges that children with cochlear implants must manage. These include: acoustic, academic, attention, associative, and adjustment. An understanding of each of these, how they impact performance and what can be done to mitigate them is necessary for children to receive maximal benefit from the mainstream environment.

When assessing the *acoustic* challenges of children with implants, one must consider the classroom environment in which the child is seated and the individual performance of the child with the device. New standards set forth by American National Standards Institute, (ANSI, 2002) require that classrooms have ambient noise levels no greater than 35 dBA and a reverberation time of no greater than 0.6 msec in order to be deemed acoustically reliable. In order to meet these standards, factors including the size of the room, the number of pupils in the room and the proximity to external environmental noise must be considered.

In addition to the physical issues of the classroom, the perceptual abilities of the child with the cochlear implant must also be taken into consideration. Although the child is capable of hearing sound at normal conversational speech levels, individual perceptual differences contribute to performance that can be maximal, minimal, and all points in between. In addition, children with cochlear implants in one ear only are provided with unilateral input. This places them at distinct disadvantages in noisy environments and when attempting to localize speech that is related to classroom discussion. Clearly, as academic content becomes more rigorous, the ability to follow teacher instruction and classroom dialog is compromised and often can result in misunderstanding.

The present day cochlear implant processing schemes are all capable of providing access to speech at normal conversational levels. In addition, most implant users are supplied with important high-frequency information that eluded them through traditional amplification. This is one of the key features that set the electrical stimulation of the implant apart from the acoustic stimulation of hearing aids which, in turn, makes overall performance superior. However, the implant does not restore normal hearing nor is it able to override any central processing problems that the implant recipient might demonstrate. Therefore, it is important to recognize that the implanted child in a classroom will still be presented with a myriad of listening challenges. To assist in controlling the acoustic challenges for children with cochlear implants, the major emphasis should be on improving the environment so that signal delivery and reception is maximized. This can be accomplished in a number of ways. First, the classroom itself should be treated to ensure it meets ANSI standards. Treatment can include carpeting, acoustic tiles, and the addition of absorptive materials to decrease reverberation. Also, auditory enhancement through sound field amplification systems and personal FM systems should be considered. For more information regarding model classrooms for maximizing listening, the reader is directed to the website www.arthurboothroyd.com . Finally, as evidence regarding performance improvement in bilaterally implanted children is reported (Galvin, Mok, & Dowell, 2007; Litovsky, Johnstone, & Godar, 2006a; Tyler et al., 2006) parents should consider bilateral implantation as best practice for all deaf children. In cases of residual hearing in the un-implanted ear, the use of a hearing aid should be strongly recommended. (Ching, van Wanrooy, Hill, & Incerti, 2006; Litovsky et al., 2006a; Litovsky, et al., 2006b).

In the same way that many hearing children demonstrate difficulties in learning classroom content, the implanted child may also exhibit *academic* challenges. These can be divided into two major groups: English language development and literacy development.

Suboptimal development in either of these areas will negatively affect learning. Poor language development can be a result of a multiplicity of factors that range from the presence of a spoken language other than English in the home, to the mode of communication that the child utilizes. The ability to use language to learn language is key to children throughout the educational process. Any breakdown in language learning may result in widespread issues in the classroom. In addition, today's focus on literacy depends on an intact language system to support reading with comprehension. Fortunately, studies have demonstrated that children who received cochlear implants at young ages, are enrolled in auditory oral programs and have no other disabilities can perform on par with their hearing age-mates (Connor, Craig, Raudenbush, Heavner, & Zwolan, 2006; Nicholas & Geers, 2006; Tobey, Rekart, Buckley, & Geers, 2004). Recall that it was suggested earlier that a child with an implant can process language simultaneously with the acoustic event thereby allowing language to develop in a less contrived manner. Furthermore, the opportunity for incidental learning contributes to a more efficient language acquisition experience. Language accrual in this way permits the child to have immediate access to vocabulary, syntax and complex linguistic forms in "real time" similar to hearing children, often resulting in commensurate performance outcomes. But, the mere presence of the cochlear implant does not ensure that this development will take place. As children are implanted at older ages, language learning is not as efficient as for the younger child.

Furthermore, children who wear their devices on a limited basis will not have a consistent auditory model from which to learn new skills. As noted previously, in those households where English is not the primary language, the child's ability to "lock in" to the vocabulary and grammar specific to English will be compromised. In other households in which English is spoken, parents may be unwilling or unable to provide a model that fosters continuous language growth. Finally, one must remember that like hearing children, those with cochlear implants can be diagnosed with specific language impairment (SLI) thereby creating a situation in which the child requires intervention to assist in learning. These children have been identified above as the capable performers. It is important to remember that despite the best candidacy profile prior to implantation, there is no guarantee that a deaf child who receives a cochlear implant will reach linguistic parity with his or her hearing peers. Nonetheless, early implantation and appropriate intervention can place the child on a path that has a positive trajectory toward learning and competing in the mainstream.

Regardless of whether a child has an implant or is hearing, one of the most important aspects of learning is related to *attention*. Studies of children with hearing loss demonstrate decreased amount of short term memory thereby affecting their ability to hold onto immediate information that is required to support comprehension (Wingfield & Tun, 2007). Additionally, whether a child is using speechreading or an interpreter (or cued speech transliterator), attention must be maintained and redirected on a regular basis. This creates a learning environment that is extremely tiring and can vary widely from child to child as well as situation to situation. The amount of effort required to maintain a high level of communicative interaction can affect attention over time with many children. Finally, competing noise, both acoustic and visual, can disrupt concentration, not only for the implanted child but for children with deficits in the area of attention.

With the superior high-frequency sound delivery of the cochlear implant, access to speech cues unavailable through traditional amplification augments the ability to listen as well as speechread thereby making communication flow easier—but not perfect. Children with implants may have difficulty understanding rapid classroom content especially as higher levels of subject-related vocabulary are provided. As noted earlier, competing background noise must be addressed by providing FM transmission directly to the implant to make attention to the primary signal (teacher's voice) easier. Attention disorders unrelated to hearing loss may also contribute negatively to overall classroom success. These are superfluous to the implant itself and may not be easily amenable to intervention.

One of the educational challenges not directly related to learning addresses the *associative* factors that children with hearing loss often confront. Self esteem, socialization with peers, social maturity, and cultural identity create a context for every child in the classroom that can make school attendance something to be embraced or feared. These extraneous features of schooling can change an interactive learner into a quiet non participant or vice versa. The ability to communicate in an appropriate manner is often the basis for an internalization of a positive self-image. The more compromised the communicative ability, the greater the risk for decreased confidence.

As many children with implants can often enjoy commensurate spoken language skills, communication with the larger general school population is eased. Nonetheless, daily communication activities outside the classroom may still present a variety of challenges that the implant recipient must accept. As adolescence is a period in which most children often question, rebel and define, the issue of personal identity (deaf or hearing) makes the school experience difficult in its own right. The cochlear implant may help to ease some uncertainties but will not eradicate what is a normal growth phenomenon for school-aged children. Interestingly, as more children with implants enter the mainstream environment the likelihood of these children meeting each other increases thereby permitting them to address their own cultural identities as a group.

Finally, children with hearing loss must face what can be termed *adjustment* issues throughout their school careers and lives. Like other children with learning challenges, children with implants must understand their limitations and how these will affect them daily. Embracing and accepting their differences will permit implant recipients to attain their personal best in and outside school. The child with a cochlear implant passes through a multiplicity of adjustment periods. From the early days of initial switch-on of the device to changes in technology that require relearning of sound, implanted children must adjust in order to maintain themselves. They must learn to manage their deafness and become capable of advocating for themselves in the classroom as well as the school yard. Those that adjust well will have an advantage over those who do not. However, the mere fact that the cochlear implant provides them with a means to adjust as they move through life only underscores the importance of this technology.

Final Thoughts

Despite the educational challenges that remain, more children with cochlear implants are successfully graduating from district high schools with their hearing peers. Indeed many of these students will continue their education in colleges and universities of their choice. No longer limited to choosing between Gallaudet University and the National Technical Institute for the Deaf, these students have broader access due to their personal accomplishments as well as changes in higher education. Even though choices are plentiful, the idea of a good match between a child and the college eventually chosen works for all those planning to continue their education. The size of the institution, the public or private nature of the school, the geographic location, the availability of majors that are of interest to the student, and the extent of extracurricular activities are features that will take precedence over the hearing loss. The mandate for providing accommodations will ensure that the student will have access to academic instruction at whatever college is the right match. As young adults, the advocacy skills that have been nurtured over time will assist them in negotiating college life. The work begun by parents must now be transferred to the student so that they can become independent and productive citizens in society. The years of focused listening and spoken language development begun in preschool, come to fruition in the college years and can be fully appreciated as performance outcomes validate the parents' and professionals' investment in students with implants.

References

American National Standards Institute (ANSI). (2002). *ANSI S12.60-2002. Acoustical performance criteria, design requirements, and guidelines for schools*. Melville, NY: Author.

Archbold, S., & O'Donoghue, G. (2007). Ensuring the long-term use of cochlear implants in children: The importance of engaging local resources and expertise. *Ear and Hearing, 28* (Suppl. 2), 3S–6S.

Beck, I., McKeown, M., & Kucan, L. (2002). *Bringing words to life. Robust vocabulary instruction*. New York: Guilford Press.

Berliner, D. (1978). *Changing academic learning time: Clinical interventions in four classrooms*. San Francisco: Far West Laboratory for Educational Research and Development.

Ching, T. Y., van Wanrooy, E., Hill, M., & Incerti, P. (2006). Performance in children with hearing aids or cochlear implants: Bilateral stimulation and binaural hearing. *International Journal of Audiology, 45* (Suppl. 1), S108–S112.

Chute, P. M., & Nevins, M. E. (2003). Educational challenges for children with cochlear implants. *Topics in Language Disorders, 23*, 57–67.

Chute, P. M., & Nevins, M. E. (2006). *School professionals working with children with cochlear implants*. San Diego, CA: Plural.

Connor, C. M., Craig H. K., Raudenbush, S. W., Heavner, K., & Zwolan, T. A. (2006). The age at which young deaf children receive cochlear implants and their vocabulary and speech-production growth: Is there an added value for early implantation? *Ear and Hearing, 27*, 628–644.

Firszt, J., & Reeder, R. (1996). *Classroom G O A L S: Guide to Optimizing Auditory Learning Skills*. Washington, DC: A. G. Bell Association.

Fountas, S., & Pinnell, G. S. (2001). *Guiding readers and writers*. Portsmouth, NH: Heinemann Press.

Galvin, K. L., Mok, M., & Dowell, R. C. (2007). Perceptual benefit and functional outcomes for children using sequential bilateral cochlear implants. *Ear and Hearing, 4*, 470–482.

Geers, A. E. (1997). Comparing implants with hearing aids in profoundly deaf children. *Otolaryngology-Head and Neck Surgery, 117*, 150–154.

Geers, A. E., & Moog, J. S. (1987). Predicting spoken language acquisition of profoundly hearing-impaired children. *Journal of Speech and Hearing Disorders, 52*, 84–94.

Gibbons, P. (2002). *Scaffolding language, scaffolding learning: Teaching second language learners in the mainstream classroom.* Portsmouth, NH: Heinemann Press.

Gunning, T. (1996). *Creating reading instruction for all children.* Boston: Allyn and Bacon.

Harrigan, S., & Nikolopoulos, T. P. (2002). Parent interaction course in order to enhance communication skills between parents and children following pediatric cochlear implantation. *International Journal of Otorhinolaryngology, 66,* 161–166.

Johnson, D. (2001). *Vocabulary in the elementary and middle school.* Boston: Allyn and Bacon.

Litovsky, R. Y., Johnstone, P. M., & Godar, S. P. (2006a). Benefits of bilateral cochlear implants and/or hearing aids in children. *International Journal of Audiology, 45* (Suppl. 1), S78–S91.

Litovsky, R. Y., Johnstone, P. M., Godar, S., Agrawal, S., Parkinson, A., Peters, R., et al. (2006b). Bilateral cochlear implants in children: Localization acuity measured with minimum audible angle. *Ear and Hearing, 27,* 43–59.

McGuinness, D. (2004). *Growing a reader from birth: Your child's path from language to literacy.* New York: Norton and Company.

Moog, J. S., & Biedenstein, J. (2003). *Teacher assessment of spoken language.* St. Louis, MO: Moog Center for Deaf Education.

Moog, J. S., Biedenstein, J., & Davidson, L. (1995). *Speech perception instructional curriculum and evaluation.* St. Louis, MO: Central Institute for the Deaf.

Nicholas, J. G., & Geers, A. E. (2006). Effects of early auditory experience on the spoken language of deaf children at 3 years of age. *Ear and Hearing, 27,* 286–298.

Nicholas, J. G., & Geers, A. E. (2007). Will they catch up? The role of age at cochlear implantation in the spoken language development of children with severe to profound hearing loss. *Journal of Speech, Language, and Hearing Research, 50,* 1048–1062.

No Child Left Behind Act of 2001 (NCLB). (2001). Public Law 107–110.

Robbins, A. M., Kirk, K. I., Osberger, M. J., & Ertmer D. (1995). Speech intelligibility of implanted children. *Annals of Otology, Rhinology, and Laryngology, 104*(Suppl. 166), 399–401.

Simser, J. (1999). Parents, the essential partners in the habilitation of children with hearing impairment. *Australian Journal of the Education of the Deaf, 5,* 1–13.

Spencer, L., Barker, B., & Tomblin, J. (2003). Exploring the language and literacy outcomes of pediatric cochlear implant users. *Ear and Hearing, 24,* 236–248.

Stacey, P. C., Fortnum, H. M., Barton, G. R., & Summerfield, A. Q. (2006). Hearing-impaired children in the United Kingdom: Auditory performance, communication skills, educational achievements, quality of life, and cochlear implantation. *Ear and Hearing, 27,* 161–186.

Stanovich, K. E. (1986). Matthew effects in reading: Some consequences of individual differences in the acquisition of literacy. *Reading Research Quarterly, 21,* 360–406.

Stout, G., & Windle, J. (1992). *The Developmental Approach to Successful Listening II (DASL).* Englewood, CO: Resource Point.

Tobey, E. A., Rekart, D., Buckley, K., & Geers, A. E. (2004). Mode of communication and classroom placement impact on speech intelligibility. *Archives of Otolaryngology-Head and Neck Surgery, 130,* 639–643.

Trelease, J. (2001). *The read aloud handbook.* New York: Penguin Books.

Tyler, R. S., Parkinson, A. J., Wilson, B. S., Witt, S., Preece, J. P., & Noble, W. (2002). Patients utilizing a hearing aid and a cochlear implant: Speech perception and localization. *Ear and Hearing, 23,* 98–105.

van Kleeck, A. (2006). *Sharing books and stories to promote language and literacy.* San Diego, CA: Plural.

van Kleeck, A., & Schuele, M. (1987). Precursors to literacy: Normal development. *Topics in Language Disorders, 7,* 13–31.

Vockell, E. *Educational psychology: A practical approach.* Retrieved March 28, 2008 from http://education.calumet.purdue.edu/vockell/EdPsyBook/

Vygotsky, L. S. (1962). *Thought and language.* Cambridge, MA: MIT Press.

Wie, O. B., Falkenberg, E. S., Tvete, O., & Tomblin, B. (2007). Children with a cochlear implant: Characteristics and determinants of speech recognition, speech-recognition growth rate, and speech production. *International Journal of Audiology, 46*, 232–243.

Wilkes, E. (1999). *Cottage Acquisition Scales of Listening, Language and Speech.* San Antonio, TX: Sunshine Cottage for Deaf Children.

Wingfield, A., & Tun, P.A. (2007). Cognitive supports and cognitive constraints on comprehension of spoken language. *Journal of the American Academy of Audiology, 18*, 548–558.

APPENDIX 16–A
The Food Pyramid

I. Content and Language for Children at the Commensurate Level

The Food Pyramid represents a model for making choices for healthy eating.

There are six major food groups represented in four levels within the food pyramid.

Food groups include grains, vegetables, fruits, dairy, proteins, and fats and sweets.

Eight servings of water form the base of the food pyramid.

Nutritionists recommend the number of daily servings for each food group by considering total dietary consumption for a healthy lifestyle.

Six servings of fortified-cereal, bread, rice, and pasta are recommended each day.

Three servings a day are recommended for both the milk group and the vegetable group.

We should eat two servings of both the fruit group and the meat, fish, bean, and nut group.

The tip of the pyramid contains sweets and fats and we are encouraged to use them sparingly.

Planning meals that follow pyramid guidelines will keep us healthy.

II. Adapted Content and Language for Children in the Capable Range

The Food Pyramid helps us choose the right foods to eat.

There are six food groups in the food pyramid.

They are: grains, vegetables, fruits, dairy, proteins, and fats and sweets.

You should drink eight glasses of water a day.

Nutritionists tell us how many servings we can have in each food group.

You can eat six servings of foods in the grains group.

You can eat three servings from the milk group and three servings from the vegetable group.

You can eat two servings from the fruit group and two servings from the protein group.

You can only eat a small amount from the fats and sweets group.

If you think about the food pyramid each day you will make good choices.

III. Adapted Content and Language for Children in the Challenged Range

Some foods are good to eat.

You should eat vegetables like carrots and peas.

You should eat fruit like apples and strawberries.

You can eat fish and eggs and meat and peanut butter.

You can eat bread and cereal and rice.

Drink lots of water everyday.

Don't eat a lot of candy, cookies, or chips.

Eat right and stay healthy.

CHAPTER 17

Empowering Families of Children with Cochlear Implants: Implications for Early Intervention and Language Development

JEAN L. DESJARDIN

Introduction

Lynnette and John, parents of an 18-month-old deaf child with a cochlear implant, turned, with tears in their eyes, to the professional team gathered around a table to discuss the results of their daughter, Julia's, recent 6-month post-cochlear implant assessment. "We see that Julia now responds to our voices, but what do we do now?" Julia's father asked. "What can our family do to help Julia talk?" and "How can we help guide Julia's early intervention and future language development?" Julia's mother added.

Families play a critical role in the lives of young deaf children who receive a cochlear implant. Although some parents experience considerable anxiety and concerns for their child's future prior to and during the surgery (Allegretti, 2002; Burger et al., 2005; Zaidman-Zait, 2007), many parents hold relatively high expectations for their children's future outcomes (Beadle, Shores, & Wood, 2000; Chmiel, Sutton, & Jenkins, 2000; Nikolopoulos, Lloyd, Archbold, & O'Donoghue, 2001; Weisel, Most, & Michael, 2007) and positive views regarding their child's communication skills, social relationships, and overall functioning post-cochlear implantation (Meadow-Orlans, Mertens, & Sass-Lehrer,

2003; Nicholas & Geers, 2006). During this time, some parents can be highly resourceful (Spencer, 2001; Zaidman-Zait & Most, 2005) and capable to utilize specific techniques that enrich their children's language (DesJardin & Eisenberg, 2007) and literacy skills (Aram, Most, & Mayafit, 2006; DesJardin, Ambrose, & Eisenberg, 2009). Both indirect and direct parental involvement is essential for successful cochlear implantation in a young child.

In order for families to be involved in their child's early intervention, however, parents and key caregivers need to acquire a considerable amount of knowledge and skills related to the child's educational program. Such information pertains to the cochlear implant itself, whereas other skills relate to their child's auditory and communication development (Christiansen & Leigh, 2002; Watson, Hardie, Archbold, & Wheeler, 2007). Resources related to the child's social and emotional needs are also important to families (Most & Zaidman-Zait, 2003; Zaidman-Zait & Jamieson, 2004). Obtaining support services for the family can, at times, be overwhelming (Incesulu, Vural, & Erkam, 2003; Sach & Whynes, 2005), especially for parents who experience high levels of stress (Beadle et al., 2000). A highly stressful situation for families can create more communication challenges with the child and a less satisfactory relationship between parents and professionals (Zaidman-Zait & Most, 2005).

What does a parent-professional relationship entail for families of young children with cochlear implants? How can professionals work with families to create a less stressful and more positive home environment as parents guide their child's development post cochlear implantation? How can professionals tap into families' strengths to optimize their children's educational and social experiences? Understanding the the-

oretical and clinical implications of early intervention and the critical role that parents play in their children's development is at the heart of best practices in guiding families of pediatric implant users.

This chapter first presents a description of the philosophy and empirical research that is embedded in current early intervention practices for families and their young children. Intervention constructs (e.g., parental self-efficacy and parental involvement) that positively influence children's language outcomes are thoroughly discussed with recent findings from studies of mothers and young children with cochlear implants. The importance of father involvement (and other key caregivers) and the issues of working with families who are culturally and linguistically diverse also are highlighted. This chapter concludes with a proposed "coaching model" for professionals to employ with parents during the early years post-cochlear implantation with practical educational practices for professionals and strategies for families to employ while guiding their child's auditory and communication development.

Theoretical Perspective

Early intervention programs for families with young children are founded on the premise that the development of the child can only be fully understood within a family context (Bronfenbrenner, 1974; Bruder, 2000; Shonkoff & Meisels, 2000). Both child and family exist within a broader framework of the child's school and community environment (Bronfenbrenner, 1979). The philosophy of promoting child development in the context of the family is founded in an ecological model of learning and development with the child at the center of the family system. This philosophical orientation recognizes the family as a dynamic social system in which the family affects the child and the child affects the family. The family system also is influenced by other broader systems such as the community, culture, and socioeconomic status.

The experience of having a child who has specific learning needs and challenges presents a significant impact on the family (Bailey & Powell, 2005). According to Bronfenbrenner (1974), active family involvement in the child's intervention program is critical and without such family participation, intervention is unlikely to be successful. Family factors that influence intervention and child development include the parents' ability to follow intervention recommendations, parent-child interaction patterns, and quality of life issues involving formal and informal sources of family support (Bruder, 2000). For theoretical and practical reasons, it is highly encouraged that early intervention programs establish family-centered practices that provide the necessary resources and support for parents. These professional services are invaluable to parents as they learn ways in which to facilitate their child's development in natural environments and within daily family activities (Trivette & Dunst, 2000).

Both the *Individuals with Disabilities Education Improvement Act* (IDEIA, 2004) legislation enacted by the federal government (Part C PL 99-457; 1986) and the *Division of Early Childhood (DEC) Recommended Practices in Early Intervention/ Early Childhood Special Education* (Sandall, Hemmeter, Smith, & McLean, 2005) support the notion that parents and other key family members play an active role in children's learning and development. Part C (birth–3 years old) and Part B (3–5 years old) of IDEIA (2004) focus on different aspects of intervention (educational terms and definitions are listed in Table 17–1). Under Part C, the family and child with a known disability or at risk for future learning deficits receive early intervention. Hence, an Individual Family Service Plan (IFSP) is developed and executed for the family and their child. Furthermore, service delivery of the IFSP must be carried out in natural environments (Walsh, Rous, & Lutzer, 2000). The IDEIA regulations define natural environments as "settings that are natural or normal for the child's age-peers who have no disabilities" (34 CFR Part 303.18). A more comprehensive definition of natural environments may include the daily routines, activities, and locations that are relevant to each family (Dunst, Bruder, Trivette, Raab, & McLean, 2001; McWilliam, 2000).

Under Part B of IDEIA, parental involvement in intervention for preschool and school-aged children is crucial and highly encouraged for all children, although parents do not necessarily receive direct services under the provision (Guralnick, 2005). This is particularly true for families of children who are deaf (DesJardin, Eisenberg, & Hodapp, 2006; Moeller, 2000). For children who receive services under Part B, parents and professionals together develop the Individual Education Plan (IEP) for the child. For preschool-age children (3–5 years old), family involvement in their child's early education plan promotes positive parent-child relationships and long-term educational and social outcomes for the child (Shonkoff & Meisels, 2000).

The central goal of family-centered early intervention services is for professionals to build a collaborative partnership with families. According to Dunst and his colleagues (2001), the best intervention strategies are those that not only encourage a family's involvement, but also strengthen

TABLE 17–1. Early Intervention Educational Terms and Definition for Each

Early Intervention Educational Term	Definition
Individuals with Disabilities Education Improvement Act (IDEIA, 2004)	A United States federal law that governs how states and public agencies provide early intervention, special education, and related services to children with disabilities. It addresses the educational needs of children with disabilities from birth–21 years.
Individualized Family Service Plan (IFSP)	A process and written document developed by a multidisciplinary and interagency team consisting of parents and other key family members, a service coordinator, and other professionals involved in the provision of early intervention services for families and their young children with disabilities from birth–3 years.
Individual Education Plan (IEP)	A process and written document developed by parents and a multidisciplinary team delineating the special education and related services (e.g., speech-language therapy) to be provided to the child from age 3–21 years.
Division of Early Childhood (DEC)	The single largest professional organization in the world devoted to early intervention and early childhood special education. Promotes scientifically based research that advances knowledge and the translation of knowledge for use in applied settings.
Natural Environments	IDEIA regulations define natural environments as "settings that are natural or normal for the child's age peers who have no disabilities" (34 CFR Part 303.18). A more comprehensive definition may include the daily locations, routines, and activities that are relevant to each individual family (Dunst, Bruder, Trivette, Raab, & McLean, 2001; McWilliam, 2000).

parents' (and other key caregivers') competence and confidence in the skills necessary to be involved in their child's intervention. Professionals' provision of information, guidance, and support will in turn, empower parents with the specific skills and self-assurance needed to be actively involved in their child's future education (McWilliam & Scott, 2001; Turnbull, Turbiville, & Turnbull, 2000; Turnbull & Turnbull, 2001). Findings from these studies have suggested that

family-centered practices necessitate consideration of the diversity of families in determining the most appropriate services for families. Culturally responsive practices take into consideration the family's customs and values, as well as the family's home language, in order to optimize the goals of the family and the child (Hanson & Lynch, 2004; Sylva, 2005; Watson, 2007).

For families with young children with cochlear implants, an effective early intervention program is one that promotes parent-professional relationships built on trust and open communication. Professional guidance that promotes emotional (e.g., active listening), informational (e.g., stages of auditory development), and concrete (e.g., how to employ specific language techniques) strategies is extremely important to families of pediatric cochlear implant users as they navigate resources for their child (Zaidman-Zait, 2007). Armed with specific knowledge and competencies, parents have the potential to facilitate their children's future educational and social skills post-cochlear implantation (Aram et al., 2006; DesJardin et al., 2008; DesJardin & Eisenberg, 2007; Hintermair, 2006). Positive parent-professional relationships are essential as families gain a sense of empowerment in order to support their child's development.

Empowering Families of Children with Cochlear Implants

How do professionals empower parents to make a difference in the lives of their young children with cochlear implants? Although the answer is complex, professionals have a perfect opportunity to collaborate with families under the guidelines set forth by family-centered early intervention (IDEIA, 2004). Through professional-parent collaboration, also referred to as the empowerment model (Dunst, 2000; Turnbull & Turnbull, 2001), parents are equal partners with early intervention professionals. Close mutual relationships between families and professionals promote positive parenting practices in the habilitation process for their children with cochlear implants (Dromi & Ingber, 1999; Zaidman-Zait, 2007).

In the professional-parent partnership, individuals work together to learn from each other about better ways to support the child's development. Mothers, fathers, and key caregivers (e.g., grandparents, aunt, and other caretakers) know the child better than anyone else. Parents and family members can share much knowledge about the child (e.g., medical history, learning style, personality, daily schedule, and listening and language skills demonstrated at home). Professionals, on the other hand, are able to provide parents with the knowledge and skills necessary to facilitate the child's auditory and communication development. Such information may include ways to maintain consistency in cochlear implant use, typical auditory and language milestones, and specific facilitative language techniques and educational strategies to enhance their child's communication and social development. Collaboration efforts among early intervention specialists such as the child's audiologist, speech-language pathologist, teacher of the deaf, and parents can assist with the development of achievable family and child goals.

The IFSP and IEP are the cornerstone documents that guide services for young children with cochlear implants. The overall goals and expected outcomes (e.g., objectives) stated on the IFSP reflect the parents' values and concerns for the child. The strategies developed to address the outcomes on the IFSP direct the early intervention professionals, family members, and other caregivers about how to achieve the stated objectives. As stated earlier, the IFSP must also include a description to which early intervention services will be provided in a natural environment. As Spagnola and Fiese (2007) note, "naturally occurring family routines and activities provide both a predictable structure that guides behavior and an emotional climate that supports early development" (p. 284). Specifying the ways in which family members can use selected strategies during family routines and activities increase the number of opportunities for the caregivers to support the child's developmental objectives (Dunst, Bruder, Trivette, & Hamby, 2006; Jung, 2007; McWilliam, 2000). For instance, family routines such as mealtime (Beals, 2001; Blum-Kulka & Snow, 2002) and storybook reading (Hart & Risley, 1995) provide rich arenas for auditory and language opportunities that can enhance children's communication and literacy development.

Parents of young children with cochlear implants require both information and skills. Knowledge of the child's cochlear implant (Incesulu et al., 2003; Most & Zaidman-Zait, 2003), specific ways to create optimal learning opportunities to practice and refine parent-child communicative exchanges at home (DesJardin, 2006), and emotional support (Spahn, Richter, Zschocke, Lohle, & Wirsching, 2001) are all necessary for families. Informational and emotional needs of family members may vary depending on the family's situation and support system. Parental social support (e.g., professional guidance) can be a beneficial resource to families of children with cochlear implants and has been shown to be a positive factor to parental well-being and adjustment (Zaidman-Zait, 2007).

Zaidman-Zait (2007) investigated several family factors (e.g., family, child, external resources) that are attributed to a parent's sense of coping while parenting their young child with a cochlear implant. Support offered by professionals (e.g., information, advice, practical guidance) was one of the most significant influences on the parents' coping process. The manner in which professionals share information with parents also is very important to families. Empathy, active listening, information sharing, and honesty are some of the professional traits that parents indicate are important to build-

ing a trustful parent-professional relationship in early intervention for families of children who are deaf (Sjoblad, Harrison, Roush, & McWilliam, 2001) and specifically, children with cochlear implants (Zaidman-Zait, 2007). The role of professionals is to thus, positively support parents (and other key family members) as they seek to gain access to the information they desire and require to become competent and confident—self-efficacious—in the skills necessary to guide their children's learning and development.

Parental Self-Efficacy

The keys to empowerment are knowledge and motivation (Turnbull et al., 2000). In order to become motivated, families need to possess high expectations, persistence, and self-efficacy. Perceived parental self-efficacy is defined as one's sense of knowledge and abilities to perform or accomplish daily parenting tasks and roles. According to self-efficacy theory (Bandura, 1977; 1997), parental self-efficacy beliefs should incorporate (1) the level of specific knowledge pertaining to the behaviors involved in child-rearing and (2) the degree of confidence in one's own ability to carry out the specific parental role. Conrad, Gross, Fogg, and Ruchala (1992) noted that mothers' increased knowledge alone did not result in better interactions with their young hearing children. Increased knowledge and confidence together, however, resulted in more effective high-quality interactions between mothers and their hearing toddlers.

A sense of self-efficacy can influence the way parents perform their daily tasks. When individuals perceive themselves as competent parents, they set higher goals for themselves and become committed to achieve those goals (Bandura, 1997). Higher parental self-efficacy is related to better parental well-being (Kuhn & Carter, 2006; Ozer, 1995; Sahu & Rath, 2003) and positive feelings of competence in the parenting role (Coleman & Karraker, 2003; Jackson & Huang, 2000; Teti, O'Connell, & Reiner, 1996). Individuals that perceive themselves as capable parents also demonstrate lower maternal stress (Gondoli & Silverberg, 1997; Raikes & Thompson, 2005) and maternal depression (Teti & Gelfand, 1991; Teti et al., 1996). Put simply, parents who report higher levels of self-efficacy are also able to better support their family.

Positive self-efficacy beliefs also are linked to certain parental practices that support their children's skills. A parent who is self-efficacious is able to take the knowledge learned and apply it to a given parental task, whereas a self-inefficacious parent may have the knowledge, yet be unable to persist due to self-doubt or family situations (e.g., parental depression, lack of financial resources). Brody, Flor, and Gibson (1999) reported that single low-income mothers who perceived that they had adequate family financial resources were more likely to believe that their parenting would be effective with their early elementary school-aged hearing children. Similarly, in a sample of mothers and their hearing infants, Teti and Gelfand (1991) found that maternal self-efficacy mediated the negative relationship between mothers' depressive symptoms and mothers' behaviors reflecting responsiveness (e.g., warmth and sensitivity) to their infants. These findings suggest a positive connection between mothers' own belief system and maternal behavior with their children.

Parental Self-Efficacy and Families of Children with Cochlear Implants

Parental perceived knowledge and confidence of specific skills must be measured for a particular population (Bandura, 1989). There are a few parenting scales that tap into parents' self-efficacy beliefs (e.g., empowerment) for populations of hearing children with disabilities (Akey, Marquis, & Ross, 2000; Trivette & Dunst, 2003). One such scale is the *Psychological Empowerment Scale* (PES) (Akey, 1996). This 32-item self-report scale was designed to assess four dimensions of psychological empowerment: attitudes of control and competence (e.g., "I believe I have the power to make positive changes for my family."), knowledge and skills (e.g., "I know where to get information about the resources that my family needs."), and participatory behaviors—participation in informal activities (e.g., "I spend time with other parents talking about my family.") and formal activities (e.g., "I am actively involved in a parent organization."). This scale was specifically designed for families of children with disabilities, and thus, can be a helpful tool to gain an overall picture of parental efficacy and informal and formal family involvement. However, the PES does not provide professionals with specific information about the knowledge and competencies generally utilized by families of children with hearing loss, and more specifically by families of pediatric cochlear implant users.

One tool specifically designed for parents of young children who are deaf or hard of hearing and can be used with families of young children with cochlear implants is the *Scale of Parental Involvement and Self-Efficacy or SPISE* (DesJardin, 2003). This instrument measures parents' perceptions of their knowledge and specific skills necessary to guide their child's auditory and communication development and the extent to which parents perceive themselves as involved in these activities (e.g., checking the child's cochlear implant and developing their child's language skills). Using this measure, DesJardin and Eisenberg

(2007) investigated mothers' self-efficacy (in terms of auditory and language development) in a sample of 32 mothers and their young children with cochlear implants (mean age = 4.8 years). Findings from this study suggest a strong positive relationship between maternal self-efficacy in terms of developing their children's language skills and mothers' linguistic input during free play and storybook interactions with their young preschoolers.

More specifically, mothers who perceived themselves higher in having the knowledge and skills to guide their children's language skills were more apt to use complex utterances (mean length of utterance or MLU; $r = 0.47$; $p < 0.01$) during interactions with their children. Similar to research in young hearing children (Chapman, 2000; Girolametto, Weitzman, Wiigs, & Pearce, 1999; Hart & Risley, 1999; Weizman & Snow, 2001), mothers' MLU emerged as a strong predictor variable for children's receptive and expressive language skills after accounting for child age. Furthermore, mothers' perceived efficacy was related to mothers' use of one higher level facilitative language technique, parallel talk ($r = 0.45$; $p < 0.05$). This particular language technique is defined as "a caregiver or parent providing a description relating to what the child is directly looking at or a child action." This language technique has been associated with greater language gains in young hearing children with language delays (Girolametto & Weitzman, 2006; Kaiser & Hancock, 2003). Consistent with Bandura's model (1997), mothers' self-efficacy beliefs in developing their children's language can positively influence language skills in children post-cochlear implantation.

With informed knowledge and confidence, some parents are also able to make their own decisions independently from professionals. Using a questionnaire format,

Watson and colleagues (2007) tapped parents' views regarding their child's mode of communication before and after cochlear implantation. Findings from this study showed that parents remained "neutral" to the proposition that they were following professional advice. For many of the families, parents changed from signed (preimplant) to spoken language (postimplant activation) due to the child's better awareness of sound and growing communication abilities. Some parents, however, continued to utilize sign language in addition to spoken language in order to meet the communication needs of their child. All families attended the same cochlear implant center and although not stated, may have received consistent supportive guidance from the professionals. In general, parents who perceive themselves as obtaining the necessary information to support their child are more apt to choose the most effective way to communicate with their child (Watson, 2007) and may even use specific language techniques to facilitate their children's emerging language skills (DesJardin & Eisenberg, 2007).

Family Involvement in Children with Cochlear Implants

Both informal and formal types of parental involvement are necessary for children with cochlear implants. Informal involvement may include the parents making important informed decisions for their child, whereas formal involvement may pertain to linguistic input during parent-child interactions. Parents and key caregivers are central figures in their child's life and can change the course of their child's development (Shonkoff & Meisels, 2000; Shonkoff & Phillips, 2000). Utilizing case studies (Allegretti, 2002) and cohorts of parent-child dyads (Des-

Jardin & Eisenberg, 2007; Geers & Brenner, 2003; Spencer, 2004), researchers have noted that parental involvement is an essential factor for children's learning and achievement from early preschool through elementary school years. As Nicholas and Geers (2006) state, "the device alone will not typically lead to spontaneous spoken language acquisition" (p. 276). Consistent involvement by parents who have the essential knowledge and skills necessary to support their children's learning and development better ensures successful implantation (Allegretti, 2002; DesJardin et al., 2006; Spencer, 2004).

Spencer (2004) examined various behavioral indicators of parental involvement relating to their children's education and development prior to and after cochlear implantation. Parental involvement was measured using an interview format. Some of the topics included the child's educational and related experiences before receiving the cochlear implant, parents' process of decision-making about the cochlear implant, parent and child experiences shortly after surgery, and parents' evaluation of child's progress with the implant. One important finding from this study was that parents differed substantially in their descriptions of the resources and processes during the decision-making period of obtaining a cochlear implant for their child. Moreover, parents of the children who performed at the highest levels in language, as measured by the *Clinical Evaluation of Language Fundamentals-Preschool* or CELF-P (Wiig, Secord, & Semel, 1992) also reported having taken much time debating the issue of whether to obtain a cochlear implant for their child. Spencer (2004) noted, "parents who reported being highly involved in learning activities at home and in advocacy roles with educational programs had also reported extended and intense involvement in making the decision about getting the cochlear implant" (p. 408). Put simply, a more rigorous, information-seeking approach to decision-making prior to cochlear implantation was associated with better parental involvement with the child's later learning.

Parental perceived involvement in their children's intervention seems to also influence the way in which parents interact with their young children post implantation. Similar to the findings related to parental self-efficacy, DesJardin and Eisenberg (2007) found that mothers' sense of involvement in their child's speech-language development (using the SPISE questionnaire) was positively related to mothers' quantitative (MLU) and qualitative (facilitative language techniques) linguistic input during interactions with their children. After controlling for child age and length of implant use, mothers' MLU and use of open-ended questions emerged as strong predictor variables for children's expressive language skills. Those same kinds of questions (wh-questions and open-ended questions) during storybook reading interactions also appear to support emergent literacy and basic reading skills in preschool and early elementary school-aged children with cochlear implants (Aram et al., 2006; DesJardin et al., 2009).

Conversely, mothers who felt less involved in their children's language program were more apt to exhibit linguistic mapping, imitations and directives. Such lower level techniques, in turn, were inversely related to their children's language skills (DesJardin & Eisenberg, 2007). These particular techniques have been shown to support hearing children at the prelinguistic stage of language development (Warren et al., 2006). Hence, variability in children's language and literacy skills, in part, may be due to quantitative and qualitative aspects of maternal linguistic input (e.g., involvement during mother-child interaction) post-cochlear implantation.

Most of the research on parental involvement in families of children with cochlear implants has involved quantitative studies showing positive relationships between various forms of parental involvement and children's developmental skills. Recently, however, Zaidman-Zait and Young (2008) carried out a qualitative study to investigate maternal involvement and its influence on the child's progress over time in two case studies of mothers and their young children with cochlear implants (ages 39 and 25 months old). Mothers and their children were videotaped during their daily activities in their home, and at the same time, interview data was used to measure the processes by which parents construct meaning from those interactions. Findings from this study suggest that mothers intentionally engaged their children in activities that they believed facilitated their children's development following cochlear implantation.

Findings from Zaidman-Zait (2007) further suggest that emotions can play an important role in parent-child joint actions. For instance, the emotion of joy drove the joint activities for one mother-child dyad and increased maternal satisfaction. On the other hand, the emotion of frustration created a challenge for the progress of the other mother-child interaction and further created maternal disappointment and feelings of incompetence. Professionals' use of active listening and reflection with families will help enable parents to capitalize on the strengths of the parent-child relationship, as well as the barriers, that can inhibit a more positive parent-child relationship, and in turn, hinder the child's progress.

The Role of Fathers and Other Key Family Members

Research in the area of families of children with cochlear implants has focused primarily on a mother's role in her child's intervention program or habilitation process. However, studies investigating children with other disabilities have shown that fathers and other key family members (e.g., grandparents) also play a critical role in offering support to the family and fostering the child's learning and development. It is important to discuss the dramatic changes in the roles that fathers and grandparents play in early intervention and how these may apply specifically to young children with cochlear implants.

Over the past 50 years, the role of fathers and father figures has changed significantly (Cabrera, Tamis-LeMonda, Bradley, Hofferth, & Lamb, 2000; Lamb & Lewis, 2004). Earlier investigations on paternal involvement focused primarily on a deficit model, highlighting families in which fathers were not present and the negative impact of a father's absence on child development. In recent years, however, the focus has shifted considerably to a strengths-based approach, investigating the positive influences of the father's involvement on child development over time (Lamb & Tamis-LeMonda, 2004; Pleck & Masciadrelli, 2004). Despite this more positive approach, there remains concern about the amount of time fathers are able to spend with their children and the ways in which fathers contribute to their children's later learning (Quesenberry, Ostrosky, & Corso, 2007). For many families, financial concerns may play a part in having other members of the family spend more time with the child, rather than the child's own father or father figure. Nevertheless, fathers are influential in a young child's life and need to be highly encouraged to participate in their child's cochlear implant habilitation intervention.

There are several ways that a father may impact his child's learning. Pleck and Masciadrelli (2004) suggest three areas to consider when involving fathers in an early intervention or habilitation program: (1) engagement and interaction, (2) availability and accessibility, and (3) responsibility for day-to-day care (as cited in Quesenberry et al., 2007).

Naturally, fathers, like mothers, have their own ways of interacting with and nurturing their children. Investigating parental engagement in young hearing children, researchers have shown that levels of paternal engagement have significantly increased over the past several decades (Lamb & Lewis, 2004). The quality of interactions in a father-child relationship has positively affected the cognitive and social development of young hearing children (Pruett, 1997). Similar findings were shown for fathers and their young deaf children (Hadadian, 1995). However, fathers' attitudes toward deafness were negatively related to their children's security of attachment within the father-child relationship.

Availability and accessibility refer to both physical and emotional presence in the family. The amount of time that a father is able to spend with his child can be highly dependent on factors such as work schedules and variations in child routines. Researchers have noted that levels of availability and accessibility have increased as fathers become more and more involved in the lives of their young typical hearing children (Pleck & Masciadrelli, 2004). However, when fathers of children with special challenges play a reduced role in childcare, the impact on mothers—both directly and indirectly—is negative and often profound (Lamb & Lewis, 2004).

Additional demands on the family exist for families of children who receive a cochlear implant. When parenting a deaf child with a cochlear implant, fathers (as well as mothers) have added responsibilities that include ongoing cochlear implant

mapping appointments, weekly professional-parent meetings, and daily teaching of explicit auditory and language skills. These added responsibilities could inhibit a father's involvement in the decision-making and execution of intervention plans. We know from literature on young hearing children with disabilities (Scorgie, Wilgosh, & McDonald, 1998) and, specifically, children with cochlear implants (Sach & Whynes, 2005) that fathers' lack of involvement can lead to familial stress and can put significant strain on the parents' marriage.

The Role of Grandparents in Families of Young Children

Much less is known about the role that grandparents play in the lives of families of children with disabilities (Mitchell, 2007; Sandler, Warren, & Raver, 1995; Trute, 2003) and, specifically, children who are deaf (Nybo, Scherman, & Freeman, 1998). Although there is some evidence that grandparents may experience a period of adjustment as they come to terms with the child's disability (Hastings, 1997), many grandparents provide invaluable support, both practical (e.g., respite care) and emotional (e.g., active listening) to the family (Baranowski & Schilmoeller, 1999). As one may expect, some grandparents provide more support than others depending on geographic location and personal health. Nevertheless, the grandparents' involvement in the child's intervention program can help guide child care practices (Mitchell, 2007) and reduce parental stress (Trute, 2003). This is especially true for fathers. The kinds of tasks that paternal grandparents perform (e.g., tasks typically performed by fathers) reduces the pressure that fathers experience (Sandler et al., 1995; Trute, 2003).

In terms of children who are deaf, the extent of the grandparents' involvement may depend on the grandparent-parent relationship. Nybo and collegues (1998) explored the role of grandparents in six hearing and deaf families, across at least three generations. Results from this study suggest that the grandparents were willing to provide a variety of support services to the parents and grandchildren. However, the support was limited depending on the grandparents' knowledge about deafness (and related issues) and the nature of the existing relationship between grandparent and parent. Grandparents of families with unresolved family issues tended to be less involved in the child's life, whereas grandparents of families with healthy open communication exchanges were more apt to be involved with the family and the needs of the deaf child. Ways to include fathers and other key family members (e.g., grandparents) in the child's early intervention program and habilitation process are highlighted later in this chapter.

Families of Children from Linguistically and Culturally Diverse Homes

Culture is the framework that guides life practices. The importance of a family's culture and early intervention practices is critical in implementing family-centered programs. Although families of the same cultural background may share the same tendencies, members' behaviors will vary depending on family socioeconomic status, gender, age, education, length of time since immigration, and cultural expectations about early intervention services and outcomes (Hanson & Lynch, 2004). Some parents identify strongly with one particular culture, whereas others may combine practices from several cultural groups. Variables such as cultural practices, ethnicity, diversity of attitudes and beliefs, and the primary language used

within the home are defining characteristics of the natural environment and, thus, need to be considered when providing supportive services to families and their young children with cochlear implants (Watson, 2007).

Cultural practices, as well as individual characteristics of the parent, may influence the parent-professional relationship and the family receiving services. Such differences can inhibit the process of developing trust and communication (Lynch & Hanson, 2004) and can create a lack of family participation in the intervention program (Zhang & Bennett, 2003). When the professional and family are from different cultures, communication barriers can arise and the parent or the professional may misunderstand the intent of the intervention plan. The professional must individualize interventions for each family to address families' concerns and priorities. Accordingly, the professional must be sensitive and knowledgeable about the families' cultural practices in order to enhance the process of the parent-professional relationship.

Cultural norms, customs, and language can also influence parental attitudes toward deafness and intervention (Salas-Provance, Erickson, & Reed, 2002). For instance, some families may believe that fathers play the primary role as decision-maker during the preimplant process, whereas the mothers' role is to participate in the habilitation process postimplantation. It also could be the case that extended family members (e.g., grandmother or aunt) play significant roles in caring for the child. It is essential for professionals to develop a common foundation of knowledge and practical strategies to address the specific needs of families with backgrounds different from their own (Hanson & Lynch, 2004; Rhoades, 2007).

Many culturally diverse families often speak more than one language. In fact, demographers project that by the year 2030 nearly 40% of the school-aged population of the United States will be learning English as a second language (Roseberry-McKibbin, Brice, & O'Hanlon, 2005). This increase raises the probability that many more culturally diverse families of children with cochlear implants will speak a language other than English. Linguistically diverse learners in the United States include children from monolingual families who speak among other languages Spanish, Korean, Cantonese, Urdu, Somali, Hmong, and Vietnamese (Kohnert, Yim, Nett, Kan, & Duran, 2005). Linguistically diverse children also include simultaneous bilingual children whose families alternate between two languages (e.g., Spanish and English). Professionals should take the opportunity to update their knowledge about typical second language acquisition, particularly the language expectations for young bilingual children with cochlear implants, including ways to optimize their children's language acquisition.

Several reports have suggested that learning a second language does not impede the acquisition of their first language for hearing children with specific language disabilities (Cheatham, Santos, & Ro, 2007; Goldstein & Kohnert, 2005; Kohnert, 2007) and specifically, cochlear implant users (El-Kashlan & Zwolan, 2008; Levi, Boyett-Solano, Nicholson, & Eisenberg, 2001; Moore, Prath, & Arrieta, 2006; Robbins, Green & Waltzman, 2004; Waltzman, Robbins, Green, & Cohen, 2003). Facilitating the home language while the child is learning English is likely to provide young children with more learning opportunities than focusing primarily on English learning. Generally speaking, home language use is emphasized in early intervention for linguistically diverse children with language delays (Genesee, Paradis, & Crago, 2004; Kohnert & Derr, 2004).

Other researchers have noted, however, that some young children have difficulty transferring language skills from the home language to the majority language (Kohnert et al., 2005). Similar to hearing children (Hart & Risely, 1999), parents can make an important contribution to their children's language development. Parents who speak their native language as well as their second language fluently (e.g., bilingual families) may be more at ease to provide optimal language input for their children. For parents who speak one language fluently (e.g., Spanish) and are learning a second language (e.g., English), facilitating rich and complex language models that would allow their children to develop native English-language skills may be more challenging. Limited linguistic input can inhibit the acquisition of the child's spoken English skills (Kohnert et al., 2005).

Parents and key family members who speak limited English benefit from intervention programs that directly teach them how to facilitate their child's language development in their native language (Kohnert et al., 2005; Lopez & Greenfield, 2004; Moore et al., 2006; Robbins et al., 2004, Tabors, 1997). It is crucial that early childhood professionals (e.g., speech-language pathologists, early interventionists, teachers of the deaf) provide parents and key family members direct instruction in language activities. Demonstrating specific techniques in the family's natural environments during natural routines will better enable the child to transfer their home language skills to the majority language.

Given the previous discussion, it seems of fundamental importance to support home language acquisition for young children with cochlear implants. Access to both home and community language is essential to social, emotional, cognitive, academic, and vocational success. Optimal home language skills can further provide smoother transitions to new learning environments such as home to preschool settings (Cheatham et al., 2007). Helping families develop their child's home language not only allows the child access to other family members and culture but also provides a means for families to support their children's development (de Valenzuela & Niccolai, 2004).

Summary

Families of young children with cochlear implants need well-designed early intervention and habilitation programs to meet the various needs of the family as well as the child. Family members may request different types of information and resources from professionals at various stages prior to and post-cochlear implantation. The ultimate goal of the parent-professional collaborative relationship is to ensure that the parents and key family members obtain a sense of empowerment—self-efficacy—in the knowledge and competencies needed to support their child's learning and development in order for families to take an active and engaging role in the child's early intervention program and habilitation process. Professionals can further nurture the professional-parent relationship by being sensitive to the families' needs, goals, culture, as well as, native language and communication modality preference.

Early Intervention Recommendations for Families of Children with Cochlear Implants

Returning to the opening vignette at the beginning of this chapter, let's now reflect on the following questions, "How can professionals guide Julia's family in order for both parents and child to prosper from an early intervention program?" and "What does an ideal early intervention program offer to Julia's parents (and extended family members) to ensure that their daughter is a successful cochlear implant user?" From a theoretical, family-centered, educational framework and cumulative research, we can apply the fundamental core aspects that are critical for professionals and the families that they serve as they nurture their young child with a cochlear implant.

The Coaching Model

One successful approach that we advocate for families and their young children with cochlear implants is the coaching model. The coaching model is a method in family-centered practices that embraces the parent-professional team as equal members. The professional or coach is a collaborative partner working alongside the parents and other key family members to enhance self-efficacy in important skills in order for the parents to support the goals for their child (Hanft, Rush, & Shelden, 2004; Rush, Shelden, & Hanft, 2003). Accordingly, the coaching model embraces a family-centered empowerment philosophy where parents and professionals learn from each other and work together to enhance the life for the family and child prior to and post-cochlear implantation.

Members of the Coaching Model

In a coaching model, the terms coach and learners describe the partners who participate in a coaching relationship, both gaining knowledge from each other. The role of the coach is to support the parent or learner when, where, and how the support is needed (Shelden & Rush, 2001). For families of children with cochlear implants, a coach could be an audiologist, speech-language pathologist, teacher of the deaf, and/or early interventionist. A professional or coach encourages and guides parents to develop their knowledge and competencies—self efficacy—regarding their child's cochlear implant and ways to support their child's auditory and language development. Parents receive hands-on training and practice with constructive and encouraging feedback based on the parent's strengths and needs. This guidance offers parents and caregivers continual feedback in order to enhance generalization of newly learned techniques across various activities and settings (Woods, Kashinath, & Goldstein, 2004).

Parents (and key family members) or learners can also provide insightful and valuable information to the professional or team in order to optimize learning experiences (Nunes, Pretzlik, & Ilicka, 2005; Zaidman-Zait, 2007). Such information may be about the child (e.g., strengths and challenges, learning style, likes and dislikes), family routines (e.g., breakfast, bathing, nighttime rituals), and real-life family situations (e.g., church, parent-me play group, library story hour) which target auditory and language intervention. Children are more apt to learn new skills during teachable moments. Such teachable moments can happen any time during a day, not only when a professional is present (Dunst, Hamby, Trivette, & Bruder, 2000; Dunst, Hamby, Trivette, Raab, & Bruder, 2002). The ultimate goal of a coaching relationship is for parents to achieve independent, confident use of knowledge and techniques that they can use in every day family occurrences to foster their child's communication and social competences in the child's natural environment (e.g., home and community settings).

Essentials of the Coaching Model

Coaching is an interactive process of observation, reflection, and action in which a coach promotes the learner's ability to support a child's learning and participation in both family and community contexts (Flaherty, 1999; Hanft et al., 2004; Kinlaw, 1999). It provides a structure for developing the competence and skills of family members and professionals to support a child's learning participation in home and community settings in meaningful ways. Professionals and parents, together, agree upon appropriate goals and objectives for the child.

Hanft and colleagues (2004) propose five interrelated constructs that are key to understanding the essential elements of the coaching process: (1) collaborative, (2) context driven, (3) performance based, (4) reflective, and (5) reciprocal. For instance, parents and professionals *collaborate* to identify naturally occurring opportunities (e.g., natural environment such as the family's home) for auditory and language instruction in a specific family routine or *context* (e.g., snack time). At snack time, for example, the professional would demonstrate ways to enhance the child's listening and language skills within that setting while also providing the parent with ample practice (*performance based*). The professional would later engage the parent in *reflective* conversation to prompt the parent to think about how the interactions between the parent and child went during the practice session. This involves active engagement and discussion between the coach (professional) and the learners (parents or key family members) to build the learner's ability to self-assess and generalize effective techniques to other family routines and situations. Finally, *reciprocal* learning emphasizes that coaching is built on shared knowledge between the professional and parent. Each partner adds specialized information and experiences to the partnership. Various early intervention specialists or coaches can share their knowledge about child development, expertise in auditory and language development, learning strategies and techniques, and how to build a trustful relationship. Similarly, learners or parents supply the professional team with knowledge about their family rules and daily routines, family culture, and their hopes or dreams for their child's future. Collectively, parents and professionals benefit from working and learning together as they support the child's auditory and language acquisition, as well as social development, post-cochlear implantation.

Coaching sessions can occur anytime during early intervention. Parents whose children participate in early childhood programs may have coaching conversations with early childhood practitioners, teachers of the deaf, and speech-language pathologists. Early childhood specialists also may coach families in their home. All coaching interactions with family members should acknowledge existing strengths of the parent and the child and offer support to key caregivers. As trust, respect, and communication develop between professionals and parents, coaching conversations will include more specific requests and recommendations for additional information and further support.

Parents of implanted children can provide a wide range of information about their child's medical, educational, and communication needs (Most & Zaidman-Zait, 2003; Spahn et al., 2001). Although parents may enter the coaching process with a vast amount of information from the Internet regarding general applications of the cochlear implant and habilitation (Zaidman-Zait & Jamieson, 2004), professionals need to guide and support parents as they process pertinent materials from the Internet and apply what is useful to their own child. Professionals also need to provide specific suggestions to related topics. Such topics may include, but are not limited to: (1) consistent use and troubleshooting of the cochlear implant, (2) checking the child's auditory and listening capabilities daily, (3) specific strategies to enrich their child's auditory learning environment and speech-language development in their home, (4) creative ways to include their children in activities that would promote pragmatic skills and socialization competencies with their hearing peers, and (5) ways to meet other families of children with cochlear implants (e.g., parent support groups). Parental stress is mitigated when families are given careful professional support and guidance continuously throughout their child's rehabilitation program (Hintermair, 2006; Weisel et al., 2007).

The Coaching Process

The coaching process in family-centered early intervention is a dynamic reciprocal process. Hanft and colleagues (2004) illustrate five components necessary for the coaching process. These include: (1) initiation, (2) observation, (3) action, (4) reflection, and (5) evaluation. Coaching is not a linear process. Each situation determines the order of the coaching components. During the coaching relationship, however, the professional and parent will move through each of the components. Definitions and specific examples for each coaching component as they pertain to families of young children with cochlear implants are offered in Table 17–2. For further discussion and a more in-depth analysis of each component, the reader is referred to Hanft, Rush, and Shelden (2004).

TABLE 17–2. Components of the Coaching Model for Families of Young Children with Cochlear Implants

Components of the Coaching Process	Definition	Examples
Initiation	• Professional invites parents into a coaching relationship (e.g., IFSP or IEP meeting) • Parents initiate a coaching conversation (e.g., seeks advice of professional such as the child's audiologist, speech-language pathologist, or teacher of the deaf).	• Professional identifies coaching opportunities. • Professional shares goals of coaching relationship in early intervention or preschool-aged program. • Professional discusses cultural values and customs, and language preference with the family. • Professional and parent identify and address any barriers for an effective coaching process. • Professional and parent discuss ways to optimize parental involvement, as well as involvement of key family members or caregivers.
Direct Observation	• Professional observes parent interactions or strategies in a natural environment during a family or child routine or activity. • Parent or key caregiver observes a professional demonstration to promote optimal child development or behavior. • Professional and parent observe an intervention or therapy/preschool program together.	• Audiologist observes parent put on cochlear implant and utilize the Ling 6-sound test with child. • Speech-language pathologist observes parent facilitate child's language during storybook reading. • Parent observes teacher of the deaf using specific language techniques during free play with child. • Parent observes early interventionist during a language activity in child's preschool program. • If appropriate, professional demonstrates ways to support the child's early literacy learning (e.g., rhyming, phonemic awareness, print knowledge). • Professional and parent observe a new preschool program for the child for the child's transition from IFSP to IEP program.

continues

529

TABLE 17–2. *continued*

Components of the Coaching Process	Definition	Examples
Action	• Professional and parent brainstorm ways to embed listening and language activities within the family's life. Family events may be going to church, an outdoor event, a parent-me group, and/or a family celebration. Daily events or routines could be at mealtimes, hand washing, playing with toys, storybook reading, riding in the car, when a parent arrives home from work, and/or bedtime rituals.	• Parent practices specified language techniques (e.g., parallel talk and expansion) during storybook reading. • Parent reinforces new vocabulary with child while taking a walk in the park (e.g., "Squirrel," "I see a squirrel," "There he is!," "The squirrel is going up the tree," "Do you see the squirrel?"). • Professional models the language techniques, open-ended question and recast, while making cookies with grandma and child in their home. • Parent reinforces targeted sounds in the home with child (e.g., "I hear a car in the driveway, "listen, beep beep," "daddy's car!," "Daddy's home from work," "Do you hear daddy's car? It goes, 'beep-beep'").
Reflection	• Professional assists the parents in reviewing or reflecting on parental knowledge and skills during or shortly after the interaction with the child. • Parents reflect on the knowledge and competencies that they have gained through the coaching process. • Professional uses open-ended questions to elicit additional parental strengths and accomplishments. • Parents discuss new ways for other key members of the family and caregivers to be involved in their child's intervention program. • Professional and parent plan new observations and/or techniques to implement during the action stage.	• Parents brainstorm and make a list of the strengths and skills learned from the coaching process. • Professionals and parents brainstorm ways to include other family members (e.g., siblings, cousins, grandparents) in the child's intervention. • Parents discuss with professional what techniques or activities are working in terms of the child's listening and language development and/or brainstorm new ideas to increase the child's auditory or communication skills.

Components of the Coaching Process	Definition	Examples
Evaluation	• Professional and parents review the coaching relationship and process; continuation or resolution. • Professional and parents analyze the strengths or challenges of the coaching relationship. • Professional and parents determine whether progress is being made to achieve desired family and child goals and objectives (e.g., IFSP or IEP).	As part of the evaluation, professionals and parents address questions such as: 1. Are there additional resources (e.g., language programs, workshops, support groups) that the family needs? 2. Does the family need access to other families of young or older children with cochlear implants? 3. Does the family need any additional emotional or social support networks for the parents (e.g., parenting classes, counseling) or child (e.g., social skills training, behavior therapy, related services for additional disabilities or challenges)?

531

Initiation

During initiation, either the professional invites the learner into a coaching relationship (e.g., the IFSP or IEP meeting) or the parent initiates the coaching conversation or seeks the advice and experience of the professional. In the opening vignette, Julia's mother and father sought out information from the professional on how to further support their child's listening and language skills. This is an important time in the coaching process where the professional can share the goals of a collaborative relationship, the role of each participant, and the ultimate goal in intervention or habilitation for families and their children. Professionals need to emphasize that the ultimate goal for intervention is for parents to obtain the competencies and skills to guide their children's development in the context of their family and community. After the professional establishes clear goals and family issues (e.g., parent work schedules, other family supports), the professional and parent can set up a time for the professional to visit the family and child in their natural environment (e.g., home, early intervention program, therapy session, or mapping appointment).

At the initial contact appointment with the family, it is an ideal time for a professional to discuss cultural norms and customs, as well as language preferences, to better ensure parent participation. Several studies have reported that culturally linguistically diverse (CLD) families exhibit lower levels of participation than European American families in early intervention (Zhang & Bennett, 2003). Thoughtful ways of how to better support parental involvement need to be considered for CLD families of children with cochlear implants. Taking time to understand the families concerns, needs, and priorities will help in developing a trusting professional-parent relationship which will,

in turn, put the parents at ease and ensure more parental participation. Moreover, providing additional time to explain newly acquired terms prior to and post-cochlear implantation (e.g., audiogram, mapping, listening versus language activities) and unfamiliar early intervention terminology (e.g., IDEA, IFSP, IEP) will ensure better communication between parent and professional. Better understanding of the various educational terms can lead to parents taking a active part in the IFSP or IEP process and become better advocates for their child in future discussions related to early intervention needs and goals for the entire family (see Zhang & Bennett, 2003 for a more thorough review of research and strategies to enhance participation for CLD families).

Resources for professionals (Barrera, Corso, & Macpherson, 2003; Goldstein, 2000) as well as checklists (Goode, 2006; Rhoades, 2007) are now available to better promote professional cultural competency in early intervention settings. One such tool is the "Caregiver Intake Interview" (Rhoades, 2007). This tool was designed to guide professionals as they provide culturally competent services to families of children with cochlear implants. Some of the issues that are addressed through the interview format are: family customs and culture, religious practice, beliefs about the child's role in life and the family, and family support systems. One approach, however, may not be successful with all cultural groups. Therefore, professionals need to examine a range of strategies to enhance professional-parent relationships with families from a variety of cultural and linguistic backgrounds.

During initiation, a professional can further discuss ways to optimize parental involvement, and more specifically, father participation (and other key family members) in the child's habilitation post-cochlear implantation. Because parental involvement is a crucial factor in a child's habilitation process (DesJardin et al., 2006; Geers & Brenner, 2003; Spencer, 2004), professionals should take note of parents who may not understand the importance of their role and provide additional supports as necessary. Professionals wishing to enhance parental involvement could make programs and home visits more consistent with family preferences. For instance, fathers are more likely to participate in activities that are play-based, occur at home, and are inclusive of the entire family (Turbiville, Turnbull, & Turnbull, 1995).

With regard to a father's participation, Quesenberry and colleagues (2007) suggest a framework in which there is a logical fit between the specific needs of the father and the stated outcomes of the program. To develop this framework, professionals should first assess the needs of the father (e.g., evening or weekend workshops, flexible meeting places or times, strategies to become more confident in skills). Consistent evaluation of the program is critical to make sure that it is addressing the father's needs and concerns. Although John, in the opening vignette, wishes to be involved in his daughter's cochlear implant habilitation process, other fathers might not be as comfortable in this role. Fathers, mothers, and other key caregivers such as grandparents also may benefit from spending time with other families of children with cochlear implants (Nunes et al., 2005). Care must be taken to determine the unique strengths and concerns of each parent as professionals provide family-centered services to families and their young children.

Direct Observation

The second component of the coaching model involves direct observation. There are various ways that observations can occur. One way it could occur is for a pro-

fessional to watch a parent interacting with the child while practicing a new skill previously discussed in a coaching session. Observing a parent during a naturally occurring family routine serves as an ideal way to see how newly acquired parental skills are being generalized into the family's life. For example, the early intervention specialist could observe Julia's father using a new facilitative language technique (parallel talk) while playing with Julia. A speech-language pathologist might observe how Julia's mother engages her daughter during storybook interactions and utilizes specific facilitative language techniques (e.g., label, expansion) tailored to Julia's language level. Observations should be directly followed by a specific constructive comment by the professional that focuses on the parent's strengths.

An observational situation might also occur with the parent observing the professional demonstrate a particular skill, technique, or strategy. Demonstration of listening-language activities by the intervention professional or therapist could positively influence mothers' use of language techniques when communicating to their child. DesJardin and Eisenberg (2007) suggested that mothers who felt that they were provided with visual models and "hands on" practice with language techniques were more apt to utilize language techniques that were positively related to their child's language skills. Conversely, mothers who felt that they did not receive such practice were more apt to use techniques that did not necessarily support their child's language level. Providing parents and key caregivers with various ways to engage the child in listening and language opportunities, and then modeling appropriate facilitative language techniques in the context of the family's home, will enhance the coaching process.

A third possible way direct observation may occur is by joint observation. Joint observation is when parents and a professional observe an educational program together. During joint observation, the professional and parent can provide important information to the early childhood specialist (e.g., preschool or daycare teacher) regarding optimal listening and language learning opportunities within the classroom or childcare setting.

Action

An action is an experience that is planned or spontaneous. Actions require specific events that occur in real-life family activities. Family-centered early intervention programs highlight the importance of embedding listening and language techniques in naturally occurring interactions with children within the family's daily routines and activities (Dunst, 2006; Roper & Dunst, 2003; Woods et al., 2004). Everyday occurrences such as mealtime, hand washing, playing with toys, joint storybook reading, and bedtime routines are common in most families of young children. In the action phase, parents incorporate a new skill such as a language technique previously learned in the observation portions of the coaching process. Auditory or language activities embedded in early family routines provide the foundation for children's later language, social-emotional, and academic development (Rosenkoetter & Barton, 2002; Spagnola & Fiese, 2007).

Parental Facilitation of Children's Audition. The first step in facilitating auditory development in children with cochlear implants is to ensure the children are hearing on a consistent basis. Parental understanding of the importance of continual audition is critical for the child's listening success after cochlear implantation. Issues pertaining to cochlear implant troubleshooting and use may arise (Incesulu et al., 2003; Most & Zaidman-Zait, 2003). Profes-

sionals may need to brainstorm with parents to find effective ways for the child to use the cochlear implant consistently at home, school, and community settings. Key caregivers also will need to understand the importance of daily cochlear implant monitoring and checking the child's listening capabilities using the device.

Families also can benefit from examples of sounds that their child can detect in their home. For instance, early intervention professionals can guide parents as they identify loud sounds (e.g., ringing of the telephone, car horns, a knock at the door, dog barking) and soft sounds (e.g., father whispering "sh," dishwasher running, soft music) and how they can facilitate the child's ability to distinguish between sound patterns (auditory discrimination skills). Making new sounds meaningful to the child is critical for later development of auditory identification (e.g., the child recognizes a sound without prompting) and comprehension (e.g., the child can process and use auditory information for meaning) skills. Parents will need explicit instances and ways to provide their children with intentional meaningful daily auditory experiences.

Parental Facilitation of Children's Spoken Language. Parents are their children's first and most enduring teachers and have the ability to support their children's language, social, and academic development. The Division of Early Childhood (DEC) (Sandall et al., 2005) and resources on habilitation for children with cochlear implants (Estabrooks, 2007; Garber & Nevins, 2007; Lim & Simser, 2005) highlight the importance of parental responsiveness to children's linguistic attempts for facilitating optimal spoken language development. These guidelines are based on the social interactionist theory of language development, which postulates that young children learn language in the contexts of their daily experiences and particularly, through interactions with their family or caregivers (Chapman, 2000; Hoff, 2000). Generally, the adult's role is to provide linguistic input that is appropriate for the child's developmental level. As the child's language skills increase, the adult provides more complex input and less support, allowing the child to take more control of the learning process.

Variation observed in language skills for young hearing children (Fewell & Deutscher, 2004; Hart & Risley, 1995; Weizman & Snow, 2001) and children with cochlear implants (DesJardin & Eisenberg, 2007) are strongly linked to parental linguistic input; both (1) quantity (e.g., number of different words or vocabulary diversity, MLU) and (2) quality (e.g., facilitative language techniques). Generally speaking, children who are provided with a variety of words and phrases (e.g., utterances) slightly above their language level develop better language skills. These linguistic constructs have been shown to correlate positively with important indicators for later school achievement (Catts, Fey, Tomblin, & Zhang, 2002; Hart & Risely, 1999). Furthermore, although some language techniques (e.g., linguistic mapping, imitation) enhance language learning in young hearing children at the single-word stage of language development (Warren et al., 2006), other language techniques (e.g., recast, open-ended questions) better support children at the two-to-three-word language level (Fey, Krulik, Loeb, & Proctor-Williams, 1999; Girolametto & Weitzman, 2006; Kaiser & Hancock, 2003; McNeil & Fowler, 1999). Parental linguistic input that is "fine-tuned" to their child's language level can accelerate spoken language development (Chapman, 2000; Yoder & Warren, 1998).

Professionals in the field should be knowledgeable about empirically based language programs that optimize language learning for young children with language delays. Language intervention programs listed in Table 17–3 all emphasize parents and family members as key agents in the acquisition of their child's language development. McCauley and Fey (2006) note that "those interventions that train parents to act as language facilitators in the home and elsewhere are intended to capitalize on parents' potential to be exceptional interventionists because of their unique knowledge of, access to, and commitment to their children" (p. 21). Although language programs for young children vary in terms of specific facilitation techniques (e.g., linguistic mapping, imitation, expansion, recast) and various kinds of instructional methods (e.g., demonstration, coaching, role-play, videotaped example, constructive feedback), they all have a common critical factor— parental involvement. The specific facilitative language technologies are described later in this chapter (also refer to Figure 17–5 for definitions). Kaiser and Hancock (2003) state, however, that parent teaching of specific techniques will only be successful if professionals have the expertise in the intervention procedures, are skilled in teaching parents, and collaborate with parents in terms of goals and outcomes. For a more in-depth discussion on intervention programs for children with language challenges, and ways to support parental teaching of language techniques, the reader is referred to Estabrooks (2007), Kaiser and Hancock (2003), and McCauley and Fey (2006).

Within each language intervention program, professionals teach parents how to employ interactive strategies and specific language techniques tailored to their child's language level. For young hearing children, Warren and his colleagues (2006) suggest that the first year of life is the time for building auditory and receptive language skills. Language intervention programs such as prelinguistic milieu teaching (Warren et al.,

TABLE 17–3. Evidence-Based Interactive Language Interventions for Families of Children with Cochlear Implants

Interactive Language Intervention	Description	Target Age	Parental Aspect	Facilitative Language Techniques
Auditory-Verbal (A-V) Therapy	The Auditory-Verbal philosophy is a set of principles that are designed to be implemented by the child's parents and key caregivers in order to achieve maximum use of hearing for learning.	Children with hearing loss (birth–school age).	Parents and family members are provided with education, guidance, family support, and specific skills to develop the child's listening and language skills by participating in weekly-individualized parent guided A-V sessions. Goals and skills are incorporated into family daily routines and activities.	Parallel Talk Label Expansion Expatiation Open-ended question
It Takes Two To Talk: The Hanen Program	Program for parents of children with receptive and expressive language delays. Clinician and parents jointly select communication goals and use focused techniques during naturalistic interactions (e.g., family routines and activities).	Hearing toddlers (18–30 months) and preschool children with specific language disorders.	Promotes caregivers' use of optimal language input with their children to increase frequency of caregiver-child conversational interactions and joint engagement. Caregivers learn: • child-centered strategies, • interaction promoting techniques, and • language modeling techniques.	Parallel Talk Imitation Linguistic mapping Label Expansion Expatiation
Focused Stimulation Approach	Deliberate manipulation of preselected language targets and child's environment (e.g., child interest) to elicit target language objective (e.g., form, content, or use of language).	Toddlers through early school-age children with specific language disorders.	Professional-directed language sessions with supplemented information to parents in order for caregivers to carry over the techniques in the home.	Arranging the environment Parallel Talk Label Using multiple repetitions of a variety of questions and statements to target a specific language objective.

Interactive Language Intervention	Description	Target Age	Parental Aspect	Facilitative Language Techniques
Language Is the Key	Designed to optimize language and literacy development for children with communication needs by training professionals and family members to facilitate language, preliteracy skills, and play activities during free play and storybook interactions. Strategies are appropriate for a variety of cultures and ethnic groups.	Children with typical language development or children with language delays below 4 years of age.	Parents are taught to use wait time, parallel talk, questions, and expansions during naturally occurring free play and storybook interactions.	Parallel Talk Closed-ended question Open-ended question Expansion Recast Expatiation
Responsivity Prelinguistic Milieu Teaching	Professional implemented and parent training intervention of techniques designed to facilitate nonverbal communication development.	Children with language delays (2–3 year old children who are functioning developmentally between 9–18 months of age).	Professionals train parents to use specialized strategies and techniques designed to increase the frequency and complexity of nonverbal communication as a precursor for language.	Environmental arrangement Following child's lead Turn-taking Parallel talk Linguistic mapping Imitation Adequate response time
Enhanced Milieu Teaching	Promotion of communication using the family environment and responsive interaction techniques.	Preschool–early school-aged children (MLUs between 1.0–3.5 years).	Parents are trained by clinicians to use responsive interaction techniques and milieu teaching procedures to prompt language production in naturalistic parent-child interactions.	Environment arrangement Contingent feedback (e.g., prompting, reinforcement) Parallel talk Expansion Balanced turn-taking Modeling language targets

537

2006) focus on teaching parents techniques to facilitate language learning in hearing infants and toddlers with language delays (developmentally between 9- and 18-months old). The prelinguistic milieu teaching program is designed to increase children's early gestures and vocalizations. At the initial stage of linguistic development, responsive interaction techniques, such as following the child's lead, turn-taking, linguistic mapping, and imitation, have been shown to support emerging language skills in young hearing children (Yoder, McCathren, Warren, & Watson, 2001). Most importantly, parent training of these types of techniques enhances the way parents respond to their hearing toddlers (Yoder & Warren, 2002). Although only one intervention program listed in Table 17–3 (Auditory-Verbal Therapy) and several facilitative techniques (e.g., Aram et al., 2006; DesJardin & Eisenberg, 2007) have been studied in pediatric implant populations, each of the programs listed in Table 17–3 can add value to well-designed intervention programs for families and their children with cochlear implants.

Although some programs are designed to support children at the prelinguistic stage of development, other programs are more appropriate to support children's emerging vocabulary and syntactic abilities. Two such programs that are designed for hearing children from preschool- to early school-age are (1) *It Takes Two to Talk: The Hanen Program* or HP (Girolametto & Weitzman, 2006; Pepper & Weitzman, 2004; Weitzman, 1994) and (2) *Language Is the Key* or LIK (Cole, Maddox, & Lim, 2006). Both programs teach parents how to facilitate their children's language development in natural occurring interactions (e.g., free play, storybook interactions). Within each program, child-centered strategies (e.g., following the child's lead), interaction techniques (e.g., wait time, asking questions to elicit child response), and facilitative language techniques (e.g., label and expansion for HP; recast and open-ended question for LIK) are highlighted. Higher level techniques such as recast and open-ended question provide children with a diversity of words and phrases to better support their emerging vocabulary and syntactic skills (Ard & Beverly, 2004; Bradshaw, Hoffman, & Norris, 1998; Camarata & Nelson, 2006; Ezell, Justice, & Parsons, 2000, Justice & Pence, 2007; Nelson, Camarata, Welsh, Butkovsky, & Camarata, 1996; Proctor-Williams, Fey, & Loeb, 2001). Tables 17–4 and 17–5 provide definitions and examples of facilitative language techniques.

It is important that early intervention professionals observe the language techniques used by parents and other key caregivers as they interact with their child with a cochlear implant. According to Vygotskian theory (1962), children develop linguistically through caregiver interactions that reflect children's zone of proximal development (ZPD). A child's ZPD is defined as the distance between a child's current level of development and the level in which the child can function with adult assistance. Depending on age at implantation, length of implant use, and intervention goals, children require parental linguistic input tailored to their needs. For a young child with six months cochlear implant experience (similar to Julia in the earlier vignette), parental use of lower level language techniques (e.g., linguistic mapping, label, imitation) may be essential. Once a child demonstrates the use of a variety of vocabulary and begins to put words together into two- and three-word phrases, higher level techniques (e.g., recast, open-ended question) are necessary to promote more advanced language (DesJardin & Eisenberg, 2007).

TABLE 17–4. Description and Examples of Parental Facilitative Language Techniques for Children <12 Months Post Cochlear Implant

Facilitative Language Technique	Definition	Examples
Linguistic mapping	Putting into words or interpreting the child's intended message using the context as a clue (child uses a preceding vocalization that is not recognizable as an approximation of a word).	Child hands mother a toy dog and vocalizes—mother says, "doggie." Child pushes the storybook away and vocalizes—father says, "all done."
Imitation	Repeating verbatim the child's preceding vocalization or verbalization without adding any new words.	Child says, "hat" and mother says, "yeah hat." Child says, "yellow car" and mother says, "yes, yellow car."
Label	Stating the name for a toy, picture, or object.	Grandmother says, "There is the moon" or "I see the stars."
Closed-ended question	Stating a question in which the child can only answer with a one-word response.	Father asks child, "Is that your book?" or "Do you like that book?"

Higher level techniques encourage a child's participation during the interaction and facilitate conversational exchanges eliciting more complex vocabulary and syntactic skills of the child. When parents use language techniques that are fine-tuned to their child's language level, they are helping their children gain communicative competence and confidence.

Families of children from linguistically diverse homes also benefit from explicit language techniques and activities. Through daily interactions, young children can experience the value of their home language as the basic linguistic tool used within their home with family members. Storybook and free play interactions are rich environments for communication development across cultures (Johnston & Wong, 2002; Lim & Cole, 2002). Similar to children learning English only, however, parents need to do more than just speak to their children using the language used in the home (Tabors, 1997). Direct instruction of facilitative language techniques has been shown to maximize children's home language learning and in turn, children's second language acquisition (Cole et al., 2006; Kohnert et al., 2005).

Some limitations to the utilization of language techniques with culturally and linguistically diverse families must be noted. First, an essential issue arises if the professional is not proficient in the family's home language. In this situation, utilizing a paraprofessional who is skilled in the home language might be a more effective means to teach parents specific language techniques

TABLE 17–5. Description and Examples of Parental Facilitative Language Techniques for Children >12 Months Post Cochlear Implant

Facilitative Language Technique	Definition	Examples
Parallel Talk	Caregiver talks aloud about what the child is directly doing, looking at, or referencing.	Child is looking directly at a bird outside the window and caregiver says, "The little bird is looking for food."
Open-ended question/phrase	Caregiver provides a phrase/question in which the child can answer using more than one word.	While looking at a storybook, caregiver says, "What is happening in this picture?" or "What do you think will happen on the next page?"
Expansion	Caregiver repeats child's verbalization providing a more grammatical and complete language model without modifying the child's word order or intended meaning.	Child says, "car go fast," and the caregiver says, "The car is going fast."
Expatiation	Similar to expansion except caregiver adds new information.	While driving in the car—child says, "go store" and mother says, "Yes, we are going to the store. We are going to the grocery store to buy milk."
Recast	Caregiver restates the child's verbalization into a question format.	Child says, "grandma here" and the caregiver says, "Is grandma here? or "Do you think grandma is here?"

(Hancock, Kaiser, & Delaney, 2002; Leseman & van Tuijl, 2001). Second, empirical evidence of facilitative techniques is limited in terms of their application to culturally and linguistically diverse families. Although empirical evidence suggests that the language program, *Language Is the Key*, can promote language learning in Korean (Lim & Cole, 2002) and Mexican families (Valdez-Menchaca & Whitehurst, 1992), and *The Hanen Program* has been translated into several languages, most of the research has focused primarily on English-speaking populations. Techniques embedded within each of these programs may or may not be consistent with cultural values of other linguistically diverse families (Johnston & Wong, 2002; van Kleeck, 1994). For instance, Chinese parents may be more willing to create explicit language lessons rather than embedding their teaching in play with their young children (Johnston & Wong, 2002). Similarly, Japanese (Fernald & Morikawa, 1993) and Korean mothers (Lim & Cole, 2002) are more apt to focus on the development of affect and the emotional bond between mother and child during storybook reading, and less on information-orientated activities than American mothers. Please refer to the following resources for more explicit information on the cultural considerations needed for effective professional-parent collaboration for optimal parent-child interactions (e.g., Brice, 2002; Goldstein, 2000; Lynch & Hanson, 2004; Moore & Perez-Mendez, 2003; Wyatt, 2002).

Reflection

Reflection is one of the most important components to the coaching process. Reflection aligns well with recommended practices in family-centered intervention (Dunst, 2000; Turnbull & Turnbull, 2001; McWilliam & Scott, 2001; Guralnick, 2005). This is the time when parents can think about the knowledge and competencies that they have gained through the use of discussion. The role of the coach or professional is to ask open-ended questions rather than closed-ended questions in order to elicit reflections from the parent on his or her current strengths and skills that positively support the child's listening and language abilities. The ultimate goal is for the parents or caregivers to identify and believe that they have the specific knowledge and competencies—self-efficacy—to guide their child's listening and language acquisition. The professional's role is to affirm the parent throughout the coaching process by acknowledging his or her strengths, competence, and mastery of skills.

Throughout reflection, professionals also can highlight the contribution that parents made in their various kinds of involvement during their child's habilitation. For example, perhaps for one mother, presenting material to the staff at the child's preschool was beneficial. For another father, learning ways to engage his child in play and demonstrating appropriate language techniques showed significant results. At this point, parents also can reflect on new innovative ways to be involved with their child's intervention based on the child's developmental level or emerging communication or social needs. Furthermore, families also may feel a need to be more connected with other families with shared experiences. Connecting with other families of children with cochlear implants may reduce parents' social isolation, strengthen emotional connections with the child, and can help parents to better respond to their children during parent-child interactions (Zaidman-Zait, 2007).

Evaluation

The last component of the coaching model is to evaluate the coaching relationship and the coaching process. This requires the professional and parents to review the effectiveness of the professional-parent relationship. This can occur at anytime during the coaching process such as at a weekly or monthly coaching session, a 6-month IFSP team meeting or annual IEP conference, and/or at the child's transition meeting from early intervention (IFSP) to preschool-age program (IEP). Continuation or termination of the coaching relationship is determined between professional and parent through open and honest discussions.

Educational provisions for families need to be flexible as professionals evaluate family needs and concerns. Issues relating to the family support and services need to be addressed at the evaluation meeting. For instance, although some families may only need a biweekly or a monthly coaching session, other families may require a weekly meeting with a professional to obtain ongoing support. Similarly, some families may need more contact with other families of children with cochlear implants depending on their geographic location, whereas other families might need additional resources and services due to the child's age (e.g., transition from IFSP to IEP programs) or the child's on-going behavioral or communication needs. Moreover, due to the child's communication abilities or special needs, some parents may require additional sign language classes (Watson et al., 2007). These are only some of the issues that may arise during an evaluation meeting. It is important for professionals to keep in mind that family needs can vary in terms of the amount of information, skills, and resources required to support their child's listening and language skills. Table 17–6 provides a list of resources for professionals and parents.

Summary

Families are central figures in the lives of children's development prior to and following cochlear implant activation. The theoretical and practical importance for family-centered early intervention practices for families and their young children with cochlear implants have been described in this chapter. Current early intervention federal mandates (IDEIA, 2004) not only invite parents to participate in their child's habilitation after cochlear implantation, but under these regulations, parents also are expected to be an integral part in their child's early intervention program. It is the ultimate goal of family-centered early intervention for parents to gain the sense of self-efficacy and advocacy in order to steer their children's future course in the optimal direction. As culturally competent professionals support parents' sense of self-efficacy and parental involvement in the knowledge and skills necessary to guide their child's development, parents offer professionals invaluable information regarding the family and child in order to optimize the habilitation process. Through collaborative parent-professional relationships, families are empowered with the tools needed to make significant contributions to their children's future learning and education. Early language intervention programs that utilize the most effective intervention strategies and parental facilitative language techniques—tailored to a child's language level and occurring in the child's natural environment—are most likely to positively impact children's later communication and social performance. For Julia's parents, Lynnette and John, a family service plan that incorporates a coaching model will better ensure that her parents and family members obtain the informational and emotional guidance necessary to support their young daughter's auditory and language development with the use of a cochlear implant.

TABLE 17–6. Resources for Professionals and Families of Young Children with Cochlear Implants

Resource	Description	Phone/Web Site
Alexander Graham Bell Association for the Deaf (AG Bell)	An organization for parents and professionals working with families of children with hearing loss. Through advocacy, education, and research, AG Bell helps to ensure that every child with hearing loss has the opportunity to listen, talk, and thrive in mainstream society.	(800) HEAR-KID (202) 337-5220; www.agbell.org
American Academy of Audiology	An organization that provides information to audiologists and speech-language pathologists.	(800) 222-2336; www.audiology.org
American Speech-Language-Hearing Association (ASHA)	An organization that promotes the interests of and provides services for professionals in audiology, speech-language pathology, and speech and hearing science. It also advocates for children with communication disabilities.	(800) 638-8255; www.asha.org
Auditory-Verbal International	Auditory-Verbal International is now integrated with the AG Bell Association. This particular philosophy supports the option for children with all degrees of hearing loss to develop the ability to listen and to use verbal communication with their family.	For additional information: http://www.listen-up.org/oral/a-v.htm
My Baby's Hearing	A Web site supported by Boys Town National Research Hospital that provides information for families regarding hearing and amplification, language and learning development, and parent resources.	www.babyhearing.org
Beginnings: For Parents of Children Who Are Deaf or Hard of Hearing	A nonprofit agency that provides information and emotional support as a central resource for families with children who are deaf or hard-of-hearing (age birth–21) and the professionals who serve them. The mission of BEGINNINGS is to inform and empower parents as they make decisions about their child.	www.ncbegin.org Raleigh, N.C. office: (800) 541-4327

continues

TABLE 17–6. *continued*

Resource	Description	Phone/Web Site
The Listen–Up Web	A Web site that provides many resources for professionals and families of children with hearing loss. It offers extensive links to other sites about cochlear implants.	www.listen-up.org
The Hanen Centre	A program that provides family-focused early language intervention and learning resources for parents and professionals around the world.	www.hanen.org
Laurent Clerc National Deaf Education Center Gallaudet University	A Web site for professionals and families to navigate a variety of cochlear implant information including many links to parent resources for oral language habilitation for children with cochlear implants.	http://clerccenter.gallaudet.edu/
Bringing Sound to Life: Principles and Practices of Cochlear Implant Rehabilitation	A systematic approach to spoken language habilitation for children of all ages. It includes a video training series, a manual, and curriculum. The video training series includes four videotapes: (1) Building Blocks of Spoken Language; (2) Understanding Hearing and Hearing Loss; (3) Cochlear Implants and Children: An Opportunity, Not a Cure; and (4) Principles and Practices of Cochlear Implant Rehabilitation. The videos are an excellent resource for family education and/or teacher training.	Available through Advanced Bionics: http://www.bionicear.com/printables/AB_Rehab_Materials_2006.pdf
Learn To Talk Around The Clock	An early intervention program designed for professionals who work with families of children who are deaf or hard of hearing (birth-3 years). It focuses on oral language learning in the child's home environment. It provides materials for professionals to maximize the caregiver's language development techniques by encouraging interactions during everyday activities.	http://www.learntotalkaroundtheclock.com/Welcome.html

Resource	Description	Phone/Web Site
Listen, Learn, and Talk	An auditory habilitation program for young deaf and hard of hearing children who are learning to listen and talk. Consists of a manual and three videotapes (Babies Babble, Toddlers Talk, and Children Chatter). Videos provide practical ways that families can provide spoken language enhancement in their home. The manual provides information on the importance of parent participation in the habilitation process, strategies for facilitating spoken language development and the theory behind auditory development. It also provides integrated scales for monitoring and documenting development in listening, language, speech, cognition, and social communication.	http://www.cochlearamericas.com/ Support/170.asp
Listen Little Star (A Listening Program)	A series of parent-child activities designed to help young children with hearing loss develop listening and speaking skills. The techniques it uses are based on the Auditory-Verbal approach. The program includes a manual with handouts about hearing loss and a step-by-step plan of sequential activities for the professional and family.	Materials offered by Auditory-Verbal Learning Institute, Inc. http://avli.org/Merchant2/merchant.mv? Screen=PROD&Store_Code=AS& Product_Code=K1&Category_Code=K
My Baby and Me	A notebook-style resource for parents (and professionals) that provides strategies and tips for helping a child learn to listen and talk in an easy-to-use "baby book" format that is personalized for each family and child. This resource provides detailed information about language learning and hearing loss and provides space for families to document their child's individual development.	Developed by: Betsy Moog Brooks http://www.hearingexchange.com/store/ 1.html

References

Akey, T. M. (1996). *Exploratory factor analysis and item analysis of the Psychological Empowerment Scale.* Unpublished manuscript, Auburn University, AL.

Akey, T. M., Marquis, J. G., & Ross, M. E. (2000). Validation of scores on the Psychological Empowerment Scale: A measure of empowerment for parents of children with a disability. *Educational and Psychological Measurement, 60,* 419–438.

Allegretti, C. M. (2002). The effects of a cochlear implant on the family of a hearing-impaired child. *Pediatric Nursing, 28,* 614–620.

Aram, D., Most, T., & Mayafit, H. (2006). Contributions of mother-child storybook telling and joint writing to literacy development in kindergartners with hearing loss. *Language, Speech, and Hearing Services in Schools, 37,* 209–223.

Ard, L. M., & Beverly, B. L. (2004). Preschool word learning during joint book reading: Effect of adult questions and comments. *Communication Disorders Quarterly, 26*(1), 17–28.

Bailey, D. B., & Powell, T. (2005). Assessing the information needs of families in early intervention. In M. J. Guralnick (Ed.), *The developmental systems approach to early intervention* (pp. 151–183). Baltimore: Paul H. Brookes.

Bandura, A. (1977). Self-efficacy: Toward a unifying theory of behavioral change. *Psychological Review, 84,* 191–215.

Bandura, A. (1989). Regulation of cognitive processes through perceived self-efficacy. *Developmental Psychology, 25,* 729–735.

Bandura, A. (1997). *Self-efficacy: The exercise of control.* New York: W. H. Freeman.

Baranowski, M. D., & Schilmoeller, G. L. (1999). Grandparents in the lives of grandchildren with disabilities: Mothers' perceptions. *Education and Treatment of Children, 22,* 427–446.

Barrera, I., Corso, R. M., & Macpherson, D. (2003). *Skilled dialogue: Strategies for responding to cultural diversity in early childhood.* Baltimore: Paul H. Brookes.

Beadle, E. A., Shores, A., & Wood, E. J. (2000). Parental perceptions of the impact upon the family of cochlear implantation in children. *Annals of Otology, Rhinology, and Laryngology, 109*(Suppl. 185), 111–114.

Beals, D. E. (2001). Eating and reading: Links between family conversations with preschoolers and later language and literacy. In D. K. Dickinson & P. O. Tabors (Eds.), *Beginning literacy with language: Young children at home and school* (pp. 75–92). Baltimore: Paul H. Brookes.

Blum-Kulka, S., & Snow, C. E. (2002). *Talking to adults: The contribution of multiparty discourse to language acquisition.* Mahwah, NJ: Lawrence Erlbaum Associates.

Bradshaw, M. L., Hoffman, P. R., & Norris, J. A. (1998). Efficacy of expansions and cloze procedures in the development of interpretations by preschool children exhibiting delayed language development. *Language, Speech, and Hearing Services in Schools, 29,* 85–95.

Brice, A. E. (2002). *The Hispanic child: Speech, language, culture, and education.* Boston: Allyn & Bacon.

Brody, G. H., Flor, D. L., & Gibson, N. M. (1999). Linking maternal efficacy beliefs, developmental goals, parenting practices, and child competence in rural single-parent African-American families. *Child Development, 70*(5), 1197–1208.

Bronfenbrenner, U. (1974). *Is early intervention effective?* (Publication No. CDH 74-25). Washington, DC: Department of Health, Education, and Welfare, Office of Child Development.

Bronfenbrenner, U. (1979). *The ecology of human development: Experiments by nature and design.* Cambridge, MA: Harvard University Press.

Bruder, M. B. (2000). Family-centered early intervention: Clarifying our values for the new millennium. *Topics in Early Childhood Special Education, 20,* 105–115.

Burger, T., Spahn, C., Richter, B., Eissele, S., Lohle, E., & Bengel, J. (2005). Parental distress: The initial phase of hearing aid and cochlear implant fitting. *American Annals of the Deaf, 150,* 5–10.

Cabrera, N. J., Tamis-LeMonda, C. S., Bradley, R. H., Hofferth, S., & Lamb, M. E. (2000). Fatherhood in the twenty-first century. *Child Development, 71,* 127–136.

Camarata, S. M., & Nelson, K. E. (2006). Conversational recast intervention with preschool and older children. In R. J. McCauley & M. E. Fey (Eds.), *Treatment of language disorders in children* (pp. 237–264). Baltimore: Brookes.

Catts, H., Fey, M., Tomblin, J., & Zhang, X. (2002). A longitudinal investigation of reading outcomes in children with language impairments. *Journal of Speech, Language, and Hearing Research, 45,* 1142–1157.

Chapman, R. S. (2000). Children's language learning: An interactionist perspective. *Journal of Child Psychology and Psychiatry: Annual Research Reviews, 41,* 33–54.

Cheatham, G. A., Santos, R. M. & Ro, Y. E. (2007). Home language acquisition and retention for young children with special needs. *Young Exceptional Children, 11*(1), 27–39.

Chmiel, R., Sutton, L., & Jenkins, H. (2000). Quality of life in children with cochlear implants. *Annals of Rhinology and Laryngology, 109*(Suppl. 185), 103–105.

Christiansen, J. B., & Leigh, I. W. (2002). *Cochlear implants in children–Ethics and choices.* Washington, DC: Gallaudet University Press.

Cole, K. N., Maddox, M. E., & Lim, Y. S. (2006). Language is the key: Constructive interactions around books and play. In R. J. McCauley & M. E. Fey (Eds.), *Treatment of language disorders in children* (pp. 149–173). Baltimore: Paul H. Brookes.

Coleman, P. K., & Karraker, K. H. (2003). Maternal self-efficacy beliefs, competence in parenting, and toddlers' behavior and developmental status. *Infant Mental Health Journal, 24,* 126–148.

Conrad, B., Gross, D., Fogg, L., & Ruchala, P. (1992). Maternal confidence, knowledge, and quality of mother-toddler interactions: A preliminary study. *Infant Mental Health Journal, 13,* 353–362.

DesJardin, J. L. (2003). Assessing parental perceptions of self-efficacy and involvement in families of young children with hearing loss. *Volta Review, 103*(4), 391–409.

DesJardin, J. L. (2006). Family empowerment: Supporting language development in young children who are deaf or hard of hearing, *Volta Review, 106,* 275–298.

DesJardin, J. L., Ambrose, S. A., & Eisenberg, L. S. (2009). Literacy skills in children with cochlear implants: The importance of early oral language and joint storybook reading. *Journal of Deaf Studies and Deaf Education, 14,* 22–43.

DesJardin, J. L., & Eisenberg, L. S. (2007). Maternal contributions: Supporting language development in children with cochlear implants. *Ear and Hearing, 28,* 456–469.

DesJardin, J. L., Eisenberg, L. S., & Hodapp, R. M. (2006). Sound beginnings: Supporting families of young deaf children with cochlear implants. *Infants and Young Children, 19,* 179–189.

de Valenzuela, J. S., & Niccolai, S. L. (2004). Language development in culturally and linguistically diverse students with special education needs. In L. M. Baca & H. T. Cervantes (Eds.), *The bilingual special education interface* (pp. 124–156). Upper Saddle River, NJ: Pearson Prentice-Hall.

Dromi, E., & Ingber, S. (1999). Israeli mothers' expectations from early intervention with their preschool deaf children. *Journal of Deaf Studies and Deaf Education, 4,* 50–68.

Dunst, C. J. (2000). Revisiting "Rethinking Early Intervention." *Topics in Early Childhood Special Education, 20*(2), 95–104.

Dunst, C. J. (2006). Parent-mediated everyday child learning opportunities: Foundations and operationalization. *CASEinPoint, 2*(2), 1–10.

Dunst, C. J., Bruder, M. B., Trivette, C. M., & Hamby, D. W. (2006). Everyday activity settings, natural learning environments, and early intervention practices. *Journal of Policy and Practice in Intellectual Disabilities, 3,* 3–10.

Dunst, C. J., Bruder, M. B., Trivette, C. M., Raab, M., & McLean, M. (2001). Natural learning opportunities for infants, toddlers, and preschoolers. *Young Exceptional Children, 4*(3), 18–25.

Dunst, C. J., & Hamby, D., Trivette, C. M., & Bruder, M. B. (2000). Everyday family and community life and children's naturally occurring learning opportunities. *Journal of Early Intervention, 23,* 151–164.

Dunst, C. J., Hamby, D., Trivette, C. M., Raab, M., & Bruder, M. B. (2002). Young children's participation in everyday family and community activity. *Psychological Reports, 91,* 875–897.

El-Kashlan, T. E., & Zwolan, T. A. (2008). Children with cochlear implants who live in monolingual and bilingual homes. *Otology and Neurotology, 29,* 230–234.

Estabrooks, W. (2007). The Auditory-Verbal approach: A professional point of view. In S. Schwartz (Ed.), *Choices in deafness* (3rd ed.). Bethesda, MD: Woodbine House.

Ezell, H. K., Justice, L. M., & Parsons, D. (2000). Enhancing the emergent literacy skills of preschoolers with communication disorders: A pilot investigation. *Child Language Teaching and Therapy, 16,* 121–140.

Fernald, A., & Morikawa, H. (1993). Common themes and cultural variations in Japanese and American mothers' speech to infants. *Child Development, 64,* 637–656.

Fewell, R. R., & Deutscher, B. (2004). Contributions of early language and maternal facilitation variables to later language and reading abilities. *Journal of Early Intervention, 26*(2), 132–145.

Fey, M. E., Krulik, T. E., Loeb, D. F., & Proctor-Williams, K. (1999). Sentence recast use by parents of children with typical language and children with specific language impairment. *American Journal of Speech-Language Pathology, 8,* 273–286.

Flaherty, J. (1999). *Coaching: Evoking excellence in others.* Boston: Butterworth-Heinemann.

Garber, A. S., & Nevins, M. E. (2007). The Newly Implanted Infant/Toddler. HOPE Notes Online Library, from http://www.cochlearamericas.com/Support/1837.asp

Geers, A., & Brenner, C. (2003). Background and educational characteristics of prelingually deaf children implanted by five years of age. *Ear and Hearing, 24*(Suppl. 1), 2S–14S.

Genesee, F., Paradis, J., & Crago, M. B. (2004). *Dual language development and disorders: A handbook on bilingualism and second language learning.* Baltimore: Paul H. Brookes.

Girolametto, L., & Weitzman, E. (2006). It takes two to talk—The Hanen Program for parents: Early language intervention through caregiver training. In R. J. McCauley & M. E. Fey (Eds.), *Treatment of language disorders in children* (pp. 77–103). Baltimore: Paul H. Brookes.

Girolametto, L., Weitzman, E., Wiigs, M., & Pearce, P. S. (1999). The relationship between maternal language measures and language development in toddlers with expressive vocabulary delays. *American Journal of Speech-Language Pathology, 8,* 364–374.

Goldstein, B. (2000). *Cultural and linguistic diversity resource guide for speech-language pathologists.* San Diego, CA: Singular/Thompson Learning.

Goldstein, B., & Kohnert, K. (2005). Speech, language, and hearing in developing bilingual children: Current findings and future directions. *Language, Speech, and Hearing Services in Schools, 36,* 264–267.

Gondoli, D. M., & Silverberg, S. B. (1997). Maternal emotional distress and diminished responsiveness: The mediating role of parenting efficacy and parental perspective taking. *Developmental Psychology, 33*(5), 861–868.

Goode, T. D. (2006). *Promoting cultural diversity and cultural competency: Self-assessment checklist for personnel providing behavioral health services and supports to children, youth, and their families.* Washington, DC: Georgetown University Center for Child & Human Development.

Guralnick, M. J. (2005). Early intervention for children with intellectual disabilities: Current knowledge and future prospects. *Journal of Applied Research in Intellectual Disabilities, 18,* 313–324.

Hadadian, A. (1995). Attitudes toward deafness and security of attachment relationships among young deaf children and their parents. *Early Education and Development, 6,* 181–191.

Hancock, T. B., Kaiser, A. P., & Delaney, E. M. (2002). Teaching parents of preschoolers at high risk: Strategies to support language and positive behavior. *Topics in Early Childhood Education, 22*, 191–212.

Hanft, B. E., Rush, D. D., & Shelden, M. L. (2004). *Coaching families and colleagues in early childhood intervention.* Baltimore: Paul H. Brookes.

Hanson, M. J., & Lynch, E. W. (2004). *Understanding families: Approaches to diversity, disability and risk.* Baltimore: Paul H. Brookes.

Hart, B., & Risley, T. R. (1995). *Meaningful differences in the everyday experience of young American children.* Baltimore: Paul H. Brookes.

Hart, B., & Risley, T. R. (1999). Observing children and families talking. In B. Hart & T.R. Risley (Eds.), *The social world of children learning to talk* (pp. 7–29). Baltimore: Paul H. Brookes.

Hastings, R. (1997). Grandparents of children with disabilities: A review. *International Journal of Disability, Development and Education, 44*, 329–340.

Hintermair, M. (2006). Parental resources, parental stress, and socioemotional development of deaf and hard of hearing children. *Journal of Deaf Studies and Deaf Education, 11*(4), 493–513.

Hoff, E. (2000). *Language development.* Pacific Grove, CA: Brooks/Cole.

Incesulu, A., Vural, M., & Erkam, U. (2003). Children with cochlear implants: Parental perspective. *Otology and Neurotology, 24*, 605–611.

Individuals with Disabilities Education Improvement Act of 2004. (2004). Amendments to the Individual with Disabilities Education Act. Public Law 108-446. Retrieved March 18, 2008, from http://www.copyright.gov/legislation/pl108-446.pdf

Jackson, A. P., & Huang, C. C. (2000). Parenting stress and behavior among single mothers of preschoolers: The mediating role of self-efficacy. *Journal of Social Service Research, 26*, 29–42.

Johnston, J. R., & Wong, M. (2002). Cultural differences in beliefs and practices concerning talk to children. *Journal of Speech, Language, and Hearing Research, 45*(5), 916–926.

Jung, L. A. (2007). Writing individualized family service plan strategies that fit into the routine. *Young Exceptional Children, 10*(3), 2–9.

Justice, L. M., & Pence, K. (2007). Parent-implemented interactive language intervention: Can it be used effectively? *EBP Briefs, 2*(1), 1–13.

Kaiser, A. P., & Hancock, T. B. (2003). Teaching parents new skills to support their young children's development. *Infants and Young Children, 16*, 9–21.

Kinlaw, D. C. (1999). *Coaching for commitment: Interpersonal strategies for obtaining superior performance from individuals and teams.* San Francisco: Jossey-Bass/Pfeiffer.

Kohnert, K. (2007). Supporting two languages in bilingual children with primary developmental language disorders. *Bilingual children and adults.* San Diego, CA: Plural.

Kohnert, K., & Derr, A. (2004). Language intervention with bilingual children. In B. Goldstein (Ed.), *Bilingual language development and disorders in Spanish-English speakers* (pp. 315–343). Baltimore: Paul H. Brookes.

Kohnert, K., Yim, D., Nett, K., Kan, P. F., & Duran, L. (2005). Intervention with linguistically diverse preschool children: A focus on developing home languages. *Language, Speech, and Hearing Services in Schools, 36*, 251–263.

Kuhn, J. C., & Carter, A. S. (2006). Maternal self-efficacy and associated parenting cognitions among mothers of children with autism, *American Journal of Orthopsychiatry, 76*(4), 564–575.

Lamb, M. E., & Lewis, C. (2004). The development and significance of father-child relationships in two parent families. In M. E. Lamb (Ed.), *The role of the father in child development* (4th ed., pp. 272–306). New York: Wiley.

Lamb, M. E., & Tamis-LeMonda, C. S. (2004). The role of the father: An introduction. In M. E. Lamb (Ed.), *The role of the father in child development* (4th ed., pp. 272–306). New York: Wiley.

Leseman, P., & van Tuijl, C. (2001). Home support for bilingual development of Turkish 4- to 6-year-old immigrant children in the Netherlands: Efficacy of a home-based educational programme. *Journal of Multilingual and Multicultural Development, 22,* 309–324.

Levi, A, V., Boyett-Solano, J., Nicholson, B., & Eisenberg, L. S. (2001). Multilingualism and children with cochlear implants. *Hearing Review.* Retrieved from http://www.hearing review.com/issues/articles/2001-06_02.asp

Lim, Y. S., & Cole, K. N. (2002). Facilitating first language development in Korean children through parent training in picture book interactions. *Bilingual Research Journal, 26,* 213–227.

Lim, S. Y. C., & Simser, J. (2005). Auditory-verbal therapy for children with hearing impairment. *Annals of Academy of Medicine Singapore, 34*(4), 307–312.

Lopez, L. M., & Greenfield, D. B. (2004). The cross-language transfer of phonological skills of Hispanic Head Start children. *Bilingual Research Journal, 28,* 1–18.

Lynch, E. W., & Hanson, M. J. (Eds.). (2004). *Developing cross-cultural competence: A guide for working with children and their families* (3rd ed.). Baltimore: Paul H. Brookes.

McCauley, R. J., & Fey, M. E. (2006). *Treatment of language disorders in children.* Baltimore: Paul H. Brookes.

McNeil, J., & Fowler, S. (1999). Let's talk: Encouraging mother-child conversations during story reading. *Journal of Early Intervention, 22,* 51–69.

McWilliam, R. (2000). It's only natural . . . to have early intervention in the environments where it's needed. In S. Sandall & M. Ostrosky (Eds.), *YEC Monograph Series: Natural environments and inclusion* (pp. 17–26). Longmont, CO: Sopris West.

McWilliam, R., & Scott, S. (2001). A support approach to early intervention: A three-part framework. *Infants and Young Children, 13,* 55–66.

Meadow-Orlans, K. P., Mertens, D. M., & Sass-Lehrer, M. A. (2003). *Parents and their deaf children: The early years.* Washington, DC: Gallaudet University Press.

Mitchell, W. (2007). Research review: The role of grandparents in intergenerational support for families with disabled children: A review of the literature. *Child and Family Social Work,* 12, 94–101.

Moeller, M. P. (2000). Early intervention and language development in children who are deaf and hard of hearing. *Pediatrics, 106*(3), 1–9.

Moore, J. A., Prath, S., & Arrieta, A. (2006). Early Spanish speech acquisition following cochlear implantation, *Volta Review, 106,* 321–341.

Moore, S. M., & Perez-Mendez, C. (2003). *Cultural contexts for early intervention: Working with families.* Rockville, MD: American Speech-Language-Hearing Association.

Most, T., & Zaidman-Zait, A. (2003). The needs of parents of children with cochlear implants. *Volta Review, 103,* 99–113.

Nelson, K. E., Camarata, S. M., Welsh, J., Butkovsky, L., & Camarata, M. (1996). Effects of imitative and conversational recasting treatment on the acquisition of grammar in children with specific language impairment and younger language-normal children. *Journal of Speech and Hearing Research, 39,* 850–859.

Nicholas, J. G., & Geers, A. E. (2006). The process and early outcomes of cochlear implantation by three years of age. In P. E. Spencer & M. Marschark (Eds.), *Advances in the spoken language development of deaf and hard-of-hearing children* (pp. 271–297). Oxford: Oxford University Press.

Nikolopoulos, T. P., Lloyd, H., Archbold, S., & O'Donoghue, G. M. (2001). Pediatric cochlear implantation: The parents' perspective. *Archives of Otolaryngology-Head and Neck Surgery, 127,* 363–367.

Nunes, T., Pretzlik, U., & Ilicka, S. (2005). Validation of a parent outcome questionnaire from pediatric cochlear implantation. *Journal of Deaf Studies and Deaf Education, 10*(4), 330–356.

Nybo, W. L., Scherman, A., & Freeman, P. (1998). Grandparents' role in family systems with a deaf child: An exploratory study. *American Annals of the Deaf, 143,* 260–267.

Ozer, E. M. (1995). The impact of childcare responsibility and self-efficacy on the psychological health of professional working mothers. *Psychology of Women Quarterly, 19,* 315–335.

Pepper, J., & Weitzman, E. (2004). *It takes two to talk: A practical guide for parents of children with language delays.* Ontario, Canada: The Hanen Centre.

Pleck, J. H., & Masciadrelli, B. P. (2004). Paternal involvement by U.S. residential fathers: Levels, sources, and consequences. In M. E. Lamb (Ed.), *The role of the father in child development* (4th ed., pp. 272–306). New York: Wiley.

Proctor-Williams, K., Fey, M. E., & Loeb, D. F. (2001). Parental recasts and production of copulas and articles by children with specific language impairment and typical language. *American Journal of Speech-Language Pathology*, *10*, 155–168.

Pruett, K. D. (1997). How men and children affect each other's development. *Zero to Three Journal*, *18*, 1–10.

Quesenberry, A., Ostrovsky, M. M., & Corso, R. (2007). Skilled and knowledgeable caregivers: The role of fathers in supporting young children's development. *Young Exceptional Children*, *10*(4), 11–19.

Raikes, H. A., & Thompson, R. A. (2005). Efficacy and social support as predictors of parenting stress among families in poverty. *Infant Mental Health Journal*, *26*(3), 177–190.

Rhoades, E. A. (2007). Setting the stage for culturally responsive intervention. *Volta Voices*, *14*(4), 10–13.

Robbins, A. M., Green, J. E., & Waltzman, S. B. (2004). Bilingual oral language proficiency in children with cochlear implants, *Archives of Otolaryngology-Head and Neck Surgery*, *130*, 644–647.

Roper, N., & Dunst, C. J. (2003). Communication intervention in natural learning environments: Guidelines for practice. *Infants and Young Children*, *16*(3), 215–226.

Roseberry-McKibbin, C., Brice, A., & O'Hanlon, L. (2005). Serving English language learners in public school settings: A National Survey. *Language, Speech, and Hearing Services in Schools*, *36*, 48–61.

Rosenkoetter, S., & Barton, L. R. (2002). Bridges to literacy: Early routines that promote later school success. *Zero to Three*, *22*(4), 33–38.

Rush, D. D., Shelden, M. L., & Hanft, B. E. (2003). Coaching families and colleagues: A process for collaboration in natural settings. *Infants and Young Children*, *16*(1), 33–47.

Sach, T. H., & Whynes, D. K. (2005). Pediatric cochlear implantation: The views of parents. *International Journal of Audiology*, *44*, 400–407.

Sahu, F. M., & Rath, S. (2003). Self-efficacy and wellbeing in working and non-working women: The moderating role of involvement. *Psychology and Developing Societies*, *15*, 187–200.

Salas-Provance, M. B., Erickson, J. G., & Reed, J. (2002). Disabilities as viewed by four generations of one Hispanic family. *American Journal of Speech-Language Pathology*, *11*(2), 151–162.

Sandall, S., Hemmeter, M. L., Smith, B. J., & McLean, M. E. (Eds.). (2005). *DEC recommended practices: A comprehensive guide for practical application in early intervention/early childhood special education*. Longmont, CO: Sopris West.

Sandler, A. G., Warren, S. H., & Raver, S. A. (1995). Grandparents as a source of support for parents of children with disabilities: A brief report. *Mental Retardation*, *33*, 248–250.

Scorgie, K., Wilgosh, L., & McDonald, L. (1998). Stress and coping in families of children with disabilities: An examination of recent literature. *Developmental Disabilities Bulletin*, *26*, 22–42.

Shelden, M. L., & Rush, D. D. (2001). The ten myths about providing early intervention services in natural environments. *Infants and Young Children*, *14*(1), 1–13.

Shonkoff, J. P., & Meisels, S. J. (Eds.). (2000) *Handbook of Early Childhood Intervention* (2nd ed.). Cambridge: Cambridge University Press.

Shonkoff, J. P., & Phillips, D. A. (Eds.). (2000). *From neurons to neighborhoods: The science of early childhood development*. Washington, DC: National Academy Press.

Sjoblad, S., Harrison, M., Roush, J., & McWilliam, R. A. (2001). Parents' reactions and recommendations after diagnosis and hearing aid fitting. *American Journal of Audiology*, *10*, 24–31.

Spagnola, M., & Fiese, B. H. (2007). Family routines and rituals: A context for development in the lives of young children. *Infants and Young Children*, *20*(4), 284–299.

Spahn, C., Richter, B., Zschocke, I., Lohle, E., & Wirsching, M. (2001). The need for psychosocial support in parents with cochlear implant children. *International Journal of Pediatric Otorhinolaryngology, 57,* 45–53.

Spencer, P. E. (2001, March). *Language performance of children with early cochlear implantation: Child and family factors.* Paper presented at the 8th Symposium on Cochlear Implants in Children, Los Angeles, CA.

Spencer, P. E. (2004). Individual differences in language performance after cochlear implantation at one to three years of age: Child, family, and linguistic factors. *Journal of Deaf Studies and Deaf Education, 9,* 395–412.

Sylva, J. A. (2005). Issues in Early Intervention: The impact of cultural diversity on service delivery in natural environments. *Multicultural Education, 13*(2), 26–29.

Tabors, P. O. (1997). *One child, two languages: Children learning English as a second language.* Baltimore: Paul H. Brookes.

Teti, D. M., & Gelfand, D. M. (1991). Behavioral competence among mothers of infants in the first year: The mediational role of maternal self-efficacy. *Child Development, 62,* 918–929.

Teti, D. M., & O'Connell, M. A., & Reiner, C. D. (1996). Parenting sensitivity, parental depression, and child health: The mediational role of parental self-efficacy. *Early Development and Parenting, 5*(4), 237–250.

Trivette, C. M., & Dunst, C. J. (2000). Recommended practices in family-based practices. In S. Sandall, M. E. McLean, & B. J. Smith (Eds.), *DEC recommended practices in early intervention/early childhood special education* (pp. 39–46). Longmont, CO: Sopris West.

Trivette, C. M., & Dunst, C. J. (2003). *Parenting Experiences Scale.* Morganton, NC: Orelena Hawks Puckett Institute.

Trute, B. (2003). Grandparents of children with developmental disabilities: Intergenerational support and well-being. *Families in Society: Journal of Contemporary Human Services, 84,* 119–126.

Turbiville, V. P., Turnbull, A. P., & Turnbull, H. (1995). Fathers and family-centered intervention. *Infants and Young Children, 7,* 12–19.

Turnbull, A. P., Turbiville, V., & Turnbull, H. R. (2000). Evolution of family-professional partnerships: Collective empowerment as the model for the early twenty-first century. In J. P. Shonkoff & S. J. Meisels (Eds.), *Handbook of early childhood intervention,* (2nd ed., pp. 630–650). New York: Cambridge University Press.

Turnbull, A. P., & Turnbull, H. R. (2001). *Families, professionals, and exceptionality: Collaborating for empowerment* (4th ed.). Upper Saddle River, NJ: Merrill Prentice Hall.

Valdez-Menchaca, M. C., & Whitehurst, G. J. (1992). Accelerating language development through picture book reading: A systematic extension to Mexican daycare. *Developmental Psychology, 28,* 1106–1114.

van Kleeck, A. (1994). Potential cultural bias in training parents as conversational partners with their children who have delays in language development. *American Journal of Speech-Language Pathology, 3,* 67–78.

Vygotsky, L. (1962). *Thought and language.* Cambridge, MA: MIT Press.

Walsh, S., Rous, B., & Lutzer, C. (2000). The federal IDEA natural environments provisions. In S. Sandall & M. Ostrosky (Eds.), *Young Exceptional Children Monograph Series No. 2* (pp. 3–15). Denver, CO: Division for Early Childhood of the Council for Exceptional Children.

Waltzman, S. B., Robbins, A. M., Green, J. E., & Cohen, N. L. (2003). Second oral language capabilities in children with cochlear implants. *Otology and Neurotology, 24,* 757–763.

Warren, S. F., Bredin-Oja, S. L., Escalante, M. F., Finestack, L. H., Fey, M. E., & Brady, N. C. (2006). Responsivity education/Prelinguistic milieu teaching. In R. J. McCauley & M. E. Fey (Eds.), *Treatment of language disorders in children* (pp. 47–75). Baltimore: Brookes.

Watson, K. (2007). Language, education and ethnicity: Whose rights will prevail in an age of globalisation? *International Journal of Educational Development, 27*(3), 252–265.

Watson, L. M., Hardie, T., Archbold, S. M., & Wheeler, A. (2007). Parents' views on changing communication after cochlear implantation.

Journal of Deaf Studies and Deaf Education, 13, 104-116.

Weisel, A., Most, T., & Michael, R. (2007). Mothers' stress and expectations as a function of time since child's cochlear implantation. *Journal of Deaf Studies and Deaf Education, 12*(1), 55-64.

Weitzman, E. (1994). The Hanen Program for early childhood educators: Inservice training for child care providers on how to facilitate children's social, language, and literacy development. *Infant-Toddler Intervention: The Transdisciplinary Journal, 4,* 173-202.

Weizman, Z. O., & Snow, C. E. (2001). Lexical input as related to children's vocabulary acquisition: Effects of sophisticated exposure and support for meaning. *Developmental Psychology, 37,* 265-279.

Wiig, E., Secord, W., & Semel, E. (1992). *Clinical Evaluation of Language Fundamentals-Preschool.* San Antonio, TX: Psychological Corporation, Harcourt Brace.

Woods, J., Kashinath, S., & Goldstein, H. (2004). Effects of embedding caregiver-implemented teaching strategies in daily routines on children's communication outcomes. *Journal of Early Intervention, 26*(3), 175-193.

Wyatt, T. A. (2002). Assessing the communicative abilities of clients from diverse cultural and language backgrounds. In D. E. Battle (Ed.), *Communication disorders in multicultural populations* (3rd ed., pp. 415-459). Boston: Butterworth-Heinemann.

Yoder, P. J., McCathren, R. B., Warren, S. F., & Watson, A. L. (2001). Important distinctions in measuring maternal responses to communication in prelinguistic children with disabilities. *Communication Disorders Quarterly, 22*(3), 135-147.

Yoder, P. J., & Warren, S. F. (1998). Maternal responsivity predicts the prelinguistic communication intervention that facilitates generalized intentional communication. *Journal of Speech, Language, and Hearing Research, 41,* 1207-1219.

Yoder, P. J., & Warren, S. F. (2002). Effects of prelinguistic milieu teaching and parent responsivity education on dyads involving children with intellectual disabilities. *Journal of Speech, Language, and Hearing Research, 45*(6), 1158-1174.

Zaidman-Zait, A. (2007). Parenting a child with a cochlear implant: A critical incident study. *Journal of Deaf Studies and Deaf Education, 12*(2), 221-241.

Zaidman-Zait, A., & Jamieson, J. R. (2004). Searching the cochlear implant information of the internet maze: Implications for parents and professionals. *Journal of Deaf Studies and Deaf Education, 9,* 413-426.

Zaidman-Zait, A., & Most, T. (2005). Cochlear implants in children with hearing loss: Maternal expectations and impact on the family. *Volta Review, 105,* 129-150.

Zaidman-Zait, A., & Young, R. A. (2008). Parental involvement in the habilitation process following children's cochlear implantation: An action theory perspective. *Journal of Deaf Studies and Deaf Education, 13*(2), 193-214.

Zhang, C., & Bennett, T. (2003). Facilitating the meaningful participation of culturally and linguistically diverse families in the IFSP and IEP process. *Focus on Autism and Other Developmental Disabilities, 18*(1), 51-59.

CHAPTER 18

Working with Children from Lower SES Families: Understanding Health Disparities

DANA L. SUSKIND
SARAH GEHLERT

Introduction

Socioeconomic status (SES) has been demonstrated to be a significant determinant of health in children and adults (Shavers, 2007). There also is evidence that medical advances, especially those involving complex regimens, preferentially benefit higher SES individuals (Goldman & Lakdawall, 2005). Although the field of pediatric cochlear implantation (CI) is relatively new, SES increasingly is observed to be a significant factor in both rates of implantation and postimplant outcomes (Geers, 2006; Hodges, Eilers, & Cobo-Lewis, 1994; Hyde & Power, 2006; Sorkin & Zwolan, 2008). In fact, often the greatest challenge to the professional caring for the low SES implanted child is not the operation itself, but instead surmounting the psychosocial obstacles postimplantation. Although many children of low SES thrive after implantation, a significant subset fail to reach their full potential due to the obstacles presented by the world in which they live.

Successful implantation has a tremendous impact on the life trajectory of children and produces significant societal cost-savings (Cheng et al., 2000; Easterbrooks, O'Rourke, & Todd, 2000; Francis, Koch, Wyatt, & Niparko, 1999; Mohr et al., 2000). Addressing the disparities in rates of implantation and postimplantation success, therefore, has important benefits for individuals, families, and society as a whole. The challenge of professionals in the field of cochlear implantation is to discern the factors, individual and environmental, that affect outcomes in order to develop strategies to effect positive change.

This chapter provides information on health disparities in general as well as in pediatric implantation. We attempt to provide a framework from which to study and address inequities.

Health Disparities as a Critical Factor

Health disparities are described as the "unequal burden in disease morbidity and mortality rates experienced by ethnic/racial groups as compared to the dominant group" (U.S. Department of Health and Human Services [USDHHS], 2004, p. 3). The profound, widening health care gap in the United States is of great concern to the medical community. The U.S. Department of Health and Human Services *Healthy People 2010* has designated the elimination of health disparities as one of its essential goals (USDHHS, 2000). Studies are being conducted in all areas in which disparities occur, from pediatric asthma to breast cancer; almost no area is unaffected. One target of Healthy People

2010 is improving the "hearing health of the nation through prevention, early detection, treatment and rehabilitation" (National Institute on Deafness and Other Communication Disorders [NIDCD], 2004). The plan is to increase the proportion of infants undergoing the 1-2-3 6 guidelines (screening, diagnosis and intervention for hearing loss) and the number of individuals with severe to profound hearing loss who use cochlear implants (NIDCD, 2004).

Although the etiology of health disparities is complex, SES appears to be both the most frequently cited and most consistent contributor (Adler & Rehkopf, 2008). SES, usually defined by income, education, wealth, or a combination of the three, essentially translates into people having the requisite resources to receive and sustain good healthcare (Shavers, 2007). Seventeen percent of children in the United States live at or below the federal poverty line (i.e., below 150% of poverty), *more than in any other segment of the population* (U.S. Census Bureau [USCB], 2006). As shown in Table 18-1, this percentage increases significantly along racial and ethnic lines. Thirty-three percent

TABLE 18–1. Poverty and Health Insurance Coverage: Disparities Along Racial and Ethnic Lines

Race	Below 100% of Poverty**	Below 150% of Poverty**	Health Insurance (Hi)		
			Private Hi*	Public Hi*	Uninsured*
White	13.8%	24.3%	71.6%	20.5%	7.9%
African American	32.6%	46.9%	40.5%	48.3%	11.3%
Asian	11.3%	18.9%			
Hispanic	26.6%	45.6%	30.5%	49.9%	19.7%
All children	16.9%	28.1%	57.8%	31.0%	11.7%

*Percentages from 2005 data.
**Percentages from 2006 data.

of African American children and 27% of Hispanic children live in poverty. Almost 50% of African American and 50% of Hispanic children are on public insurance (USDHHS, 2003). An additional 11% of African American and almost 20% of Hispanic children have no insurance at all. Robust SES gradients clearly indicate this socioeconomic stratum suffers the most ill health compared to the highest, which enjoys the best (Minkler, Fuller-Thomson, & Guralnik, 2006).

The actual modes of influence, however, are not entirely understood (Adler & Rehkopk, 2008). Adler hypothesizes that SES affects health outcomes via three fundamental mechanisms: health care, environmental exposure, and health behavior/lifestyle (Adler & Newman, 2002). In other words, health outcomes will be influenced societally via the lack of available health care and/or toxins such as lead exposure or poor housing conditions and, individually, because of health/lifestyle behavior, which itself is influnced by societal factors, such as placement of grocery stores that sell fresh fruits and vegetables. The chronic stress related to poverty, for example, "uncertainty, conflict, and threats" and feelings of hopelessness/helplessness in controlling one's destiny also is believed to result in physiologic and behavioral "adaptions" which negatively affect health (Adler & Newman, 2002; Adler & Rehkopf, 2008; Harper et al., 2002; McEwen & Seeman, 1999). This chronic stress, that is, "allostatic load," has been seen in children of poverty where it has been shown to mediate the relationship of school absences to illness and poor housing conditions (Evans, 2003; Johnston-Brooks, Lewis, Evans, & Whalen, 1998). Interestingly, advances in medical technology initially often widen the health care gap by preferentially benefitting higher SES individuals (Goldman & Lakdawall, 2005). This is especially true when the advances entail complex regimens, such as postimplant habilitation.

Health Disparities in Pediatric Cochlear Implantation

Although the field of pediatric cochlear implantation still is relatively young, there already are strong indications that a disparity exists in both rates of implantation and outcomes between lower SES and minority children and their more affluent counterparts (Geers & Brenner, 2003; Hoff & Tian, 2005; Hyde & Power, 2006; Sorkin & Zwolan, 2008).

Disparities in Hearing-Impaired Ethnic Minorities: A Double Jeopardy

The disparities among deaf children of low SES compared to children of affluence are not unlike the disparities found in their hearing counterparts. The tragedy is compounded, however, by the fact that, isolated from the hearing world, deaf children have much less chance to break through the barrier and reach their true potential. Deaf children of poverty are more likely to be incorrectly diagnosed as learning disabled, less likely to be mainstreamed, and much more likely to drop out of school (Bowen, 2000; Kluwin, 1994; Nuru, 1993; Stewart & Benson, 1988; Wolbers, 2002). This results in deaf minorities being more likely to be unemployed or, if employed, working at vocational jobs earning significantly less than their white or Asian deaf counterparts (MacLeod-Gallinger, 1997).

Early Hearing Detection and Intervention (EHDI)

The universal newborn hearing screening (UNHS) and the "1-3-6 guidelines," which became federal mandates in 1999, are critical for early diagnosis and implantation (Joint Committee on Infant Hearing, et al., 2000). The best practice guidelines recommend hearing screening by one month, diagnosis by three months and intervention by six months has significantly decreased the average age of diagnosis and intervention. Although UNHS represents a tremendous advancement for the field of hearing loss, there continues to be a signficant loss to follow-up after failed initial screening in 59.9% of the children (U.S. Department of Health and Human Services, 2005). Among children living in poverty, however, the rate is significantly higher (Brach et al., 2003; Liu, Farrell, MacNeil, Stone & Barfield, 2005; Liu et al., 2008; Sommers, 2005; Vohr, Moore, & Tucker, 2002). Massachusetts, for example, despite having an excellent follow-up and intervention record for failed newborn hearing screening, found that children who were ethnic minorities or publicly insured were one and a half to two times more likely to be lost to follow-up for audiologic evaluation after failing the newborn screening (Liu et al., 2008). These data are significant indicators for the ultimate disparity in implantation rates.

Implantation Rates

Implantation rates based on income and ethnicity have been noted by a number of investigators (Fortnum, Marshall, & Summerfield, 2002; Stern, Yueh, Lewis, Norton, & Sie, 2005; Sorkin & Zwolan, 2008). Stern's initial report demonstrated that white children were implanted at "relative rates" 5 to 10 times that of Hispanic and African American children (Stern et al., 2005). Sorkin and Zwolan (2008) found that African American children comprised only 1.4% of a randomized sample from a CI manufacturer's database, although comprising 12.3% of the U.S. population. White children, on the other hand, made up 88.5% of the sample although comprising only 75.1% of the U.S. population. An income disparity also was noted. Children living in poverty (<$25,000) made up only 12.8% of the sample versus their U.S. population levels of 28.7%; those with incomes >$100,000 made up 23.6% of the sample versus a U.S. population level of 12.3%. These statistics were supported by Wiley, Meinzen-Derr, and Arjmand (2007), who noted that deaf children who were of lower SES, of single parents and/or nonwhite were signficantly less likely than their more affluent counterparts to be referred for cochlear implant evaluation. Fortnum et al. (2002) noted a similar situation in the United Kingdom where, theoretically, the issue of implant coverage does not exist because of the National Health Care Service.

Auditory, Speech, and Language Outcomes

Successful outcome in pediatric cochlear implantation is dependent on postimplantation habilitation. From the beginning, the literature indicated the role of SES in this success (Hodges et al., 1994). In their presentation, "The Effects of Socioeconomic Status on Pediatric Cochlear Implant Users," Hodges et al. (1994) reported that children's performances educationally were correlated with their SES. Several years later, Hodges et al. (1999) noted that SES significantly contributed to speech perception abilities. In "Cochlear Implants in Children: What Constitutes a Complication?" Luetje and Jackson (1997) noted that SES was one of the four predictors of postimplantation success. The literature continues to demonstrate the effect of SES on postimplantation success. Tobey, Geers, Brenner, Altuna, and Gabbert (2003) found that SES was a significant independent factor in speech production in children implanted by age five years. Geers (2006) noted that higher parental income and education are important 'family factors' influencing language outcomes in children undergoing early implantation. In another study, Geers (2003) also found that reading competence was associated with higher family income level. Connor and Zwolan (2004) reported that low SES status significantly affected reading comprehension scores in implanted children.

Although the effect of SES is undeniable, it is important to explore the components that produce the effects. It has become apparent that the inequities noted are not the result of lack of potential in the children, but from forces preventing them from reaching that potential. Although we have evidence of existing inequities, a true understanding of their root causes has yet to be explored. Connor and Zwolan (2004) concluded that research on the effects of SES on outcomes with cochlear implants in children is important.

What Next? Understanding and Addressing Disparities in Pediatric Implantation

Disparities in cochlear implantation mirror the more global problem of poverty. Professionals in our field are in a unique position; we understand both the clinical problems attached to cochlear implantation and the habilitation necessary to make the implantation a success. We also are able to analyze the reasons for lack of success and to devise programs to correct problems. As professionals, it is our mandate to point out discrepancies in access to cochlear implantation and to help devise guidelines and national policies to eliminate disparities so that

income level is not a factor in a child's being given access to the world of sound. Above all, we must advocate for the population of children that cannot speak for itself and may have no one else to speak for it.

Horn and Beal (2004) designed a three staged approach to childhood health disparities: (1) identification of the health disparity, (2) determination of its root causes, and (3) development of effective interventions with a continual two directional association between steps two and three (Figure 18–1).

Understanding the Root Causes of Pediatric Implant Disparities

"Child health disparities research is integral to all areas of child research" (Horn & Beal, 2004, p. 269)

Research is an essential first step in understanding of the causes of cochlear implantation disparities. Factors, such as income, educational level, environment, health behaviors and governmental, health system and societal components, including their synergistic interactions must be explored.

Audiologists' Experiences: A National Survey

A recent study by Kirkam et al. (2008) surveyed pediatric cochlear implant audiologists throughout the United States to better understand *perceptions* of outcome disparities in lower SES implanted children. Questions included the perceived importance of patient insurance status, access to habilitation resources, role of parents in the CI process, and potential support strategies. One hundred and four (44%) pediatric audiologists responded to the survey. Several

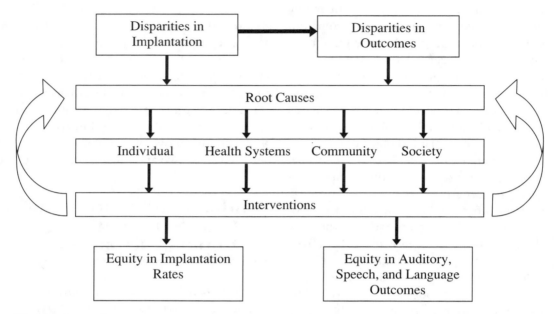

Figure 18–1. Eliminating health disparities in cochlear implantation is a multistep process. Adapted from Horn and Beal, 2004, p. 273.

interesting themes emerged, including the negative impact of SES on CI outcomes (78%), adherence to treatment recommendations as an issue in low SES families (89%) and limited parental involvement as a contributor to outcome disparities. Overwhelmingly, *increasing parental involvement* was seen as having the greatest potential for positive change.

Implications for Professionals Caring for Implanted Children

It is well known that health promotions that do not directly target individuals of low SES

background will widen rather than lessen health group differences in health (Adler, 2003). Antismoking initiatives, for example, more successfully decreased smoking in the educated versus uneducated, leading to a significant disparity in smoking rates and to smoking-related morbidity and mortality (Adler, 2003). This lesson should not be lost on those designing strategies for increasing awareness and participation among lower SES parents of implanted children.

Delineating a research agenda is beyond the scope of this chapter. Table 18-2, however, lays out potential areas that may be targeted and potential strategies to improve outcomes.

TABLE 18–2. Multilevel Examples of Potential Root Causes and Strategies to Address Implantation and Outcome Disparities*

Levels		Potential Causes	Potential Strategies
Individual	Child	Late Age of Implantation	1. Increased coordination and funding of UNHS & EHDI to lower age of implantation
	Parent-child	1. Limited Parental Self-Efficacy, Involvement in and Understanding of Habilitation; 2. Nonfacilitative Parental Linguistic Characteristics	1. Incorporate Education, Empowerment, Self-Efficacy Training Programs into EI/preschool and Implant Programs, 2. Comprehensive Social Services
	Family	1. Health Behaviors Negatively Affecting Adherence to Medical and educational recommendations	1. Incorporate Education, Empowerment, Self-Efficacy Training Programs into EI/preschool Programs, 2. Comprehensive Social Services
Health systems	Provider	1. Sociocultural and Language Barriers 2. Access barriers and wait times for Quality Habilitation 3. Distance/Number of Implant Centers	1. Define and implement standards for bias-free option discussion by early providers 2. Improved Reimbursement of Implant-related Services 3. Cultural Competent Health care 4. Increased Training and Community Partnership to allow for service provision in Critical need areas
	Local	1. Fragmentation of EHDI education and coordination 2. Limited reimbursement of surgery and habilitation services	1. Implement evidence-based standards of care for coordination of EI services 2. Improved reimbursement for services
	National	Inadequate workforce (both quantity and training) for post implant habilitation	National Training Programs directed toward local service providers (i.e., PPCI)

continues

561

TABLE 18–2. *continued*

Levels		Potential Causes	Potential Strategies
Community	Neighborhood	Isolation of Low SES families with implanted children	Parent Networking Opportunities Facilitated through EHDI and EI
	Local government	1. Limited Quality and Access of Listening and Spoken Language Development Programs in Early Intervention and Public School Systems; 2. Poor transition between EI programs and Preschool	1. Increased partnership between implant teams and community CI service providers 2. Increased funding of professional training programs 3. Develop and implement policy and procedures to ensure seamless transitions
Societal	Community and Federal government	Inadequate Funding and Public Support for Early Intervention Programs and Medicaid Reimbursement	Public health initiatives to increase awareness of Societal Cost Savings/ Benefit of Successful Implantation in Children

*SES indicates socioeconomic status.

Universal Newborn Hearing Screen (UNHS) and Early Hearing Detection Intervention (EHDI)

UNHS and EHDI are monumental milestones in the diagnosis and treatment of children with hearing loss. Both are crucial for giving all children the potential to auditory access. Although health promotions may improve *overall* health, specific strategies are essential to decrease or prevent the widening health disparities between groups with different SES in the United States (Adler, 2003). One method of mitigating EHDI disparities is to initiate evidence-based practices that

decrease the loss to follow-up which is significantly more common in underprivileged children (Liu et al., 2008; Vohr et al., 2002).

The Liu et al. (2008) recommendations for Massachusetts SES-related disparities in EHDI " . . . include(d) modification of the data system to flag high-risk families for priority contact, collaboration with other state programs, development of culturally and linguistically sensitive outreach and educational materials, and improvement in transportation and in the number and location of ADCs" (Liu et al., 2008, p. e342). Francozo Mde, Fernandes, Lima, and Rossi (2007) found that an intensive education program by hospital social workers aimed at mothers from "economically underprivileged populations" prior to hospital discharge significantly decreased their "loss to follow-up" after failure of UNHS.

In addition, an evidence-based, bias-free consultation regarding the habilitation options for children diagnosed with deafness is necessary. Individuals with health literacy and Internet savvy are able to research in greater depths the options available to their children. In contrast, those limited by inadequate health literacy and the "digital divide" are completely reliant on the counsel of their pediatrician and early interventionists.

Access to Quality Habilitation: Early Intervention and Preschool Programs

Excellent early intervention (EI) and preschool programs are essential to postimplantation success. Affluential parents of implanted children are able to pay for private, after-school, programs that supplement those given in schools (Barton, Fortnum, Stacy, & Summerfield, 2006; Sach, Whynes, Archbold, & O'Donoghue, 2005; Sorkin & Zwolan, 2008). Low SES children, however, are completely dependent on government-sponsored, often less than adequate, programs. Nobel Laureate economist James Heckman has stated that early, accessible to all intervention programs are both the "just" approach and the pragmatic one based on cost-benefit analyses (Heckman, 2006). This "just," economically sound approach for early, excellent intervention applies to all children, including those who are deaf.

Specialized listening and spoken language programs incorporated into early intervention programs are critical to successful postimplantation. Approximately only half of children with hearing loss are enrolled in

EI programs. In addition, in order to secure excellent programs, including those outside of schools, many parents have to pay "out of pocket." These challenges make outcome differentials much less surprising (Barton et al., 2006; Sach et al., 2005; Sorkin & Zwolan, 2008).

Archbold and O'Donoghue (2007), in discussing how to expand cochlear implant services to all and to sustain these services in the long term, stressed the importance of moving from a specialist who is clinic-based to service providers who are community-based by harnessing the potential of parents and teachers. This community partnership, in which professionals most familiar with the child are trained and educated to provide quality, socioculturally sensitive listening and spoken language habilitation, would allow services to be centered at home and at school. This is especially critical for individuals living in remote areas, where the advantages of telemedicine have been discussed. Charles Grim, assistant surgeon general, discussed the objective of elevating health status of Native Americans and Native Alaskans, noting that audiology telepractice for aural rehabilitation and cochlear implant programming/mapping may offer a practical solution for these gaps in service (Grim, 2006).

For optimum programs, both in terms of quality and quantity, to be developed, a significant increase in a properly trained and educated workforce is necessary. Programs such as Professional Preparation in Cochlear Implants (PPCI) have developed in response to the significant need for trained professionals in underserved regions, including rural areas and inner city neighborhoods. Developing a strong partnership between implant and educational centers is critical. Encouraging workforce diversity is crucial for encouraging cultural competence. Agencies such as the NIDCD, in conjunction with the National Center on Minority Health and Health Disparities, currently are recruiting and training individuals from underrepresented backgrounds (NIDCD, 2004).

Supporting and Educating Families: Education, Empowerment, Self-Efficacy Training Programs

Support and education of families are key for early intervention programs. Parents are ultimately the first and most influential teachers. The Pediatric CI literature is replete with discussion of the essential importance of parental involvement, parental self-efficacy, and parental adherence (DesJardin & Eisenberg, 2007; Spencer, 2004; Zaidman-Zait, 2007; Zaidman-Zait & Young, 2008). As the pediatric implant population grows and the habilitation burden shifts from implant centers to educational centers, parental involvement will be the critical factor to successful outcomes (Archbold & O'Donoghue, 2007). It is critical then that early intervention programs caring for children who are deaf or hard-of-hearing should focus on the education and guidance of parents (Simser, 1999; Zaidman-Zait, 2007).

Unfortunately, the tremendous psychosocial and financial struggles that vulnerable families grapple with may significantly impact their ability to adequately support their implanted children. Low health literacy, prevalent throughout the U.S. population, but perhaps more so among low SES adults, acts as a barrier to understanding, navigating and advocating in the health care environment (Porterfield & McBride, 2007).

Negotiating the health care/rehabilitation system remains a long-term reality for parents of deaf children with cochlear implants, making lack of health literacy even more critical. In addition, parents living in poverty often report lower levels of self-efficacy in surveys, which similarly is a critical factor in advocating for their children (Hughes & Demo, 1989; Johnston-Brooks, Lewis, & Garg, 2002; Raikes & Ross, 2005; Wolf et al., 2007). Jackson (1998) found that low SES parents with higher levels of self-efficacy had less parental stress and more positive parenting behavior. Interventions aimed at increasing social support and improving self-efficacy positively affect parental adherence (Luszczynska, Sarkar, & Knoll, 2007).

Parent-directed interventions have a positive effect on pediatric implantation, including low SES populations. Harrigan and Nikolopoulos (2002) describe a program in which they were able to enhance an implanted child's language development by affecting the communication skills of his parents. Most, Aram, and Andorn (2006), in a comparison of literacy performances among hearing-impaired children in Israel, noted the suprising lack of expected SES differential. They hypothesized that equity likely occurred because all children and parents were involved in the concentrated early intervention program, MICHA. The MICHA program recognizes the role that parents play in promoting their child's habilitation. The MICHA program teaches the parents strategies on how to interact with their child in order to promote communication, academic, and social development. This philosophy may have contributed to the reduced influence of SES (Most et al., 2006). Parent-directed programs developed for families of deaf children must be culturally sensitive to be effective for parents from a diversity of backgrounds.

Culturally Competent Healthcare: The Potential to Relate, Empower, and Improve Adherence

Cultural competence is key to decreasing health disparities (U.S. Census Bureau, 2000). By 2020, 44.5% of U.S. children will be from racial and/or ethnic minorities. Cultural competence is not merely providing language interpreters for non-English-speaking families, but represents the health systems' sensitivity to diverse cultural backgrounds and their influence on health beliefs and behaviors. Its goal is to help patients to become empowered and equal partners in their own care. Culturally competent health care requires a multifaceted approach on the organizational, structural and clinical levels (Betancourt, Green, Carrillo, & Ananeh-Firempong, 2003). It is critical for addressing sociocultural barriers at each step of care, from the initial UNHS/EHDI to audiology/implant center evaluations and treatment, to postimplant habilitation.

Adherence remains a challenge for all aspects of health care and for all strata of society, especially in individuals of lower SES backgrounds. In the *Proceedings of the National Academy of Sciences*, Goldman and Smith (2002) identified adherence to be a significant variable for SES gradients in health outcomes in both clinical trials and population-based settings.

Although adherence is undoubtedly a complicated issue, one encouraging aspect of Goldman and Smith's study (2002) was their finding that issues of adherence were amenable to intervention. In this regard, the dynamic interrelationship of culturally competent health care, health literacy, and self-efficacy should not be underestimated. When we are able to communicate with parents in ways that they can understand, to connect with and to foster within them the feeling they can be effective partners in their children's health care, adherence becomes more attainable. Betancourt (2006), a leading authority in the field of cultural competence, describes the ESFT (explanatory/social/fears/treatment) method as a tool that ascertains adherence obstacles and addresses specific strategies to combat these obstacles. Developing and testing culturally appropriate and empowering interventions specifically to improve adherence and patient satisfaction is a worthwhile endeavor in delivering high quality care and improving outcomes.

Public Policy and Advocacy

The UNHS/EHDI represents a significant public policy advance, with the goal that all children receive early identification and treatment of hearing loss. It was the result of the advocacy of professionals who spoke up for the children being diagnosed too late for optimum care. This chapter is but a continuation of the goals of UNHS/EHDI, which will require similar evidence-based research and strong advocacy. Increased funding is necessary for surgery to be accessible to the many children who meet criteria for cochlear implants. Adequate programs for habilitation must be funded to assure that implantation will succeed. In addition, the children most likely to be left behind, those from lower SES backgrounds, must be targets of specific health promotion initiatives that are evidenced-based, extending seamlessly from early intervention to public school programs. These initiatives will require local, state, and national governmental support, which will come with the government's understanding that each investment in a deaf child's future is a sound financial and societal investment overall. Although most of us are not advocates on the policy stage, we may each be advocates for those children and families who need the help we can give them and are powerless to advocate for themselves.

Project ASPIRE: Efforts to Address Pediatric Implant Disparities

Health promotions must target and develop strategies to help their intended populations. We have been in the process of developing Project ASPIRE (*Achieving Superior Parental Involvement for Rehabilitative Excellence*), a parent-directed educational intervention for children in lower SES strata. Its goal is to empower and educate parents to become effective collaborators in their child's aural habilitation. Project ASPIRE is an interactive multimedia DVD program. It is presented within group settings utilizing a "best-practices" curriculum and an iterative process which adapts information from established curricula, scientific literature reviews, and the clinical expertise of consultants from the fields of deaf education, audiology, speech and language pathology, linguistics, health disparities, interactive multimedia development, and evaluation criteria for interventions targeting vulnerable populations. The core curriculum was designed to increase parental understanding of the components necessary for a child's postimplant success, to demonstrate their own importance to that success, and to supply the knowledge and skills to help ensure that success. The Project ASPIRE team identified those steps most critical to postimplant success, determined their appropriate sequence and worked them into a user-friendly program with sequenced modules. Initial modules concentrate on proper care and maintenance of the device and the need for consistent use. Successive modules include language development and learning to understand, an important adjunct to audition. All modules include ways to help a child achieve each step and, most importantly, ways to achieve the critically important positive parent-child relationship. Although the DVDs will be produced to "stand alone" (e.g., for use by families in remote areas), they are intended to be watched in professionally led group sessions which adds the support from other parents as well as feedback from the professional.

Project ASPIRE is created to be entertaining in order to be more effectively informative. The weekly interactive DVD program will include an animated introduction, parent-child videos which demonstrate methods "in action" and a simple video game to solidify the lesson. The initial 3-D animated module introduces the concept of ASPIRE and the skills which will be taught in successive modules. The ongoing seven characters include the central characters, Star and Stella, a mother and her implanted daughter. Each animated module will have its own appropriate song to help concept recall: for example, "The Ling-Six Song." In addition to its entertainment value, animation allows the modules to be translated into any language. Parent-child videos illustrating "real parents" will include families of diverse ethnicity and children at different ages. In addition, in order to enhance participation, professionals leading the sessions will utilize a motivational interview technique at the beginning of each group session. This brief intervention (5 to 10 min) has been shown, in psychotherapy literature, to increase parental motivation, attendance, and adherence to treatment (Nock & Kazdin, 2005).

A successful intervention results in the desired change in health behavior. It is dependent on the accurate insight and appraisal of the target population. Project ASPIRE has been developed by optimal research methods. These methods, including formal focus groups and semistructured interviews, have been utilized to examine and respond to barriers to participation, understanding, and overall acceptability and feasibility. ASPIRE programs have been examined for factors such as cultural appropriateness, enjoyment, and to assess the clarity and ease of use of module media content including the animated characters, storyboards, music, and games. During the final development process, each component will undergo beta testing for acceptability, feasibility, comprehensibility (health literacy), and educational effectiveness. Modifications of the interactive multimedia components will be ongoing based on results of the testing described. The ultimate goal of Project ASPIRE is to educate and empower parents so they can help their children reach their listening, speaking, and understanding potential.

Conclusion

We are currently in a golden age with tremendous opportunities for children with hearing loss to have access to the world of sound and spoken language. It is a worthy and pragmatic goal that all children with hearing loss have access to an auditory environment. Awareness of disparities among different SES groups and designing initiatives to mitigate them can prevent widening disparities. When all deaf children have equal access to cochlear implantation accompa-

nied by excellent habilitation, all implanted children will have a chance to optimize their potential.

References

Adler, N. E. (2003). Community preventive services. Do we know what we need to know to improve health and reduce disparities? *American Journal of Preventive Medicine*, *24*(Suppl. 3), 10–11.

Adler, N. E., & Newman, K. (2002). Socioeconomic disparities in health: Pathways and policies. *Health Affairs (Project Hope)*, *21*, 60–76.

Adler, N. E., & Rehkopf, D. H. (2008). U.S. disparities in health: Description, causes, and mechanisms. *Annual Review of Public Health*, *29*, 235–252.

Archbold, S., & O'Donoghue, G. M. (2007). Ensuring the long-term use of cochlear implants in children: The importance of engaging local resources and expertise. *Ear and Hearing*, *28*(Suppl. 2), 3S–6S.

Barton, G. R., Fortnum, H. M., Stacey, P. C., & Summerfield, A. Q. (2006). Hearing-impaired children in the United Kingdom, III: Cochlear implantation and the economic costs incurred by families. *Ear and Hearing*, *27*, 563–574.

Betancourt, J. R. (2006). Cultural competency: Providing quality care to diverse populations. *Consultant Pharmacist*, *21*, 988–995.

Betancourt, J. R., Green, A. R., Carrillo, J. E., & Ananeh-Firempong, O., II. (2003). Defining cultural competence: A practical framework for addressing racial/ethnic disparities in health and health care. *Public Health Reports*, *118*, 293–302.

Bowen, S. (2000, March). *Hispanic deaf students in rural education settings: Complex issues*. Paper presented at the meeting of Capitalizing on Leadership in Rural Special Educations: Making a Difference for Children and Families Conference Proceedings, Alexandria, VA (ERIC Document Reproduction Service No. ED439875).

Brach, C., Lewit, E. M., VanLandeghem, K., Bronstein, J., Dick, A. W., Kimminau, K. S., et al. (2003). Who's enrolled in the State Children's Health Insurance Program (SCHIP)? An overview of findings from the Child Health Insurance Research Initiative (CHIRI). *Pediatrics, 112,* e499.

Cheng, A. K., Rubin, H. R., Powe, N. R., Mellon, N. K., Francis, H. W., & Niparko, J. K. (2000). Cost-utility analysis of the cochlear implant in children. *Journal of the American Medical Association, 284,* 850–856.

Connor, C. M., & Zwolan, T. A. (2004). Examining multiple sources of influence on the reading comprehension skills of children who use cochlear implants. *Journal of Speech, Language, and Hearing Research, 47,* 509–526.

DesJardin, J. L., & Eisenberg, L. S. (2007). Maternal contributions: Supporting language development in young children with cochlear implants. *Ear and Hearing, 28,* 456–459.

Easterbrooks, S. R., O'Rourke, C. M., & Todd, N. W. (2000). Child and family factors associated with deaf children's success in auditory-verbal therapy. *American Journal of Otology, 21,* 341–344.

Evans, G. W. (2003). A multimethodological analysis of cumulative risk and allostatic load among rural children. *Developmental Psychology, 39,* 924–933.

Fortnum, H. M., Marshall, D. H., & Summerfield, A. Q. (2002). Epidemiology of the UK population of hearing-impaired children, including characteristics of those with and without cochlear implants—audiology, aetiology, comorbidity and affluence. *International Journal of Audiology, 41,* 170–179.

Francis, H. W., Koch, M. E., Wyatt, J. R., & Niparko, J. K. (1999). Trends in educational placement and cost-benefit considerations in children with cochlear implants. *Archives of Otolaryngology-Head and Neck Surgery, 125,* 499–505.

Françozo Mde, F., Fernandes, J. C., Lima, M. C., & Rossi, T. R. (2007). Improvement of return rates in a Neonatal Hearing Screening Program: The contribution of social work. *Social Work in Health Care, 44,* 179–190.

Geers, A. E. (2003). Predictors of reading skill development in children with early cochlear implantation. *Ear and Hearing, 24*(Suppl. 1), 59S–68S.

Geers, A. E. (2006). Factors influencing spoken language outcomes in children following early cochlear implantation. *Advances in Otorhinolaryngology, 64,* 50–65.

Geers, A., & Brenner, C. (2003). Background and educational characteristics of prelingually deaf children implanted by five years of age. *Ear and Hearing, 24*(Suppl. 1), 2S–14S.

Goldman, D. P., & Lakdawall, D. N. (2005). A theory of health disparities and medical technology. *Contributions to Economic Analysis and Policy, 4,* 1–30.

Goldman, D. P., & Smith, J. P. (2002). Can patient self-management help explain the SES health gradient? *Proceedings of the National Academy of Sciences of the United States of America, 99,* 10929–10934.

Grim, C. Addressing the audiology needs of Indian County. Paper presented at the Albuquerqe Area Indian Health Board Audiology Meeting. Retrieved March 25, 2008, from http://www.ihs.gov/PublicInfo/PublicAffairs/Director/2006_Statements/ABQ_Audiology_Meeting-April_25-Web_version.pdf

Harper, S., Lynch, J., Hsu, W. L., Everson, S. A., Hillemeier, M. M., Raghunathan, T. E., et al. (2002). Life course socioeconomic conditions and adult psychosocial functioning. *International Journal of Epidemiology, 31,* 395–403.

Harrigan, S., & Nikolopoulos, T. P. (2002). Parent interaction course in order to enhance communication skills between parents and children following pediatric cochlear implantation. *International Journal of Pediatric Otolaryngology, 66,* 161–166.

Heckman, J. (2006). Skill formation and the economics of investing in disadvantaged children. *Science, 312,* 1900–1902.

Hodges, A. V., Dolan Ash, M., Balkany, T. J., Schloffman, J. J., & Butts, S. L. (1999). Speech perception results in children with cochlear implants: Contributing factors. *Otolaryngology-Head and Neck Surgery, 121,* 31–34.

Hodges, A. V., Eilers, R. E., & Cobo-Lewis, A. B. (1994, October). The effects of socioeconomic status on pediatric cochlear implant users. *Proceedings of the International Cochlear*

Implant, Speech, and Hearing Symposium. Melbourne, Australia.

Hoff, E., & Tian, C. (2005). Socioeconomic status and cultural influences on language. *Journal of Communication Disorders, 38,* 271–278.

Horn, I. B., & Beal, A. C. (2004). Child health disparities: Framing a research agenda. *Ambulatory Pediatrics, 4,* 269–275.

Hughes, M., & Demo, D. H. (1989). Self Perceptions of Black Americans: Self-esteem and personal efficacy. *American Journal of Sociology, 95,* 132–159.

Hyde, M., & Power, D. (2006). Some ethical dimensions of cochlear implantation for deaf children and their families. *Journal of Deaf Studies and Deaf Education, 11,* 102–111.

Jackson, A. P. (1998). The role of social support in parenting for low-income, single, black mothers. *Social Service Review, 72,* 365–389.

Johnston-Brooks, C. H., Lewis, M. A., Evans, G. W., & Whalen, C. K. (1998). Chronic stress and illness in children: The role of allostatic load. *Psychosomatic Medicine, 60,* 597–603.

Johnston-Brooks, C. H., Lewis, M. A., & Garg, S. (2002). Self-efficacy impacts self-care and HbA1c in young adults with Type I diabetes. *Psychosomatic Medicine, 64,* 43–51.

Joint Committee on Infant Hearing; American Academy of Audiology; American Academy of Pediatrics; American Speech-Language-Hearing Association; Directors of Speech and Hearing Programs in State Health and Welfare Agencies. (2000). Year 2000 position statement: Principles and guidelines for early hearing detection and intervention programs. *Pediatrics, 106*(4), 798–817.

Kirkham, E., Du, E., Perry, T., Baroody, F., Nevins, M. E., & Suskind, D. (2008, April). P*ediatric CI outcome disparities: An audiologic perspective.* 10th International Conference on Cochlear Implants and Other Implantable Auditory Technologies. San Diego, CA.

Kluwin, T. N. (1994). The interaction of race, gender and social class effects in the education of deaf students. *American Annals of the Deaf, 139,* 465–471.

Liu, C. L., Farrell, J., MacNeil, J. R., Stone, S., & Barfield, W. (2008). Evaluating loss to follow-up in newborn hearing screening in Massachusetts. *Pediatrics, 121,* e335–e343.

Liu, C. L., Zaslavsky, A. M., Ganz, M. L., Perrin, J., Gortmaker, S., & McCormick, M. C. (2005). Continuity of health insurance coverage for children with special health care needs. *Maternal and Child Health Journal, 9,* 363–375.

Luetje, C. M., & Jackson, K. (1997). Cochlear implants in children: What constitutes a complication? *Otolaryngology-Head and Neck Surgery, 117,* 243–247.

Luszczynska, A., Sarkar, Y., & Knoll, N. (2007). Received social support, self-efficacy, and finding benefits in disease as predictors of physical functioning and adherence to antiretroviral therapy. *Patient Education and Counseling, 66,* 37–42.

MacLeod-Gallinger, J. (1993, April). *Deaf ethnic minorities: Have they a double liability?* Paper presented at the Annual Meeting of the American Educational Research Association, Atlanta, GA.

MacLeod-Gallinger, J. (1997). Deaf adults who are ethnic minorities: How do they fare? *NTID Research Bulletin, 2,* 2–7.

McEwen, B. S., & Seeman, T. (1999). Protective and damaging effects of mediators of stress. Elaborating and testing the concepts of allostasis and allostatic load. *Annals of the New York Academy of Sciences, 896,* 30–47.

Minkler, M., Fuller-Thomson, E., & Guralnik, J. M. (2006). Gradient of disability across the socioeconomic spectrum in the United States. *New England Journal of Medicine, 355,* 695–703.

Mohr, P. E., Feldman, J. J., Dunbar, J. L., McConkey-Robbins, A., Niparko, J. K., Rittenhouse, R. K., & Skinner, M. W. (2000). The societal costs of severe to profound hearing loss in the United States. *International Journal of Technology Assessment in Health Care, 16,* 1120–1135.

Most, T., Aram, D., & Andorn T. (2006). Early literacy in children with hearing loss: A comparison between two educational systems. *Volta Review, 106,* 5–28.

National Institute on Deafness and other Communication Disorders. (2004). *Healthy People 2010: Hearing health progress review.*

Retrieved March 4, 2008, from http://www .nidcd.nih.gov/health/healthyhearing/what _hh/progress_review_04.asp

Nock, M. K., & Kazdin, A. E. (2005). Randomized controlled trial of a brief intervention for increasing participation in parent management training. *Journal of Consulting and Clinical Psychology*, 73, 872–879.

Nuru, N. (1993). Multicultural aspects of deafness. In D. E. Battle (Ed.), *Communication disorders in multicultural populations* (pp. 287–305). Boston: Andover Medical.

Porterfield, S. L., & McBride, T. D. (2007). The effect of poverty and caregiver education on perceived need and access to health services among children with special health care needs. *American Journal of Public Health*, 97, 323–329.

Raikes, A. H. T., & Ross, A. (2005). Efficacy and social support as predictors of parenting stress among families in poverty. Michigan Association for Infant Mental Health. *Infant Mental Health Journal*, 26, 177–190.

Sach, T. H., Whynes, D. K., Archbold, S. M., & O'Donoghue, G. M. (2005). Estimating time and out-of-pocket costs incurred by families attending a pediatric cochlear implant programme. *International Journal of Pediatric Otorhinolaryngology*, 69, 929–936.

Shavers, V. L. (2007). Measurement of socioeconomic status in health disparities research. *Journal of the National Medical Association*, 99, 1013–1023.

Simser, J. (1999). Parents: The essential partner in the habilitation of children with hearing impairment. *Australian Journal of Education of the Deaf*, 5, 55–62.

Sommers, B. D. (2005). From Medicaid to uninsured: Drop-out among children in public insurance programs. *Health Services Research*, 40, 59–78.

Sorkin, D. L., & Zwolan, T. A. (2008). Parental perspectives regarding early intervention and its role in cochlear implantation in children. *Otology and Neurotology*, 29, 137–141.

Spencer, P. E. (2004). Individual differences in language performance after cochlear implantation at one to three years of age: Child, family, and linguistic factors. *Journal of Deaf Studies and Deaf Education*, 9, 395–412.

Stern, R. E., Yueh, B., Lewis, C., Norton, S., & Sie, K. C. (2005). Recent epidemiology of pediatric cochlear implantation in the United States: Disparity among children of different ethnicity and socioeconomic status. *Laryngoscope*, 115, 125–131.

Stewart, D. A., & Benson, G. (1988). Dual cultural negligence: The education of black deaf children. *Journal of Multicultural Counseling and Development*, 16, 98–109.

Tobey, E. A., Geers, A. E., Brenner, C., Altuna, D., & Gabbert, G. (2003). Factors associated with development of speech production skills in children implanted by age five. *Ear and Hearing*, 24(Suppl. 1), 36S–45S.

U.S. Census Bureau. (2000). Population division, population projections program, projections of the total resident population by 5-year age groups, race, and Hispanic origin with special age categories. Middle series, 2016–2020. Retrieved March 4, 2008, from http://www .census.gov/population/projections/nation/ summary/np-t3-e.txt

U.S. Census Bureau, Poverty. (2006). Income, poverty and health insurance coverage in the United States: 2006. Retrieved March 4, 2008, from http://www.census.gov/hhes/www/ poverty/poverty06.html

U.S. Department of Health and Human Services. (2000). Health Resources and Services Administration, *Healthy People 2010: Understanding and improving health* (2nd ed.). (DHHS Publication No. S/N 017-001-00550-9). Washington, DC: U.S. Government Printing Office.

U.S. Department of Health and Human Services. (2003). Agency for Healthcare Research and Quality. MEPS Statistical Brief, No. 28: Health insurance status of children in America: 1996–2002 estimates for the non-institutionalized population under age 18. Retrieved July 24, 2008, from http://www.ahrq.gov/child/Find ings/childins.htm

U.S. Department of Health and Human Services. (2005). Centers for Disease Control and Prevention, Early Hearing Detection and Intervention (EHDI) Program. Annual EHDI data, 2005, final summary of 2005 National EHDI data (version 6). Retrieved March 25, 2008, from http://www.cdc.gov/ncbddd/ehdi/data.htm#Survey

Vohr, B. R., Moore, P. E., & Tucker, R. J. (2002). Impact of family health insurance and other environmental factors on universal hearing screen program effectiveness. *Journal of Perinatology, 22*, 380–385.

Wiley, S., Meinzen-Derr, J., & Arjmand, E. (2007, April). *Children with moderately severe or worse SNHL: Audiometric referral criteria for CI*. Paper presented at the 11th International Conference on Cochlear Implants in Children, Charlotte, NC.

Wolbers, K. A. (2002). Cultural factors and the achievement of black and hispanic deaf students. *Multicultural Education, 10*, 43–48

(ERIC Document Reproduction Service No. EJ654876).

Wolf, M. S., Davis, T. C., Osborn, C. Y., Skripkauskas, S., Bennett, C. L., & Makoul, G. (2007). Literacy, self-efficacy, and HIV medication adherence. *Patient Education and Counseling, 65*, 253–260.

Zaidman-Zait, A. (2007). Parenting a child with a cochlear implant: A critical incident study. *Journal of Deaf Studies and Deaf Education, 12*, 221–241.

Zaidman-Zait, A., & Young, R. A. (2008). Parental involvement in the habilitation process following children's cochlear implantation: An action theory perspective. *Journal of Deaf Studies and Deaf Education, 13*, 193–214.

CHAPTER 19

Cochlear Implantation in Children with Multiple Disabilities

KAREN C. JOHNSON
SUSAN WILEY

Introduction

The number of deaf children with additional disabilities receiving cochlear implants (CI) is on the increase. A decade ago, the percentage of CI children with multiple disabilities was reported in the 5 to 8% range (Lesinski, Hartrampf, Dahm, Bertram, & Lenarz, 1995; Uziel, Mondain, & Reid, 1995). However, more recent surveys have put the number at one-quarter (27%; Pyman, Blamey, Lacy, Clark, & Dowell, 2000) to nearly one-half (46%; Wiley, Meinzen-Derr, & Choo, 2004) of children implanted in some clinical programs. This range likely represents differences in referral bias and variability in comfort level among cochlear implant centers with implanting this population of children.

A number of factors have contributed to this significant increase in CI children with additional disabilities over the past 10 years. First, early pediatric clinical trials of cochlear implants tended to exclude deaf children who had other conditions that could adversely impact CI success, with success being defined as the development of spoken language (Berliner & Eisenberg, 1985; Northern et al., 1986; Tiber, 1985). Once the implant was approved for use in children by the Food and Drug Administration (FDA), many CI centers, noting the impressive gains being reported for otherwise typically developing children, began to implant children with additional developmental and/or learning disabilities. A second contributing factor has been the development of physiologically based techniques using electrical stimulation to evoke compound action potential (ECAP) (Brown, 2003; Brown et al, 2000; Hughes, Brown, Abbas, Wolaver, & Gervais, 2000) and stapedius reflex (ESR) (Bresnihan, Normal,

Scott, & Viani, 2001; Hodges et al., 1997; Shallop & Ash, 1995; Spivak & Chute, 1994). These tools have enabled clinicians to estimate important programming parameters in children not fully able to participate in mapping. Although physiologic estimates do not take the place of behavioral responses, they may be very useful in setting threshold and comfort levels in very young children and children with developmental disabilities, particularly in the initial stages of programming. A third factor has been the implementation of newborn hearing screening programs across this country and around the world. With emphasis on early detection and intervention, a greater number of very young children are being referred for CI consideration. Coupled with the FDA's lowering of the recommended age for implanting children with profound hearing loss from 2 years to 1, an increasing number of children are being implanted before other conditions such as autism are diagnosed or confirmed. Given contemporary trends toward even earlier implantation (ages 1 year or younger) (Coletti et al., 2005; Dettman, Pinder, Briggs, & Dowell, 2007; Luxford, Eisenberg, Johnson, & Mahnke, 2004; Waltzman & Roland, 2005), it is certain that more deaf children with yet to be diagnosed developmental delays or disabilities will be implanted.

Despite the dramatic increase in CI children with multiple disabilities over the past decade, there remains little consensus regarding the benefit such children receive from implantation. Evidence on outcomes in this population is severely lacking. The majority of what has been reported comes from retrospective studies, small case series, and case reports, most of which represent a wide variety in type and extent of disability. This stems largely from the fact that deaf children with additional disabilities remain a low incidence population (Edwards, 2007;

Holt & Kirk, 2005). However, combining many types of disability into one report makes it difficult to apply outcomes to specific groups and most centers do not have enough children of specific disability types to be able to make more substantive recommendations. In addition, there have been no consistent criteria as to what constitutes "benefit" and how it should be quantified. Thus, previous reports of CI outcomes in this population have varied considerably, ranging from minimal measurable gains (e.g., Hamzavi, Baumgartner, Egelierler, Franz, Schenk, & Gstoettner, 2000; Pyman et al., 2000) to "significant" benefit (e.g., Hamzavi et al., 2000; Waltzman, Scalchunes, & Cohen, 2000). For these reasons, the literature to date has been limited in providing clinicians with information to guide clinical decisions or postimplant care for this complex population.

The purpose of this chapter is to summarize the current literature on outcomes in CI children with multiple disabilities and to outline some of the clinical considerations in candidacy determination, evaluation, and management of this population. In doing so, the authors attempt to combine experience from two pediatric programs with historically differing philosophies regarding the implantation of children with known disabilities in addition to hearing loss. As stated elsewhere in this volume, the Children's Auditory Research and Evaluation (CARE) Center at the House Ear Institute, where the first author (KCJ) is located, has been the more conservative of the two when considering implantation of children whose potential for development of spoken language was in question. In recent years, however, this point of view has begun to undergo some change, as our perspective on post-CI "benefit" has broadened. In contrast, the Ear and Hearing Center at Cincinnati Children's Hospital

Medical Center, where the second author (SW) is located, has routinely implanted children with a wide variety of additional developmental and behavioral disabilities for a number of years. The authors also represent two professional disciplines involved in the evaluation and management of deaf children with additional disabilities; those of a pediatric audiologist and a developmental behavioral pediatrician. It is hoped that by combining these perspectives, a balanced representation of a number of issues regarding CI candidacy, assessment, and management is achieved.

Prevalence of CI Children with Additional Disabilities

It is estimated that 30 to 40% of deaf and heard-of-hearing (deaf/HOH) children have co-occurring conditions (Fortnum & Davis, 1997; Gallaudet Research Institute [GRI], 2005a, 2005b; Schildroth & Hotto, 1996; Van Naarden, Decoufle, & Caldwell, 1999). These prevalence estimates have remained fairly consistent over the past decade, despite differences among studies with regard to the population sampled, the nature of additional conditions included, and the purpose for which the data were collected.

A pair of epidemiologic studies conducted in the 1990s yielded prevalence rates of 38.7% and 30.4%, respectively, for the presence of additional conditions in children with permanent hearing loss and living in the Trent Region of the UK (Fortnum & Davis, 1997) and metropolitan Atlanta (Van Naarden et al., 1999). The Trent study included children with clinical conditions such as craniofacial abnormalities, syndromes, and other systemic disorders, but did not ascertain their severity or

disabling effect. The most prevalent condition reported for this cohort was cognitive deficit (13.9%). Approximately half of the children identified with other conditions were reported to have at least two additional medical or developmental issues. In contrast, the Atlanta study drew solely from cases enrolled in the Metropolitan Atlanta Developmental Disabilities Surveillance Program (MADDSP), which was designed specifically to track children with selected developmental disabilities. These include hearing impairment, vision impairment, mental retardation, seizure disorders, and cerebral palsy. Twenty-six percent of all cases in the Atlanta cohort were dually diagnosed with hearing loss and mental retardation. Two-thirds of hearing-impaired children with other conditions exhibited more than one additional disability.

The annual surveys conducted by the Gallaudet Research Institute (GRI) have also been used estimate the prevalence of conditions requiring additional support services for children with hearing loss in educational settings (Holden-Pitt & Diaz, 1998). The Annual Survey of Deaf and Hard-of-Hearing Children and Youth, which constitutes the largest ongoing database of this population in the United States, represents approximately 60% of all HOH students receiving special education services in this country. In these surveys, additional disabilities are categorized according to functional domain and their impact on the need for support services (e.g., orthopedic impairment, learning disability, mental retardation). Over the years, specific categories have been redrawn and refined according to prevailing trends in disability assessment. Nevertheless, the estimated proportion of deaf/HOH children with additional educationally significant conditions has remained around 40% in the surveys spanning the 1999–2000 to 2004–2005 school years

(GRI, 2001, 2002, 2003a, 2003b, 2005a, 2005b). Mental retardation and learning disabilities (LD) have consistently accounted for the highest percentage of conditions listed, with prevalence rates around 9% and 10%, respectively. Due to the manner in which the data are reported, however, it cannot be determined how many children represented in these surveys presented with more than one condition in addition to deafness. The issue is further complicated by the fact that Public Law 108-446 (Individuals with Disabilities Education Improvement Act; IDEIA, 2004) continues to exclude problems with learning that may be secondary to hearing loss in its definition of LD. In the past this has resulted in a reluctance to refer deaf/HOH students for LD assessment and to diagnose LD in deaf/HOH children (Mauk & Mauk, 1998; Plapinger & Sikora, 1990; Roth, 1991).

Among children who meet audiologic criteria for cochlear implantation, proportionally fewer children with additional disabilities receive implants than children who present with hearing loss alone (Fortnum, Marshall, & Summerfield, 2002; Fortnum, Stacey, & Summerfield, 2006; Holden-Pitt, 1997). Using data drawn from the 1996 GRI survey, Holden-Pitt (1997) compared the characteristics of a group of 816 prelingually deaf children who had been implanted to an age-matched group of deaf children who had not received implants. Eighteen percent of the implanted group had disabilities in addition to deafness, compared with 30% of the nonimplanted group. Furthermore, only 2% of the implanted group had more than one disability, compared to 8% of the nonimplanted group. Fortnum et al. (2002) reported similar differences in children with and without implants in their ascertainment study of all children with permanent hearing loss in the UK. Of the children with profound hearing loss, 22% of the children who received CIs were reported to have at least one additional disability, compared to 27.8% of the children who were not implanted. Among the additional conditions accounted for, significantly smaller percentages of children with LD, cognitive deficits, vision problems, psychosocial problems, and epilepsy were represented amont those who were implanted than those who were not. However, there were no significant differences in the rate of implantation for children identified with conditions such as respiratory problems, cardiac/circulatory anomalies, cerebral palsy, neuromotor disabilities, musculoskeletal disorders, brain abnormalities, and developmental delay, to name a few. In a survey involving a more recent cohort of children with permanent hearing loss, Fortnum and colleagues (Fortnum et al., 2006; Stacey, Fortnum, Barton, & Summerfield, 2006) reported that children with CIs were less likely to have two or more disabilities compared to children without CIs.

Multiple Disabilities Defined

Clearly, prevalence estimates and post-CI outcomes in deaf children with additional needs will be impacted by definitions specifying those conditions that, coupled with hearing loss, constitute "additional disability." In past studies these have included: intellectual disabilities, autism spectrum disorders, visual impairments, motor impairments, learning disabilities, attention deficit disorders, behavioral and emotional disorders, as well as a number of syndromes and clinical conditions.

Recently, distinctions have begun to be made between deaf children with additional needs who may require special adaptation(s) to facilitate learning versus those children who are truly multiply disabled

(Daneshi & Hassanzadeh, 2007; Knoors & Vervloed, 2003). The former group includes children with specific learning disabilities and attention deficit/hyperactivity disorders who are likely to require additional support in the form of classroom accommodations, modified intervention and teaching strategies, or adaptations in academic curricula. Not to minimize the impact of such conditions, the educational accommodations and supports that may be required for children with learning or behavioral disabilities typically complement those considered appropriate for deaf/HOH children. For example, the use of structured classrooms to focus attention and manage behavior, individualized instruction, and teaching approaches designed to reduce memory demands and supplement audition are all accommodations routinely enlisted in support of deaf/HOH as well as learning disabled students (Samar, Paranis, & Berent, 1998; Soukup & Feinstein, 2007; Stewart & Kluwin, 2001). Furthermore, collaboration with educators who have expertise in the fields of learning disabilities and/or behavioral problems should serve to identify and tailor additional strategies to enhance learning and development for the individual child.

In the case of the multiply disabled child, however, the combination of two or more disabling conditions early in life creates a unique and complex situation that differs from that typically associated with any one disability. These combinations include deafness in association with blindness, mental retardation, autism, and/or physical impairment, in which methods of intervention and support appropriate for one disability may not be entirely applicable in the presence of the second disability. For example, in a child who is both deaf and blind, the vision loss limits the degree to which that modality can be used to compensate for the loss of hearing, whereas the

hearing loss limits use of that sensory system to compensate for the loss of vision (Chen, 2004; McInnes, 1999). For the child with combined hearing loss and motor impairment, interventions that address the hearing loss (e.g., sensory device use, sign-supported language) may reduce barriers to receptive communication; however, they may not address those imposed by motor limitations to expressive communication (Beukelman & Mirenda, 2005). As Knoors and Vervleod (2003, page 82) suggest, "It is the reduction in possibilities for compensation, whether spontaneously or after intervention, that makes a child multiply disabled."

In the overview of etiologies and summary of reported outcomes that follow, we touch on a variety of additional conditions that can co-occur with hearing loss and impact a child's ability to make use of the sound afforded by the CI. For the remainder of the chapter, however, we focus on children who are truly multiply disabled, as defined above, because it is with regard to these children that most questions about CI efficacy and how to maximize benefit arise.

Postimplant Outcomes in Children with Multiple Disabilities

Early Surveys and Case Reports

Accounts of CI children with additional disabilities began to appear in the literature in the mid-1990s. In the first large scale survey of cochlear implantation in children with multiple disabilities, Uziel and colleagues (1995) reported that 31 (5%) out of a total of 601 children implanted in 22 European clinics exhibited disabilities in addition to deafness. Blindness was most common

(35%), whereas intellectual disabilities (19%) and developmental disabilities (16%) were listed as second and third, respectively. Other handicaps included conditions such as autism and VATER syndrome, both of which may include intellectual and developmental delays as part of their clinical presentation. The same year, Lesinski et al. (1995) reported that 108 (19%) out of the 569 children evaluated for implantation in their program exhibited handicaps in addition to deafness. Of these 108 children, 47 were implanted and 30 were postponed in order to undergo further training and evaluation. Children who were implanted tended to be those with medical conditions such as heart disease, endocrine disorders, anatomic or muscle abnormalities, or other physical disabilities that could complicate surgery or postoperative rehabilitation, but that were not considered to be of major consequence with regard to auditory perception. Children who were postponed tended to be those diagnosed with "neuropsychiatric" conditions considered to be more likely to impact auditory perception (e.g., sensorimotor integration disabilities, intellectual delay, visual impairment, motor delay, cerebral palsy, and cognitive dysfunction).

A number of case reports and small case series also appeared describing outcomes in CI children with genetic syndromes likely to impact development (Chute & Nevins, 1995; Jorgensen, Chmiel, Clark, & Jenkins, 1995; Young, Johnson, Mets, & Hain, 1995). Chute and Nevins (1995) published a research note on three children with Usher syndrome (US), two of whom already had markedly restricted peripheral vision. One of the two children with significant vision impairment (age at CI = 6.5 years) achieved open-set speech recognition after 3 years of implant use. Furthermore, her ability to navigate through familiar environments was considerably improved. A second child (age

at CI = 9.5 years), whose vision was not yet significantly compromised, achieved only pattern perception after 2 years of device use. However, her ability to speech-read was considerably improved and her performance was considered on par with other children with similar duration of deafness. The third child had been implanted for less than 6 months, but was already beginning to show attention to environmental sound and respond to his name. Young and colleagues (1995) reported on 4 children with Usher syndrome type I (USH1) implanted at age 5 years or under, following the diagnosis of US, but well before the onset of associated vision loss. At the time of the report, all four children had 12 months or less of implant experience; thus, results were limited. Nevertheless, each of the children had demonstrated some improvement in auditory skills post-CI, ranging from consistent phoneme detection for one child implanted for 6 months to emerging open-set recognition for another child implanted for 11 months. Jorgensen et al. (1995) described 3-year outcomes for a 13-year-old girl with CHARGE syndrome. Implanted at the age of 9.75 years, after 9 years of consistent sensory device use (hearing aids, FM system, tactile aid), this child was reported to make dramatic gains in speech perception abilities over the next 3 years, with no signs of plateau in any area of learning. Her developmental, intellectual, and neurologic status prior to implantation were not described, however, thus limiting the extent to which these observed outcomes could be considered representative of other children with CHARGE.

Isaacson, Hasenstab, Wohl, and Williams (1996) published the first study comparing outcomes in CI children with and without additional disabilities. They reviewed post-CI speech perception and language abilities in five pairs of children with deafness secondary to meningitis; one child in each pair presented with a learning disability (LD) in addition to hearing loss, the other child did not. The presence of LD in children identified with this disability was confirmed by both the child's educational program as well as an independent evaluator. Children were closely matched along a number of parameters, including: age of deafness onset, age at implantation, ear implanted, number of electrodes activated, nonverbal mode of communication, and type of placement in classroom. Outcome measures included tests of auditory perception, receptive language, and sequential organization. All children were reported to improve on all tasks over time. However, the child with the LD diagnosis in each pair showed slower progress, demonstrated lower scores overall in auditory perception and linguistic competence, and was more inconsistent in performance.

Retrospective Studies in CI Children with Mixed Additional Disabilities

Over the next few years, a number retrospective studies and case reports appeared from centers around the world describing CI outcomes in clinical patients with a wide variety of co-occuring conditions. Waltzman, et al. (2000) published one of the largest such studies to date, examining outcomes in 29 deaf children with additional disabilities who had been implanted for at least one year. The additional conditions represented ranged from global developmental delay and pervasive developmental disorder at one end of the disability spectrum to learning disabilities and oral motor deficits at the other end. No data or only minimal data could be obtained from 11 of the 29 subjects tested out to 3 years postimplant. Not surprisingly, these tended to be the

children with the conditions most likely to compromise overall development, with or without the additional disability of deafness. In contrast, 12 children appeared to achieve some degree of open-set word recognition by 2 to 3 years postimplant. These tended to be the children with the least disabling conditions of those included in the series. The course of development in the study group overall, however, was slower and less stable than in a comparison group of 38 congenitally deaf children the authors had reported on previously (Waltzman et al., 1997).

Hamzavi and colleagues (2000) reported on a smaller series of 10 children described as multihandicapped, emphasizing the need to focus on individual outcomes in this population. Formal speech perception results could only be reported for 3 of the 10 children in their sample; children for whom "moderate learning difficulties" were listed as the additional condition. For these 3 children, open-set word recognition ranged from 83% at 18 months post-CI to 100% at 3 years post-CI. Six of the seven remaining children were listed as demonstrating severe intellectual deficits or severe psychomotor retardation, in isolation or combination with other conditions. The remaining child was identified with "severe learning difficulties." In these seven children, results were limited to anecdotal reports of behavioral changes with the implant activated. These changes included increased auditory awareness in all but one child, with rudimentary sound differentiation in two children and evidence of device bonding in another two. Five children demonstrated increased phonation, with emerging speech production in two. In addition, four children, all with sensorimotor integration deficits and/or psychomotor retardation, were noted to demonstrate improved motor skills and/or a reduction in hyperactivity or stereotypic behaviors.

Filipo, Bosco, Mancini, and Ballantyne (2004) described a number of "special cases" implanted at their facility in whom the presence of additional disabilities and/or social issues (e.g., family factors, bilingual households, cultural differences) added to the complexity of both candidacy determination and assessment of benefit. Among these special cases were 11 children with additional sensory, cognitive/developmental, or psychiatric disabilities. Age of implant ranged from 2 to 12 years (mean age at CI = 7.1 years). Length of implant use ranged from 13 to 53 months (mean length of CI use = 3 years). With the exception of a child diagnosed with psychosis, all remaining children showed improved speech perception following implantation by advancing in the hierarchy of auditory skills (Erber, 1982). Nevertheless, the amount of improvement and the duration over which it occurred varied widely among children. The child with psychosis had showed improved auditory perception for the first year following implantation. However, with no identifiable precipitating event, this child began to show new signs of self-destructive behavior and isolation, rejecting her implant in the presence of any kind of discomfort.

In 2004, Winter, Johnson, and Vranisic described outcomes in 10 children with additional disabling conditions, the severity of which became apparent only after implantation. Disabilities included: autistic-like behavior following meningitic hearing loss ($n = 2$), congenital cytomegalovirus (CMV) ($n = 3$), sensory integration disorders ($n = 4$), and seizure disorder with soft neurologic signs ($n = 1$). Mean age at CI was 3.2 years. Retrospective analysis of speech perception abilities and educational placement at 2 to 5 years post-CI showed that most of the children had made only minimal progress in developing functional listening skills and spoken communication.

Vlahovic and Sindija (2004) reported on four children with a range of additional disabilities, implanted at or prior to 4 years of age. One child exhibited a communication disorder, two children demonstrated moderate psychomotor retardation, and a fourth child was diagnosed with atrophy of the left side of the brain. The length of postimplant follow-up ranged from 12 to 58 months. The two children who had been followed between 4 to 5 years were reported to have achieved level 5 on the Categories of Auditory Performance (CAP) (Archbold, Lutman, & Marshall, 1995), corresponding to the understanding of common phrases without lipreading. A third child reached level 4 after 2.5 years of follow-up, corresponding to discrimination of some speech sounds. For these three children, speech production lagged far behind. The fourth child, who had been followed for only 12 months, achieved level 2 on the CAP, consistent with the ability to perform a response to a spoken signal (e.g., "go"). This child's speech was reported as unintelligible speech at the single word level.

In view of the considerable variability in outcomes demonstrated by CI children with such a wide array of additional conditions, a number of investigators have attempted to narrow their focus to outcomes in children sharing a common category of disability.

Cognitive and Developmental Delays

Pyman, et al. (2000) conducted a retrospective chart review of 75 children implanted consecutively at their facility. Based on medical examinations and detailed parent interviews taken prior to implantation, 20 of the 75 children (26.6%) were considered to show evidence of cognitive delay ($n = 6$), motor delay ($n = 3$), or both

($n = 11$). The remaining 55 (73.4%) children were reported to have achieved normal developmental milestones. Speech perception outcomes were classified according to the performance levels, ranging from detection to open-set word recognition (Dowell, Blamey, & Clark, 1995). Not surprisingly, children with delays tended to start at a lower level of performance than the more typically developing children. Although all children in the delayed group achieved detection within the first 3 months post-CI, their ability to discriminate supra-segmental features, vowels, and consonants in closed sets developed at a significantly slower rate than children without delays. Furthermore, 40% of the delayed children had not achieved open-set speech recognition after four years of implant experience

In a second study from this center, Dettman et al. (2004) investigated the association between the severity of cognitive impairment and speech perception outcomes in CI children. They identified 49 children who had undergone psychological evaluation prior to implantation for various reasons. In view of the wide range of ages and developmental abilities represented by the children, a variety of cognitive measures was employed. Each of these measures used different descriptors to categorize results. Children were divided into three groups based on the cognitive outcome. Group 1 was composed of the 27 children who had been described as "normal," "average," "mid-average," "high-average," and "superior." Group 2 was composed of the 14 children who were considered to be "borderline-normal," "low-average," or demonstrating "mild" delay. Group 3 was composed of the 8 children who demonstrated "moderate" delay, "significant" delay or who were considered "intellectually disabled." Groups showed no statistically significant differences with respect to age of hearing aid fit-

ting, residual hearing, duration of hearing loss, age at implant, or device experience at the time of assessment. Twenty-five children (51%) were able to complete at least one formal closed-set or open-set speech measure, including 16 (59%) Group 1 children, 6 (43%) Group 2 children, and 2 (25%) Group 3 children. For the remaining 24 children, speech perception skills were rated by two clinicians familiar with the child based on a variety of detection and speech perception tasks appropriate for young children and/or those with limited verbal skills. Results for all children were then assigned to one of seven categories of performance ranging from detection to open-set recognition (Dowell et al, 1995; Dowell & Cowan, 1997). The majority of Group 1 children, with normal or above average cognition, achieved a median category of 7 after an average of 2.5 years of CI experience, corresponding to open-set recognition of sentence material with greater than 50% phoneme recognition. Group 2 children, with mild delays, achieved a median category of 5.5 after and average of 2.77 years of experience, corresponding to performance mid-way between open-set recognition of familiar key words (5% to 20% phoneme recognition; category 5) and open-set recognition of familiar words and phrases (20% to 50% phoneme recognition; category 6). Group 3 children, with moderate to significant delays, achieved a median category of 2 after an average of 4 years of device experience, corresponding to discrimination of pattern perception in closed-set tasks. Although degree of cognitive delay was associated with general category of postimplant speech perception attained, results were highly variable with at least one child in each group achieving some degree of word recognition in open-set sentences. With regard to communication mode, a greater proportion of children in Group 3

(50%) were enrolled in total communication (TC) educational programs following implantation compared to children in Group 1 (14%) and Group 2 (21%).

In an attempt to isolate the impact of mild cognitive delays on postimplant outcomes, Holt and Kirk (2005) conducted a retrospective analysis on speech perception and speech and language outcomes in 69 children, 19 of whom had mild cognitive delays but no other disabilities. The remaining 50 children demonstrated no cognitive delays, nor any other disability apart from hearing loss. These 50 typically developing children, who served as controls, were further stratified by communication mode: 25 of whom were primarily oral communicators (OC) and 25 of whom communicated through total communication (TC). Children were assessed on the basis of structured parent report, closed-set speech perception, modified open-set word and sentence recognition, and multimodal word recognition. Prior to implantation, similar performance was noted for all groups in auditory skill development, word, and sentence recognition. All three groups also were well below age level on three measures of receptive and expressive language. Following implantation, similar improvements were observed in auditory-only word recognition for children with and without cognitive delays over the course of 2 years following CI. In multimodal testing, all three groups showed improved word recognition in the auditory-only, auditory-visual and combined modalities over the course of the first year, although the delayed children tended to score somewhat lower than the non-delayed children in the auditory-only condition. At the level of auditory-only sentence recognition, however, an interaction was noted in which improvement in children with cognitive delays occurred later than in the typically developing group. Significant improvements in receptive vocabulary and expressive language skills were noted for all three groups of children following implantation. Nevertheless, the children with cognitive delays had significantly lower scores on two out of three measures of receptive and expressive language as compared to the children without delays. Taken together, these investigators concluded that deaf children with mild cognitive impairment derive benefit from cochlear implantation. However, their post-CI gains may be tempered somewhat compared to those made by their typically developing peers, particularly with respect to aspects of speech perception and language requiring higher level cognitive abilities.

Citing the difficulties inherent in cognitive assessment of very young children, Edwards, Frost, and Witham (2006) explored the association of more generalized developmental delay and postimplant outcomes in a series of 32 children implanted under the age of 3.5 years. Of these 32 children, 11 were identified as delayed on the basis of developmental testing conducted prior to implantation (mean age of assessment; 1.9 years). The remaining 21 children (66%) showed no delays. Significant differences were found between the delayed and the nondelayed groups in speech perception and speech intelligibility at 1 and 2 years postactivation. Regression analysis showed developmental delay to be an important predictor of postimplant progress, whether expressed in terms of global development (using an index including motor development) or a subset of skills relating more specifically to cognitive development. It is important to note that the eight children with mild delays did make progress in both speech perception and speech production, though not to the same extent as the typically developing children. The three children identified with significant delays, however, showed almost no progress in either domain. Furthermore, these three children showed no behavioral evidence of sound awareness and one of the children consistently rejected the device. As Edwards and colleagues have suggested, "There may be a point where the developmental delay is such that the potential benefits are not sufficient to outweigh the surgical risks, emotional, physical and financial pressures placed on the family" (p. 1599).

Wiley, Meinzen-Derr, and Choo (2008) examined auditory skill growth post-CI as a function of developmental level as well as the presence versus absence of additional disabilities. They used the Auditory Skills Checklist© (ASC) (Meinzen-Derr, Wiley, Choo, & Creighton, 2004) to track the acquisition of early auditory skills in a group of 35 CI children implanted under the age of 36 months, 14 of whom demonstrated additional disabilities. The ASC is a criterion-referenced tool designed to monitor progress in the development of functional auditory behaviors in very young children with sensorineural hearing loss. Based on Erber's (1982) hierarchical model, the checklist uses structured parent interview and clinician observation to rate the child's acquisition of skills at the levels of detection, discrimination, identification, and comprehension. When grouped according to disability status, the children identified with additional disabilities were observed to progress through the hierarchy of skills at a similar rate to that shown by the group of children without additional disabilities, although the children in the former group tended to start at lower baseline skill sets. However, when grouped on the basis of developmental quotient (i.e., developmental age divided by chronological age; DQ <80 versus ≥80) irrespective of disability status, the differences among children were more notable. In children with a DQ ≥80, the rate of progress was twice as steep as for children with a DQ <80. Interestingly, the mean DQ in the delayed group was half that of the typically developing deaf children. Further-

more, the children with a DQ <80 were less likely to move much beyond detection and some discrimination to identification and comprehension over the first year post-CI.

Autism Spectrum Disorders (ASDs)

As of this writing there has been one study published on postimplant outcomes in children with autism spectrum disorders (ASDs). Donaldson, Heavner, and Zwolan (2004) conducted a retrospective review of speech perception and communication outcomes in seven children with ASDs, which they reported as affecting 1.7% of their total clinical population. Two of the children were diagnosed with pervasive developmental disorder (PDD); they were the only children who could be assessed with formal measures at more than one post-CI test interval. One child, implanted at 4 years of age, achieved 100% recognition of familiar sentences by 24 months post-CI and significant growth in receptive and expressive vocabulary by 5 yrs post-CI. He was also the only child to develop spoken language to communicate. The other child, implanted at 9 years of age, showed a 25% improvement in word recognition by 6 months post-CI, a modest gain in expressive vocabulary, and a significant growth in receptive vocabulary (per parental inventory) by 12 months post-CI. For the five children diagnosed with autism, outcome data were obtained almost entirely from parent-report measures. Improvements in auditory skill development and/or receptive vocabulary were noted for three of the four children on whom these measures were obtained. One child showed no change in auditory skills and no comprehension of spoken words by 12 months post-CI. No change in behaviors associated with autism were reported following CI.

Deaf-Blindness and Low Vision

Most published accounts of CI use in the deaf-blind children involve those diagnosed with Usher syndrome (US), an autosomal recessive disorder, with an estimated prevalence of 4.4 per 100,000 (Boughman, Vernon, & Shaver, 1983) and which is considered to account for 66% of deaf-blindness in the United States (Merlin & Auerbach, 1976). Of the three most widely recognized clinical types (Kumar, Fishman, & Torok, 1984), Usher type 1 (USH1) is the most severe. This variant is characterized by congenital sensorineural hearing loss (SNHL), vestibular hypofunction, and progressive pigmentary retinopathy (RP). The hallmark of vestibular hypofunction in these children is a significant delay in their ability to walk independently (Mets, Young, Pass, & Lasky, 2000). Usher type 2 (USH2) is characterized by moderate to severe SNHL, normal vestibular function, and RP. Usher type 3 (USH3), which is relatively rare, is characterized by postlingual progressive SNHL, variable vestibular findings, and adult-onset night blindness in some individuals.

To date, at least seven chromosomal loci have been mapped and five causative genes identified for USH1, thus allowing for early diagnosis and intervention of children with this disorder (Loundon et al., 2003). Early identification is made all the more imperative by the dual sensory deficit that will ultimately occur. In children diagnosed with USH1, the goal of early cochlear implantation is to provide the child with an auditory foundation for developing oral communication before blindness sets in (Loundon et al., 2003; Mets et al., 2000; Young et al., 1995).

In addition to the case reports by Chute and Nevins (1995) and Young et al. (1995) summarized earlier in this chapter, a few CI children with USH1 have been included in larger series of deaf-blind patients (El-Kashian, Boerst, & Telian, 2001; Saeed, Ramsden, & Axon, 1998). Saeed et al. (1998) described the post-CI course of an 8-year-old girl with USH1. Prelingually deaf, she also had begun to lose peripheral and nocturnal vision, a contributing factor to the decision to implant before the age of 5 years. At the time of the report, more than 3 years following implantation, she was able to identify the Ling six sounds (Ling, 1989) across the frequency spectrum. Her lip-reading skills and ability to perceive environmental sounds were considerably enhanced, along with her self-confidence. Her auditory memory also was reported to have improved to the point where she was able to follow two- and three-item instructions. The case described by El-Kashian et al. (2001) was that of a 12-year-old girl implanted at the age of 3.5 years. Diagnosed with profound hearing loss at the age of 1 year, she showed little benefit from amplification, including no pattern perception and limited language development. By 1-year postimplant, she was scoring 75% open-set recognition of familiar words and her expressive vocabulary had grown to approximately 100 words. At 7 years of age, her peripheral vision began to deteriorate, followed by decreases in visual field and acuity. Nine years after implantation she had developed excellent open-set speech recognition, scoring 100% on common phrases and 88% on sentences presented in the auditory only condition.

Loundon et al. (2003) described a series of 13 children diagnosed with US on the basis of genetic testing. USH1 was identified in 11 of the 13 cases, USH3 was identified in 1 case, and an unclassified variant accounted for the final case. Grouped according to age at implant, the speech perception and speech production outcomes did not differ significantly from CI children with non-US diagnoses at comparable ages of implantation.

Considerably fewer reports involve children with blindness due to other etiologies. In their report, Saeed et al. (1998) described a 9-year-old boy with retinopathy, glaucoma, and cataracts, as sequelae to congenital rubella. The duration of device use was not specified. Nevertheless, he was reported to be able to identify Ling sounds and follow two-item instructions presented in closed sets. The child was communicating in sign. El-Kashian et al. (2001) described a 3.5-year-old boy with multiple central nervous system (CNS) anomalies who had been implanted only 6 months prior to the time of report. Born with Chiari Type I malformation requiring decompression, this child also presented with hydrocephalus requiring multiple shunt revisions, seizure disorder, visual impairment, and significant developmental delay. After 6 months of device experience, he was reported to be showing interest in noise-producing toys with which he did not play prior to implantation. His mother also reported that he was more alert with the implant on and activated, and that he used a greater number of phonemes during vocal play.

Specific Etiologies and Syndromes

There are many causes of hearing loss that result in additional disabling conditions as well. However, certain etiologies are frequently represented among the deaf children with multiple disabilities referred for CI. These include children with CHARGE and congenital CMV infection, about which a number of studies describing CI outcomes have been published.

CHARGE Syndrome

CHARGE syndrome is an autosomal dominant disorder resulting most often from mutations in the chromodomain helicase DNA-binding protein-7 (CHD7) gene (Vissers et al., 2004). The acronym CHARGE is used to describe a specific constellation of multiple congenital malformations that include: "ocular coloboma, heart defect, "choanal atresia, retarded growth, development and/or CNS anomalies, genital hypoplasia or hypogonadism, and ear anomalies or deafness (Hall, 1979; Hittner, Hirsh, Kreh, & Rudolph, 1979; Pagon, Graham, Zonana, & Yong, 1981). The diagnosis of CHARGE is based on the presence of at least four of the major features above (Pagon et al., 1981; Blake et al., 1998) or three major plus at least three minor features, which include facial clefting, dysmorphic facies, tracheoesophageal fistula, short stature, and developmental delay (Blake et al, 1998).

The incidence of CHARGE is only about 1 in 8,500 to 12,000 births (Issekutz, Graham, Prasad, Smith, & Blake, 2005). However, because hearing loss is one of the common features of the syndrome, children with CHARGE are routinely referred for otologic and audiologic management, including cochlear implantation if indicated. Cognitive and developmental sequelae are also common. In the one of the earliest descriptions of the syndrome (Pagon et al., 1981), 53 out of the 54 patients demonstrated some degree of developmental delay or intellectual disability.

In addition to the case report by Jorgensen et al. (1995) summarized previously, there have been three published studies describing CI outcomes in children with CHARGE. Developmental delays or mental retardation was identified in all but one child across the three studies. Bauer, Wippold, Goldin, and Lusk (2002) summarized post-CI results in five children, four of whom were identified with retarded development or CNS abnormalities. All five showed various degrees of improvement by structured parent report. Three children who had been implanted 1 year or longer showed improvement on either the closed-set or modified open-set word and sentence recognition. One child, implanted for 4 years, achieved 50% open-set word and sentence recognition. Au, Hui, Tsang, and Wei (2004) reported a case study involving a child diagnosed with CHARGE, global developmental delay and mild mental retardation, who was implanted at the age of 2.5 years. At 4 years post-CI, this child was able to identify syllable patterns with 95% accuracy and Ling sounds with 80% accuracy. However, identification of vocabulary items (task not specified) was reported to be only 40%, with sentence comprehension at 35%. At the age of 7 years, this child's expressive and receptive language age-equivalents were 2.05 and 2.04 years, respectively. Lanson, Green, Roland, Lalwani, and Waltzman, (2007) described outcomes in the series of 10 CI children implanted between the ages of 1 and 3.5 years, each of whom showed developmental retardation. All 10 children showed varying, but limited degrees of benefit, as assessed though soundfield detection and structured parent report. None of the children were reported to have developed spoken language, including one child with 15 years of implant experience. Another child was reported to be receiving communication in the auditory-oral mode, but using sign for expressive communication.

Congenital Cytomegalovirus (CMV)

CMV infection is the most common intrauterine viral infection, affecting approximately 0.6 to 0.7% of live births worldwide (Dollard, Grosse, & Ross, 2007; Kenneson & Cannon, 2007). Sensorineural hearing loss (SNHL) is reported to be the most common sequela of CMV infection in utero (Dahle et al., 2000; Fowler & Boppana, 2006). Symptoms of congenital CMV infection include intrauterine growth retardation, microcephaly, hepatosplenomegaly, thrombocytopenia, petechiae, and intracerebral calcifications (Pass, Stagno, Myers, & Alford, 1980; Williamson et al., 1982). Hearing loss is estimated to affect 22 to 65% of symptomatic children (Fowler & Boppana, 2006). In addition to deafness, congenital CMV infection can result in a host of developmental disabilities, including blindness, cognitive impairment, and motor impairments. However, only 10 to 15% of infected children are symptomatic (Dollard et al, 2007; Kennison & Cannon, 2007; Pass et al., 1980). In the 85 to 90% of infected children who show no symptoms at birth, 6 to 23% are likely to develop hearing loss (Fowler & Boppanna, 2006).

Rameriz Inscoe and Nikolopoulos (2004) compared postimplant speech perception and production in 16 children whose deafness was attributed to CMV with the average outcome for a group of 131 CI children with non-CMV congenital deafness. The average ages of implantation were similar between groups, with a mean age of 3.9 years for the CMV children versus 4.1 years for the children without the CMV diagnosis. No specifics regarding the diagnosis of CMV were provided. Apart from the mention that three of the CMV children also were diagnosed with ASD, the cognitive status and/or presence of other disabilities were not described for either group. Median scores on measures of speech intelligibility (production) and closed-set sentence perception tended to be lower for CMV children as compared to the non-CMV children. However, a wide range of performance was noted for both groups and no statistically significant differences between the CMV and non-CMV groups were identified in two out of three measures assessed.

Lee, Lustig, Sampson, Chinnici, and Niparko (2005) described outcomes in 13

CI children with CMV-related deafness, implanted at a mean age of 5.6 years. The diagnosis of CMV infection was made on the basis of positive anti-CMV titers for the mother and positive titers or CMV in the urine for the child. Five of the children presented with other symptoms of CMV infection; seven were asymptomatic. Speech perception outcomes on a number of routine clinical measures were expressed in terms of level achieved on modification of the Speech Perception Categories described by Geers and Moog (1987). Outcomes were highly variable, with some children making minimal progress through the hierarchical categories and others making substantial gains. Nevertheless, all but three children had achieved a minimum of consistent closed-set word recognition 48 months post-CI; seven children had advanced to open-set word recognition during this postoperative interval. In this small series, no significant differences were noted between those children with additional symptoms of CMV and without such symptoms.

Communication Mode

In the studies summarized above, a greater proportion of the children with multiple disabilities were reported to use some form of sign-supported communication following cochlear implantation than children without additional developmental conditions. In the relatively large scale studies by Waltzman and colleagues, 100% of typically developing children were able to use oral communication (Waltzman et al., 1997); compared to only 59% of children with additional disabilities (Waltzman et al., 2000). Pyman et al. (2000) reported that only one-third of children in their study with cognitive and/or motor delays were in oral education placements, compared to two-thirds of the children without delays. Mode of communication was the only factor known to impact speech perception outcomes on which the two groups differed. These investigators posed two explanations for this difference between groups. On the one hand, they suggested that placement in total or other manual communication programs may have slowed the development of oral/aural speech perception skills in some children, most of whom belonged to the group with cognitive and/or motor delays. Alternatively, they suggested that such placement for the majority of delayed children might have reflected postimplant decisions made by their families in view of their relatively slow progress in the auditory-only mode. The communication outcomes reported by Winter and colleagues (2004) were in keeping with this second account. Although nine of the children in their study began in oral educational placements, most did not make sufficient gains in oral language development to remain in oral programs and only two children could be classified as functional oral communicators.

Wiley et al. (2004) reported that 66% of the 32 children with only one additional disability implanted in their program used TC, compared to 47% of 37 children with no additional disabilities. However, all 10 children with cognitive involvement used TC. Furthermore, children with >1 additional disability were more likely to use TC compared to children with only one additional disability (91% versus 52%, respectively).

Other Perceived Benefits of Implantation

Despite the caution regarding minimal measurable gains reported for many of the children, most authors attested to benefits that could not be assessed using routine clinical tools. Lesinski and colleagues (1995) suggested that ability to identify the difference through audition alone between speech and environmental sound might be one parameter by which to judge "success." Other investigators have alluded to increased "connectedness" with the environment and improved opportunities for enhanced social relationships (Bauer et al., 2002; Hamzavi et al., 2000; Waltzman et al., 2000).

Donaldson and colleagues (2004) surveyed the families in their study of the children with ASDs who had been implanted. Although little impact was observed on the behaviors most closely associated with ASDs, parents did report changes in responsiveness to sound, including increases in vocalization, eye contact, and interest in music following implantation. Also reported was the increased use of sign language and response to requests. Five of the six families in their study indicated that they would recommend a CI to another family member in a similar situation. Vlahovic and Sindija (2004) also obtained parental impressions of CI benefit via questionnaire in their study reported above. Parents reported improved sound awareness and speech perception, but slower progress in the development of speech production. Nevertheless, on average, parents reported that their children tended to use speech in communication during play and that the CI had improved their children's peer interactions.

Wiley, Jahnke, Meinzen-Derr, and Choo (2005) examined the qualitative benefits of CIs in children with a mixed array of additional disabilities. They interviewed 19 families of 20 children using a structured interview technique. Open- and closed-set questions were adapted for this purpose from other existing instruments not designed for this population. All of the families reported that their child had made progress in developing communication skills. Furthermore, they believed that their children were more attentive and aware of the world around them. All families reported that, if they were asked to make the decision again, they would still elect to have their child implanted.

Implantation of Children with Multiple Disabilities: Clinical Considerations

Considerations for Candidacy

In considering cochlear implantation for any deaf child, the anticipated benefits must be weighed against the surgical risks. Candidacy decisions are not always straightforward, even for otherwise typically developing children, and a large number of variables come into play. For most children, however, spoken language is the goal in sight and the decision to implant is based largely on a child's potential for developing oral language skills.

Access to sound, however, is not synonymous with access to language (Knoors & Vervleod, 2003). The use of language requires knowledge about its structure (grammar) and the rules governing its use. It also calls into play the development of higher level information processing skills, including working memory, speed of verbal rehearsal, and patterns of lexical access (Dawson, Busby, McCay, & Clark, 2002; Pisoni & Cleary, 2003; Pisoni, Cleary, Geers, & Tobey, 2000; Pisoni & Geers, 2000). Whereas improved auditory access may aid in the growth of these skills, there also is likely to be a limit to the degree to which they may develop in the presence of cognitive disabilities. Furthermore, even with an implant, audition will continue to be an imperfect channel through which to learn language. Although postoperative detection may be brought to within what is generally considered the "mild hearing loss" range, electrical stimulation is not equivalent to acoustic stimulation and the child is still required to map meaning onto these new sensations. In fact, on average, CI children with detection thresholds in the "mild loss" range function more like children with moderately-severe to severe hearing losses using amplification in terms of their speech perception, speech production, and language (Blamey et al., 2001; Boothroyd & Boothroyd-Turner, 2002; Eisenberg, Kirk, Martinez, Ying, & Miyamoto, 2004). Thus, for some children with cognitive disabilities, the improved ability to detect and perhaps understand speech at the single word level may or may not translate to the ability to comprehend spoken language.

Conditions such as cognitive impairment, autism, and specific learning disabilities also can compromise a child's ability to receive or process information through the visual channel (Jones & Jones, 2003; Knoors & Vervloed, 2003). For some children the grammar of sign language itself may be too difficult to comprehend (Kahn, 1996). In such cases, communication might be supported by use of a more limited set of highly relevant signs. Other children, including those who are deaf-blind, may need the use of objects, graphic or tactile symbols, or natural gestures, at least in the beginning stages of communication development (Chen, 2004; Stillman & Battle, 1986). Thus, for some CI children with additional disabilities, multimodal communication approaches may continue to be more effective than approaches that emphasize one sensory channel over the other. Finally, large asymmetries between a child's perception and production capabilities may exist.

For example, in children with motor impairments, spoken or sign-supported language may be viable modes for receiving communication, but augmentative systems and devices might still be required for expressive communication (Beukelman & Mirenda, 2005).

Clearly, the nature and extent of additional conditions are likely to have a sustained influence on post-CI outcomes, even if other variables are favorable. Although cochlear implantation may mitigate the overall impact of the hearing loss, it does not result in "normal" hearing in the implanted ear. Furthermore, providing a child access to sound does not change the nature or the extent of other underlying disabilities and their impact on communication development. In many instances it may be difficult to ascertain to what extent the communication delay or impairment can be ascribed to the hearing loss versus other conditions, the impact of which may become more apparent only after implantation has taken place. In other cases, co-existing conditions may not be diagnosed until after implantation, when the child is not making the expected amount of progress. Thus, decisions about the implantation of any given deaf child with multiple disabilities should be based, in part, on developmental expectations for a hearing child with comparable ability/disability. In this context, the acquisition of auditory skills to the extent allowed by the other disabilities is a reasonable goal and should be supported.

Objectives for Implantation

Although pediatric selection criteria have relaxed over the past two decades, there is no widespread agreement among CI centers as to which children with additional needs may be suitable candidates for implantation. During FDA clinical trials and the initial period that followed, behavioral, psychological, or cognitive conditions considered likely to limit spoken language development or the ability to participate in testing and mapping were contraindications to implantation. Many centers have continued to use similar exclusionary criteria. At these centers children with additional disabilities known to impact language learning, even in the presence of normal auditory sensitivity, might not be considered CI candidates on the basis of questionable prognoses for spoken language development.

There is some evidence for this. As born out in most of the studies reviewed earlier in this chapter, deaf children with intellectual and developmental disabilities are at a disadvantage compared to more typically developing deaf children with respect to the acquisition of oral language following cochlear implantation. It can be argued, however, that the latter group does not provide the appropriate comparison group and that expectations for postimplant benefit should be based on reasonable goals for hearing children with similar disabilities. In addition, most studies have involved very small numbers and many of the variables known to impact pediatric CI outcomes in general could not be controlled. These variables include well-established child factors (duration of deafness, age of implantation, residual hearing and aided benefit pre-CI, and consistency of device use), family factors (parent interaction style, home language, socioeconomic variables, and other family stressors), and education/habilitation factors (mode of communication, access to services, educational setting, and hours of therapy). Finally, the variability in reported outcomes has been large, with some CI children at the milder end of the disability spectrum developing some spoken language skills. The majority of children reported as multiply disabled, however, have not developed similar skills.

Other CI centers have adopted the position that cochlear implantation opens up an additional sensory channel to children whose overall developmental potential is already compromised by other conditions. In addressing deafness as the additional disability, it is anticipated that the combined developmental impact of disabling conditions will be lessened. From this perspective, the goal of implantation appears to be general auditory awareness, allowing the child to participate more fully in his or her environment. As the studies reviewed earlier suggest, when auditory detection is the goal for implantation, this objective likely will be met.

Even when other factors work against the development of spoken language, the capacity to detect sound in one's environment is not trivial. Awareness of sound supports growth in a number of skills and pre-cursors to child development. These include social attachment, behavioral regulation, attention, and turn-taking. The association of sound with meaning (recognition of familiar voices, sound-object association) lays important groundwork at the prelinguistic stage of communication development. In addition, sound awareness provides an important safety function in potentially dangerous environments and, along with vision, provides cues to orientation in space. For children with dual sensory impairment (deafness and vision impairment), awareness of sound may impart better safety awareness when teaching mobility and orientation skills. For children with significant motor impairments or delays, greater sound awareness may encourage exploration of the environment, thereby increasing mobility and motor skills. Thus, sound awareness is not just important for development of communication, but supports child development and safety as a whole. Furthermore, parents and therapists of deaf/HOH children have reported notable improvements in child participation in a wide range of therapies (e.g., physical, occupational, and feeding) when using sensory devices (implant or hearing aid) to access sound. Other parents of multiply disabled CI children whose primary communication mode is sign have reported that their ability to communicate with their child is noticeably enhanced when using the device. These anecdotal accounts, in combination with other qualitative benefits reported by parents (Wiley et al., 2005), suggest a number of ancillary benefits that might be provided by CI use in this population, even when spoken language development is unlikely.

Thus, *minimum objectives* for cochlear implantation in children with multiple disabilities might be:

1. Improved auditory awareness, including the ability to detect the voices of family members and other significant individuals.
2. Improved communication, supported by access to sound, in the modality or combination of modalities most appropriate for the child.
3. Improved ability to participate in the world around them through perception of environmental sound relevant for their development and safety.

To these objectives, others may be added within the context of the child's pre-CI auditory skills and communication abilities, availability of communication and educational resources, and what might be considered reasonable expectations for hearing children with similar disabilities. It is important to state, however, that these minimum goals should serve merely as starting points rather than final benchmarks. Establishing postimplant objectives within the context of a hierarchical skill set can guide families and clinicians in monitoring progress and identifying the appropriate next goal to attain.

"Realistic" Expectations

Along with well-defined objectives by the CI center, the family's goals in pursuing implantation for their child should be explored. As a start, it is important that families understand that cochlear implantation does not result in "normal" hearing and that any gains achieved come only with intensive intervention and consistent device use over time. Families of children with multiple disabilities should be aware that although improved sound awareness may be evident within the first few weeks or months following implantation, further development in auditory skills may emerge only after a prolonged period of device use or may not develop at all.

Although "realistic expectations" on the part of the family have been long established as part of candidacy criteria (Mecklenberg, Demorest, & Staller, 1991; Northern et al., 1986; Tiber, 1985), large variability in outcomes has consistently been noted, even among otherwise typically developing children (Miyamoto et al., 1989; Nikolopoulos, O'Donoghue, & Archbold, 1999; Svirsky, Robbins, Kirk, Pisoni, & Miyomoto, 2000). Thus, it is not always clear what "realistic" may mean (Zaidman-Zait & Most, 2005). Furthermore, beyond the general caveat that progress would likely be "slow" for children with multiple disabilities, there have been limited data with which to guide families in developing appropriate expectations regarding the benefit their children might achieve.

As a point of illustration, Figure 19–1 summarizes speech perception outcomes observed over a 3-year period in 34 CI children, 8 of whom have additional developmental disabilities. These 8 children (developmentally delayed, or DD, group; mean age at CI = 37 months; range = 13 to 72 months),

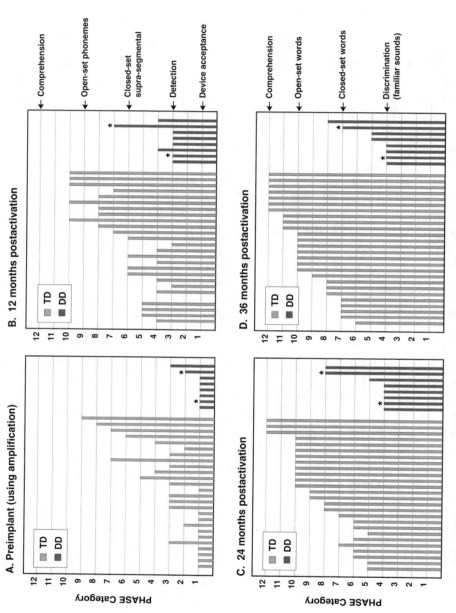

Figure 19–1. Auditory skill development in 34 CI children over 36 months postactivation as categorized according to the Pediatric Hierarchy of Auditory Skill Emergence (PHASE). TD = typically developing; DD = developmental delay/disability; * = child with autism diagnosed after implantation. Categories refer to the following: 1 = device acceptance (hearing aid prior to implantation); 2 = change in vocal behavior with device on; 3 = auditory detection; 4 = discrimination/familiar sounds; 5 = discrimination, able to choose between two alternatives; 6 = closed-set identification, suprasegmental; 7 = closed-set identification, words (segmental); 8 = closed-set identification, sentences; 9 = open-set recognition, phonemes; 10 = open-set recognition, words; 11 = open-set recognition, sentences; 12 = comprehension.

are part of an ongoing study at the House Ear Institute (HEI) CARE Center tracking CI outcomes in special populations (Johnson, Winter, Visser-Dumont, Martinez, & Eisenberg, 2008). Their additional disabilities include: cerebral palsy ($n = 1$), autism ($n = 3$), and cognitive/developmental delay ($n = 4$). Two of the children with autism (designated in Figure 19–1 with asterisks) were diagnosed with the disorder after implantation. The remaining 26 CI children with no known additional disabilities were implanted over a similar range of ages (typically developing, or TD, group; mean age at CI = 33 months; range = 13 to 61 months) and time period and are generally representative of the clinical population served by the HEI CARE Center. Auditory development was examined using the Pediatric Hierarchy of Auditory Skill Development (PHASE) (Johnson & Eisenberg, 2007). Originally developed to track the auditory progress of pediatric auditory brainstem implant (ABI) recipients (Eisenberg et al., 2008), the PHASE classifies auditory and speech perception milestones ascending from device acceptance (Level 1) through comprehension (Level 12). Category assignment is made on the basis of both parental report and clinical observations and measures, particularly at the very early stages of auditory acquisition. Similar to other categorical approaches, outcomes are expressed in terms of achieving general levels of performance (e.g., open-set speech recognition) rather than attaining stimulus-bound scores (e.g., % correct).

Figure 19–1A shows the categories achieved by each of the children using amplification prior to implantation; the TD children are shown in the left side of the panel (lighter bars) and the DD children are shown in the right side (darker bars). Even in the preimplant period, variability in skill level was large. Nine TD children and six DD children fell at the minimum level (Level 1), indicating a willingness to wear their hearing aids, but not much more. Ten children, including two children from the DD group, were showing a consistent change in vocal behavior (Level 2) or consistent sound detection (Level 3) with amplification. A few of the more TD children were showing varying degrees of closed-set or emerging open-set abilities, ranging from pattern perception (Level 6) to phoneme recognition (Level 8). These children tended to be those with more residual hearing. By the end of the first year postactivation (see Figure 19–1B), all children from both groups had achieved, at a minimum, consistent sound detection (Level 3). One-third of all children, including one child with as-yet undiagnosed autism, were at the level of closed-set word identification (Level 7) or beyond. Although five of the remaining children with additional disabilities stayed at the detection level (Level 3), two were beginning to recognize familiar sounds (Level 4), as were five children in the TD group. Notably, two of the children without additional disabilities also remained at the level of detection (one child from the TD group was not evaluated at this time interval).

By 24 months postactivation (see Figure 19–1C), a little over half of the TD children had achieved open-set recognition for phonemes, words, or sentences, although nearly as many were still working their way through the lower level closed-set measures. These data for the TD group are consistent with previous research that suggests it takes, on average, 2 to 3 years to achieve open-set recognition (Cheng, Grant, & Niparko, 1999). A second child from the DD group was demonstrating closed-set word identification (Level 7), whereas the remaining children with additional disabilities had not progressed further in recognition of familiar sounds (Level 4) by observation or parent report. By 36 months postactivation (see Figure 19–1D), 17 of the TD children were at the level of open-set word recognition (Level 10) or higher, with the remaining 8 TD children ranging between discrimination on a two-alternative forced-choice task and emerging open-set phoneme recognition. Although the variability among the typically developing children remains large, measurable auditory skill development continued to be observed even among those at the lower end of the range of performance. In contrast, only two children from the group with additional developmental disabilities have been able to demonstrate speech perception abilities beyond simple discrimination by 3 years postactivation when assessed using traditional pediatric test batteries.

These data serve to illustrate several important points: (1) variability in skill acquisition is large, even among children without additional disabilities, (2) skills are acquired over years, even among otherwise typically developing children, (3) children with additional developmental disabilities can and do demonstrate improved sound detection fairly soon following implantation, (4) some children with additional developmental disabilities are able to participate in formal speech perception testing, demonstrating skills commensurate with those shown by some children without known additional disabilities at the same assessment interval, but (5) for most children with additional developmental disabilities, progression through this hierarchy of auditory skills lags behind their more typically developing peers.

As argued previously, CI children without additional disabilities may not form the most appropriate group with which to compare progress for CI children from special populations. However, the expectations that parents (and many others) bring to the initial CI assessments are likely to be influenced by a number of factors, including what is portrayed about CIs in the media (including the Internet), what appears in manufacturer's literature, and any previous experience with more typically developing CI children. Even with early identification and intervention, by the time their child is being considered for CI, most parents have spent a substantial amount of time in the waiting rooms of otologists, audiologists, and therapists, observing other children and talking with their families. Thus, CI children without additional disabilities may be the primary frame of reference for many parents seeking out cochlear implantation for their own multiply disabled child.

Educational Setting and Support for Auditory Skill Growth

Although most of the formal assessments conducted to determine candidacy, map the device, and monitor progress are likely to take place at the CI center, the vast majority of the child's use of the device will be at home and at school. Research has shown that for CI children without additional disabilities, better outcomes are associated with placement in educational settings that emphasize an oral-aural mode of communication, whether benefit is assessed in terms of speech perception, speech production or language development (Geers et al., 2002). For deaf children with multiple disabilities with or without CIs, however, studies examining educational variables associated with better outcomes, including mode of communication, is largely lacking (Jones & Jones, 2003; Knoors & Vervloed, 2003). Nevertheless, even when spoken language development is not the primary CI goal, it is reasonable to predict that educational settings supportive of auditory skill growth will be associated with greater gains than those that emphasize visual communication with little or no voicing. Thus, auditory goals and opportunities for learning to listen should be balanced among the broader developmental goals established for the child.

The Cochlear Implant Team

The above considerations should be evaluated and weighed by a multidisciplinary team in making the decision about whether to proceed with implantation. Although the team concept has been integral to the CI process since the earliest days of implantation (e.g., American Speech-Language-Hearing Association, 1986; Beiter, Staller, & Dowell, 1991; Downs, Campos, Firemark, Martin, & Myers, 1986; Northern et al., 1986), some centers have come to base CI candidacy solely on audiologic and surgical criteria, leaving the outcomes sought in the case of an individual child largely undefined. Although it may be argued that if audiological and surgical criteria are not met other candidacy considerations are irrelevant, input from other members of the team is vital in articulating what might constitute postimplant "benefit" in children with vastly differing developmental and ability profiles. Furthermore, these same team members are likely to assume a central role in pulling together the postimplant habilitation program, many of the components of which should be in place prior to surgery (see Winter and Phillips, Chapter 2 this volume).

The composition of the implant team is likely to vary from center to center and perhaps from child to child. Core team members typically include a surgeon, an audiologist, and a speech-language pathologist, whose customary roles as part of the team are described elsewhere in this volume. In the case of children with additional disabilities, some of these roles may expand or change to accommodate the needs of a specific child, as described in sections below. The educational specialist also should be considered a vital component of the pediatric CI team, especially in the case of children with multiple disabilities being considered for implantation. Whether this role is filled by a center-based educational liaison or a community-based teacher of the deaf who consults with the team, the educational specialist can assess the educational setting into which the child likely will be placed following implantation and identify the availability of options and services to support auditory skill growth. Of equal importance is the role of this specialist in serving as a resource for community-based educators and therapists, providing information about the device and developing expectations for its use. Furthermore, it is the educational specialist who is likely to have the most contact with a child's teachers and other service providers outside the center and who thus are critical to the successful implementation of the educational/habilitation program should the child be implanted. Archbold (1994) has used the term "local team" to describe these providers in the community. Including, but not limited to, the child's early interventionist or classroom teacher (who may or may not be a teacher of the deaf), educational audiologist or aural habilitation therapist and itinerant speech-language specialist, these professionals are in unique positions to supply important information about the child and the family during the preimplant workup and throughout the postimplant period.

If not a routine member of the team, access to a psychologist who is skilled in the assessment of deaf children would be important to consider for this population. Not only can the psychologist provide input with regard to the general cognitive and learning abilities of the young children under consideration for cochlear implantation, he or she may also play an important role in identifying child and family behaviors and issues that could impact successful CI use. In some centers, social workers are part of the team, consulting with family about their expectations and the support systems that they have or need. Social workers also may assist to identify barriers to compliance in the case of families who are not following through with appointments, as well as developing strategies for improving compliance.

In view of the complexity of some developmental disabilities or combinations thereof, it may be relevant to seek input from other sources outside the CI center-based team on a case-by-case basis. These include physical therapists, occupational therapists, vision therapists, behavioral intervention therapists, and feeding therapists, who can contribute important information about how the child's other developmental or sensory conditions might impact device use or the post-CI services. These specialists can identify potential obstacles to consistent device use or full participation in educational/habilitation programs, as well as suggest accommodations or solutions to minimize their impact. They also may be helpful in identifying some of the child's strengths, and abilities that can be capitalized upon in implementing the program.

Some CI centers have begun to include developmental pediatricians as part of their team. A relative subspecialty of pediatric medicine, the development pediatrician has specific training in assessing and managing children with a wide range of developmental and behavioral disabilities (Wiley, 2004). Although not a substitute for the psychologist, whose role it is to conduct the cognitive, developmental, and behavioral assessments, the developmental pediatrician may assist the team in understanding the impact of any additional disabilities coupled with the hearing loss. Furthermore, he or she may identify areas of concern in children as yet unrecognized developmental delay. Thus, access to this pediatric specialist may be particularly helpful for teams assessing large numbers of children with multiple disabilities or at risk for developmental delay. The developmental pediatrician also may assist in monitoring and managing these children in the postimplant period.

Of course, parents and/or primary caregivers play a critical role as members of the team, not only by outlining their goals in seeking the implant for their child, but also informing the group about how their child communicates and functions on a day-to-day basis. Furthermore, it is the parents or caregivers who are largely responsible for the follow-through necessary to achieve any benefit, including assuring consistent device use, taking the child to his or her various appointments and advocating for their child in educational planning.

Thus far the discussion has centered on children with known disabilities at the time of candidacy determination and implantation. However, with earlier implantation comes the increased possibility that developmentally relevant conditions exist that may not become apparent until after implantation. In addition to those described earlier in this chapter, these conditions may include specific learning disabilities, sensory issues, oral-motor disorders or behavioral disorders that impact language learning and/or speech production that may not be suspected until the child fails to make the expected progress with the device. Thus, in the case of any deaf child presented for candidacy determination, it is incumbent on the team to discuss with the family the possibility that as-yet undiagnosed conditions may impact outcomes, especially with respect to spoken language development.

Contraindications for Cochlear Implantation in Children with Multiple Disabilities

Even in the context of well-defined postimplant goals, realistic expectations on the part of the family and educators, and access to appropriate habilitation services, there are some sensory or behavioral conditions that may contraindicate cochlear implantation. Although the numbers are small, poor outcomes have been reported for implanted children with severe intellectual disability (Hamzavi et al., 2000), severe behavioral disturbances with autoaggression (Hamzavi et al., 2000), and psychosis (Filipo et al., 2004).

Some children with cognitive disabilities, deaf-blindness, and autism show extreme patterns of disruptive behavior (e.g., self-injurious behaviors, acting-out behaviors) (McClintock, Hall, & Oliver, 2003; Richman, 2008; Schroeder, Reese, Hellings, Loupe, & Tessel, 1999). If present, these behaviors need to be addressed prior to implantation. Self-injurious behaviors that could result in device failure, such as repetitive head-banging, would contradict implantation until brought under control. In some cases, these behaviors may serve a communication function for children who have no other means to express themselves and improvements in the ability to communicate can lead to a reduction of such behavior (Durand, 1993a, 1993b). In other cases, they may represent attention-seeking or avoidance behaviors that have become socially reinforced (Kurtz et al., 2003). Functional behavioral analysis, conducted by a behavioral specialist, can help uncover the purpose of problem behaviors and suggest function-based interventions. For some children, medication or intensive psychotherapy may be required as an adjunct to behavioral therapy (Baumeister, Todd, & Sevin, 1993; Carvill & Marston, 2002; Farber, 1986).

It also has been suggested by some that conditions including therapy-resistant seizure disorder, neural and/or central deficits, severe learning disabilities and hyperactivity be considered possible contraindications (Bertram, 2004; Bertram, Lenarz, & Lesinski, 2000). However, no specific evidence has been brought to bear for such disorders, and because these conditions present over a range of severity it is up to each CI center to establish its own guidelines.

An example of a condition that ranges in severity is autism spectrum disorder. Some centers have included the diagnosis of autism on the list of contraindications for cochlear implantation (e.g., Bertram et al., 2000); other centers have not (e.g., Hayman & Franck, 2005). In making the decision as to whether to implant a child with diagnosed or suspected autism, Hayman and Franck (2005) describe the use of an expanded version of the Children's Implant Profile (ChIP) (Hellman et al., 1991) to weigh other factors known to contribute to successful implant outcomes. At their center (The Children's Hospital of Philadelphia, CHOP), age, parental expectations, other disabilities, and child behavior were weighted more heavily than the other factors on the list. For example, this team is more likely to implant a younger child, with no disabilities beyond hearing loss and autism, and who does not demonstrate severe hyperactivity, aggression, self-stimulation, or repeated disengagement during therapy. Input regarding the child's behavior is obtained not only from the parents and the CI team, but is actively sought from other professionals working with the child on a routine basis. Furthermore, the team has stipulated that the child have some type of formal language system in place (oral, cued speech, signed English, American Sign Language or ASL, Picture Exchange Communication System, other augmentative communication, or any combination thereof) before the decision is made to implant.

Employed in similar manner, any of the candidacy profiles in current use could be applied to rate concerns in weighted fashion regarding implantation in the presence of other types of disabilities in the development of center-specific guidelines. These profiles, which are all variants of the ChIP, include the Graded Profile Analysis (GPA) (Daya et al., 1999), the Nottingham Children's Implant Profile (NChIP) (Nikolopoulos, Dyar, & Gibbin, 2004), and another modified version of Children's Implant Profile (Edwards, 2003). It is still not known, however, whether such strategies are effective in determining candidacy, particularly with regard to special populations. To date, there have been few studies comparing developmental outcomes in deaf children with specific types of additional disabilities who have been implanted versus those who have not. Furthermore, the weighting of specific criteria by a given CI team may shift over time, as the center gains more expertise in implanting children from special populations and putting into place their post-CI habilitation plan. For example, the CI team at Cincinnati Children's Hospital (where the second author is located) used to have a similar criterion to that described above, wherein a language system needed to be in place in order for a child with ASD to be considered a candidate in their program. However, they have since relaxed this criterion, adopting the position that the language approach needs to be individualized based on the child's current level of communication and/or presymbolic communication, no matter what the child's functional hearing with an implant. In that building a language base is key to the cognitive development in hear-

ing children with autism, an implant should not detract from these tenets.

In the past, degenerative diseases or conditions with shortened life expectancy have been considered contraindications to implantation (Bertram, 2004; Bertram et al., 2000; Uziel et al., 1995). At the time of this writing, however, anecdotal reports of children with Infantile Refsum disease (IRD) receiving cochlear implants have begun to appear (Royal Institute for Deaf and Blind Children, 2008; The Ear Foundation, 2008). One child with this diagnosis has been implanted at Cincinnati Children's Hospital Medical Center. IRD is a rare inborn error of phytanic acid, a substance found commonly in food. Toxic buildup of this substance results in damage to the white matter of the brain, leading to blindness (retinitis pigmentosa), hearing loss, motor impairment, and mental and growth retardation. Symptoms begin in infancy and progress into early childhood. The disease is ultimately fatal, but some children survive into their teens and sometimes beyond (National Institute of Neurological Disorders and Stroke, 2007). This willingness on the part of some CI teams to implant children with such poor long-term prognoses signals a dramatic shift in candidacy criteria among some of the more experienced pediatric CI centers and the increasing importance of quality of life considerations in determining when to proceed. As in the case of any child being considered for a cochlear implant, appropriate expectations should be in place and each child should be considered on a case-by-case basis.

Preimplant Multidisciplinary Assessment

In considering the preimplant assessment, the CI center might take one of two philosophical approaches. The first approach would be to determine whether the child meets the candidacy criteria for that center. This puts the primary decision-making capacity in the hands of the cochlear implant team. Although it is important to establish that the child meets basic surgical and audiological criteria for implantation, implant centers are likely to differ with respect to the additional criteria for moving forward, particularly in considering children with additional disabilities. Thus, if the child is determined not to be a candidate at the first center, referral to another pediatric CI center with differing criteria may be appropriate. A second approach assumes that the child who meets basic audiologic and surgical criteria is a CI candidate and that the remaining assessments are conducted to determine what types of supports a child and family may need after receiving a CI in order to achieve the maximum benefit.

The specifics of the process are likely to vary from center to center, particularly with respect to point of entry, the order in which evaluations are carried out, and the person on the team who serves as coordinator. In general, however, preimplant evaluation consists of the same core components, including: otologic, audiologic, communication, cognitive/developmental, social/family support and expectations, and educational evaluations. Referrals for further evaluations may be made on a case-by-case basis, upon recommendations of team members. In the event it is determined that the child is not a CI candidate by the center, the information obtained in the multidisciplinary assessment may be used as a basis for further referrals and recommendations for other therapeutic interventions.

Otologic Assessment

The otologic workup consists of a medical evaluation to assess general health status and radiologic imaging of the temporal bone to examine the anatomy of the cochlea and auditory nerve. In children with known additional disabilities, it also may be important to image the central nervous system (brain), which may shed light on the origin and, perhaps, extent of a specific disability. Because it is much more difficult to obtain magnetic resonance imaging (MRI) of the brain once the implant is in place, such imaging should at least be considered prior to proceeding with cochlear implantation.

The CI surgeon also may need to communicate with other pediatric specialists to determine whether the child is a surgical candidate from a broader perspective. For some children with complex medical issues, additional workups and presurgical clearances (e.g., cardiac, respiratory, anesthesiology) may be necessary and additional personnel may need to be available at the time of surgery or during postoperative recovery (e.g., pediatric anesthesiologist, cardiologist, neurologist, respiratory therapist). In some cases, these requirements may dictate where the surgery should take place (e.g., a pediatric hospital versus a general outpatient surgical facility). In the presence of conditions or diseases that render the child medically fragile or at increased surgical risk (e.g., cardiac anomalies or significant lung disease), cochlear implantation needs to be carefully considered. Furthermore, in the case of conditions that are likely to necessitate access to MRI, the risks imposed by the surgery and limited access to MRI must be weighed against the benefits of even minimum audition, the ability to participate more fully in treatment, and the potential for improved quality of life.

If the etiology of the hearing loss has not been determined, referral for genetic evaluation may be indicated. Of the nearly 600 syndromes that have now been identified as associated with hearing loss (Joint Committee on Infant Hearing, 2007), many include cognitive, developmental, sensory, or motor impairments in their constellation of features. In most cases, determination of hearing loss etiology will not alter the course of otologic or audiologic management; however, it may provide a larger context within which to consider additional referrals or the plan of follow-up that might be indicated. In other cases, knowing the etiology of hearing loss might impact the timing or course of otologic intervention (e.g., the diagnosis of USH1). Furthermore, there are many combinations of genetic and environmental factors that can influence developmental outcomes. Thus, the identification of one set of factors that could well explain a given child's clinical presentation (e.g., prematurity) does not preclude the possibility of other etiologies for the hearing loss (e.g., GJB2 mutations). Recent studies have identified GJB2 mutations in a number of children with additional developmental delays and/or structural abnormalities (Kenna et al., 2007; Wiley, Choo, Meinzen-Derr, Hilbert, & Greinwald, 2006), some of whom had been diagnosed with other hearing loss etiologies prior to GJB2 screening. Mutations in the GJB2 gene, which encodes the gap junction protein connexin 26 and is important in maintaining inner ear homeostasis, has been estimated to cause up to 50% of autosomal recessive nonsyndromic hearing loss (Cohn et al, 1998). In the past, children with connexin-26 related hearing loss were considered to have no other developmental issues as the GJB2 mutation only impacts hearing (Cohn & Kelley, 2000). Although the GJB2 mutations are not considered to underlie these non-auditory clinical findings, such a diagnosis would be important information for the families given the prevalence of GJB2-related hearing loss.

Beyond these considerations for special populations, the same presurgical precautions warranted for any child being considered for cochlear implantation apply to children with additional disabilities. Thus, it is important to identify and, if necessary, treat any middle ear disease that might be present in preparation for surgery (Fayad, Tabaee, Micheletto, & Parisie, 2003). Children with craniofacial anomalies and certain syndromes (e.g. CHARGE, trisomy 21) are particularly susceptible to middle ear disease. It also is important to ensure that immunization for streptococcus pneumoniae is up to date, particularly if there is evidence of cochlear malformation (Cohen, Roland, & Marrinan, 2004).

Audiologic Assessment

The preimplant audiologic assessment serves a number of objectives, including: (1) determination of the child's audiologic candidacy with regard to the center's criteria for cochlear implantation, (2) assessment of the adequacy of the child's current sensory device fitting and the benefit derived from its use, and (3) counseling the family about CI technology and the range of possible post-CI outcomes. In some cases, the child may have been receiving audiological services, including the fitting and monitoring of amplification, at the CI center for some time before the CI referral is made. When this is the case, the pre-CI evaluation is largely a matter of updating the clinical record and providing parents with information about CI technology in general and the features of various devices in particular. In other cases, the child will be new to the center and, in conjunction with a review of previous records, an audiologic and hearing aid assessment must be undertaken prior to counseling.

The assessment of aided and unaided auditory function typically proceeds in the same manner as it would for a child at a similar developmental level. The test battery should consist of a combination of behavioral and physiologic measures that cross-check and complement one another (Johnson & Winter, 2003; Roush, Holcomb, Roush, & Escolar, 2004). For a given child, the relative emphasis placed on physiologic versus behavioral measures in defining degree and configuration of the loss will depend on the child's age, developmental level, and other physical and sensory abilities. Thus, in infants, children with developmental delays, and children who are otherwise unable to participate fully for behavioral testing, physiologic procedures (auditory brainstem response, auditory steady-state response, acoustic immittance measures, and otoacoustic emissions) are likely to play the larger role in assessment. In children with the motor skills and cognitive ability to participate in the tasks required, including some children with milder developmental delays, behavioral measures (visual reinforcement or conditioned play audiometry) are likely to assume the major role. Nevertheless, behavioral findings should always be supplemented with physiologic measures (at a minimum acoustic immittance measures and otoacoustic emissions) and physiologic estimates of auditory sensitivity should be supported by observations of the child's behavior in response to sound (Jerger & Hayes, 1976).

To some extent, the child's degree of loss and audiological history may also be a factor in the degree to which behavioral testing techniques can be used to obtain consistent and reliable information about the child's minimal detection thresholds. A child whose hearing loss was identified early, monitored frequently, and has at least some experience with sound (even if only at higher intensity levels) may be better able to be conditioned for behavioral tasks than a child who was identified more recently, has not been tested frequently, and/or for whom the degree of loss affords little to no auditory access, even with well-fit amplification. In either case, it is important to ascer-

tain the degree to which a child is capable of providing consistent behavioral responses to sound as this will impact the determination of hearing aid benefit prior to implantation and the programming of the device if implanted.

Assessment of children with multiple disabilities often requires adaptations in conditioning, testing setup, and technique. Many of these adaptations are well known to pediatric audiologists experienced in the assessment of infants and young children with and without developmental delays. These may include the use of tactile-auditory conditioning for children unable to condition to air-conducted stimuli alone, the incorporation of longer response intervals, and the use of tangible or edible reinforcers. Other adaptations for children with specific types of disabilities include the use of infant seats to support young children with low muscle tone while testing (Roush et al., 2004) and, in the case of children with visual impairment, positioning the child close to illuminated reinforcement toys or moving the reinforcers close to the child (Gravel, 1989; Moore, 1995). For some children conditioning may take place over time using a series of short sessions at the clinic, combined with reinforcement at home and in therapy. Input from families and interventionists who work with the child on a regular basis can be invaluable in identifying what has worked in the past, what behaviors might constitute a response, and potential barriers to testing.

With the progress made in early hearing detection and intervention (EHDI) programs over the last decade, pediatric audiologists also have grown well accustomed to fitting amplification on very young children. For the most part, techniques that have been developed for the fitting and verification of amplification for young infants and toddlers have application for children with additional disabilities. That is to say, the use of audibility-based pediatric prescriptive procedures and real-ear measures should play a central role in selecting and verifying the electroacoustic characteristics of the hearing aid (American Academy of Audiology, 2003).

There are some important exceptions, however. Children with severe hearing and visual loss use acoustic cues to obtain important information about the environment (De l'Aune, 1980; Tharpe, 2000). These include: (1) loudness cues to estimate distance, (2) sound shadow (sound absorption by an object) and change in spectral shape to locate objects between listener and sound source, and (3) resonances from reflected sound to enable the avoidance of large obstacles. For this reason, optimization of hearing aid characteristics for speech perception (e.g., relative emphasis on higher frequencies over lower frequencies, compression schemes that alter loudness cues) may fail to provide important acoustic information for such children trying to develop orientation and mobility skills (Tharpe, 2000; Tharp, Ashmead, & Rothplet, 2002). Thus, the additional functions that audition might serve in special populations and how amplification (and ultimately the CI) fits into that scheme should be considered carefully. McCracken and Bamford (1995) also have pointed out that for children with multiple disabilities, real-ear measures that require use of a probe microphone in the ear canal may be especially difficult to obtain in the presence of excessive movement or tactile defensiveness. Nevertheless, it is in this population that such measures may be particularly important. In the case of craniofacial anomalies, for example, ear canal volumes may be unusually small compared to other children of similar chronologic age and use of average real-ear-to-coupler differences (RECD) may be significantly underestimated.

In the preimplant period, assessment of the functional benefit derived from the use of amplification is typically limited to soundfield detection thresholds and parent report. For the latter purpose, the Infant-Toddler Meaningful Integration Scale, (IT-MAIS) (Zimmerman-Phillips, Robbins, & Osberger, 2000) and the older Meaningful Auditory Integration Scale, or MAIS (Robbins, Renshaw, & Berry, 1991) have well-established histories among CI centers. These tools also have been recommended for functional auditory assessment of young children with severe and profound hearing loss using amplification (American Speech-Language-Hearing Association, 2004). The IT-MAIS is a 10-probe parent-report scale, designed to evaluate developing auditory behavior in CI children ages 1 to 3 years. Obtained through structured interview, parents rate how often their child engages in specific vocal behavior and auditory behaviors using a 5-point scale (0 to 4). Items probe vocal behavior with the sensory device on (probes 1 and 2), alerting to sound in environment (probes 3 through 6), and ability to derive meaning from sound (probes 7 through 10). The MAIS is appropriate for use in CI children that have attained a developmental age of 4 years and above. The MAIS is identical to the IT-MAIS, with the exception of the first two items, which assess evidence of device bonding on the part of the older child.

With the successful implementation of EHDI programs has come the development of a number of new tools for assessing auditory skill acquisition in very young preverbal children using sensory devices. These include, but are not limited to, the Auditory Skills Checklist (Meinzen-Derr, et al., 2004; Meinzen-Derr, Wiley, Creighton, & Choo, 2007), the Checklist of Auditory Communication Skills (MED-EL Corporation & Caleffe-Schenck, 2006), the LittlEARS Auditory Questionnaire (Kuhn-Inacker, Weichbold, Tsiakpini, Coninx, & D'Haese, 2003), and the Functional Auditory Performance Indicators (FAPI: Stredler-Brown & Johnson, 2001, 2003, 2004). Each of these measures is based on hierarchical models of auditory development (e.g., Erber, 1982; Stout & Windle, 1992). Although not all were developed for use with multiply disabled or CI children, these tools can provide a baseline against which to compare further auditory skill growth in the postimplant period. A summary of these questionnaires and checklists is provided in Table 19–1.

Psychological Assessment

A child's cognitive abilities, information processing, and problem-solving skills and learning style may be important variables to consider in formulating expectations for CI benefit (Geers, Brenner, & Davidson, 2003a; Geers, Nicholas, & Sedey, 2003b; Nikolopoulos et al., 2004; Pisoni, 2000; Tobey, Geers, Brenner, Altuna, & Gabbert, 2003). Thus, an assessment by a licensed psychologist with experience in the evaluation deaf children can contribute significantly to discussions about the range of outcomes that might be expected and the time it may take for such outcomes to emerge. This input would be particularly pertinent in the case of a child with multiple disabilities. Nevertheless, psychological assessment prior to pediatric cochlear implantation raises a number of issues. These include questions about the relationship between intelligence and post-CI outcomes. They also include concerns about the appropriateness of using standardized instruments with deaf children in general and deaf children with additional disabilities in particular.

A number of investigators have shown relationships between measured IQ and CI outcomes in otherwise typically developing deaf children (Dawson et al., 2002; Geers et al., 2003a; Geers et al., 2003b; Tobey et al., 2003); others have not (Knutson, Ehlers, Wald, & Tyler, 2000a). However, in studies that spe-

cifically compared outcomes in CI children to those without cognitive or developmental delays, it generally has been observed that children with delays progress more slowly and demonstrate fewer gains than those without such delays (Dettman et al., 2004; Edwards et al., 2006; Holt & Kirk, 2005).

As discussed by Knutson and Stika (Chapter 13 this volume), the use of standardized instruments can provide important information about the child's basic cognitive and psycho-social development, as well as areas of strength and weakness that may be addressed in post-CI habilitation. Furthermore, preimplant assessment using standardized measures can provide a baseline against which to evaluate postimplant benefit. Nevertheless, substantial caution should be used when interpreting results obtained on young deaf children, in view of the linguistic, auditory, and/or attentional demands entailed in most of these instruments.

Measures of adaptive behavior and functional skills may be particularly relevant for this subset of children. Adaptive behaviors refer to those skills required for adapting to and participating in one's everyday environment. Unlike cognition, which is generally considered to be stable, adaptive behavior is modifiable and responsive to intervention (Sparrow, Cicchetti, & Balla, 2005). As such, measurement of adaptive behavior is becoming an increasingly important component in the psychoeducational assessment of children with disabilities. One of the most commonly used functional measures is the Vineland Adaptive Behavior Scales (Second Edition) (Vineland-II; Sparrow et. al., 2005). The Vineland-II assesses personal and social skills within the domains of communication, socialization, motor skills and daily living skills. It has an extensive normative database in children and adults with a variety of developmental disabilities, although it has not been used extensively with young children with hearing loss.

TABLE 19–1. Checklists and Questionnaires for Tracking Development of Functional Auditory Skills in Young Deaf and Hard-of-Hearing (Deaf/HOH) Children Using Sensory Devices

Questionnaire or Checklist	Purpose & Targeted Population	Description	Response Format
Auditory Skills Checklist (ASC) Meinzen-Derr, Wiley, Choo, & Creighton, 2004)	Purpose: Developed to serve as a bridge in assessing functional skill growth between those evaluated by the IT-MAIS and more formal measures of auditory comprehension. Target group: Any young child with sensorineural hearing loss.	35-item checklist of auditory skills progressing from detection, through discrimination, identification, and comprehension. For each item, the child is assigned one of three scores 0—"does not have the skill," 1—"emerging skill development", 2—"consistently demonstrates the skill".	Structured parent report and clinician observation
Checklist of Auditory Communication Skills (MED-EL Corporation & Caleffe-Schenck, 2006)	Purpose: Developed for use in multiple settings to track auditory skill growth and develop auditory goals. Only those skills observed in the auditory-condition are to be noted. Targeted Group: Children of all ages and skill levels.	27-item checklist of auditory skills that support development of spoken communication. Items range from awareness of sound to understanding in background noise. The majority of items can be marked as having been demonstrated: never, sometimes (25%), often (50%), or always (75% or more).	Structured parent report and teacher or therapist observation.

Questionnaire or Checklist	Purpose & Targeted Population	Description	Response Format
LittlEARS Auditory Questionnaire (Kuhn-Inacker, Weichbold, Tsiakpini, Coninx, & D'Haese, 2003)	Purpose: Developed to track attainment of preverbal auditory milestones in typically hearing children and deaf/HOH children using sensory devices. Targeted Group: Normal hearing children from birth to two years; Deaf/HOH children over the first two years following sensory device fitting (i.e., first two years "hearing age").	35 questions relating to auditory milestones observed in typically hearing and developing children during the first two years. Items range from response to familiar voice to child's attempts to sing along with familiar songs. For each item parents answer "yes" (behavior observed at least once) or "no" (behavior never observed or "not sure"). Validated in 218 normally hearing children in Europe (Tsiakpini, Weichbold, Coninx, & D'Haese, 2002).	Parent questionnaire
Functional Auditory Performance Indicators (FAPI) (Stredler-Brown & Deconde Johnson, 2001, 2003)	Purpose: Developed to serve as a tool for quantifying a child's competencies in each of seven categories of auditory skill development and provide means for creating individualized intervention plans. Targeted Group: Young children with hearing loss enrolled in early intervention programs.	31 skills within a hierarchical framework of 7 categories of auditory development, from sound awareness through linguistic auditory processing. Each skill rated as "not present," "emerging," "in process," or "acquired" under a variety of conditions (e.g., in quiet, with visual cues, when prompted). Although categories are hierarchical, it is assumed that child may be working on many skills at the same time. Detailed scoring and weighting system that results in profile of individual strengths and needs.	Rating scales in each of seven categories completed by parent, early interventionists, and clinicians.

For some children, criterion-referenced measures, such as the Developmental Assessment for Students with Severe Disabilities (DASH-2; Dykes & Erin, 1999) may provide additional information about functional domains and incremental changes in skill level that traditional assessment batteries are not intended to measure. Developed for use with individuals who are functioning developmentally between the ages of birth to 6 years, 11 months, the DASH-2 consists of five scales that assess language skills, sensorimotor skills, social-emotional skills, basic academic skills, and activities involved in daily living. Within each scale, skills are rated according the amount of assistance required in performing each task. The sequence of skills acquisition and the nature of the child's attempts to complete a task are considered more important than the age equivalents or total scores in identifying emerging skills, monitoring skill development and identifying areas that should be targeted during teaching and in therapy.

Preoperative assessment also provides the psychologist with the opportunity to discuss parental expectations, observe family interactions, and identify factors that may impact successful CI use. These factors include behavioral and emotional issues, diagnosed or otherwise, on the part of the child. They also may include issues related to parental acceptance of the hearing loss and other disabilities, along with the social and emotional resources upon which the parents have to draw in raising a multiply disabled child. If indicated, the psychologist may recommend referrals for further assessment or counseling.

Developmental Assessment

As stated earlier, some CI centers have begun to enlist the expertise of developmental pediatricians as part of their preimplant evaluation process and postoperative follow-up.

Many CI centers do not and among those that do, there can be wide variability in exposure to typically developing deaf/HOH children. There also is some overlap between developmental behavioral pediatrics and psychology; however, the input provided by the two disciplines can be complementary. This may particularly be true in the case of children with complex medical as well as developmental needs. Developmental pediatricians have training in a multitude of specific disabilities and thus can contribute to the discussion about developmental expectations and likely CI outcomes. This includes reinforcing the concept that although the device may allow access to sound, the way deaf children with additional disabilities process and use what they hear can be quite variable.

In the initial assessment, the developmental pediatrician takes a comprehensive family, medical, and developmental history and performs a thorough physical examination that includes a neurologic assessment. In collaboration with other team members, he or she can identify, in a broad sense, the child's strengths and needs in a variety of domains including cognitive, self-help, fine motor, gross motor, and communication. During follow-up care, the developmental pediatrician can play an important role in assuring that all aspects of a child's development are being addressed in educational and therapeutic planning.

Communication Assessment

One of the primary motives for all parents of deaf children seeking cochlear implantation is to be able to communicate more effectively with their child. Although the communication goal of implantation for most typically developing deaf children is to acquire spoken language, for the multiply disabled child it is to foster communication in whatever modality or combination of modalities may be most appropriate. Thus, for these children, the purpose of the preimplant communication assessment is to determine: (1) whether and how the child is attempting to communicate, and (2) the likelihood that communication can be further developed through access to sound via a CI. The data obtained also provide a baseline against which to monitor skill growth if the child is implanted.

Frequently, the deaf child who presents for CI assessment is at the prelinguistic stage of communication. This is particularly the case in very young children and children with developmental disabilities. Among the latter group, the problem may be compounded by other conditions (e.g., motor disorders such as cerebral palsy) that impact the child's expressive abilities. Because most standardized clinician-elicited language measures are not designed to tap into the skills observed in children below the age of 1 year (Table 11–1C, Ambrose, Hammes-Ganguly, & Lehnert, Chapter 11 this volume), their use can be limited in the preimplant stage. Thus, measures based on parent report are typically required to provide important information about the child's communication abilities. Examples include the SKI*HI Language Development Scale (Watkins & Tonelson, 2004) and the Rossetti Infant-Toddler Language Scale (Rossetti, 2006), both of which are criterion-referenced measures. Ambrose and colleagues have discussed each of these measures, including the strengths and limitations of each with the young deaf/HOH population, and the reader is referred to their chapter for more detail.

A parent-report instrument increasingly being adopted by CI teams to assess communication skills before and after cochlear implantation is the MacArthur-Bates Communicative Development Inventories (CDI) (Fenson et al., 2007). The CDI is a set of checklists in which patients indicate the gestures, words, and syntax forms their child understands or produces. Unlike the SKI*HI and Rossetti, the CDI is a norm-referenced measure that may be used to compare a child's communication abilities to normally hearing, typically developing children in the same age range. The current version has recently been validated for assessing the early language development in deaf children with CIs (Thal, Desjardin, & Eisenberg, 2007). Furthermore, normative data have been developed for an earlier version of the CDI (Fenson et al., 1993) for deaf/HOH children using a range of communication modalities (Mayne, Yoshinaga-Itano, & Sedey, 2000a; Mayne, Yoshinaga-Itano, Sedey, & Carely, 2000b). The sample upon which these latter data are based include children who range in degree of both hearing loss and cognitive ability. A version of the CDI also has been adapted for use with children using ASL (Anderson & Reilly, 2002), as well as 45 other spoken languages, including three forms of Spanish (Moreno, 2007).

Two CDI forms reflect language skills acquired by children in different age ranges. CDI-Words and Gestures (W/G) provides norms for normal hearing children ages 8 to 18 months and probes vocabulary comprehension, production and the use of gestures; the CDI-Words and Sentences (W/S), extends the list of vocabulary words produced and surveys a number of aspects of grammatical development typically acquired by 30 months of age. Of particular relevance in the assessment of very young children and those with developmental delays in the pre-verbal, prelinguistic stages of development, are the inventories of gestures and play behaviors included in CDI-W/G. Items included in early gestures reflect many of those associated with the onset of intentional communication and emerging joint attention abilities. Items included under late gestures and play behaviors reflect some of those associated with development of representational abilities. Communicative intent, joint attention, turn-taking, and symbolic play are important predictors of subsequent language development in normally hearing and typically developing children (Tait, Lutman, & Robinson, 2000; Watt, Wetherby, & Shumway, 2006; Wetherby, Cain, Yonclas, & Walker, 1988). In general, typically developing deaf/HOH children acquire the same repertoire of pre-linguistic behaviors (Adamson, 1995; Lederberg & Everhart, 1998; Prezbindowski, Adamson, & Lederberg, 1998; Spencer, 2000; Yoshinaga-Itano & Stredler-Brown, 1992), with some minor variations between deaf children of deaf parents versus deaf children of hearing parents (Waxman & Spencer, 1997). However, altered patterns of pre-linguistic communication have been observed in children with a range of developmental disabilities (Arens, Cress, & Marvin, 2005; Calandrella & Wilcox, 2000; Wetherby, Yonclas, & Bryan, 1989).

Information about the child's communicative behavior provided by the parents can be supplemented by observation of the child, either informally or through the use of structured activity. Another instrument that combines direct behavioral observation of child and parent input is the Communication and Symbolic Behavior Scales (CSBS) (Wetherby & Prizant, 1993, 2003). The CSBS is a standardized tool designed to assess the communicative, social-affective, and symbolic abilities of infants through preschool-aged children. It uses natural play routines and other adult interactions to assess functional communication skills in typically developing children between 8 and 24 months of age and atypically developing children up to 72 months of age. The child's behavior is sampled during structured interaction with both clinician and parent, using activities designed to elicit spontaneous communication and play

behavior. Nonverbal and early verbal behaviors are scored on 18 scales that measure 6 aspects of communicative behavior and on 4 scales that measure symbolic development. In a study investigating the relationship between prelinquistic communication behavior and subsequent language learning in young CI children (Kane, Schopmeyer, Mellon, Wang, & Niparko, 2004), positive, but weak correlations were found between CSBS scores obtained around the time of device activation and scores on the Reynell Developmental Language Scales (RDLS) (Reynell & Gruber, 1990) obtained after an average of 20 months of CI experience. Although high scores on the CSBS did not predict high scores on the RDLS; poor performance on the CSBS appeared to be a "red flag" with regard to the later acquisition of spoken language this group of children. In this sample no gross motor delays were observed; however, cognitive status was not assessed. These investigators concluded that the quality of prelinguistic communicative behaviors as measured on the CSBS provided important predictive information about later language development. Furthermore, they suggested that this type of assessment could offer insight into strategies for therapeutic and parent-based interventions and assist in setting parental expectations about communication outcomes.

As orginally developed, the CSBS has been used primarily as a research tool for evaluating prelinguistic communication in typically developing children (e.g., Prior et al., 2008; Reilly et al., 2006) and children with specific types of disability (e.g., Kane et al., 2004; McCathren, Yoder, & Warren, 1999, Wetherby, Prizant, & Hutchinson, 1998). A shorter version of the CSBS, the Communication and Symbolic Behavior Scales Developmental Profile (CSBS-DP) (Wetherby & Prizant, 2002) has been adapted for clinical use, specifically in the screening and evaluation of children at risk for communication and developmental delays. In the CSBS-DP, the number of scales of communication and symbolic behaviors assessed has been decreased to 20 (compared to a total of 22 scales in the CSBS) and the scoring procedures for the behavioral sample (BS) have been simplified. Furthermore, the BS has been shortened from between 45 and 60 minutes for the original CSBS to approximately 30 minutes for the DP version. In addition to the BS, the CSBS-DP includes two parent-report measures, an Infant-Toddler Checklist and a Caregiver Questionnaire (CQ), both of which target the same seven language predictors as measured in the BS. These language predictors include: emotion and use of eye gaze, communication, gestures, sounds, use of words, understanding of words, and object use. The parent-report measures were normed on a large sample of children ages 6 to 24 months with no known disabilities, whereas the BS was normed on a smaller subset of the same children between the ages of 12 and 24 months. The one-page Infant-Toddler Checklist consists of 24 multiple-choice questions that can be used independently from the CQ and BS to screen for developmental delays. At the time of this writing, the Checklist was available in a number of languages in addition to English, including Spanish, Chinese, German, and Slovenian (Florida State University Research Foundation, 2007). The four-page CQ consists of 41 multiple-choice items on which parents rate the frequency ("not yet," "sometimes," "often") with which they observe specific behaviors. In addition the CQ includes a recognition list consisting of the 36 words reported by Fenson et al. (1994) to be those that parents reported with the highest frequency on the MacArthur-Bates CDI. Although developed for screening and identification purposes, the CSBS-DP has been used in recent studies involving chil-

dren with known disabilities, in order to examine the communication profiles yielded by children representing different disability groups (e.g., Wetherby, Watt, Morgan, & Shumway, 2007; Wetherby et al., 2004) and to track early communication development in a pair of fraternal twins with communication delay, one with normal hearing and the other with sensorineural loss who received a CI (Seung, Holmes, & Colburn, 2005).

In cases where communicative intent is not observed on the part of the child or when there are concerns about the parent's ability to build on the child's prelinguistic behaviors, a short period of diagnostic therapy may be used. As discussed by Ambrose et al. (Chapter 11), the purpose of diagnostic therapy is to assess the child's responsiveness to external stimulation in general, as well as demonstrating more facilitative language techniques for the family. Such observations may provide insight into the family's willingness and ability to learn and implement therapy goals once the child is implanted.

As part of the candidacy evaluation process and continued monitoring thereafter, it is important to determine the modality or combination of modalities likely to be most effective for the child. Communication mode is, of course, the parents' choice, with the team's role being to provide information and support to help the parents make an informed decision. Furthermore, the selection of a mode of communication for a child with multiple disabilities enrolled in early intervention and/or other educational programs may have already been made, based on the child's abilities and/or limitations in the context of the other developmental, sensory, and mobility issues. In other instances, the choice may have been put on hold by the parents, while they pursue the possibility of implantation. In any event, input from and collaboration with other professionals and educators working with these children will be crucial in evaluating the child's communicative potential and the best means of tapping into that potential.

Although speech development may not be the primary goal in implanting a given child with multiple disabilities, some can and do develop speech over time (Nikolopoulos, Archbold, Wever, & Lloyd, 2008). Thus, factors that can impact speech production also should be taken into consideration. Taking a good history regarding feeding skills and advancing through the stages of baby foods as well as performing an oral motor evaluation can provide some insight into a child's skills and needs for the foundation of speech production.

Educational Setting and Communication Options

The identification of a child's educational needs prior to implantation informs the process of developing an educational/habilitation program that will support auditory skill growth and foster communication in the mode or modes that may be most appropriate. In forming this plan, the complexity of all the child's developmental needs should be taken into account, so as not to shift the focus from the whole child. Information about the child should be actively sought from the educators, interventionists, and therapists who work with the child in the community. Because they interact with the child and the family on a more routine basis, these professionals are in a position to provide invaluable information about how the family interacts and communicates in more natural settings, as well as added insight into the parental expectations for benefit with device use. Furthermore, they are likely to have insight about the child's learning style, ability to use new information, and the sensory mode or combination thereof that might be the most efficient route for the child's subse-

quent learning. Thus, in addition to being key to consistent and successful use of the device across different settings, input and support from community-based professionals is crucial in developing and implementing the post-CI habilitation/education plan.

The educational setting into which the child is likely to return following implantation also should be assessed. Even though other forms of communication may be used, it is critical that some part of the habilitation plan include intervention to develop auditory and listening skills using the device. The ability of the program and school district to support such skill development should be evaluated by individuals experienced with postimplant habilitation. If needed, alternatives or additional resources within the local education area (LEA) should be identified and enlisted to provide support and training to current educators and service providers.

Access to an educational audiologist knowledgeable in cochlear implants should also be part of the child's individualized education plan. In conjunction with the team's educational specialist, the educational audiologist can provide a bridge between the CI center and the school. This process can and should start prior to implantation. Once the family begins to undergo the pre-evaluation process for cochlear implantation, written notification should be provided to the school stating that fact and a plan for a new Individualized Family Service Plan (IFSP) or Individualized Educational Program (IEP) should be drawn up.

Family Expectations and Support

It has been suggested that among parents of children with additional disabilities seeking cochlear implantation, it must be assumed that expectations are too high, in spite of the team's attempts to counsel otherwise (Bertram, 2004; Bertram et al., 2000). Thus, they are likely to be disappointed if their child shows little or no signs of benefit. We have found this to be especially true during the first year post-CI, despite parents' claims to be satisfied with their decision to pursue implantation for their child. Linking families with those of other CI children with similar types of disabilities may be particularly helpful to parents during the preimplant assessment period. Parents are often eager to speak with other parents, who are in a better position than most professionals to appreciate the complexity of raising a deaf child with additional needs. Exchange between families can assist those parents contemplating a CI for their child in anticipating not only the potential benefits of implantation, but also potential challenges that may lie ahead. In some centers, families may already be available from among those whose children have been implanted. Other resources include the implant manufacturers, each of which has a mechanism for parent-to-parent interaction.

Consistent device use has been linked with long-term outcomes (e.g., Fryauf-Bertchy, Tyler, Kelsay, Gantz, & Woodworth, 1997). Thus, the family's dedication to keeping a sensory device on the child and functioning appropriately, even in the absence of overt signs of progress, may be one of the most telling indicators of the family's ability to commit to the post-CI process. In this way, the family's history with regard to their child's hearing aid use in the pre-CI period is important to consider when assessing the family's ability to fulfill their role in supporting consistent and effective device use in the long run. As in the case of any potential CI family, the ability to follow through with appointments and other recommendations prior to considering CI candidacy are additional indications of the family's capacity to do what it takes to maximize their child's opportunities for growth. This pertains to all family members

and caregivers, with whom the child may be expected to spend extended time. Furthermore, all significant family members involved in the child's routine care should be in agreement to move forward with implantation. This is especially important when the parents are separated or divorced and the child is likely to be spending time in two households. It is also the case when the child is being reared by relatives other than the parents (e.g., grandparents).

Postimplant Programming and Monitoring

Initial Activation and Device Programming

Device activation usually takes place 3 to 4 weeks following the surgery. As in the case of any young child, it is helpful to schedule the initial stimulation and mapping over several days. Device programming proceeds in much the same manner as with other children of similar developmental ages and abilities. The ultimate objective is to develop a map that will allow the child to experience audible and comfortable stimulation over the maximum number of available electrodes and an optimum dynamic range. A well-fitted map, characterized by an up-to-date speech processing strategy and a dynamic range that supports loudness growth with increasing stimulus intensity, has been shown to be a significant factor in speech perception and oral communication outcomes (Geers et al., 2003a; Tobey et al., 2003). Even when spoken language is not the immediate goal for a given child, the importance of establishing a quality map for the purpose of auditory learning cannot be understated.

On the first day of implant activation and programming the primary objective is to get the device on the child, set low enough so that he or she will not reject it. For those children known to be defensive to tactile stimulation or anxious in response to change (e.g., children with autism or cognitive delay), reintroducing the hearing aid (turned off) to the implanted ear in the weeks prior to actual CI activation may enable the child to accept the new device more readily. If the speech processor is body-worn, it may be helpful to have the child become accustomed to the device (or just the harness) as well, even though the device has not yet been programmed and activated. The period between surgical implantation and activation also can be used to continue developing a conditioned response to sensory input, using tactile or visual stimuli. Involving the child's family and community-based therapists at this stage can be of particular assistance in establishing consistent response behaviors and preparing the child to be ready to listen across a number of environments.

For those children in whom a reliable conditioned response can be established, minimum response levels (MRLs) are obtained for as many available electrodes as possible (i.e., those that are fully inserted and fall within compliance standards). At the time of device activation, a child's MRLs to electrical stimulation are likely to be well above "true" threshold, particularly if he or she has had limited experience with sound. Thus, for the initial maps it is customary to set the upper limit of electrical stimulation (i.e., "C" or "M" levels, depending on the device) at the child's MRL and, if required by the programming software, setting the threshold or T-levels lower still. This ensures audibility while minimizing the likelihood of discomfort when the entire array is switched on. For those children not yet able to provide a reliable behavioral response or who do not have the attention to

continue to participate beyond the programming of the first couple of electrodes, electrophysiologic measures can be very helpful in estimating the stimulation parameters. These measures include obtaining thresholds for the electrically evoked compound action potential (ECAP) and the electrically evoked stapedius reflex (ESRT). Both measures can be recorded in awake children.

Currently, all three manufacturers of CI devices approved in the United States incorporate bidirectional telemetry within their programming software, allowing for measurement of the ECAP from an intracochlear electrode. Previous research on the relationship between the ECAP and psychophysical judgments in adults and children have demonstrated that ECAP thresholds tend to lie within the dynamic range between the threshold and the maximum T- and C/M-levels, although individual variability does not allow for the accurate prediction of either behavioral threshold and comfort levels (Brown, Abbas, & Gantz, 1998; Brown et al., 2000; Eisen & Franck, 2004; Franck & Norton, 2001; Hughes et al., 2000). Nevertheless, ECAP thresholds do provide useful starting points for delivering electrical stimuli likely to be audible, yet comfortable. Because a stimulus presented at or above the ECAP threshold can be presumed to be perceptible to the child, conditioning can be attempted to establish a consistent behavioral detection response. Furthermore, a number of protocols have been developed that incorporate the combination of behavioral data and ECAP thresholds to fit a map across the electrode array (Franck & Norton, 2002; Gordon, Papsin, & Harrison, 2004a; Hughes et al., 2000; Smoorenburg, Willeboer, & van Dijk, 2002) or that use a combination of objective measures when behavioral data cannot be obtained (Gordon, Papsin, & Harrison, 2004b). Intraoperative ECAPs obtained at the time of surgery can also be used to establish some upper boundaries for stimulation in initial programming (Lai & Dillier, 2000).

Consistent relationships between the ESRTs and perceptual judgments of maximum comfortable listening levels in experienced adult and pediatric implant users have been reported by a number of investigators (Bresnihan et al., 2001; Hodges et al., 1997; Shallop & Ash, 1995). Thus, when present, ESRTs can be used to establish maximal levels of stimulation (C/M-levels) along the electrode array, while minimizing the likelihood of overstimulation (Gordon et al, 2004a, 2004b). To record the ESRT the child needs to have a normal tympanogram in the measurement ear. He or she also needs to be sitting quietly with a minimum of head movement. For this purpose we often have the child sit on the parent's lap while watching a video. We have found it useful to have the parent bring in the child's favorite video for this purpose. Alternatively, an attempt can be made to schedule these measures to coincide with the child's naptime.

Because behavioral thresholds, once established, tend to decrease with the child's implant experience and ESRTs tend to increase (Gordon et al., 2004a), the processor should be remapped frequently during the first 6 months. These visits also can be used to obtain feedback from the parents, teachers, and therapists as to how the child is progressing in developing listening skills.

Audiologic Follow-up and Monitoring

During the first few months following implantation, the focus likely will be on the child's adaptation to device use and observations of his or her auditory behavior with the device. In most children sound awareness will be noted fairly quickly. However, further noticeable auditory development in CI children with multiple disabilities may be incremental and, for some children, may take a year or more to observe. As in the case of very young implanted children, parental feedback will be the primary source of information about how the child uses audition for the first year or more. For this purpose, the use of parent diaries, structured questionnaires, and hierarchical checklists can be helpful in tracking the emergence of functional auditory behaviors in the child's routine environment. Continued input from teachers and therapists also is important, especially with regard to the child's consistency of device use and any difficulties encountered keeping the device on and functioning.

With increased experience to sound, it may be possible to obtain a conditioned response in some children who could not be conditioned prior to implantation. This is useful not only in further refining the map, but also in beginning to obtain sound-field detection thresholds. Imperfect as they are, such thresholds offer some verification that the minimal stimulation levels have been set to allow audibility across the frequency range. Detection responses using the Ling six-sound test (Ling, 1989; 2002/03) also may serve to confirm that the child has auditory access across the speech spectrum and provides a means for behavioral device checks at home.

As important as audibility is to auditory skill development, detection is not synonymous with perception. Thus, auditory detection thresholds do not provide information about the degree to which a child is able to use acoustic-phonetic information to distinguish the sound patterns of spoken language. Typically, we rely on behavioral measures of speech perception to provide such evidence. Speech perception measures that may be introduced when a child is 2 or 3 years of age or its developmental equivalent include the Early Speech Perception (ESP) Test (Moog & Geers, 1991), the Northwestern University-Children's Perception of Speech (NU-CHIPS) (Elliott & Katz, 1980), and the Pediatric Speech Intelligibility (PSI) Test (Jerger & Jerger, 1984). All are closed-set identification tasks that require the child to make a choice among a number of alternatives, usually through a picture-pointing response. Furthermore, all require that the child have sufficient vocabulary and syntactic knowledge to identify the pictured word and sentence targets.

As illustrated earlier (see Figure 19–1), many children with developmental delays and disabilities cannot be assessed using formal speech perception measures because they are not able to perform the response task required (make a deliberate choice among alternatives) or they do not have the representational and/or vocabulary skills required to identify word pictures. Such task- and vocabulary-related related concerns are similar to those posed by infants and very young children being fit with sensory devices. At the House Ear Institute, a test battery has been under development for the purpose of assessing speech pattern contrast perception in children 6 months to 5 years of age. Derived from the Speech Pattern Contrast Test (SPAC) (Boothroyd, 1984), the battery is composed of four tests: VRASPAC, PLAYSPAC, OLIMSPAC, and VIDSPAC (Eisenberg, Martinez, & Boothroyd, 2007; Martinez, Eisenberg, Boothroyd, & Visser-Dumont, 2008). All four measures use the same phonetic contrasts, which include: vowel height ("oodoo" versus "aadaa"), vowel place ("oodoo" versus "eedee"), consonant voicing ("oodoo" versus "ootoo"), consonant continuance or manner ("oodoo" versus "ooshoo"), consonant place in the

front or bilabial-alveolar position ("oodoo" versus "ooboo"), and consonant place in the back or alveolar-palatal position ("oodoo" versus "oogoo"). However the behavioral response task used to identify phonetic change is based on the developmental level and abilities of the child. Performance is quantified not only by percent-correct identification of speech pattern contrasts, but also by the level of confidence that responses are not random.

At the House Ear Institute, we have found two tests in this battery, VRASPAC and PLAYSPAC, to be useful in assessing children with additional disabilities. VRASPAC (Visual Reinforcement Assessment of the Perception of Speech Pattern Contrasts) uses a child's visually reinforced head turn response to indicate that he or she has detected a phonetic change in a series of repeated syllables. Adapted from techniques originally described by Eilers, Wilson, and Moore (1977), the child is first conditioned to look toward the speaker/reinforcer when the contrast occurs. VRASPAC is generally appropriate for infants and very young children between the ages of 6 months and 2 years or the developmental equivalent who can provide a head-turn response. PLAYSPAC (Play Assessment of Speech Perception Contrasts) uses conditioned play audiometric techniques to assess the ability to detect phonetic change. Modeled after the Speech Feature Test (Dawson, Nott, Clark, & Cowan, 1998), PLAYSPAC is appropriate for children reaching the developmental equivalent of about 3 years of age and older. In both cases test trials begin as soon as the child is responding to the change consistently. A preset stopping rule is used to terminate the task once the a priori confidence level (e.g., 90%) has been reached, indicating that the head-turn or motor responses are not random. The algorithm underlying the stopping rule, which is based on probability theory, takes into account the number of trials, deviant utterances, hits, and false positives. Trials can also be terminated by the tester (for example, if the child is losing interest in the task).

Figure 19–2 shows results obtained for a CI child with developmental delay of unknown etiology. Identified with a severe-to-profound bilateral hearing loss, she was fit with amplification by 3 months of age. A developmental assessment conducted at the age of 13 months suggested significant global delays, as evaluated using the Bayley Scales of Infant Development (BSID-II) (Bayley, 1993). She was implanted at 1 year, 5 months of age and activated 1 month later. The left panel (see Figure 19–2A) shows the profile of confidence levels for each of the speech contrasts obtained at 12 months postactivation (child age: 2 years, 6 months); the right panel (see Figure 19–2B) shows profile of confidence levels obtained at 16 months postactivation (child age: 2 years, 10 months). At the 12-month visit, five out of six possible contrasts were assessed. Of these five, three were identified with 90% or greater confidence, including: vowel height, vowel place, and consonant continuance/manner. When she returned 4 months later, we were able to assess consonant place in the rear position after re-establishing the conditioned response using vowel height. Furthermore, a couple of responses were evident for consonant place in the frontal position, although perception of this contrast did not meet 50% confidence, due to a high false positive rate. Thus, we have evidence that this little girl was not only detecting the presence of sound 12 to 16 months following device activation, but she was beginning to discriminate consistently between a number of speech pattern contrasts.

Figure 19–3 shows results for a boy with autism implanted at the age of 4 years, 4 months. Born in another country, this child received no newborn hearing screening. He was diagnosed with a severe loss in the right ear and profound loss in the left ear the age of 2 years, 11 months, after failing to develop speech and language. He was fit with amplification at the age of 3 years. A developmental assessment conducted at the age of 3 years, 11 months estimated his nonverbal cognitive abilities in the lower half of the 3-year-old age range. Although autism was suspected prior to implantation, his neurologist was hesitant to make this diagnosis in the presence of deafness until after the child had had some experience with sound. Thus, the final diagnosis of autism was not made until 6 months following CI. Panel 19–3A shows results obtained at 24 months postactivation using VRASPAC (child age: 6 years, 4 months), the first post-CI interval for which we attempted this task. At this visit, he was able to identify three contrasts with 90% confidence, including: vowel height, vowel place, and consonant place in the front position, before his attention waned. Figure 19–3B shows the results obtained 6 months later using PLAYSPAC (child age: 6 years, 10 months). At this interval we were able to assess two additional contrasts, consonant voicing and consonant continuance. Although he met the 90% confidence criterion for consonant voicing, he did not meet criterion for consonant continuance (confidence = 63%).

To date we have attempted to use the VRASPAC or PLAYSPAC with eight developmentally disabled CI children and have been able to successfully test at least one contrast (vowel height) in five children. The remaining three children could not yet be conditioned for the behavioral task.

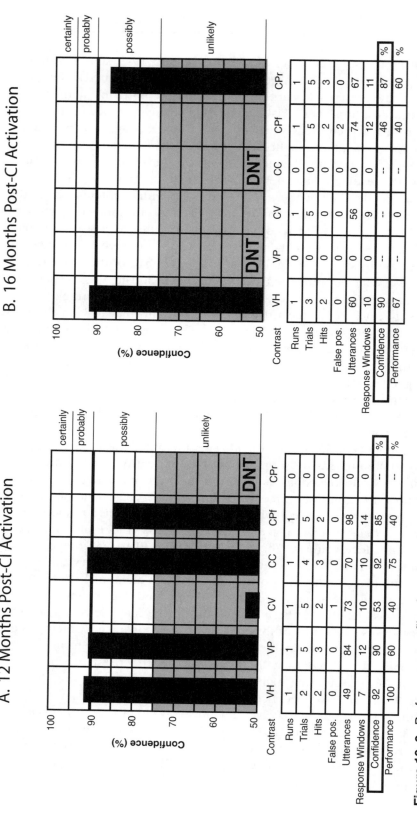

Figure 19–2. Performance profiles for a CI child with developmental delay assessed using VRASPAC at 12 months postactivation (**A**) and 16 months postactivation (**B**).

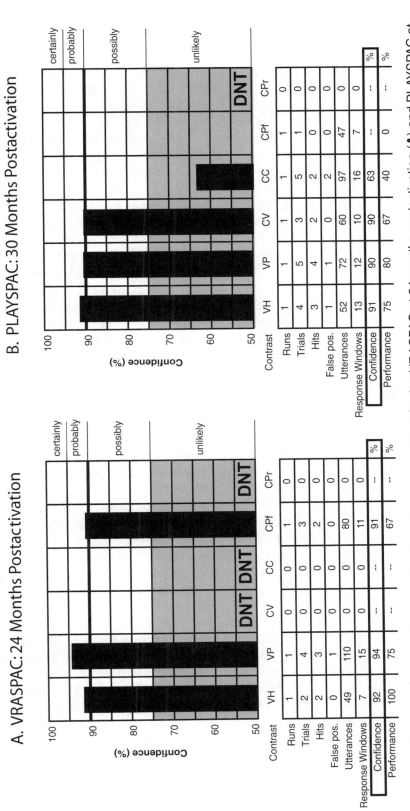

Figure 19–3. Performance profiles for a CI child with autism assessed using VRASPAC at 24 months postactivation (**A**) and PLAYSPAC at 30 months postactivation (**B**).

Communication Follow-up and Monitoring

Continued contact with the team's speech language specialist over the first few months following device activation can serve to address any new questions the family may have about how best to foster their child's communication. It has been our experience that when CI children who begin to show sound awareness shortly following device activation, many families assume that speech and language will soon follow, despite the extent of other disabilities. Thus, when possible, touching base with the family when they return for mapping sessions opens the door for ongoing discussions about their expectations regarding the auditory, speech, and language development of their child.

At the HEI CARE Center, a formal counseling session with the speech-language pathologist on the team is scheduled as part of the 6-month follow-up to review what the family has observed and to allow them to raise any concerns that may have developed since device activation. Depending on their child's preimplant abilities and stated progress in communication, the parent may be asked to complete some communication or vocabulary checklists. The MacArthur Bates CDI/Words and Gestures can be particularly helpful in this regard. Even if vocabulary (spoken or sign) has not changed, the child's current use of early and later gestures, along with evidence of symbolic play, can provide a developmental context in which to consider the child's emerging communication abilities. This information can be used to further guide families in supporting their child's language learning (Johnson, DesJardin, Barker, Quittner, & Winter, 2008).

It also is helpful to have the family bring a copy of their child's most recent IEP or IFSP to the 6-month follow-up visit. This allows for review of the auditory and communication goals that have been established and the mode of communication that is being used. Information about the skills that are being addressed in the classroom and in therapy, as well about any other services the child is receiving, may also provide the center-based staff with insight into additional supports the team can make available. For example, the speech-language pathologist might be able to recommend additional activities that the parent can carry out at home to reinforce what is being done in therapy and at school. He or she may also point to other resources available to families, many of which are available on-line.

More formal assessment of communication skills typically is made at annual intervals following device activation, at least through the first couple of years postimplant. Depending on the child's skill growth, standardized clinician-elicited language measures may or may not yet be appropriate. Thus, parent-report measures are likely to continue to serve a central role in monitoring the communication development of these children. Regardless of metric used, communication should be assessed in the mode or combination of modes in place for the child. As stated previously, a number of variables may come into play in moving forward with development of functional communication, whereby the child is able to express his or her thoughts, feelings, and needs. Even among CI children with similar constellations of co-occurring conditions (e.g., deafness plus cognitive impairment, vision impairment, autism, or other learning and behavioral disabilities), one mode does not fit all. Thus, it is important to revisit communication choices on a regular basis to make sure they are meeting the needs (receptive and expressive) of the child. Furthermore, it is important not to set the bar too low. With functional communication in place, goals should be established to further linguistic development.

Educational Follow-up and Monitoring

In the postimplant period, continuing communication with the educational providers is critical to ensuring that the teachers, therapists and classroom aids are comfortable with the equipment and that the child is using the CI consistently. The degree to which the auditory channel is tapped to facilitate learning in a given classroom likely will depend on whether the teacher or interventionist was trained in special versus deaf education. Teachers from both types of background may have limited experience in working with deaf children or with children who use cochlear implants. In this regard, they may be uncomfortable with the implant technology and unfamiliar with the possibilities or limitations that might be expected with device use (Archbold, 1994; Archbold & O'Donoghue, 2007; Moog & Geers, 1991). When this is the case, the team-based educational specialist or the school-based educational audiologist can provide training in managing the equipment, including supervised practice in putting the implant on and taking it off the child. Training can also address use of auxiliary classroom amplification systems (e.g., classroom tower speaker systems). For teachers in a non-deaf special education setting, recommendations can be made about how to maximize the acoustic environment and promote auditory skill growth. For teachers in a deaf education setting, connecting with educators knowledgeable in the additional

disability may suggest further modifications to the educational curriculum based on the child's individualized needs.

A new IFSP or IEP may need to be written that incorporates new educational goals and services related to the child's use of the new device. Ideally, this should be done prior to surgery so that the plan can be initiated as soon as the child's implant is activated. Elements to be considered include auditory training goals, self-help goals related to the implant, and the incorporation of classroom amplification systems. The educational specialist on the CI team can serve as a variable resource for both the family and interventionists in formulating some of these short and long-term goals, along with identifying supports that may need to be put into place. The educational specialist also can continue to consult with parents and child's educational personnel about appropriate expectations for auditory and communication skill growth following implantation and the length of time it may take for such skills to emerge.

Developmental Assessments and Monitoring

CI children with multiple disabilities may benefit from ongoing follow-up by a developmental pediatrician. Such contact would support overall monitoring of a child's developmental needs across all domains. In addition to documenting the child's progress, these visits can serve to provide guidance with regard to further therapy, educational interventions, and equipment that may be warranted. Periodic reassessment of the child's skill levels can also help identify the next set of developmental goals to consider in educational planning. It can reassure families, therapists, and educators that the therapy strategies that have been put into place are helpful or indicate that some adjustment of these strategies is needed for continued progress. Educational advocacy is another role many developmental pediatricians play, which can be important for children with such complexity.

General Considerations in Assessing and Monitoring CI Children with Multiple Disabilities

For children with multiple disabilities, assessment may not proceed as smoothly as with typically developing deaf children. Deaf children in general often need additional processing time, may fatigue due to processing demands, and may require supplemental nonlinguistic cues (e.g., nonverbal communication, picture support, and demonstration) to comprehend the task at hand. In the evaluation of some deaf children with multiple disabilities, standardized assessment batteries may not even be appropriate. Although children with cognitive issues may need more practice opportunities to understand what they are being asked to do, some testing measures do not allow for multiple practice opportunities. The number of items on a testing battery may overload children who need more processing time. Breaking up testing into multiple sessions and settings may allow for a more accurate representation of what the child can accomplish. Although it is important to obtain objective results from measurements that permit the evaluation of progress over time, sometimes we must rely on alternative assessment strategies.

Teachers, therapists, and parents can provide insight into strategies that have worked or not worked for a specific child in the past and their expertise should be tapped. Combining formal and informal approaches to assessment is also important in this population. Using functional measures and checklists can provide information about a child in settings outside the clinical domain. Furthermore, such measures can help the clinician determine the most appropriate starting point for more formal assessment based on general cognitive and language level. Providing the time and opportunity for diagnostic teaching, incorporating appropriate environmental adaptations, and individualizing the evaluation process can increase the likelihood that the assessment will yield a valid representation of the child's abilities and potential.

Recently a new tool has been introduced that provides a means for documenting functional change and benefit following cochlear implantation in this complex population. The Champions–Evaluation Profiles for Paediatric Cochlear Implant Users with Additional Disabilities (Herrmannova, Phillips, O'Donohue, & Ramsden, 2008) is a compilation of brief scales designed for tracking progress across time in communication, listening, psychosocial development, and preacademic/educational skills, integrating input from a variety of sources in one tool. It also provides a mechanism to record parents' or caregivers' perceptions of progress in each of these domains, as well as perspectives of their child's overall quality of life.

Final Thoughts and Future Directions

There is reason to be cautiously optimistic about future trends in cochlear implantation in deaf children with multiple disabilities. Given the contemporary emphasis on early detection and identification of at-risk and special needs children, those with known and as yet unknown disabilities are likely to be brought in for assessment and intervention at earlier ages. As CI centers gain increasing experience in implanting children from special populations, they will be more likely to implant those children with special needs at younger ages as well. This is a far different picture than that of just a few years ago when the presence of developmental disabilities was likely to delay identification and intervention for hearing loss, including the consideration of cochlear implantation.

The relaxing of audiologic candidacy criteria also means children with greater amount of residual hearing will be considered as CI candidates; children with additional disabilities are not likely to be different in this regard. Furthermore, improvements in hearing aid technology are likely to provide access to a higher quality of auditory input for all infants in the preimplant period. Thus, many deaf/HOH children with additional disabilities will not only present for CI consideration at earlier ages, but may also have had more auditory experience on which to build in the postimplant period.

References

Adamson, L. B. (1995). *Communication development during infancy*. Madison, WI: Brown & Benchmark.

Aiken-Forderer, M. (1988). Home and school support for physically handicapped deaf children. In H. T. Pricket & E. Duncan (Eds.), *Coping with the multi-handicapped hearing impaired* (pp. 29–36). Springfield, IL: Charles C. Thomas.

American Academy of Audiology. (2003). *Pediatric amplification protocol*. Retrieved October 10, 2008. from: http://www.audiology.org/NR/rdonlyres/53D26792-E321-41AF-850F-CC253310F9DB/0/pedamp.pdf

American Speech-Language-Hearing Association. (1986, April). Report of the Ad Hoc Committee on Cochlear Implants. *Asha*, pp. 29–52.

American Speech-Language-Hearing Association. (2004). *Guidelines for the audiological assessment of children from birth to 5 years of age*. Retrieved October 10, 2008: from http://www.asha.org/docs/pdf/GL2004-00002.pdf

Anderson, D., & Reilly, J. (2002). The MacArthur Communicative Development Inventory: Normative data for American Sign Language. *Journal of Deaf Studies and Deaf Education*, 7, 83–106.

Archbold, S. (1994). The specialist cochlear implant team for deaf children. In I. J. Hochmair-Desoyer & E. S. Hochmair (Eds.), *Advances in cochlear implants* (pp. 539–545). Manz, Germany: Wien.

Archbold, S., Lutman, M. E., & Marshall, D. H. (1995). Categories of auditory performance. *Annals of Otology, Rhinology, and Laryngology*, 104(Suppl. 166), 312–314.

Archbold, S., & O'Donoghue, G. M. (2007). Ensuring the long-term use of cochlear implants in children: The importance of engaging local resources and expertise. *Ear and Hearing*, 28 (Suppl.), 3S–6S.

Arens, K., Cress, C. J., & Marvin, C. M. (2005). Gaze-shift patterns of young children with developmental disabilities who are at risk for being nonspeaking. *Education and Training in Developmental Disabilities*, 40, 158–170.

Au, D. K. K., Hui, Y., Tsang, A. W. C., & Wei, W. I. (2004). ENT management of a child with CHARGE association. *Asian Journal of Surgery*, 27, 141–143.

Bauer, P. W., Wippold, F. J., Goldin, J., & Lusk, R. P. (2002). Cochlear implantation in children with CHARGE Association. *Archives of Otolaryngology-Head and Neck Surgery*, 128, 1013–1017.

Baumeister, A. A., Todd, M. E., & Sevin, J. A. (1993). Efficacy and specificity of pharmacological therapies for behavior disorders in persons with mental retardation. *Clinical Neuropharmacology*, 16, 271–294.

Bayley, N. (1993). *Bayley Scales of Infant Development* (2nd ed.). San Antonio, TX: The Psychological Corporation.

Beiter, A. L., Staller, S. J., & Dowell, R. C. (1991). Evaluation and device programming in children. *Ear and Hearing*, 12(Suppl.), 25S–33S.

Berliner, K. I., & Eisenberg, L. S. (1985). Methods and issues in the cochlear implantation of children: An overview. *Ear and Hearing, 6*(Suppl.), 6S-13S.

Bertram, B. (2004). Cochlear implantation for children with hearing loss and multiple disabilities: An evaluation from an educator's perspective. *The Volta Review, 104* (Monograph), 349-359.

Bertram, B., Lenarz, T., & Lesinski, A. (2000). Cochlear implant for multi-handicapped children: Pedagogic demands and expectations. In S. B. Watzman & N. L. Cohen (Eds.), *Cochlear implants* (pp. 247-249). New York: Thieme.

Beukelman D. R., & Mirenda, P. (2005). *Augmentative and alternative communication: Supporting children and adults with complex communication needs* (3rd ed.). Baltimore: Paul H. Brookes.

Blake, K. D., Davenport, S. L , Hall, B. D., Hefner, M. A., Pagon, R. A., Williams, M. S., et al. (1998). CHARGE association: An update and review for the primary pediatrician. *Clinical Pediatrics, 37*, 159-173.

Blamey, P. J., Sarant, J. Z., Paatsch, L. E., Barry, J. G., Bow, C. P., Wales, R. J., et al. (2001). Relationships among speech perception, production, language, hearing loss, and age in children with impaired hearing. *Journal of Speech, Language, and Hearing Research, 44*, 264-285.

Boothroyd, A. (1984). Auditory perception of speech contrasts by subjects with sensorineural hearing loss. *Journal of Speech and Hearing Research, 27*, 134-144.

Boothroyd, A., & Boothroyd-Turner, D. (2002). Postimplantation audition and educational attainment in children with prelingually acquired profound deafness. *Annals of Otology, Rhinology, and Laryngology, 111*(Suppl. 189), 79-84.

Boughman, J. A., Vernon, M., & Shaver, K. A. (1983). Usher's syndrome: Definition and estimate of prevalence from two high-risk populations. *Journal of Chronic Diseases, 36*, 595-603.

Bresnihan, M., Norman, G., Scott, F., & Viani, L. (2001). Measurement of comfort levels by mean of electrical stapedial reflex in children. *Archives of Otolaryngology-Head and Neck Surgery, 127*, 963-966.

Brown, C. (2003). Clinical uses of electrically evoked auditory nerve and brainstem responses. *Current Opinion in Otolaryngology-Head and Neck Surgery, 11*, 383-387.

Brown, C. J., Abbas, P. J., & Gantz, B. (1998). Preliminary experience with neural response telemetry in the Nucleus CI24M cochlear implant. *American Journal of Otology, 19*, 320-327.

Brown, C. J., Hughes, M. L., Luk, B., Abbas, P. J., Wolaver, A., & Gervais, J. (2000). The relationship between EAP & EABR thresholds and levels used to program the Nucleus 24 speech processor: Data from adults. *Ear and Hearing, 21*, 151-163.

Calandrella, A. M., & Wilcox, M. J. (2000). Predicting language outcomes for young prelinguistic children with developmental delay. *Journal of Speech, Language, and Hearing Research, 43*, 1061-1071.

Carvill, S., & Marston, G. (2002). People with intellectual disability, sensory impairments and behaviour disorder: A case series. *Journal of Intellectual Disability Research, 46*, 264-272.

Chen, D. (2004). Young children who are deaf-blind: Implications for professionals in deaf and hard of hearing services. *Volta Review, 104*(Monograph), 273-284.

Cheng, A. K., Grant, G. D., & Niparko, J. K. (1999). Meta-analysis of pediatric cochlear implant literature. *Annals of Otology, Rhinology, and Laryngology, 108*(Suppl. 177), 124-128.

Chute, P. M., & Nevins, M. E. (1995, May-June). Cochlear implants in people who are deaf-blind. *Journal of Visual Impairment and Blindness*, pp. 297-301.

Cohen, N. L, Roland, J. T., Jr., Marrinan, M. (2004). Meningitis in cochlear implant recipients: The North American experience. *Otology and Neurotolgy, 25*, 275-281.

Cohn, E. S., & Kelley, P. M. (1999). Clinical phenotype and mutations in connexin 26 (DFNB1/GJB2), the most common cause of childhood hearing loss. *American Journal of Medical Genetics Part C: Seminars in Medical Genetics, 89*, 130-136.

Cohn, E. S., Kelley, P. M., Fowler, T. W., Gorga, M. P., Lefkowitz, D. M., Kuehn, H. J., et al.

(1999). Clinical studies of families with hearing loss attributable to mutations in the connexin 26 gene (GJB2/DFNB1). *Pediatrics*, *103*, 546–550.

Colletti, V., Carner, M., Miorelli, V., Guida, M., Colletti, L., & Fiorino, F. G. (2005). Cochlear implantation at under 12 months: Report on 10 patients. *Laryngoscope*, *115*, 445–449.

Dahle, A. J., Fowler, K. B., Wright, J. D., Boppana, S. B., Britt, W. J., & Pass, R. F. (2000). Longitudinal investigation of hearing disorders in children with congenital cytomegalovirus. *Journal of the American Academy of Audiology*, *11*, 283–290.

Daneshi, A., & Hassanzadeh, S. (2007). Cochlear implantation in prelingually deaf persons with additional disability. *Journal of Laryngology and Otology*, *121*, 635–638.

Dawson, P. W., Busby, P. A., McCay, C. M., & Clark, G. M. (2002). Short-term auditory memory in children using cochlear implants and its relevance to receptive language. *Journal of Speech, Language, and Hearing Research*, *45*, 789–801.

Dawson, P. W., Nott, P. E., Clark, G. M., & Cowan, R. S. C. (1998). A modification of play audiometry to assess speech discrimination ability in severe-profoundly deaf 2-to-4 year old children. *Ear and Hearing*, *19*, 371–384.

Daya, H., Figueirido, J. C., Gordon, K. A., Twitchell, K., Gysin, C., & Papsin, B. (1999). The role of a graded profile analysis in determining candidacy and outcome for cochlear implantation in children. *International Journal of Pediatric Otorhinolaryngology*, *49*, 135–142.

De l'Aune, W. R. (1980). Hearing: Its evolution and ways of compensating for its loss. *Journal of Visual Impairment and Blindness*, *74*, 19–23.

Dettman, S. J., Fiket, H., Dowell, R. C., Charlton, M., Williams, S. S., Tomov, A. M., et al. (2004). Speech perception results for children using cochlear implants who have additional special needs. *Volta Review*, *104*(Monograph), 361–392.

Dettman, S. J., Pinder, D., Briggs, R. J. S., & Dowell, R. C. (2007). Communication development in children who receive the cochlear implant younger than 12 months: Risks versus benefits. *Ear and Hearing*, *28*(Suppl.), 11S–18S.

Dollard, S. C., Grosse, S. D., & Ross, D. S. (2007). New estimates of the prevalence of neurological and sensory sequelae and mortality associated with congenital cytomegalovirus infection. *Reviews in Medical Virology*, *17*, 355–363.

Donaldson, A. I., Heavner, K. S., & Zwolan, T. A. (2004). Measuring progress in children with autism spectrum disorder who have cochlear implants. *Archives of Otolaryngology-Head and Neck Surgery*, *130*, 666–671.

Dowell, R. C., Blamey P. J., & Clark, G. M. (1995). Potential and limitations of cochlear implants in children. *Annals of Otology, Rhinology, and Laryngology*, *104*(Suppl. 166), 324–327.

Dowell, R. C., & Cowan, R. S. C. (1997). Evaluation of benefit: Infants and children. In: G. M. Clark, R. S. C. Cowan, & R. C. Dowell (Eds.), *Cochlear implantation for infants and children: Advances* (pp 171–190). San Diego, CA: Singular.

Downs, M. P. (Chairperson), Campos, C. T., Firemark, R., Martin, E., & Myers, W. (1986). Psychological issues surrounding children receiving cochlear implants. *Seminars in Hearing*, 7, 383–405.

Durand, V. M. (1993a). Problem behaviour as communication. *Behaviour Change*, *10*, 197–226.

Durand, V. M. (1993b). Functional communication training using assistive devices: Effects on challenging behavior and affect. *Augmentative and Alternative Communication*, *9*, 168–176.

Dykes, M. K., & Erin, J. N. (1999). *DASH-2: A Developmental Assessment for Students with Severe Disabilities—Second Edition*. Austin, TX: Pro-Ed.

Edwards, L. C. (2003). Candidacy and the Children's Implant Profile: Is our selection appropriate? *International Journal of Audiology*, *42*, 426–431.

Edwards, L. C. (2007). Children with cochlear implants and complex needs: A review of outcome research and psychological practice. *Journal of Deaf Studies and Deaf Education*, *12*, 256–268.

Edwards, L. C., Frost, R., & Witham, F. (2006). Developmental delay and outcomes in paediatric cochlear implantation: Implications for candidacy. *International Journal of Pediatric Otorhinolaryngology, 70,* 1593–1600.

Eilers, R. E., Wilson, W. R., & Moore, J. M. (1977). Developmental changes in speech discrimination in infants. *Journal of Speech and Hearing Research, 20,* 766–780.

Eisen, M. D., & Franck, K. H. (2004). Electrically evoked compound action potential amplitude growth functions and HiResolution programming levels in pediatric CII implant subjects. *Ear and Hearing, 25,* 528–538.

Eisenberg L. S., Johnson, K. C., Martinez, A. S., DesJardin, J. L., Stika, C. J., Dzubak, D., et al. (2008). Comprehensive evaluation of a child with an auditory brainstem implant. *Otolology and Neurotology, 29,* 251–257.

Eisenberg, L. S., Kirk, K. I., Martinez, A. S., Ying, E. A., & Miyamoto, R. T. (2004). Communication abilities of children with aided residual hearing: Comparison with cochlear implant users. *Archives of Otolaryngology-Head and Neck Surgery, 130,* 563–569.

Eisenberg, L. S., Martinez, A. S., & Boothroyd, A. (2007). Assessing auditory capabilities in young children. *International Journal of Pediatric Otorhinolaryngology, 71,* 1339–1350.

El-Kashian, H. K., Boerst, A., & Telian, S. A. (2001). Multi-channel cochlear implantation in visually impaired patients. *Otology and Neurotology, 22,* 53–56.

Elliot, L., & Katz, D. (1980). *Development of a new children's test of speech discrimination* (Technical manual). St. Louis, MO, Auditec.

Erber, N. (1982). *Auditory training.* Washington, DC: Alexander Graham Bell Association for the Deaf.

Farber, J. M. (1987). Psychopharmacology of self-injurious behavior in the mentally retarded. *Journal of the American Academy of Child and Adolescent Psychiatry, 26,* 296–302.

Fayad, J. N., Tabaee, A., Micheletto, J. N., & Parisier, S. C. (2003). Cochlear implantation in children with otitis media. *Laryngoscope, 113,* 1224–1227.

Fenson, L., Dale, P. S., Reznick, J. S., Bates, E., Thal, D., & Pethick, S. J. (1994). Variability in early communicative development. *Monographs of the Society for Research in Child Development, 59,* 1–173.

Fenson, L., Dale, P. S., Reznick, J. S., Thal, D., Bates, E., Hartnung., J., et al. (1993). *The MacArthur Communicative Development Inventories.* San Diego, CA: Singular.

Fenson, L., Marchman, V. A., Thal, D. J., Dale, P. S., Reznick, J. S., & Bates, E. (2007). *MacArthur-Bates Communicative Development Inventories: User guide and technical manual* (2nd ed.). Baltimore: Paul H. Brookes.

Filipo, R., Bosco, E., Mancini, P., & Ballantyne, D. (2004). Cochlear implants in special cases: Deafness in the presence of disabilities and/or associated problems. *Acta Oto-Laryngologica, 124*(Suppl. 552), 74–80.

Florida State University Research Foundation. (2007). *FIRST WORDS® Project.* Tallahassee FL: Florida State University. Retrieved December 11, 2008, from http://firstwords.fsu.edu/toddlerChecklist.html

Fortnum, H. M., & Davis, A. (1997). Epidemiology of permanent childhood hearing impairment in Trent Region, 1985–1993. *British Journal of Audiology, 31,* 409–446.

Fortnum, H. M., Marshall, D. H., & Summerfield, A. O. (2002). Epidemiology of the UK population of hearing-impaired children, including characteristics of those with and without cochlear implants—Audiology, aetiology, comorbidity and affluence. *International Journal of Audiology, 41,* 170–179.

Fortnum, H. M., Stacey, P.C., & Summerfield, A. O. (2006). An exploration of demographic bias in a questionnaire survey of hearing-impaired children: Implications for comparisons of children with and without cochlear implants. *International Journal of Pediatric Otorhinolaryngology, 70,* 2043–2054.

Fowler, K. B., & Boppana, S. B. (2006). Congenital cytomegalovirus (CMV) infection and hearing deficit. *Journal of Clinical Virology, 35,* 226–231.

Franck, K. H., & Norton, S. J. (2001). Estimation of psychophysical levels using the electrically evoked compound action potential measured with neural response telemetry capabilities of Cochlear Corporation's CI24M Device. *Ear and Hearing, 22,* 289–299.

Fryauf-Bertschy, H., Tyler, R. S., Kelsay, D. M., Gantz, B. J., & Woodworth, G. G. (1997). Cochlear implant use by prelingually deafened children: The influences of age at implant and length of device use. *Journal of Speech, Language, and Hearing, 40,* 183-199.

Gallaudet Research Institute. (2001, January). *Regional and national summary report of data from the 1999-2000 annual survey of deaf and hard of hearing children and youth.* Washington, DC: GRI, Gallaudet University. Retrieved January 11, 2008, from http://gri.gallaudet.edu/Demographics/2000-National_Summary.pdf/

Gallaudet Research Institute. (2002, January). *Regional and national summary report of data from the 2000-2001 annual survey of deaf and hard of hearing children and youth.* Washington, DC: GRI, Gallaudet University. Retrieved January 11, 2008, from http://gri.gallaudet.edu/Demographics/2001-National_Summary.pdf/

Gallaudet Research Institute. (2003a, January). *Regional and national summary report of data from the 2000-2001 annual survey of deaf and hard of hearing children and youth.* Washington, DC: GRI, Gallaudet University. Retrieved January 11, 2008, from http://gri.gallaudet.edu/Demographics/2002-National_Summary.pdf/

Gallaudet Research Institute. (2003b, December). *Regional and national summary report of data from the 2002-2003 annual survey of deaf and hard of hearing children and youth.* Washington, DC: GRI, Gallaudet University. Retrieved January 11, 2008, from http://gri.gallaudet.edu/Demographics/2003-National_Summary.pdf/

Gallaudet Research Institute. (2005a, January). *Regional and national summary report of data from the 2003-2004 annual survey of deaf and hard of hearing children and youth.* Washington, DC: GRI, Gallaudet University. Retrieved January 11, 2008, from http://gri.gallaudet.edu/Demographics/2004-National_Summary.pdf/

Gallaudet Research Institute. (2005b, December). *Regional and national summary report of data from the 2004-2005 annual survey of deaf and hard of hearing children and youth.* Washington, DC: GRI, Gallaudet University. Retrieved January 11, 2008, from http://gri.gallaudet.edu/Demographics/2005_National_Summary.pdf

Geers, A., Brenner, C., & Davidson, L. (2003a). Factors associated with development of speech perception skills in children implanted by age five. *Ear and Hearing, 24*(Suppl.), 24S-35S.

Geers, A., Brenner, C., Nicholas, J., Uchanski, R., Tye-Murray, N., & Tobey, E. (2002). Rehabilitation factors contributing to implant benefit in children. *Annals of Otology, Rhinology, and Laryngology, 111*(Suppl. 189), 127-130.

Geers, A., & Moog, J. (1987). Predicting spoken language acquisition of profoundly hearing-impaired children. *Journal of Speech and Hearing Disorders, 52,* 84-94.

Geers, A., Nicholas, J. G., & Sedey, A. L. (2003b). Language skills of children with early cochlear implantation. *Ear and Hearing, 24*(Suppl.), 46S-58S.

Gordon, K. A., Papsin, B. C., & Harrison, R. V. (2004a). Toward a battery of behavioral and objective measures to achieve optimal cochlear implant stimulation levels in children. *Ear and Hearing, 25,* 447-463.

Gordon, K. A., Papsin, B. C., & Harrison, R. V. (2004b). Programming cochlear implant stimulation levels in infants and children with a combination of objectives measures. *International Journal of Audiology, 43*(Suppl.), 28-32.

Gravel, J. S. (1989). Behavioral assessment of auditory function. *Seminars in Hearing, 10,* 216-228.

Hall, B. D. (1979). Choanal atresia and associated anomalies. *Journal of Pediatrics, 95,* 395-398.

Hamzavi, J., Baumgartner, W. D., Egelierler, B., Franz, P., Schenk, B., & Gstoettner, W. (2000). Follow-up of cochlear implanted handicapped children. *International Journal of Pediatric Otorhinolaryngology, 56,* 169-174.

Hartrampf, R., Lesinski, A., Allum, D. J., Dahm, M. C., & Lenarz, T. (1995). Reasons for rejected candidacy for cochlear implantation in children. *Advances in Oto-Rhino-Laryngology, 50,* 14-18.

Hayman, C. D., & Franck, K. H. (2005). Cochlear implant candidacy in children with autism. *Seminars in Hearing, 26,* 217–225.

Hellman. S. A., Chute, P. M., Kretschmer, R. E., Nevins, M. E., Parisier, S. C., & Thurston, L. C. (1991). The development of a children's implant profile. *American Annals of the Deaf, 136,* 77–81.

Herrmannova, D., Phillips, R., O'Donohue, G., & Ramsden, R. (n.d.). *Champions: Evaluation profiles for paediatric cochlear implant users with additional disabilities.* Nottingham, UK: The Ear Foundation. Available through: www.earfoundation.org.uk

Hittner, H., M., Hirsh, N., J., Kreh, G., M., & Rudolph, A. J. (1979). Colobomatous microphthalmia, heart disease, hearing loss, and mental retardation—a syndrome. *Journal of Pediatric Ophtalmologic Strabismus, 16,* 122–128.

Hodges, A. V., Balkany, T. J., Ruth, R. A., Lambert, P. R., Dolan-Ash, M. S., & Schloffman, J. J. (1997). Electrical middle ear muscle reflex: Use in cochlear implant programming. *Otolaryngology-Head and Neck Surgery, 117,* 255–261.

Holden-Pitt, L. (1997, November). *Who and where are our children with cochlear implants?* Paper presented at the Annual Convention of the American Speech-Language-Hearing Association, Boston. Retrieved January 25, 2008, from http://gri.gallaudet.edu/Cochlear/ASHA.1997/sld001

Holden-Pitt, L., & Diaz, J. A. (1998). Thirty years of the annual survey of deaf and hard of hearing children & youth: A glance over the decades. *American Annals of the Deaf, 143,* 72–76.

Holt, R. F., & Kirk, K. I. (2005). Speech and language development in cognitively delayed children with cochlear implants. *Ear and Hearing, 26,* 132–148.

Hughes, M. L., Brown, C. J., Abbas, P. J., Wolaver, A. A., & Gervais, J. P. (2000). Comparison of EAP thresholds with MAP levels in the Nucleus 24 cochlear implant: Data from children. *Ear and Hearing, 21,* 164–174.

Isaacson, J. E., Hasenstab, S., Wohl, D. L., & Williams, G. H. (1996). Learning disability in children with postmeningitic cochlear implants. *Archives of Otolaryngology-Head and Neck Surgery, 122,* 929–936.

Individuals with Disabilities Education Improvement Act of 2004. (2004). Public Law 108-446. 20, U. S. C. 1400 note. 10.

Issekutz, K. A., Graham, J. M., Jr., Prasad, C., Smith, I. M., & Blake, K. D. (2005). An epidemiological analysis of CHARGE syndrome: Preliminary results from a Canadian study. *American Journal of Medical Genetics, Part A, 133A,* 309–317.

Jerger, J., & Hayes, D. (1976). The cross-check principle in pediatric audiology. *Archives of Otolarygology, 102,* 614–620.

Jerger S., & Jerger J. (1984). *Pediatric Speech Intelligibility (PSI) test.* St. Louis, MO: Auditec.

Jerger, S., Lewis, S., Hawkins, J., & Jerger, J. (1980). Pediatric Speech Intelligibility Test. I. Generation of test materials. *International Journal of Pediatric Otorhinolaryngology, 2,* 217–230.

Johnson, K. C., DesJardin, J. L., Barker, D. H., Quittner, A. L., & Winter, M. E. (2008). Assessing joint attention and symbolic play in children with cochlear implants and multiple disabilities: Two case studies. *Otology and Neurotology, 29,* 246–250.

Johnson, K., & Eisenberg, L. (2007). *Pediatric Hierarchy of Auditory Skill Emergence.* Los Angeles: House Ear Institute.

Johnson, K. C., & Winter, M. E. (2003). Audiologic assessment of infants and toddlers. *Volta Review, 103*(Monograph), 221–251.

Johnson, K. C., Winter, M. E., Visser-Dumont, L., Martinez, A. S., & Eisenberg, L. S. (2008, April). *Auditory outcomes in CI children with and without additional disabilities at two years postimplantation.* Paper presented at the 10th International Conference on Cochlear Implants and other Implantable Auditory Technologies, San Diego, CA.

Joint Committee on Infant Hearing. (2007). Year 2007 position statement: Principles and guidelines for early hearing detection and intervention programs. *Pediatrics, 120,* 898–921.

Jones, T. W., & Jones, J. K. (2003). Educating young deaf children with multiple disabilities. In B. Bodner-Johnson & M. Sass-Lehrer (Eds.), *The young deaf or hard of hearing child: A family-centered approach to early education* (pp. 297–327). Baltimore: Paul H. Brookes.

Jorgensen, S. K., Chmiel, R. A., Clark, J. G., & Jenkins, H. A. (1995). Cochlear implantation in a multihandicapped child. *Annals of Otology, Rhinology, and Laryngology, 104*(Suppl. 166), 329–332.

Kahn, J. V. (1996). Cognitive skills and sign language knowledge of children with severe and profound mental retardation. *Education and Training in Mental Retardation and Developmental Disabilities, 31,* 162–168.

Kane, M. O., Schopmeyer, B., Mellon, N. K., Wang, N-Y., & Niparko, J. K. (2004). Prelinquistic communication and subsequent language acquisition in children with cochlear implants. *Archives of Otolaryngology-Head and Neck Surgery, 130,* 619–623.

Kenna, M. A., Rehm, H. L., Robson, C. D., Frangulov, A., McCallum, J., Yaeger, D., & et al. (2007). Additional clinical manifestations in children with sensorineural hearing loss and biallelic GJB2 mutations: Who should be offered GJB2 testing? *American Journal of Medical Genetics, Part A, 143A,* 1560–1566.

Kenneson, A., & Cannon, M. J. (2007). Review and meta-analysis of the epidemiology of congenital cytomegalovirus (CMV) infection. *Reviews in Medical Virology, 17,* 253–276.

Knoors, H., & Vervloed, M. P. J. (2003). Educational programming for deaf children with multiple disabilities: Accommodating special needs. In M. Marschark & P. E. Spencer, (Eds.), *Oxford handbook of deaf studies, language, and education* (pp. 82–94.) New York: Oxford University Press.

Knutson, J. F., Ehlers, S. L., Wald, R. L., & Tyler, R. S. (2000a). Psychological predictors of pediatric cochlear implant use and benefit. *Annals of Otology, Rhinology, and Laryngology, 109*(Suppl. 185), 100–103.

Knutson, J. F., Wald, R. L., Ehlers, S. L., & Tyler, R. S. (2000b). Psychological consequences of pediatric cochlear implant use. *Annals of Otology, Rhinology, and Laryngology, 109* (Suppl. 185), 109–111.

Kuhn-Inacker, H., Weichbold, V., Tsiakpini, L., Coninx, S., & D'Haese, P. (2003). *LittleEars Auditory Questionnaire: Parents questionnaire to assess auditory behavior.* Innsbruck, Austria: Med-El.

Kumar, A., Fishman, G., & Torok, N. (1984). Vestibular and auditory function in Usher's syndrome. *Annals of Otology, Rhinology, and Laryngology, 93,* 600–608.

Kurtz, P. F., Chin, M. D., Huete, J. M., Tarbox, R. S., O'Connor, J. T., Paclawskyj, T. R., et al. (2003). Functional analysis and treatment of self-injurious behavior in young children: A summary of 30 cases. *Journal of Applied Behavior Analysis, 36,* 205–219.

Lai, W. K., & Dillier, N. (2000, June). *Long-term monitoring of NRT data.* Presented at the 5th European symposium on paediatric cochlear implantation, Antwerp, Belgium.

Lanson, B. G., Green, J. E., Roland, J. T., Lalwani, A. K., & Waltzman, S. B. (2007). Cochlear implantation in children with CHARGE syndrome: Therapeutic decisions and outcomes. *Laryngoscope, 117,* 1260–1266.

Lederberg, A. R., & Everhart, V. S. (1998). Communication between deaf children and their hearing mothers: The role of language, gesture, and vocalizations. *Journal of Speech, Language, and Hearing Research, 41,* 887–899.

Lee, D. J., Lustig, L., Sampson, M., Chinnici, J., & Niparko, J. K. (2005). Effects of cytomegalovirus (CMV) related deafness on pediatric cochlear implant outcomes. *Otolaryngology-Head and Neck Surgery, 133,* 900–905.

Lesinski, A., Hartrampf, R., Dahm, M. C., Bertram, B., & Lenarz, T. (1995). Cochlear implantation in a population of multihandicapped children. *Annals of Otology, Rhinology, and Laryngology, 104*(Suppl. 166), 332–334.

Ling, D. (1989). *Foundations of spoken language for hearing impaired children.* Washington, DC: Alexander Graham Bell Association for the Deaf.

Ling, D. (2002/03, Winter). The six-sound test. *The Listener,* pp. 52–53.

Lounden, N., Marlin, S., Busquet, D., Denoyelle, F., Roger, G., Renaud, F., et al. (2003). Usher syndrome and cochlear implantation. *Otology and Neurotology, 24,* 216–221.

Luxford, W. M., Eisenberg, L. S., Johnson, K. C., & Mahnke, E. M. (2004). Cochlear implantation in infants younger than 12 months. In R. Miyamoto (Ed.), *Proceedings of the 8th International Cochlear Implant Conference.*

International Congress Series, 1273, (pp. 376–379). Netherlands: Elsevier.

Martinez, A. S., Eisenberg, L. S., Boothroyd, A., & Visser-Dumont, L. (2008). Assessing speech pattern contrast perception in infants: Early results on VRASPAC. *Otology and Neurotology, 29*, 183–188.

Mauk, G. W., & Mauk, P. P. (1998). Considerations, conceptualizations, and challenges in the study of concomitant learning disabilities among children and adolescents who are deaf or hard of hearing. *Journal of Deaf Studies and Deaf Education, 3*, 15–34.

Mayne, A. M., Yoshinaga-Itano, C., & Sedey, A.L. (2000a). Receptive vocabulary development of infants and toddlers who are deaf and hard of hearing. *Volta Review, 100*,(Monograph), 29–52.

Mayne, A. M., Yoshinaga-Itano, C., Sedey, A. L., & Carely, A. (2000b). Expressive vocabulary development of infants and toddlers who are deaf and hard of hearing. *Volta Review 100*(Monograph), 1–28.

McCathren, R. B., Yoder, L. H., & Warren, S. F. (1999). The relationship between prelinguistic vocalization and later expressive vocabulary in young children with developmental delay, *Journal of Speech, Language, and Hearing Research, 42*, 915–924.

McClintock, K., Hall, S., & Oliver, C. (2003). Risk markers associated with challenging behaviours in people with intellectual disabilities: A meta-analytic study. *Journal of Intellectual Disability Research, 47*, 405–416.

McCracken, W. M., & Bamford, J. M. (1995). Auditory prostheses for children with multiple handicaps. *Scandinavian Audiology, 24*(Suppl. 41), 51–60.

McInnes, J. M. (1999). Deafblindness: A unique disability. In J. M. McInnes (Ed.), *A guide to planning and support for individuals who are deafblind* (pp. 3–33). Toronto: University of Toronto Press.

Mecklenberg, D. J., Demorest, M. E., & Staller, S. J. (1991). Scope and design of the clinical trial of the Nucleus multichannel cochlear implant in children. *Ear and Hearing, 12*(Suppl.), 10S–14S.

MED-EL Corporation, & Caleffe-Schenck, N. S. (2006). *Checklist of auditory communication skills*. Durham, NC: MED-EL Corp.

Meinzen-Derr, J., Wiley, S., Choo, D., & Creighton, J. (2004). *Auditory Skills Checklist" (ASC)*. Cincinnati, OH: Cincinnati Children's Hospital Medical Center.

Meinzen-Derr, J., Wiley, S., Creighton, J., & Choo, D. (2007). Auditory Skills Checklist: Clinical tool for monitoring functional auditory skill development in young children with cochlear implants. *Annals of Otology, Rhinology, and Laryngology, 116*, 812–818.

Merlin, S., & Auerbach, E. (1976). Retinitis pigmentosa. *Survey of Ophthalmology, 20*, 303–346.

Mets, M. B., Young, N. M., Pass, A., & Lasky, J. B. (2000). Early diagnosis of Usher syndrome in children. *Transactions of the American Ophthalmologic Society, 98*, 237–245.

Miyamoto, R. T., Osberger, M. J., Robbins, A. J., Renshaw, J., Myres, W. A., Kessler, K., et al. (1989). Comparison of sensory aids in deaf children. *Annals of Otology, Rhinology, and Laryngology, 98*(Suppl. 142), 2–7.

Moog, J., & Geers, A. (1990). *Early Speech Perception Test Battery*. St. Louis, MO: Central Institute for the Deaf.

Moog, J. S., & Geers, A. E. (1991). Educational management of children with cochlear implants. *American Annals of the Deaf, 136*, 69–76.

Moore, J. M. (1995). Behavioural assessment procedures based on conditioned head-turn responses for auditory detection and discrimination with low-functioning children. *Scandanavian Audiology, 24*(Suppl. 41), 36–42.

Moreno, M. M. (2007). *MacArthur-Bates Communicative Development Inventories: Adaptations in other languages*. San Diego, CA: CDI Advisory Board. Retrieved August 8, 2008, from: http://www.sci.sdsu.edu/cdi/adaptations.htm

Nance, W. E. (2003). The genetics of deafness. *Mental Retardation and Developmental Disabilities Research Review, 9*, 109–119.

National Institute of Neurological Disorders and Stroke (NINDS). (2007). *NINDS Infantile Ref-*

sum disease information page. Bethesda, MD: National Institutes of Health. Retrieved October 21, 2008, from http://www.ninds .nih.gov/disorders/refsum_infantile/refsum_ infantile.htm

Nikolopoulos, T. P., Archbold, S. M., Wever, C. C., & Lloyd, H. (2008). Speech production in deaf implanted children with additional disabilities and comparison with age-equivalent implanted children without such disorders. *International Journal of Pediatric Otorhinolaryngology, 72,* 1823-1828.

Nikolopoulos, T. P., Dyar, D., & Gibbin, K. P. (2004). Assessing candidate children for cochlear implantation with the Nottingham Children's Implant Profile (NChIP): The first 200 children. *International Journal of Pediatric Otorhinolarynology, 68,* 127-135.

Nikolopoulos, T. P., O'Donoghue, G. M., & Archbold, S. (1999). Age at implantation: Its importance in pediatric cochlear implantation. *Laryngoscope, 109,* 595-599.

Northern, J. L. (Chairperson), Black, F. O., Brimacombe, J. A., Cohen, N. L., Eisenberg, L. S., Kuprenas, S. V., et al. (1986). Selection of children for cochlear implantation. In D. J. Mecklenberg (Ed.), *Cochlear implants in children. Seminars in Hearing, 7,* 341-347.

Pagon, R. A., Graham, J. M., Zonana, J., & Yong, S.L. (1981). Coloboma, congenital heart disease, and choanal atresia with multiple anomalies. *Journal of Pediatrics, 99,* 223-227.

Pass, R. F., Stagno, S., A., Myers, G. J., & Alford, C. A. (1980). Outcome of symptomatic congenital cytomegalovirus infection: Results of long-term longitudinal follow-up. *Pediatrics, 66,* 758-762.

Pisoni, D. B. (2000). Cognitive factors and cochlear implants: Some thoughts on perception, learning, and memory in speech perception. *Ear and Hearing, 21,* 70-82.

Pisoni, D. B., & Cleary, M. (2003). Measures of working memory span and verbal rehearsal speed in deaf children after cochlear implantation. *Ear and Hearing, 24*(Suppl.), 106S-120S.

Pisoni, D. B., Cleary, M., Geers, A. E., & Tobey, E. A. (2000). Individual differences in effective-ness of cochlear implants in children who are prelingually deaf: New process measures of performance. *Volta Review, 101,* 111-164.

Pisoni, D. B., & Geers, A. (2000). Working memory in deaf children with cochlear implants: Correlations between digit span and measures of spoken language processing. *Annals of Otology, Rhinology, and Laryngology, 109*(Suppl. 185), 92-93.

Plapinger, D., & Sikora, D. (1990). Diagnosing a learning disability in a hearing-impaired child: A case study. *American Annals of the Deaf, 135,* 285-292.

Prezbindowski, A., K., Adamson, L. B., & Lederberg, A. R. (1998). Joint attention in deaf and hearing 22-month-old children and their hearing mothers. *Journal of Applied Developmental Psychology, 19,* 377-387.

Prior, M., Bavin, E. L., Cini, E., Reilly, S., Bretherton, L., Wake, M., et al. (2008). Influences on communicative development at 24 months of age: Child temperament, behavior problems, and maternal factors. *Infant Behavior and Development, 31,* 270-279.

Pyman, B., Blamey, P., Lacy, P., Clark, G., & Dowell, R. (2000). The development of speech perception in children using cochlear implants: Effects of etiologic factors and delayed milestones. *American Journal of Otology, 21,* 57-61.

Rameriz Inscoe, J. M., & Nikolopoulos, T. P. (2004). Cochlear implantation in children deafened by cytomegalovirus: Speech perception and speech intelligibility outcomes. *Otology and Neurotology, 25,* 479-482.

Reilly, S., Eadie, P., Bavin, E. L., Wake, M., Prior, M., Williams, J., et al. (2006). Growth of infant communication between 8 and 12 months: A population study. *Journal of Paediatrics and Child Health, 42,* 764-770.

Reynell, J. K., & Gruber, C. P. (1990). *Reynell Developmental Language Scales.* Los Angeles: Western Psychological Services.

Richman, D.M. (2008). Early intervention and prevention of self-injurious behavior exhibited by young children with developmental disabilities. *Journal of Intellectual Disability Research, 52,* 3-17.

Robbins, A. M., Renshaw, J. J., & Berry, S. W. (1991). Evaluating meaningful auditory integration in profoundly hearing impaired children. *American Journal of Otology, 12*(Suppl.), 144–150.

Rossetti, L. (2006). *The Rossetti Infant-Toddler Language Scale.* East Moline, IL: LinguiSystems.

Roth, V. (1991). Students with learning disabilities and hearing impairment: Issues for the secondary and postsecondary teacher. *Journal of Learning Disabilities, 24*, 391–397.

Roush, J., Holcomb, M. A., Roush, P. A., & Escolar, M. L. (2004). When hearing loss occurs with multiple disabilities. *Seminars in Hearing, 2*, 333–345.

Royal Institute for Deaf and Blind Children. (2003, Autumn). *Rosie's story.* North Rocks, New South Wales, Australia: RIDBC, Royal Institute for Deaf and Blind Children. Retrieved September 18, 2008, from: http://www.ridbc.org.au/news/story.asp?id = 89

Saeed, S. R., Ramsden, R. T., & Axon, P. R. (1998). Cochlear implantation in the deaf-blind. *American Journal of Otology, 19*, 774–777.

Samar, V. J., Paranis, I., & Berent, G. P. (1998). Learning disabilities, attention deficit disorders, and deafness. In M. Marschark & M. D. Clark (Eds.), *Psychological perspectives on deafness* (Vol. 2, pp. 199–242). Mahwah, NJ: Lawrence Erlbaum Associates.

Schildroth, A. N., & Hotto, S. A. (1996). Changes in student and program characteristics, 1984–85 and 1994–95. *American Annals of the Deaf, 141*, 68–71.

Schroeder, S. R., Reese, R., Hellings, J., Loupe, P., & Tessel, R. (1999). The causes of self-injurious behavior and their clinical implications (pp. 249–261). In N. Wieseler & R. Hanson (Eds.), *Challenging behavior.* Washington, DC: American Association on Mental Retardation.

Seung, H., Holmes, A., & Colburn, M. (2005). Twin language development: A case study of a twin with a cochlear implant and a twin with typical hearing. *Volta Review, 105*, 175–188.

Shallop, J. K., & Ash, K. R. (1995). Relationships among comfort levels determined by cochlear implant patient's self-programming, audiologist's programming, and electrical stapedius reflex thresholds. *Annals of Otology, Rhinology, and Laryngology, 104*(Suppl. 166), 175–176.

Smoorenburg, G. F., Willeboer, C., & van Dijk, J. E. (2002). Speech perception in Nucleus CI24M cochlear implant users with processor settings based on electrically evoked compound action potential thresholds. *Audiology and Neurotology, 7*, 335–347.

Soukup, M., & Feinstein, S. (2007). Identification, assessment, and intervention strategies for deaf and hard of hearing students with learning disabilities. *American Annals of the Deaf, 152*, 56–62.

Sparrow, S. S., Cicchettim, D. V., & Balla, D. A. (2005). *Vineland Adaptive Behavior Scales, Second Edition (Vineland-II).* Circle Pines; MN: American Guidance Service.

Spencer, P. E. (2000). Looking without listening: Is audition a prerequisite for normal development of visual attention during infancy. *Journal of Deaf Studies and Deaf Education, 5*, 291–302.

Spivak, L. G., & Chute, P. M. (1994). The relationship between electrical acoustic reflex thresholds and behavioral comfort levels in children and adult cochlear implant users. *Ear and Hearing, 15*, 184–192.

Stacey, P. C., Fortnum, H. M., Barton, G. R., & Summerfield, A. Q. (2006). Hearing-impaired children in the United Kingdom, I: Auditory performance, communication skills, educational achievements, quality of life, and cochlear implantation. *Ear and Hearing, 27*, 161–186.

Stewart, D. A., & Kluwin, T. N. (2001). *Teaching deaf and hard of hearing students. Content, strategies, and curriculum.* Boston: Allyn and Bacon.

Stillman, R. D., & Battle, C. W. (1986). Developmental assessment of communicative abilities in the deaf-blind. In D. Ellis (Ed.), *Sensory impairments in mentally handicapped people* (pp. 319–335). London: Croom Helm.

Stout, G. G., & Windle, J. V. E. (1992). *The Developmental Approach to Successful Listening* (2nd ed.). Englewood, CO: Resource Point.

Stredler-Brown, A., & DeConde Johnson, C. (2001, 2003, 2004). *Functional auditory performance indicators: An integrated approach to auditory development.* Denver,

CO: Special Education Services Unit, Colorado Department of Education. Retrieved September 20, 2008, from: http://www.cde.state.co.us/cdesped/download/pdf/FAPI_3-1-04g.pdf

Svirsky, M. A., Robbins, A. M., Kirk, K. L., Pisoni, D. B., & Miyomoto, R. T. (2000). Language development in profoundly deaf children with cochlear implants. *Psychological Science, 11*, 153-158.

Tait, M., Lutman, M. E., & Robinson, K. (2000). Preimplant measures of preverbal communication behavior as predictors of cochlear implant outcomes in children. *Ear and Hearing, 21*, 18-24.

Thal, D., DesJardin, J. L., & Eisenberg, L. S. (2007). Validity of the MacArthur-Bates Communicative Development Inventories for measuring language abilities in children with cochlear implants. *American Journal of Speech Language Pathology, 16*, 54-64.

Tharp, A. M. (2000). Service delivery for children with multiple impairments: How are we doing? In R. C. Seewald (Ed.), *A sound foundation through amplification: Proceedings of an International Conference* (pp. 175-190). Chicago: Phonak AG.

Tharp, A., Ashmead, D., & Rothpletz, A. (2002). Visual attention in children with normal hearing, children with hearing aids, and children with cochlear implants. *Journal of Speech, Language, and Hearing Research, 45*, 403-413.

The Ear Foundation. (n.d.). Life with an implant: Family experiences. In S. Archbold & A. Wheeler (Eds.), *Champions, children with additional disabilities* (pp. 32-34). Nottingham, UK: The Ear Foundation. Available at: www.earfoundation.org.uk

Tiber, N. (1985). A psychological evaluation of cochlear implant in children. *Ear and Hearing, 6*(Suppl.), 48S-51S.

Tobey, E. A., Geers, A. E., Brenner, C., Altuna, D., & Gabbert, G. (2003). Factors associated with development of speech production skills in children implanted by age five. *Ear and Hearing, 24*(Suppl.), 36S-45S.

Turner, L. M., Stone, W. L., Pozdol, S. L., & Coonrod, E. E. (2006). Follow-up of children with

autism spectrum disorders from age 2 to age 9. *Autism, 10*, 243-265.

Uziel, A., Mondain, M., & Reid, J. (1995). European procedures and considerations in children's cochlear implant program. *Annals of Otology, Rhinology, and Laryngology, 104*(Suppl. 166), 212-215.

Van Naarden, K., Decoufle, P., & Caldwell, K. (1999). Prevalence and characteristics of children with serious hearing impairment in metropolitan Atlanta, 1991-1993. *Pediatrics, 103*, 570-575.

Vissers, L. E., van Ravenswaaij, C. M., Admiraal, R., Hurst, J. A., de Vries, B. B., Janssen, I. et al. (2004). Mutations in a new member of the chromodomain gene family cause CHARGE syndrome. *Nature Genetics, 36*, 955-957.

Vlahovic, S., & Sindija, B. (2004). The influence of potentially limiting factors on paediatric outcomes following cochlear implantation. *International Journal of Pediatric Otorhinolaryngology, 68*, 1167-1174.

Waltzman, S. B., Cohen, N. L., Gomolin, R. H., Green, J. E., Shapiro, W. H., Hoffman, R. A., et al. (1997). Open-set speech perception in congenitally deaf children using cochlear implantation. *American Journal of Otology, 18*, 342-349.

Waltzman, S. B., & Roland, J. T. (2005). Cochlear Implantation in children younger than 12 months. *Pediatrics, 116*, e487-e493.

Waltzman, S. B., Scalchunes, V., & Cohen, N. L. (2000). Performance of multiply handicapped children using cochlear implants. *American Journal of Otology, 21*, 329-335.

Watkins, S., & Tonelson, S. (2004). *SKI-HI Language Development Scale* (2nd ed.). Logan, UT: HOPE.

Watt, N., Wetherby, A., & Shumway, S. (2006). Prelinguistic predictors of language outcome at 3 years of age. *Journal of Speech, Language, and Hearing Research, 49*, 1224-1237.

Waxman, R., & Spencer, P. E. (1997). What mothers do to support infant visual attention: Sensitivities to age and hearing status. *Journal of Deaf Studies and Deaf Education, 2*, 104-114.

Wetherby, A., Cain, D., Yonclas, D., & Walker, V. (1988). Analysis of intentional communication of normal children from the prelinguistic to multiword stage. *Journal of Speech and Hearing Research, 31,* 240–252.

Wetherby, A., & Prizant, B. (1993). *Communication and Symbolic Behavior Scales—Normed Edition.* Baltimore: Paul H. Brookes.

Wetherby, A., & Prizant, B. (2002). *Communication and Symbolic Behavior Scales Developmental Profile—First Normed Edition.* Baltimore: Paul H. Brookes.

Wetherby, A., & Prizant, B. (2003). *CSBS Manual: Communication and Symbolic Behavior Scales–Normed Edition.* Baltimore: Paul H. Brookes.

Wetherby, A. M., Prizant, B. M., & Hutchinson, T. A. (1998). Communicative, social/affective, and symbolic profiles of young children with autism and pervasive developmental disorders. *American Journal of Speech-Language Pathology, 7,* 79–91.

Wetherby, A. M., Watt, N., Morgan, L., & Shumway, S. (2007). Social communication profiles of children with autism spectrum disorders late in the second year of life. *Journal of Autism and Developmental Disorders, 37,* 960–975.

Wetherby, A. M., Woods, J., Allen, L., Cleary, J., Dickenson, H., & Lord, C. (2004). Early indicators of autism spectrum disorders in the second year of life. *Journal of Autism and Developmental Disorders, 34,* 473–493.

Wetherby, A. M., Yonclas, D. G., & Bryan, A. A. (1989). Communicative profiles of handicapped preschool children: Implications for early identification. *Journal of Speech and Hearing Disorders, 54,* 148–158.

Wiley, S. (2004). Developmental pediatrics and cochlear implantation. In R. Miyamoto (Ed.), *Proceedings of the 8th International Cochlear Implant Conference. International Congress Series, 1273* (pp. 324–327). Netherlands: Elsevier.

Wiley, S., Choo, D., Meinzen-Derr, J., Hilbert, L., & Greinwald, J. (2006). GJB2 mutations and additional disabilities in a pediatric cochlear implant population. *International Journal of Pediatric Otorhinolaryngology, 70,* 493–500.

Wiley, S., Jahnke, M., Meinzen-Derr, J., & Choo, D. (2005). Perceived qualitative benefits of cochlear implants in children with multi-handicaps. *International Journal of Pediatric Otorhinolaryngology, 69,* 791–798.

Wiley, S., Meinzen-Derr, J., & Choo, D. (2004). Performance of implanted children with developmental delays and/or behavioral disorders: Retrospective analysis. In R. Miyamoto (Ed.), *Proceedings of the 8th International Cochlear Implant Conference. International Congress Series, 1273* (pp. 273–276). Netherlands: Elsevier.

Wiley, S., Meinzen-Derr, J., & Choo, D. (2008). Auditory skill development among children with developmental delays and cochlear implants. *Annals of Otology, Rhinology, and Laryngology, 117,* 711–718.

Williamson, W. D., Desmond, M. M., Lafevers, N., Taber, L., Catlin, F. I., & Weaver, T. G. (1982). Symptomatic congenital cytomegalovirus: Disorders of language, learning and hearing. *American Journal of Diseases of Children, 136,* 902–905.

Winter, M. E., Johnson, K. C., & Vranisic, A. (2004). Performance of implanted children with developmental delays and/or behavioral disorders: Retrospective analysis. In R. Miyamoto (Ed.), *Proceedings of the 8th International Cochlear Implant Conference. International Congress Series, 1273* (pp. 277–280). Netherlands: Elsevier.

Yoshinaga-Itano, C., & Stredler-Brown, A. (1992). Learning to communicate: Babies with hearing impairments make their needs known. *Volta Review, 95,* 107–129.

Young, N. M., Johnson, K. C., Mets, M. B., & Hain, T. C. (1995). Cochlear implants in young children with usher syndrome. *Annals of Otology, Rhinology, and Laryngology, 104* (Suppl. 166), 342–345.

Zaidman-Zait, A., & Most, T. (2005). Cochlear implants in children with hearing loss: Maternal Expectations and impact on the family. *Volta Review, 105,* 129–150.

Zimmerman-Phillips S., Robbins, A. M., & Osberger, M. J. (2000). Assessing cochlear implant benefit in very young children. *Annals of Otology, Rhinology, and Laryngology, 109* (Suppl. 185), 42–43.

CHAPTER 20

Clinical Management of Children with "Auditory Neuropathy"

CRAIG A. BUCHMAN
PATRICIA A. ROUSH
HOLLY F. B. TEAGLE
CARLTON J. ZDANSKI

Introduction

Auditory neuropathy is a term that has been used rather commonly to describe a clinical syndrome in which gross discrepancy exists between measures of cochlear and neural function in the auditory system. Specifically, this discrepancy is most evident when oto-acoustic emissions (OAEs) and/or a cochlear microphonic (CM) (indicative of normal outer hair cell function) are present with absent or abnormal auditory brainstem responses (ABRs) (Berlin et al., 1998; Kaga et al., 1996; Rance et al., 1999; Starr, Picton, Sininger, Hood, & Berlin, 1996). In contrast to peripheral or cochlear hearing losses where hair cell activation is usually absent or severely diminished, in auditory neuropathy, hair cell activation is present, but signal transduction to the auditory nerve and through the brainstem are absent or severely disrupted. For patients with auditory neuropathy, hearing thresholds for pure tone detection can range from normal to profound levels (Madden, Rutter, Hilbert, Greinwald, & Choo, 2002b; Rance et al., 1999; Rance, Cone-Wesson, Wunderlich, & Dowell, 2002). Recent studies in older children and adults suggest that these patients' perceptual abilities can be severely impaired for both pitch discrimination in the low frequencies as well as temporal processing tasks (Rance, McKay, & Grayden, 2004; Zeng, Kong, Michalewski, & Starr, 2005). It has been hypothesized that lesions in the inner hair cells, the synapse between the inner hair cell and the auditory nerve, and the auditory nerve itself may account for the clinical findings (Berlin, Hood, Morlet,

Rose, & Brashears, 2003; Fuchs, Glowatzki, & Moser, 2003; Starr et al., 1996).

In an excellent review of the terminology and topic, Rapin and Gravel point out that generalized use of the term auditory neuropathy may be inappropriate in many cases as it lumps together a heterogeneous group of patients with a wide range of auditory dysfunctions, test results, and underlying pathologies (Rapin & Gravel, 2003; 2006). They propose that auditory neuropathy *sensu stricto* be reserved for cases where the auditory nerve and/or spiral ganglion cells and processes are affected in isolation (ganglionopathy, demyelination, or axonopathy) rather than a process that might involve the auditory system more peripherally (i.e., the inner hair cells or synapse), centrally (8th nerve nucleus or central, projections), or in a mixed fashion. As we concur with these authors' strict interpretation, we will use the term "auditory neuropathy" ("AN") in quotes to denote the inaccuracy in terminology. However, considering this group of disorders (i.e., lesion involving the inner hair cell→cochlear nucleus) together is clinically relevant since these individuals present with a similar electrophysiologic profile.

What constitutes the ideal management strategy for children with "AN" is likely unique to the individual in consideration of his or her functional manifestations. It is clear that "AN" represents a common auditory electrophysiologic profile that is present among a very heterogeneous group of disorders. Thus, it seems logical that one approach will probably not be sufficient for all children. Rather a flexible management paradigm that maximizes a child's opportunities for language development is needed. This chapter reviews the epidemiology, etiology and pathology, diagnosis, and management of children with "AN." We also include our clinical experiences and available outcome data for our diverse patient population.

Epidemiology

The precise incidence and prevalence of "AN" remains unknown and estimates are clearly dependent on the population studied and the criterion used to define the disorder. Early case reports suggested that "AN" was relatively uncommon among individuals with sensorineural hearing loss. Davis and Hirsch (1979) identified only 1 case (0.5%) out of 200 with sensorineural hearing loss that had an absent ABR. Another study suggested that the prevalence among deaf school attendees was only 3% when defined as present OAEs, absent ABR and absent middle latency responses (Lee, McPherson, Yuen, & Wong, 2001). Rance et al. (1999) found 11% of infants and young children with sensorineural hearing loss to have absent ABRs and present OAEs, whereas Madden et al. (2002b) found roughly 5% of their hearing loss database of over 400 children to have "AN." In contrast, a number of investigators have suggested that the estimates of "AN" among neonatal intensive care unit (NICU) graduates is substantially higher than those reported for the deaf population in general (Rance et al., 1999). Xoinis, Weirather, Mavoori, Shaha, and Iwamoto (2007) and Rea and Gibson (2003) reported the "AN" phenotype among hearing-impaired NICU survivors in up to 40%.

Etiology

The etiology of "AN" appears to be multifactorial and can result from a variety of lesions throughout the auditory pathway. "AN" can be congenital or acquired and might occur as a part of a known clinical syndrome (i.e., syndromic) or may be seen in isolation (i.e., nonsyndromic). Risk factors identified in association with "AN" include: family history, NICU stay, hyperbilirubinemia, birth weight <1500 g, ototoxic medication exposure, cerebral palsy, congenital malformations, visual and vestibular dysfunction, and sensory-motor neuropathy (Berg, Spitzer, Towers, Bartosiewicz, & Diamond, 2005; Madden et al., 2002b; Rance et al., 1999; Rance et al., 2002; Starr et al., 1996).

Syndromic varieties of "AN" have been associated with neurologic disorders such as Charcot-Marie-Tooth (CMT) disease, Mohr-Tranebjaerg syndrome (MTS), Refsum disease, Friedreich's ataxia, and Cockayne's disease. Leber's hereditary optic neuropathy and mitochondrial encephalomyopathies also have been associated with the "AN" phenotype. Many of these disorders have, as a hallmark, peripheral nerve involvement (Butinar et al., 1999; Ceranic & Luxon, 2004; Gandolfi, Horoupian, Rapin, DeTeresa, & Hyams, 1984; Merchant et al., 2001; Rance et al., 2008). Thus, in these cases, a primary neuropathic process may affect the auditory nerve and account for the clinical findings. In fact, in some cases, histologic examination of the temporal bones and neural tissues has confirmed demyelination and axonal loss in the presence of preserved organ of Corti structure (Bahmad, Merchant, Nadol, Jr., & Tranebjaerg, 2007; Hallpike, Harriman, & Wells, 1980; Merchant et al., 2001; Spoendlin, 1974).

Examples of genes that have been mapped in hereditary cases of "AN" include: *DDP/TIMM8A, MPZ, NDRG1, PMP22, DFNB9/OTOF, AUNA1, DFNB59* (Butinar et al., 1999; Chapon, Latour, Diraison, Schaeffer, & Vandenberghe, 1999; Delmaghani et al., 2006; Kalaydjieva, Gresham, & Calafell, 2001; Maier, Castagner, Berger, & Suter, 2003; Starr et al., 2004; Starr et al., 2003; Varga et al., 2006; Yasunaga et al., 2000; Yasunaga et al., 1999). One particularly well-documented genetic form of syndromic "AN" occurred in a group of Slovenian Roma (Gypsy) families and has been mapped to the long arm of chromosome 8 (8q24) (Butinar et al., 1999). These families are affected by an autosomal recessive, inherited sensorimotor neuropathy that is particularly severe with associated neural hearing loss and absent vestibular function. Another example of syndromic "AN" is Mohr-Tranebjaerg syndrome. This is an X-linked inherited disorder of mitochondrial metabolism that results in widespread loss of neurons in the brain, auditory and vestibular nerves, ganglion cell layer loss of the retina, and dorsal root ganglia. This syndrome results in early-onset deafness, with later blindness, dystonia, spasticity, and dementia (Bahmad et al., 2007; Merchant et al., 2001).

Nonsyndromic forms of "AN" also have been identified in patients with an autosomal recessive (DFNB59, DFNB9/OTOF) and autosomal dominant (AUNA1) mode of inheritance. In patients affected with DFNB9/OTOF mutations, abnormal production of the protein *otoferlin* can produce hearing loss that can range from mild to profound and may be early or late onset and even sensitive to changes in temperature depending on the mutation present (Varga et al., 2006). Certain missense mutations in the DFNB59 gene results in abnormalities in the protein *pejvakin,* an apparently critical protein for auditory nerve function. Affected individuals have prelingual onset deafness and electrophysiologic evidence for "AN" (Delmaghani et al., 2006). In patients affected by AUNA1 mutations, the initial phenotypic features of the hearing loss are of abnormal ABRs with normal outer hair cell functions (both OAEs and CMs present). The hearing loss progresses over 10 to 20 years, producing a profound sensorineural hearing loss with absent ABRs and OAEs (Starr et al., 2004).

Associations also have been made between infectious (measles, mumps), metabolic (diabetes, hyperbilirubinemia, hypoxia), and neoplastic processes (acoustic neuroma) as well as prematurity (Starr et al., 2001). Hyperbilirubinemia is a particularly common finding among infants with "AN" in clinical practice (Madden et al., 2002b). It has been known for some time that severe hyperbilirubinemia (i.e., kernicterus) of the newborn may result in hearing loss that can be profound (Fenwick, 1975). A number of investigators have debated the site of the lesion responsible for hearing loss in these infants. Postmortem studies have identified bilirubin staining in the basal ganglia, hippocampus, with gliosis of the cerebellar, auditory, and vestibular nuclei. Some have identified cochlear abnormalities in these infants whereas others have claimed the sensory receptors to be spared (Amatuzzi et al., 2001; Gerrard, 1952; Goodhill, 1956; Keleman, 1956; Sheykholeslami & Kaga, 2000). Animal studies of kernicterus have shown the pathology to be located in neural tissue for the most part with sparing of the organ of Corti. In a recent group of animal studies, Shaia and colleagues identified the neurotoxic effects of bilirubin in both spiral ganglion cells, large axons of the auditory nerve, and brainstem nuclei with sparing of the cochlear structures (Shaia et al., 2002; Shaia, Shapiro, & Spencer, 2005; Spencer, Shaia, Gleason, Sismanis, & Shapiro, 2002). Accepting these findings would imply that other factors beyond bilirubin toxicity might be responsible for the findings of hair cell loss and cochlear involvement identified in previous postmortem clinical studies.

Cochlear nerve deficiency (CND) is a term used to refer to those cases in which the auditory nerve is either small or absent and thus, in a strict sense, represents a severe and literal form of auditory neuropathy (Glastonbury et al., 2002). CND presumably can occur as a result of failure of the nerve to develop either partially (hypoplasia) or completely (aplasia or agenesis) or as a result of postdevelopmental degeneration. CND

has been described in studies of human temporal bones in association with inner ear malformation, internal auditory canal (IAC) stenosis, and occasionally in the presence of a normal IAC morphology (Felix & Hoffmann, 1985; Nadol & Xu, 1992; Nelson & Hinojosa, 2001; Spoendlin & Schrott, 1990; Ylikoski & Savolainen, 1984). Most recently, children with both unilateral and bilateral CND on magnetic resonance imaging (MRI) have been identified with the electrophysiologic profile of "AN" (Buchman et al., 2006). These findings are consistent with the anatomical studies which have demonstrated normal organ of Corti structure in the setting of CND in some temporal bones (Nelson & Hinojosa, 2001).

Diagnosis

For the purposes of this report, and irrespective of etiology, the diagnosis of "AN" requires (1) evidence of cochlear outer hair cell function as indicated by present OAEs and/or CM, (2) absent or severely abnormal ABR, and (3) absent middle ear muscle reflexes. Speech understanding that is worse than would be predicted from a behavioral audiogram adds credence to the diagnosis. Thus, within the context of this definition, a variety of lesions throughout the auditory system is expected and is indistinguishable based on these electrophysiologic and audiometric criteria alone. Specifically, isolated inner hair cell loss, (i.e., a cochlear [sensory] hearing loss), would manifest similarly to those with a primary auditory nerve or hair cell-dendrite synaptic disorder.

It is critical to recognize that newborn infant hearing screening protocols that use OAEs as the sole measure for detecting hearing loss will miss cases of "AN" unless a concomitant hair cell disorder exists. With this in mind, the 2007 position statement by the Joint Commission on Infant Hearing (American Academy of Pediatrics, Joint Commission on Infant Hearing, 2007) recommended that separate protocols be used for NICU and well-infant nurseries. Specifically, NICU infants admitted for more than 5 days are to have ABR included as part of their screening so that neural hearing loss will not be missed. Although these modifications will help identify infants at high risk for "AN," those without risk factors such as genetic and late onset varieties, will still be missed when OAE screening is used alone.

Audiologic Diagnostic Evaluation

No single test modality is sufficient for precisely identifying the degree of hearing impairment in a baby. Rather, a test battery is needed that might include a combination of measures such as: ABR, auditory steady-state responses (ASSR), OAE, tympanometry (immittance), and behavioral tests of hearing obtained via techniques developmentally appropriate for a child's age and ability. Although reasonably accurate, each of these testing procedures has a variety of potential shortcomings. It is paramount that the individual administering the protocol be able to recognize and interpret the various tests results within the context of these shortcomings. Our protocols have been detailed previously (Buchman et al., 2006).

Figure 20–1 shows an example of an ABR from a child with "AN." The protocol calls for single-polarity stimulation to identify the CM, if present. CM is distinguished from neural response by two criteria: (1) the polarity of the response will invert with

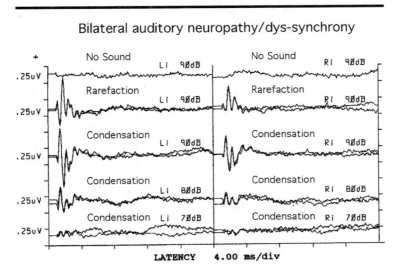

Figure 20–1. Example of a diagnostic ABR from a child with "AN." An inverting, phase-dependent response is seen in both ears that fail to increase in latency on decreasing the stimulus intensity. This is indicative of a cochlear microphonic (CM) and is confirmed not to be stimulus artifact by seeing the response disappear upon disconnecting the sound tubing.

stimulus polarity inversion; and (2) the latency of the response will remain constant with changes in stimulus level. Accordingly, when a response suspected to be the CM is noted (typically at a relatively high stimulus level), recordings are made with both rarefaction and condensation stimulus phase, and—for a constant phase—two recordings are made 10 dB apart. Special care is required in identifying the CM, because, as a consequence of monophasic stimulation, all stimulus-phase–dependent components present at the electrodes—including stimulus artifact—will emerge during the averaging process. To distinguish CM from stimulus artifact, the sound tubing coupling the transducer to the insert earphone is disconnected without altering the relative positions of the electrodes and transducers. If the stimulus-phase–dependent component disappears in this case, the response in question is the CM; if it remains, it is stimulus artifact.

Audiometric findings in patients with "AN" vary widely with thresholds ranging from normal to profound levels. The hearing loss configuration can also be quite variable. Although some investigators have reported an increased preponderance of up-sloping losses, others have shown no such association (Doyle, Sininger, & Starr, 1998; Madden et al., 2002b; Rance et al., 1999; Shivashankar, Satishchandra, Shashikala, & Gore, 2003). Fluctuation, progression and improvement in thresholds have all been reported although the latter appears to be uncommon (Madden et al., 2002b; Psarommatis et al., 2006; Rance et al., 1999). Speech perception abilities can vary widely as well. In adults, speech recognition scores that are out of proportion to the degree of pure tone hearing loss are common (Starr et al., 1996; Zeng et al., 2005). Although some children have displayed auditory perceptual skills consistent with their sensorineural

hearing loss peers, a high proportion (~50%) present with little or no ability to understand speech even when the signal is presented at clearly audible levels (Rance & Barker, 2008; Rance et al., 2007a; Rance et al., 1999; Rance et al., 2002). Listening in noise is also extremely difficult for patients with "AN," even among those with relatively good perceptual abilities in quiet (Rance et al., 2007a; Zeng et al., 2005). This poor performance in competing background noise is largely felt to reflect disordered temporal processing, especially in the low frequencies, with preserved intensity-related functions. Unfortunately, there remains very limited data regarding threshold and perceptual abilities in very young children correlated to etiology. Further research in this area is needed.

Medical Diagnostic Evaluation

The medical evaluation focuses on trying to identify an etiology for the hearing loss and associated problems that may negatively impact communication or other health issues. Implicit is the fact that a detailed understanding of the causes of hearing loss in children is needed to identify the salient issues in a particular patient. An excellent review of the potential etiologies of hearing loss previously has been published (Morton & Nance, 2006). In addition to searching for the etiology of hearing loss, careful evaluation must identify disorders in vision, craniofacial malformations, and primary speech and auditory processing disorders to allow a comprehensive approach to the communication needs of a child and his or her family. Referrals among a variety of medical professionals are often needed. For instance, many children with "AN" require an evaluation by a pediatric neurologist, pediatric geneticist, and pediatric ophthalmologist.

For the otolaryngologist, a careful history, physical examination and selective use of imaging studies and laboratory testing can identify the etiology of a child's hearing loss in many cases. In addition to knowing the details of the newborn infant screening and diagnostic auditory testing, the medical history should be thorough in the areas of pregnancy and complications, past medical/surgical history, and family history. A careful assessment of the known risk factors for "AN" should be queried (Figure 20-2).

Radiographic Imaging

Radiologic imaging is a critical aspect of the assessment of every child with newly identified hearing loss. In our program, imaging is recommended immediately after the diagnosis of hearing loss has been established by electrophysiologic measures. Early anatomic assessment of the temporal bones, auditory, vestibular, and facial nerves as well as brain may:

1. further characterize the hearing loss *etiology*,

2. identify anatomic markers for hearing loss *progression*,

3. predict *poor prognosis* from interventions such as amplification and/or cochlear implantation, and

4. *identify lesions of the central nervous system that require medical/surgical intervention* for the overall health of the patient.

There currently remains some debate regarding which of the various imaging modalities is most appropriate for assessing children with hearing loss (Adunka, Jewells, & Buchman, 2007; Adunka et al., 2006; Buchman et al., 2006; Parry, Booth, & Roland, 2005; Trimble, Blaser, James, & Papsin, 2007). This controversy stems mostly from otologists' and radiologists' familiarity in interpreting high-resolution computed tomography (HRCT) for inner ear morphologic changes. We prefer MRI rather than HRCT in all children with newly identified sensorineural hearing loss as it allows direct imaging of the cochlear nerves and brain. The consequences of missing either isolated CND or unsuspected retrocochlear/brain pathology could be profound and ultimately might

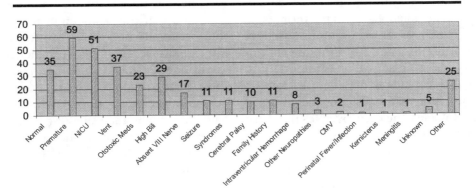

Figure 20–2. Medical diagnoses among 130 children with "AN" at UNC-Chapel Hill. NICU—neonatal intensive care unit stay, Vent—ventilator support, CP—cerebral palsy, High Bili—hyperbilirubinemia, CMV—cytomegalovirus.

result in inappropriate treatment of the child. For example, cochlear implantation in an ear without a cochlear nerve or in an ear affected by a tumor could be devastating for the child and family.

Roughly 30 to 40% of children with hearing loss will have abnormal findings on imaging of the brain, IACs, and inner ears. A variety of findings can be seen on MRI in children with "AN" that can alter treatment plans and result in a change in prognosis. Some examples of imaging findings in patients with "AN" are shown in Figures 20–3 through 20–7 and include: cochlear nerve deficiency (Figure 20–3), arachnoid cysts or neoplasms of the cerebellopontine angle and brain (Figure 20–4), developmental changes in the posterior fossa such as Dandy-Walker syndrome (Figure 20–5), white matter changes resulting from perinatal CMV infection (Figure 20–6), mitochondrial disease (Figure 20–7), and basal ganglia staining in hyperbilirubinemia.

Management

Families arrive with varying levels of knowledge regarding "AN" and its management. Some will be unfamiliar with the term while others may have strong opinions based on information obtained from the internet or from other professionals. It is important to make sure families understand the heterogeneous nature of the disorder and its underlying etiologies, the controversies that exist regarding treatment options, and the difficulty predicting outcomes during infancy. For families committed to spoken language, the process will involve diagnostic assessment combined with careful observation and a series of management decisions that may include amplification and/or cochlear

implantation. It is important for families to know that the individual strengths and needs of their child will be carefully considered and that they will be full partners in the decision-making process.

In addition to the auditory uncertainties, many children with "AN" have multiple disabilities or medical conditions that complicate management. These medical conditions can negatively impact the child's abilities to be tested, and the child's overall communication abilities. A common consideration is that of professionals being unable to assess auditory detection levels, speech perception abilities, and vocalizations because of neurologic compromise. Children with associated visual and/or motor impairment also might not be able to participate in manual modes of communication. These challenges can make evidence-based decision-making nearly impossible in some instances.

When the development of spoken language is the goal, auditory interventions might include amplification and/or cochlear implantation. For children with "AN," when hearing loss has been documented, conservative amplification has been proposed. Proponents of this approach argue that there have been a wide range of perceptual abilities demonstrated among children with "AN" and that the restoration of audibility through amplification will allow for an accurate identification of those patients who might benefit (Rance & Barker, 2008). For those who disagree with this approach, concerns regarding amplification-induced hair cell loss and the claim of nearly universally poor perceptual abilities among these patients fuel their arguments (Berlin et al., 2003). Regarding amplification-induced hearing loss, recent works seem to refute this contention (Rance, 2005; Rance et al., 2002). As previously mentioned, severely distorted perceptual abilities among patients with

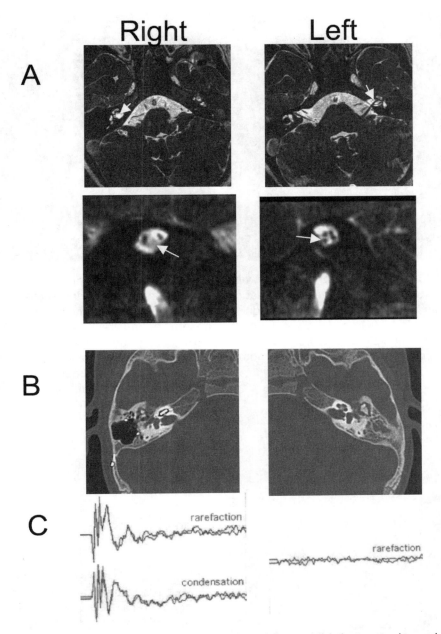

Figure 20–3. Cochlear nerve deficiency (*right ear*) in a child that experienced sudden hearing loss. MRI (**A**) shows axial and parasaggital reconstructed images in a plane perpendicular to the IAC. In the left ear, 4 nerves (superior and inferior vestibular, facial, and cochlear) are well visualized. In the right ear, the cochlear nerve is absent. The arrow points to the normal cochlear nerve on the left and the region of the absent cochlear nerve on the right. HRCT (**B**) shows normal inner ear morphology and a satisfactorily placed cochlear implant in the ear without a cochlear nerve. The ABR (**C**) shows a distinct cochlear microphonic in the right ear and no response in the ear with a normal nerve. The cochlear implant in the right ear provided limited perceptual abilities and left cochlear implantation resulted in normal, open-set speech perception.

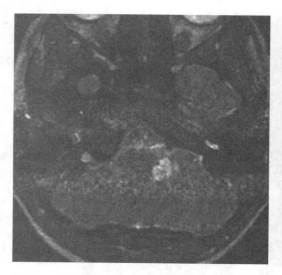

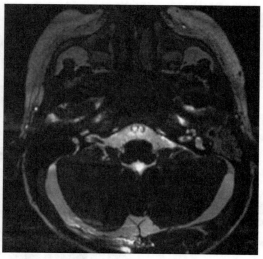

Figure 20–4. Three-year-old child with unknown age of onset unilateral, left hearing loss. Axial MRI with T2 and T1 with gadolinium demonstrates a lateral recess of the 4th ventricle/foramen of Luschka tumor that was surgically confirmed to be an ependymoma.

Figure 20–5. One-year-old child who failed a newborn infant hearing screening examination with cochlear microphonics and absent neural responses on diagnostic ABR testing consistent with "AN." Axial T2 MRI through the posterior cranial fossa demonstrates enlargement of the 4th ventricle and increased fluid spaces consistent with Dandy-Walker variant.

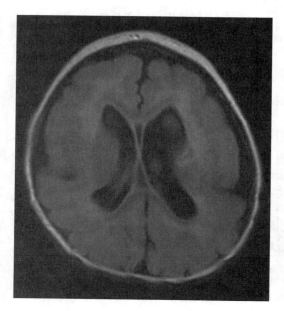

Figure 20–6. One-year-old child, born as a 27-week premature infant with failed newborn infant hearing screening examination. Diagnostic ABR demonstrates bilateral cochlear microphonics (CM) and absent neural responses consistent with "AN." Cytomegalovirus (CMV) polymerase chain reaction (PCR) testing on the Guthrie card blood spot was positive implying perinatal infection. Axial MRI FLAIR sequence (*above*) demonstrates subcortical, periventricular white matter lesions. High-resolution computed tomography shows cerebral calcifications consistent with CMV.

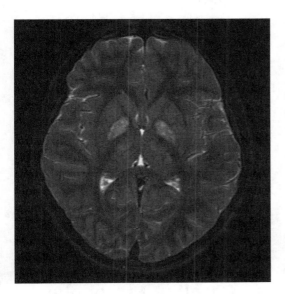

Figure 20–7. Ten-year-old child with "AN" type hearing loss, dystonia, and cardiomyopathy. T2 (and FLAIR not shown) MRI of the brain shows signal with restricted diffusion involving the globus pallidi, putamen, thalami, cerebral peduncles, and dentate nuclei bilaterally in symmetric distribution. This is consistent with mitochondrial disorder.

"AN" have, in fact, been demonstrated by a number of investigators (Rance & Barker, 2008; Rance, Barker, Sarant, & Ching, 2007b; Rance et al., 2002; Starr et al., 1996; Zeng et al., 2005; Zeng, Oba, Garde, Sininger, & Starr, 1999). A lack of benefit among patients receiving amplification supports these findings (Deltenre et al., 1999; Doyle et al., 1998; Katada, Nonaka, & Harabuchi, 2005; Starr et al., 1996). However, careful examination of these studies reveals a very limited number of subjects composed of predominantly adult subjects. Some notable exceptions are the studies by Rance and colleagues (Rance, 2005; Rance & Barker, 2008; Rance et al., 2007a; Rance et al., 2007b; Rance et al., 2002). In their landmark paper, Rance et al. (2002)

showed that for nearly 50% of a group of children with "AN," the provision of amplification resulted in significant open-set speech perception improvements. These findings have again been confirmed by this group of investigators (Rance, 2005; Rance & Barker, 2008; Rance et al., 2007a; Rance et al., 2007b). Further studies regarding the efficacy of amplification in children with "AN" are clearly needed, especially among the various groups of children and employing innovative strategies which capitalize on the unique psychoacoustic properties of these individuals' hearing loss (Narne & Vanaja, 2008; Zeng et al., 2005).

Regarding the utility of cochlear implantation in children with "AN," although data are limited, efficacy has been demonstrated in many cases, implying that electrical stimulation can improve speech perception abilities for some patients (Buss et al., 2002; Madden, Hilbert, Rutter, Greinwald, & Choo, 2002a; Madden et al., 2002b; Mason, De Michele, Stevens, Ruth, & Hashisaki, 2003; Sininger & Trautwein, 2002). Buss et al. (2002) studied 4 children with "AN" and cochlear implants. These children demonstrated robust electrically evoked ABR and middle ear muscle reflexes as well as performance levels similar to children without "AN." They concluded that in some children with "AN," electrical stimulation can result in synchronized neural impulses sufficient for auditory stimulation and reflex triggering. Other case series have demonstrated similar evidence of good speech perception in implanted children with "AN" (Madden et al., 2002a; Mason et al., 2003; Peterson et al., 2003; Rance & Barker, 2008; Shallop, Peterson, Facer, Fabry, & Driscoll, 2001; Shehata-Dieler, Volter, Hildmann, Hildmann, & Helms, 2007; Sininger & Trautwein, 2002). Nevertheless, caution should be exercised in generalizing about success with cochlear implants for all children with "AN." In a very important work, Miyamoto, Kirk, Renshaw, and Hussain (1999) reported on a child with Friedreich's ataxia, progressive hearing loss of the "AN" variety, and blindness who underwent cochlear implantation. Despite auditory awareness and enhanced closed-set understanding for vowels, open-set speech perception was extremely poor and notably no better than that measured prior to cochlear implantation. Similarly, Buchman and colleagues have implanted at least five ears with "AN" and CND on MRI. Although the implants provided some degree of sound awareness for these children, open-set speech perception has not been achieved (Adunka et al., 2007; Adunka et al., 2006; Buchman et al., 2006). Even for children with "AN" who benefit from cochlear implantation, performance may be somewhat poorer than is expected for implanted children with "typical" sensorineural hearing loss (Rance & Barker, 2008).

In these limited studies, it is safe to say that generalizations cannot be made regarding prognosis for speech perception abilities in children with "AN" irrespective of the auditory intervention employed. Some children with "AN" have reasonably preserved perceptual abilities and might benefit substantially from amplification alone while others may not. For children with a severely distorted signal despite adequate amplification, cochlear implantation might be justified. Again, whereas some children will have success with this intervention, others will not. The diversity among these results clearly points to the varying pathologic processes at work in these children and supports the implementation of a carefully observed stepwise intervention paradigm that includes obtaining reliable behavioral measures of hearing and progresses from observation to fitting of amplification and, if appropriate, moving to cochlear

implantation. A focus on identifying an objective means for selecting those children who that might benefit from amplification versus those who might be better served with other interventions is sorely needed. Some areas that might prove fruitful in this regard are imaging studies such as functional MRI and electrophysiologic measures, such as auditory and electrically evoked potentials (Patel et al., 2007; Rance et al., 2002; Santarelli, Starr, Michalewski, & Arslan, 2008; Walton, Gibson, Sanli, & Prelog, 2008; Zur, Holland, Yuan, & Choo, 2004).

University of North Carolina Protocols: Protocols and Results

Management Protocol

In an effort to achieve timely diagnosis and early intervention, we have created a timeline for the events of the first year of life following referral from a newborn hearing screen and identification of a hearing disorder (including "AN") (Figure 20–8). Although not rigidly applied, we believe this timeline provides a general framework for the events of the first year of life as they relate to the management of hearing loss. The primary goals in the first year are:

1. *identification* of hearing loss and establishing reliable estimates of auditory thresholds;
2. *diagnosis* of the etiology for the hearing impairment;
3. *intervention* through appropriate treatment and technologies; and
4. *education* by providing information for families to help make decisions.

A comprehensive diagnostic hearing evaluation is the first step following a con-

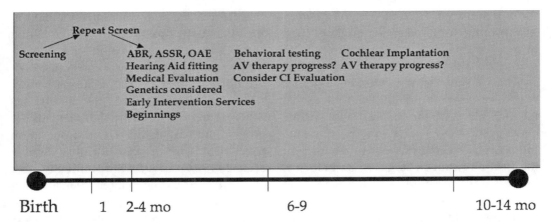

Figure 20–8. Time line for diagnostic and therapeutic intervention for infants that fail a newborn infant screen. ABR—auditory brainstem response, ASSR—auditory steady-state response, OAE—otoacoustic emissions, CI—cochlear implant.

firmed "fail" or "refer" indication by the newborn infant hearing screening examination. At our center, this evaluation is carried out by a group of experienced audiologists with expertise in pediatric hearing testing. The initial follow-up testing for each child occurs in one of three environments: natural sleep, conscious sedation, or general anesthesia. Infants younger than about 3 months of age are tested in natural sleep, if possible. Babies older than this, without other medical contraindications, are sedated prior to testing. After medical clearance by a physician, a nurse from the hospital's pediatric sedation team administers a sedative and remains at bedside to monitor the entire session. Sedation is typically accomplished with chloral hydrate delivered orally or midazolam delivered intravenously. In cases where the infant is scheduled for a procedure under general anesthesia (e.g., surgery or imaging), the evoked potential testing is incorporated into the procedure sequence, if appropriate. Some children are not deemed candidates for safe monitored conscious sedation and so testing is carried out under

the supervision of an anesthesiologist (i.e., general anesthesia). The duration of the test is usually dictated by the test environment, ranging from about 30 minutes in the operating room to over an hour under conscious sedation. Following the initial audiologic assessment, we have found that the search for the etiology of the hearing loss and for any associated medical conditions is critical and frequently impacts the treatment paradigm. This usually includes a thorough evaluation by an otolaryngologist with experience in the assessment of children with hearing loss as well as attaining appropriate laboratory testing and diagnostic imaging. Families must also begin to learn about the communicative and educational impact of their child's diagnosis. In North Carolina, once hearing loss is confirmed, referrals are made to BEGINNINGS (www.beginningssvcs.com) and the N.C. Early Intervention Program for Children who are Deaf or Hard of Hearing (www.ncoes.net/preschools.shtml). BEGINNINGS was established as a nonprofit organization, incorporated under the laws of North Carolina since 1987, to provide emotional support and access to impartial information as a resource for families with deaf or hard of hearing children, age birth through 21 years. Early intervention services encompass a variety of state agencies working together to provide services and funding for assistive technologies (AT) for children with special needs age birth to 3 years. In North Carolina, there are a growing number of teachers of the deaf and speech-language pathologists trained and certified in Auditory-Verbal Therapy. Emerging evidence suggests that in the setting of an adequate auditory signal (either through amplification or a cochlear implant), auditory-based intervention provides for better acquisition of spoken language in hearing-impaired children than communication modes that include sign language (Moog & Geers, 2003).

At UNC-Chapel Hill, we established a prospective, institutional review board (IRB)-approved protocol to study the clinical characteristics and outcomes of children with newly identified "AN." The protocol was based primarily on the work of Rance et al. described above (Rance et al., 1999; Rance et al., 2002). That is, some children might benefit from certain interventions such as amplification or cochlear implantation whereas others may not. Thus, we approach children with "AN" individually, assessing their perceptual abilities with and without amplification prior to considering cochlear implantation.

In our program, when a child is identified with the electrophysiologic characteristics of "AN," the parents are told that their child has clear evidence of an auditory disorder. We also tell them that we cannot predict their child's auditory thresholds or speech perceptual abilities and, thus, a period of careful observation ensues until an age when auditory thresholds can be determined. With experienced pediatric audiologists, thresholds are usually attainable using visual reinforcement audiometry (VRA) at approximately 7 to 9 months of age. When behavioral audiometry using VRA demonstrates stable hearing thresholds outside of the normal range, a trial of amplification is initiated. Real-ear-to-coupler differences (RECDs) are measured and hearing aids are programmed using the Desired Sensation Level (DSL) prescriptive formula (Scollie et al., 2005). Considering the difficulty most children with "AN" encounter when listening in the presence of background noise, personal FM use by parents and other caregivers is likely to be beneficial and is recommended once full-time hearing aid use is established.

Children under 3 years of age return for follow-up hearing assessment every 3 months and communication progress is closely monitored by our center-based speech and language pathologist who communicates with the child's local early intervention specialist. Speech recognition testing using developmentally appropriate closed- and open-set tests are completed as soon as the child is able to perform such testing. Should amplification prove to be of limited or no benefit in the setting of ongoing diagnostic and therapeutic speech and language therapy, cochlear implantation is considered. Although this protocol does result in minor delays, we believe the approach is justified so that children who can benefit from amplification are identified and inappropriate cochlear implantation is avoided.

One particularly challenging situation is the child who is unable to perform behavioral audiometric testing because of neurologic impairments. Both motor and cognitive delays can make reliable determination of behavioral thresholds impossible. Similarly, assessing speech perception and benefit from the various interventions can be highly subjective. As auditory thresholds and perceptual abilities can be widely ranging in children with "AN," it is difficult to make an educated guess as to what constitutes the correct intervention strategy for a particular child. In these cases, parental desires as well as professional and family observations take precedence in decision-making. In some cases, providing a unilateral cochlear implant might be considered a conservative approach so as to not miss the critical period of development.

Patient Characteristics and Results

At the University of North Carolina at Chapel Hill, more than 130 children are currently being followed for "AN." In most cases, the children are presented to our center following failure or a "refer" result on a newborn infant hearing screening examination. In all cases, the diagnostic ABR performed at our center has shown a CM with absent or severely abnormal neural responses. There has been a wide variety of CM morphologies, amplitudes, and durations observed. In many cases, although a CM was evident on ABR testing, OAEs were absent or initially present only to later disappear. Middle ear muscle reflexes are nearly always absent. One hundred four (80%) of these children are affected bilaterally while 26 have unilateral "AN." What is clear from looking at this group of children is that the electrophysiologic profile for "AN" is common among a very heterogeneous group of children. Figure 20–2 shows some of the associated diagnoses for the group of children that we are following. Many children have more than one associated finding. Our patient population has a very high rate of prematurity (nearly 50%), NICU admission, ventilatory support, and hyperbilirubinemia. In contrast, the number of children with a known syndrome or family history is relatively low (<10%). Thus, we presume that most of the children in our "AN" population have an acquired etiology rather than the inherited variety. This population appears similar to the children reported by Madden et al. (2002a, 2002b) and Rance et al. (1999) but quite different from those adults studied by Starr et al. (1996) and Zeng et al. (2005).

In terms of management, of the 26 children with unilateral "AN," 16 (59%) have normal contralateral hearing and are using no assistive device, 4 (15%) are using a contralateral hearing aid, and 6 (26%) have been fitted with a cochlear implant either unilaterally or bilaterally. Only 2 of the unilateral "AN" patients have had implants placed in their "AN" ears, in both cases as part of bilateral implantation. One postlinguistic child was initially implanted in his "AN" ear following a sudden hearing loss with unexpected poor performance. Despite sound awareness and improved lip reading, only limited closed-set abilities were evident after 16 months of consistent device usage. Re-review of his preoperative MRI revealed that his implanted "AN" ear was affected by CND (see Figure 20–3). He subsequently received a contralateral implant in his non-"AN" ear with immediate improvement and overall excellent results. The findings in this case as well as others suggest that MRI is indicated for all children diagnosed with "AN," especially in the setting of a profound sensorineural hearing loss (Adunka et al., 2007; Adunka et al., 2006; Buchman et al., 2006; Gibson & Sanli, 2007; Walton et al., 2008). Our second unilateral "AN" patient who received a sequential second side implant in their "AN" ear is currently unable to be tested.

One-hundred four children have bilateral electrophysiologic evidence of "AN" at our institution. Of these children, 18 (17%) are currently using no assistive devices, 41 (39%) are fitted with binaural amplification, and 45 (44%) have received cochlear implants. The reasons for not using assistive devices include CND ($n = 3$; 17%), parent refusal ($n = 1$; 6%), unable or too early to measure thresholds (n = 8; 44%), and normal auditory thresholds measured (n = 6; 33%). Thus, 6% of bilateral "AN" children in our center have been identified with normal auditory thresholds. Speech perception testing is underway in many of these children as age and abilities permit.

Forty-one children have been fitted with binaural hearing aids based on DSL targets using real-ear measurements at our institution. Of these children, 9 (22%) demonstrate clear benefit from amplification as evidenced by either appropriate open- or closed-set speech perception test results and/or significant gains in speech and language abilities. Three (7%) of these children show minimal to no benefit and are being considered for cochlear implantation. The remaining children that have been fit with amplification either cannot or have not been tested because they are too neurologically impaired (n = 7; 17%), too young (n = 6; 15%), lost to follow-up (n = 9; 22%), or have

only recently been fitted (n = 7; 17%) with their devices.

Forty-five children with bilateral "AN" have received cochlear implants at our institution. This represents approximately 7% (45 of 650) of the pediatric cochlear implant population at our institution. The results of 4 of these children have previously been reported (Buss et al., 2002). In general, most children that have undergone cochlear implantation in the setting of bilateral "AN" at our center have met the United States Food and Drug Administration (FDA) suggested criteria as well as the device manufacturers' indications. Thus, a severe to profound hearing loss has been documented by behavioral testing in most children and a lack of benefit from appropriately fit amplification in the setting of a strong auditory rehabilitation program is evident. Figure 20-9 shows the relationship between preoperative pure-tone average (PTA) and the age at which these children received

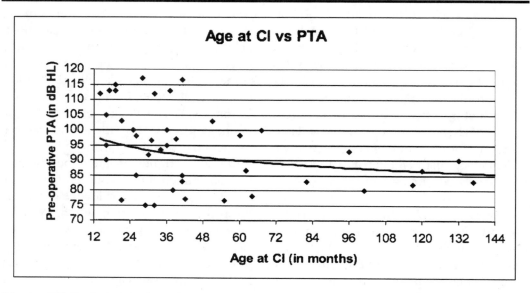

Figure 20–9. Preoperative pure-tone average (PTA) as a function of age of cochlear implantation for 45 children with bilateral "AN." There is a trend toward earlier implantation among children with greater degrees of hearing loss.

their devices. In general, children with greater degrees of hearing loss were more likely to receive their cochlear implant early.

For the 45 children that have received cochlear implants, 16 (36%) have attained open-set speech perception abilities with their devices whereas 9 (20%) have only limited open-set abilities, 11 (24%) have closed-set abilities alone and 9 (20%) are unable to be tested because of either short durations of usage or significant physical impairments. Figure 20-10 shows Phonetically Balanced-Kindergarten Word Lists (PBK) (Haskins, 1949) test scores for the 25 children with open-set speech perception results. In general, for those children that can per- form the test, a wide range of speech perception abilities is evident. Moreover, duration of device usage does not appear to explain all of the variance in this group of children. Thus, similar to previous reports, some children with "AN" that have received cochlear implants can achieve results similar to children with typical sensorineural hearing loss whereas others appear to perform more poorly (Adunka et al., 2007; Adunka et al., 2006; Buchman et al., 2006; Buss et al., 2002; Madden et al., 2002a; Mason et al., 2003; Miyamoto et al., 1999; Peterson et al., 2003; Rance & Barker, 2008; Shallop et al., 2001; Shehata-Dieler et al., 2007; Sininger & Trautwein, 2002).

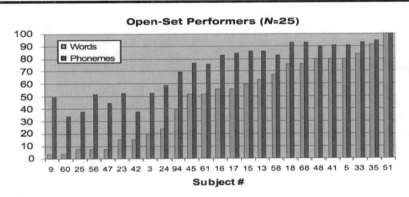

A

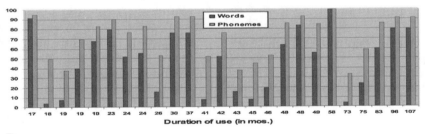

B

Figure 20–10. PBK word and phoneme scores for a group of 25 children with cochlear implants and bilateral "AN" plotted as a function of (**A**) score or (**B**) duration of implant usage. Generally, a wide range of abilities is evident and these results are not entirely explained by duration of implant use.

Conclusions

"Auditory neuropathy" ("AN") is a term used to describe a disorder in which cochlear function is spared, but afferent neural activity in the auditory nerve and central auditory pathways is impaired. It is clear that "AN" refers to a common, auditory electrophysiological profile that is present in a wide variety of medical disorders. Lesions involving the cochlear inner hair cells, hair cell-neural synapse, cochlear nerve dendrites, axons, and nucleus can all result in similar findings. When "AN" is identified on electrophysiologic testing, a careful search for a neurologic diagnosis is paramount. From a hearing perspective, generalizations should not be made regarding prognosis for speech perception abilities, and long-term speech and language development in children with "AN" irrespective of the intervention employed. The diversity of clinical findings and outcomes clearly points to the varying pathologic processes at work in these children, and supports a stepwise intervention paradigm that progresses from observation to amplification and, when indicated, to cochlear implantation. There is an urgent need for further research aimed at developing an objective means of determining optimal intervention strategies during infancy.

References

Adunka, O. F., Jewells, V., & Buchman, C. A. (2007). Value of computed tomography in the evaluation of children with cochlear nerve deficiency. *Otology and Neurotology, 28*, 597–604.

Adunka, O. F., Roush, P. A., Teagle, H. F., Brown, C. J., Zdanski, C. J., Jewells, V., et al. (2006). Internal auditory canal morphology in children with cochlear nerve deficiency. *Otology and Neurotology, 27*, 793–801.

Amatuzzi, M. G., Northrop, C., Liberman, M. C., Thornton, A., Halpin, C., Herrmann, B., et al. (2001). Selective inner hair cell loss in premature infants and cochlea pathological patterns from neonatal intensive care unit autopsies. *Archives of Otolaryngology-Head and Neck Surgery, 127*, 629–636.

American Academy of Pediatrics, Joint Commission on Infant Hearing. (2007). Year 2007 position statement: Principles and guidelines for early hearing detection and intervention programs. *Pediatrics, 120*, 898–921.

Bahmad, F., Jr., Merchant, S. N., Nadol, J. B., Jr., & Tranebjaerg, L. (2007). Otopathology in Mohr-Tranebjaerg syndrome. *Laryngoscope, 117*, 1202–1208.

Berg, A. L., Spitzer, J. B., Towers, H. M., Bartosiewicz, C., & Diamond, B. E. (2005). Newborn hearing screening in the NICU: Profile of failed auditory brainstem response/passed otoacoustic emission. *Pediatrics, 116*, 933–938.

Berlin, C. I., Bordelon, J., St John, P., Wilensky, D., Hurley, A., Kluka, E., & Hood, L. J. (1998). Reversing click polarity may uncover auditory neuropathy in infants. *Ear and Hearing, 19*, 37–47.

Berlin, C. I., Hood, L., Morlet, T., Rose, K., & Brashears, S. (2003). Auditory neuropathy/dys-synchrony: Diagnosis and management. *Mental Retardation and Developmental Disabilities Research Reviews, 9*, 225–231.

Buchman, C. A., Roush, P. A., Teagle, H. F., Brown, C. J., Zdanski, C. J., & Grose, J. H. (2006). Auditory neuropathy characteristics in children with cochlear nerve deficiency. *Ear and Hearing, 27*, 399–408.

Buss, E., Labadie, R. F., Brown, C. J., Gross, A. J., Grose, J. H., & Pillsbury, H. C. (2002). Outcome of cochlear implantation in pediatric auditory neuropathy. *Otology and Neurotology, 23*, 328–332.

Butinar, D., Zidar, J., Leonardis, L., Popovic, M., Kalaydjieva, L., Angelicheva, D., Sininger, Y., et al. (1999). Hereditary auditory, vestibular, motor, and sensory neuropathy in a Slovenian Roma (Gypsy) kindred. *Annals of Neurology, 46*, 36–44.

Ceranic, B., & Luxon, L. M. (2004). Progressive auditory neuropathy in patients with Leber's hereditary optic neuropathy. *Journal of Neurology, Neurosurgery, and Psychiatry, 75,* 626–630.

Chapon, F., Latour, P., Diraison, P., Schaeffer, S., & Vandenberghe, A. (1999). Axonal phenotype of Charcot-Marie-Tooth disease associated with a mutation in the myelin protein zero gene. *Journal of Neurology, Neurosurgery, and Psychiatry, 66,* 779–782.

Davis, H., & Hirsh, S. K. (1979). A slow brain stem response for low-frequency audiometry. *Audiology, 18,* 445–461.

Delmaghani, S., del Castillo, F. J., Michel, V., Leibovici, M., Aghaie, A., Ron, U., et al. (2006). Mutations in the gene encoding pejvakin, a newly identified protein of the afferent auditory pathway, cause DFNB59 auditory neuropathy. *Nature Genetics, 38,* 770–778.

Deltenre, P., Mansbach, A. L., Bozet, C., Christiaens, F., Barthelemy, P., Paulissen, D., & Renglet, T. (1999). Auditory neuropathy with preserved cochlear microphonics and secondary loss of otoacoustic emissions. *Audiology, 38,* 187–195.

Doyle, K. J., Sininger, Y., & Starr, A. (1998). Auditory neuropathy in childhood. *Laryngoscope, 108,* 1374–1377.

Felix, H., & Hoffmann, V. (1985). Light and electron microscopic investigation of cochlear nerve specimens from profoundly deaf patients. *Acta Oto-Laryngologica. Supplement, 423,* 67–72.

Fenwick, J. D. (1975). Neonatal jaundice as a cause of deafness. *Journal of Laryngology and Otology, 89,* 925–932.

Fuchs, P. A., Glowatzki, E., & Moser, T. (2003). The afferent synapse of cochlear hair cells. *Current Opinion in Neurobiology, 13,* 452–458.

Gandolfi, A., Horoupian, D., Rapin, I., DeTeresa, R., & Hyams, V. (1984). Deafness in Cockayne's syndrome: Morphological, morphometric, and quantitative study of the auditory pathway. *Annals of Neurology, 15,* 135–143.

Gerrard, J. (1952). Nuclear jaundice and deafness. *Journal of Laryngology and Otology, 66,* 39–46.

Gibson, W. P., & Sanli, H. (2007). Auditory neuropathy: An update. *Ear and Hearing, 28* (Suppl. 2), 102S–106S.

Glastonbury, C. M., Davidson, H. C., Harnsberger, H. R., Butler, J., Kertesz, T. R., & Shelton, C. (2002). Imaging findings of cochlear nerve deficiency. *American Journal of Neuroradiology, 23,* 635–643.

Goodhill, V. (1956). Rh child: deaf or aphasic? 1. Clinical pathologic aspects of kernicteric nuclear deafness. *Journal of Speech and Hearing Disorders, 21,* 407–410.

Hallpike, C. S., Harriman, D. G., & Wells, C. E. (1980). A case of afferent neuropathy and deafness. *Journal of Laryngology and Otology, 94,* 945–964.

Haskins, H. (1949). *A phonetically balanced test of speech discrimination for children.* Unpublished master's thesis, Northwestern University: Evanston, IL.

Kaga, K., Nakamura, M., Shinogami, M., Tsuzuku, T., Yamada, K., & Shindo, M. (1996). Auditory nerve disease of both ears revealed by auditory brainstem responses, electrocochleography and otoacoustic emissions. *Scandinavian Audiology, 25,* 233–238.

Kalaydjieva, L., Gresham, D., & Calafell, F. (2001). Genetic studies of the Roma (Gypsies): A review. *BMC Medical Genetics, 2,* 5.

Katada, A., Nonaka, S., & Harabuchi, Y. (2005). Cochlear implantation in an adult patient with auditory neuropathy. *European Archives of Oto-Rhino-Laryngology, 262,* 449–452.

Keleman, G. (1956). Erythroblastosis fetalis. *AMA Archives of Otolaryngology, 63,* 392–398.

Lee, J. S., McPherson, B., Yuen, K. C., & Wong, L. L. (2001). Screening for auditory neuropathy in a school for hearing impaired children. *International Journal of Pediatric Otorhinolaryngology, 61,* 39–46.

Madden, C., Hilbert, L., Rutter, M., Greinwald, J., & Choo, D. (2002). Pediatric cochlear implantation in auditory neuropathy. *Otology and Neurotology, 23,* 163–168.

Madden, C., Rutter, M., Hilbert, L., Greinwald, J. H., Jr., & Choo, D. I. (2002). Clinical and audiological features in auditory neuropathy. *Archives of Otolaryngology-Head and Neck Surgery, 128,* 1026–1030.

Maier, M., Castagner, F., Berger, P., & Suter, U. (2003). Distinct elements of the peripheral myelin protein 22 (PMP22) promoter regulate expression in Schwann cells and sensory neurons. *Molecular and Cellular Neurosciences, 24,* 803–817.

Mason, J. C., De Michele, A., Stevens, C., Ruth, R. A., & Hashisaki, G. T. (2003). Cochlear implantation in patients with auditory neuropathy of varied etiologies. *Laryngoscope, 113,* 45–49.

Merchant, S. N., McKenna, M. J., Nadol, J. B., Jr., Kristiansen, A. G., Tropitzsch, A., Lindal, S., et al. (2001). Temporal bone histopathologic and genetic studies in Mohr-Tranebjaerg syndrome (DFN-1). *Otology and Neurotology, 22,* 506–511.

Miyamoto, R. T., Kirk, K. I., Renshaw, J., & Hussain, D. (1999). Cochlear implantation in auditory neuropathy. *Laryngoscope, 109,* 181–185.

Moog, J. S., & Geers, A. E. (2003). Epilogue: Major findings, conclusions and implications for deaf education. *Ear and Hearing, 24*(Suppl.1), 121S–125S.

Morton, C. C., & Nance, W. E. (2006). Newborn hearing screening—a silent revolution. *New England Journal of Medicine, 354,* 2151–2164.

Nadol, J. B., Jr., & Xu, W. Z. (1992). Diameter of the cochlear nerve in deaf humans: Implications for cochlear implantation. *Annals of Otology, Rhinology, and Laryngology, 101,* 988–993.

Narne, V. K., & Vanaja, C. S. (2008). Effect of envelope enhancement on speech perception in individuals with auditory neuropathy. *Ear and Hearing, 29,* 45–53.

Nelson, E. G., & Hinojosa, R. (2001). Aplasia of the cochlear nerve: A temporal bone study. *Otology and Neurotology, 22,* 790–795.

Parry, D. A., Booth, T., & Roland, P. S. (2005). Advantages of magnetic resonance imaging over computed tomography in preoperative evaluation of pediatric cochlear implant candidates. *Otology and Neurotology, 26,* 976–982.

Patel, A. M., Cahill, L. D., Ret, J., Schmithorst, V., Choo, D., & Holland, S. (2007). Functional magnetic resonance imaging of hearing-impaired children under sedation before cochlear implantation. *Archives of Otolaryngology-Head and Neck Surgery, 133,* 677–683.

Peterson, A., Shallop, J., Driscoll, C., Breneman, A., Babb, J., Stoeckel, R., & Fabry, L. (2003).

Outcomes of cochlear implantation in children with auditory neuropathy. *Journal of the American Acadamy of Audiology, 14,* 188–201.

Psarommatis, I., Riga, M., Douros, K., Koltsidopoulos, P., Douniadakis, D., Kapetanakis, I., et al. (2006). Transient infantile auditory neuropathy and its clinical implications. *International Journal of Pediatric Otorhinolaryngology, 70,* 1629–1637.

Rance, G. (2005). Auditory neuropathy/dyssynchrony and its perceptual consequences. *Trends in Amplification, 9,* 1–43.

Rance, G., & Barker, E. J. (2008). Speech perception in children with auditory neuropathy/dyssynchrony managed with either hearing AIDS or cochlear implants. *Otology and Neurotology, 29,* 179–182.

Rance, G., Barker, E., Mok, M., Dowell, R., Rincon, A., & Garratt, R. (2007a). Speech perception in noise for children with auditory neuropathy/dys-synchrony type hearing loss. *Ear and Hearing, 28,* 351–360.

Rance, G., Barker, E. J., Sarant, J. Z., & Ching, T. Y. (2007b). Receptive language and speech production in children with auditory neuropathy/dyssynchrony type hearing loss. *Ear and Hearing, 28,* 694–702.

Rance, G., Beer, D. E., Cone-Wesson, B., Shepherd, R. K., Dowell, R. C., King, A. M., et al. (1999). Clinical findings for a group of infants and young children with auditory neuropathy. *Ear and Hearing, 20,* 238–252.

Rance, G., Cone-Wesson, B., Wunderlich, J., & Dowell, R. (2002). Speech perception and cortical event related potentials in children with auditory neuropathy. *Ear and Hearing, 23,* 239–253.

Rance, G., Fava, R., Baldock, H., Chong, A., Barker, E., Corben, L., et al. (2008). Speech perception ability in individuals with Friedreich ataxia. *Brain, 131,* 2002–2012.

Rance, G., McKay, C., & Grayden, D. (2004). Perceptual characterization of children with auditory neuropathy. *Ear and Hearing, 25,* 34–46.

Rapin, I., & Gravel, J. (2003). "Auditory neuropathy": Physiologic and pathologic evidence calls for more diagnostic specificity. *Interna-*

tional Journal of Pediatric Otorhinolaryngology, 67, 707–728.

Rapin, I., & Gravel, J. S. (2006). Auditory neuropathy: A biologically inappropriate label unless acoustic nerve involvement is documented. *Journal of the American Acadamy of Audiology, 17*, 147–150.

Rea, P. A., & Gibson, W. P. (2003). Evidence for surviving outer hair cell function in congenitally deaf ears. *Laryngoscope, 113*, 2030–2034.

Santarelli, R., Starr, A., Michalewski, H. J., & Arslan, E. (2008). Neural and receptor cochlear potentials obtained by transtympanic electrocochleography in auditory neuropathy. *Clinical Neurophysiology, 119*, 1028–1041.

Scollie, S. D., Seewald, R. C., Cornelisse, L. E., Moodie, L. S., Bagatto, M. P, Laurnagaray, D., et al. (2005). The Desired Sensation Level multistage input/output algorithm. *Trends in Amplification, 9*(4), 159–197.

Shaia, W. T., Shapiro, S. M., Heller, A. J., Galiani, D. L., Sismanis, A., & Spencer, R. F. (2002). Immunohistochemical localization of calcium-binding proteins in the brainstem vestibular nuclei of the jaundiced Gunn rat. *Hearing Research, 173*, 82–90.

Shaia, W. T., Shapiro, S. M., & Spencer, R. F. (2005). The jaundiced gunn rat model of auditory neuropathy/dyssynchrony. *Laryngoscope, 115*, 2167–2173.

Shallop, J. K., Peterson, A., Facer, G. W., Fabry, L. B., & Driscoll, C. L. (2001). Cochlear implants in five cases of auditory neuropathy: Postoperative findings and progress. *Laryngoscope, 111*, 555–562.

Shehata-Dieler, W., Volter, C., Hildmann, A., Hildmann, H., & Helms, J. (2007). Clinical and audiological findings in children with auditory neuropathy. *Laryngorhinootologie, 86*(1), 15–21.

Sheykholeslami, K., & Kaga, K. (2000). Otoacoustic emissions and auditory brainstem responses after neonatal hyperbilirubinemia. *International Journal of Pediatric Otorhinolaryngology, 52*, 65–73.

Shivashankar, N., Satishchandra, P., Shashikala, H. R., & Gore, M. (2003). Primary auditory neuropathy—an enigma. *Acta Neurologica Scandinavia, 108*, 130–135.

Sininger, Y. S., & Trautwein, P. (2002). Electrical stimulation of the auditory nerve via cochlear implants in patients with auditory neuropathy. *Annals of Otology, Rhinology, and Laryngology, 111*(Suppl. 189), 29–31.

Spencer, R. F., Shaia, W. T., Gleason, A. T., Sismanis, A., & Shapiro, S. M. (2002). Changes in calcium-binding protein expression in the auditory brainstem nuclei of the jaundiced Gunn rat. *Hearing Research, 171*, 129–141.

Spoendlin, H. (1974). Optic cochleovestibular degenerations in hereditary ataxias. II. Temporal bone pathology in two cases of Friedreich's ataxia with vestibulo-cochlear disorders. *Brain, 97*, 41–48.

Spoendlin, H., & Schrott, A. (1990). Quantitative evaluation of the human cochlear nerve. *Acta Oto-Laryngologica Supplement, 470*, 61–69; discussion 69–70.

Starr, A., Isaacson, B., Michalewski, H. J., Zeng, F. G., Kong, Y. Y., Beale, P., et al. (2004). A dominantly inherited progressive deafness affecting distal auditory nerve and hair cells. *Journal of the Association for Research in Otolaryngology, 5*, 411–426.

Starr, A., Michalewski, H. J., Zeng, F. G., Fujikawa-Brooks, S., Linthicum, F., Kim, C. S., et al. (2003). Pathology and physiology of auditory neuropathy with a novel mutation in the MPZ gene (Tyr145→Ser). *Brain, 126*, 1604–1619.

Starr, A., Picton, T. W., Sininger, Y., Hood, L. J., & Berlin, C. I. (1996). Auditory neuropathy. *Brain, 119*, 741–753.

Starr, A., Sininger, Y., Nguyen, T., Michalewski, H. J., Oba, S., & Abdala, C. (2001). Cochlear receptor (microphonic and summating potentials, otoacoustic emissions) and auditory pathway (auditory brainstem potentials) activity in auditory neuropathy. *Ear and Hearing, 22*, 91–99.

Trimble, K., Blaser, S., James, A. L., & Papsin, B. C. (2007). Computed tomography and/or magnetic resonance imaging before pediatric cochlear implantation? Developing an investigative strategy. *Otology and Neurotology, 28*, 317–324.

Varga, R., Avenarius, M. R., Kelley, P. M., Keats, B. J., Berlin, C. I., Hood, L. J., et al. (2006). OTOF mutations revealed by genetic analysis of hearing loss families including a potential temperature sensitive auditory neuropathy allele. *Journal of Medical Genetics, 43,* 576–581.

Walton, J., Gibson, W. P., Sanli, H., & Prelog, K. (2008). Predicting cochlear implant outcomes in children with auditory neuropathy. *Otology and Neurotology, 29,* 302–309.

Xoinis, K., Weirather, Y., Mavoori, H., Shaha, S. H., & Iwamoto, L. M. (2007). Extremely low birth weight infants are at high risk for auditory neuropathy. *Journal of Perinatology, 27,* 718–723.

Yasunaga, S., Grati, M., Chardenoux, S., Smith, T. N., Friedman, T. B., Lalwani, A. K., et al. (2000). OTOF encodes multiple long and short isoforms: Genetic evidence that the long ones underlie recessive deafness DFNB9. *American Journal of Human Genetics, 67,* 591–600.

Yasunaga, S., Grati, M., Cohen-Salmon, M., El-Amraoui, A., Mustapha, M., Salem, N., et al. (1999). A mutation in OTOF, encoding otoferlin, a FER-1-like protein, causes DFNB9, a nonsyndromic form of deafness. *Nature Genetics, 21,* 363–369.

Ylikoski, J., & Savolainen, S. (1984). The cochlear nerve in various forms of deafness. *Acta Oto-Laryngologica, 98,* 418–427.

Zeng, F. G., Kong, Y. Y., Michalewski, H. J., & Starr, A. (2005). Perceptual consequences of disrupted auditory nerve activity. *Journal of Neurophysiology, 93,* 3050–3063.

Zeng, F. G., Oba, S., Garde, S., Sininger, Y., & Starr, A. (1999). Temporal and speech processing deficits in auditory neuropathy. *Neuroreport, 10,* 3429–3435.

Zur, K. B., Holland, S. K., Yuan, W., & Choo, D. I. (2004). Functional magnetic resonance imaging: Contemporary and future use. *Current Opinion in Otolaryngology and Head and Neck Surgery, 12,* 374–377.

CHAPTER 21

Auditory Brainstem Implants in Children

ROBERT V. SHANNON
LILLIANA COLLETTI
LAURIE S. EISENBERG
KAREN C. JOHNSON
MARCO CARNER
VITTORIO COLLETTI

Introduction

The Auditory Brainstem Implant (ABI) was developed to provide electrical stimulation of the cochlear nucleus in the brainstem for patients with no remaining auditory nerve (Brackmann et al., 1993; Shannon et al., 1993). The ABI functions like a cochlear implant (CI) except for the placement of the electrodes (Figure 21–1). The ABI electrode consists of a 3 × 8 mm electrode array containing three rows of seven electrodes placed on a silicone carrier pad with mesh backing (Figure 21–2). The electrode array is placed within the lateral recess of the IV ventricle of the brain, usually during a surgical procedure to remove a tumor. Patients with the ABI hear different pitch percepts on the different electrodes and demonstrate

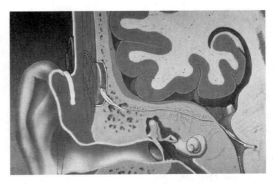

Figure 21–1. Schematic view of the placement of the ABI into the lateral recess of the IVth ventricle.

relatively normal temporal processing ability (Shannon & Otto, 1990). However, they rarely achieve a significant level of speech

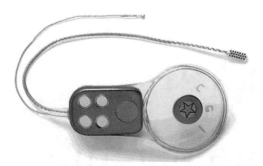

Figure 21–2. The implantable portion of the ABI is similar to a cochlear implant except for the electrode array, which has a 3 × 8 mm pad containing 21 electrode contacts in three rows of seven.

recognition without lipreading (Manrique, Cevera-Paz, Huarte, & Molina, 2004; Nevison et al., 2002; Otto, Brackmann, Hitselberger, Shannon, & Kuchta, 2002). New results from Verona, Italy have shown CI-like performance with the ABI in patients who did not have tumors—in patients who lost their auditory nerves from trauma or ossification (Colletti & Shannon, 2005). It appears that something related to the tumors, either their growth or damage to the brainstem from their removal, is limiting the performance of the ABI in tumor patients. The difference in performance between tumor and nontumor groups provides important information about the impact of pathology on outcomes. The superior results with nontumor ABIs demonstrate that open-set speech recognition is achievable even with stimulation beyond the cochlea.

Given the high level of speech recognition in nontumor adults with the ABI, clinical trials have been initiated to provide the ABI to young children who are not candidates for a cochlear implant. Is the ABI suitable for children? Is the risk of the surgery offset by a higher level of auditory performance? What etiologies are suitable or not for the ABI? This chapter addresses these issues and reports on the present data that bear on these questions.

ABI Results in NF2 and Nontumor Adults

First, let us review the results obtained with an ABI in the adult population. Initially, ABIs were implanted in patients with bilateral schwannomas on the vestibular branch of the VIIIth nerve, a condition typical of the genetic disorder neurofibromatosis type 2 (NF2) (Baser, Evans, & Gutmann, 2003; Evans et al., 1992a, 1992b). Surgery is required to remove the schwannomas before they damage the brainstem from compression. The ABI device is implanted following tumor removal, with the electrode array inserted into the lateral recess of the IVth ventricle, adjacent to the auditory cochlear nucleus. The open bars in Figure 21–3 show the percentage of patients that can recognize words in simple sentences presented in quiet listening conditions (Colletti & Shannon, 2005). More than 90% of the 210 NF2 patients could recognize less than 20% of the words in sentences correctly, and most of those scores were 0%. Although the ABI provides useful auditory information to adult patients with NF2, the level of performance has been far below that observed with cochlear implants. Only a few NF2 patients are able to recognize more than 20% of the words in sentences, a level of performance that would be expected from a CI. Adults with CIs average more than 95% correct on similar test materials (Spahr & Dorman, 2006). Although the overall level of auditory performance is low compared to a CI, the risk/benefit ratio is still highly positive in NF2 ABI adults because the surgery is performed

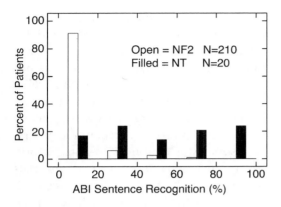

Figure 21–3. Results of sentence recognition in the sound-only condition by adults with an ABI. Open bars show results from adults with NF2 and filled bars show results from non-NF2.

to remove a life-threatening tumor and there is little additional risk of inserting the ABI device. The level of auditory benefit, although low compared to a CI, is still highly useful to patients with no hearing and who are unable to benefit from a CI.

Recently, ABI devices have been implanted in adult patients who do not have tumors or NF2–patients who lost their VIIIth, nerve from a variety of causes: skull trauma, ossification, neurologic problems, and a sporadic unilateral tumor in an only hearing ear (Colletti et al., 2005a). The profile of performance levels in this group of patients is shown as the filled bars in Figure 21–3. It can be seen that about half of the patients are able to correctly recognize 50% or more of the words in sentences. The risk/benefit ratio is different from NF2 ABIs because in nontumor ABIs the surgery is elective, but that additional risk is offset by the much higher level of auditory performance observed in this group. Many of these non-NF2 patients are able to converse on the telephone without lipreading cues.

CI Results in Children: Developmental Trajectory

When young children receive CIs they exhibit a developmental trajectory that is nearly like normal hearing children. Studies have shown improved CI performance as the age of implant decreases down to at least 2 years of age (McConkey Robbins, Koch, Osberger, Zimmerman-Phillips, & Kishon-Rabin, 2004; Svirsky, Robbins, Kirk, Pisoni, & Miyamoto, 2000). If implanted before age 2 years children appear to develop receptive and expressive language skills at a normal developmental rate, that is, 1 year of progress for each year of implant use. However, the language skills of implanted children lag behind those of normally hearing children by the length of deafness, which is equal to the age of implant in congenitally deaf children. When children are implanted at ages older than 5 years they show slower rate of language development than normally hearing children. These results suggest that there is a "critical period" for sensory development of around 5 years of age. Children implanted prior to 5 years of age can develop at a normal rate, whereas children implanted after age 5 show slower and more limited language development. Even when CIs are provided before the age of 2 years, auditory performance on complex tasks that involve speech or music identification is limited compared to normal hearing (Vongpaisal, Trehub, & Schellenberg, 2006).

These changes also are probably reflected in physiologic maturation of the auditory system, as represented by evoked auditory potentials. Ponton, Don, Eggermont, Waring, and Masuda (1996) measured auditory evoked potentials (AEP) over time in children with normal hearing and in children with CIs. In normal-hearing children the latency of wave V in the AEP decreased over time from 10s to a few msec as the child matured. In deaf children there was no AEP prior to implantation, and after implantation the electrically evoked potential (EEP) showed a long latency at first, which shortened over time. When the implanted EEPs were compared to normal hearing AEPs in terms of chronologic age, the latencies of implanted ears were longer. However, if the evoked potential latencies were compared in terms of hearing age (referenced to the age at implantation), then the trajectory of latencies as a function of age was similar between hearing and implanted children. It appears that although the deaf auditory system is immature relative to the normal system introducing the implant starts the physiologic system along a normal developmental trajectory. Sharma, Dorman, and Spahr (2002) have estimated from physiologic data that the central auditory pathways are most sensitive during the first 3.5 years, a time estimate that is consistent with the behavioral results.

ABI in Children

Although the results of CIs in children are dramatic, there are some children for whom CIs are not an option. These would include children with genetic malformations that result in an absence of a cochlea and auditory nerve, or children who have lost access to their auditory nerves as a result of head trauma or severe ossification. In some of these etiologies CIs have been attempted and failed because there has been no VIII nerve to activate. In some cases a CI was attempted and it either did not function or functioned for a short period of time and

then failed as the auditory nerve deteriorated. An ABI has not been considered a viable option for such children because it was thought that the risk/benefit ratio was not acceptable; ABI performance in NF2 adults was poor, and the surgery appeared to have higher risk than CI surgery. However, following the excellent speech recognition observed in some ABIs in non-NF2 adults, Vittorio Colletti, in Verona, Italy, initiated ABI trials in children with absent VIIIth nerves (Colletti, Fiorino, Sacchetto, Miorelli, & Carner, 2001; Colletti et al., 2005a, 2005b).

ABI Results in Children

The results by Colletti and his group show a wide range of performance outcomes across etiologies (Colletti & Zoccante, 2008; Colletti, 2007; Colletti, Colletti, Carner, Veronese, & Shannon, submitted). Some children who had hearing initially and lost their VIII nerve from trauma or ossification showed dramatic improvements with the ABI. Some children with congenital absence of the VIII nerve also showed high levels of auditory development with the ABI–levels of performance and rates of improvement similar to those observed with CIs. Some ABI children improved on the Categories of Auditory Performance (CAP) test (Archbold, Lutman, & Marshall, 1995), with performance ranging from level 1 (sound detection) to level 7 (limited open set speech recognition, ability to use the telephone with family members) over 2 years.

Other children with severe genetic malformations or auditory neuropathy, and children with multiple handicaps received limited auditory benefit, even after years of experience with the ABI. However, even those children who received limited auditory benefit with the ABI demonstrated significant improvements on tests of cognitive development (Colletti & Zoccante, 2008), including tasks that assess form completion and recognition of repeated patterns. Recent reports from the implant team in Turkey on 11 children implanted with the ABI (Sennaroglu et al., 2008) confirm the Verona results.

Several recent studies have documented the developmental trajectory of children with ABIs. Eisenberg and colleagues had the opportunity to evaluate an American child with Goldenhar Syndrome who received the ABI at age 3.5 years in Verona, Italy (Eisenberg et al., 2008). At the initial evaluation the child demonstrated detection of sound, speech pattern perception with visual cues, and inconsistent auditory-only vowel discrimination. Twelve months later, this child was able to identify speech patterns consistently; closed-set word identification was emerging. His developmental trajectory with the ABI was similar to that observed in a comparison group of congenitally deaf children implanted with a CI at a similar age.

Colletti and colleagues presented CAP results from 29 children with ABIs, representing etiologies from congenital malformations and cochlear nerve aplasia to trauma (Colletti, L. et al., submitted). Some children with congenital cochlear malformations also had multiple handicaps. Figure 21–4 replots the results from the Colletti et al. study. Note that gradual improvement is observed over time for most etiologies, but the highest performance level is less than open-set speech understanding for most children with ABI. Two children were able to achieve open-set speech recognition and telephone use after 3 years of ABI use. Three additional children are on the same trajectory, achieving CAP level 4 performance after only 2 years. These five children had diverse etiologies, so the relation between etiology and outcome remains

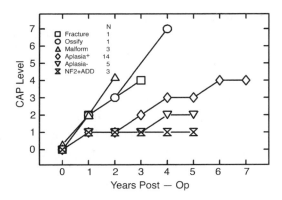

Figure 21–4. Performance of ABI children over time on the Categories of Auditory Performance (CAP) test. Category 4 indicates the ability to recognize words in a closed-set format, whereas category 7 indicates the ability to converse with family members over the telephone (moderate open-set speech recognition).

unclear. Three children who achieved CAP level 4 after 2 years of experience had severe congenital cochlear malformations. The results for children with cochlear nerve aplasia were divided into two groups based on their performance. One group ($n = 14$) made progress on auditory tasks but showed asymptotic performance at CAP level 2 even after as much as 5 years. The other group ($n = 5$) showed continued improvement over time, reaching CAP level 4 after 6 to 7 years.

Complications

Although ABIs can provide good speech recognition and auditory development to some congenitally deaf children, is the risk/benefit ratio favorable for such implantation? Not all children perform at a high level with the ABI and the surgery theoretically carries higher potential risk than the CI because the implantation site is intradural. Colletti and colleagues analyzed complication rates for 29 children with ABIs and compared them with published data from CIs and ABIs in NF2 adults (Colletti, Shannon, Carner, Veronese, & Colletti, 2008). Complications were categorized using the normal reporting system for surgical complications. They found that both major and minor complication rates of ABI surgery in children were comparable with those observed in cochlear implant surgery. The complication rates for ABIs in children were significantly lower that those observed for ABIs in NF2 adults, and similar to those of ABIs in nontumor adults. It appears that the relatively higher rate of complications observed in NF2 ABIs is due to the NF2 disease process and sequelae—not to the surgical approach or to the ABI per se. ABI in non-NF2 children and adults produce a similar complication rate to CIs.

ABI Programming and Assessment

Programming an ABI in a congenitally deaf child is considerably more difficult than programming a CI. As shown in Figure 21–2, the ABI electrodes are arranged differently from those arranged on a standard CI electrode array. Moreover, placement of the ABI electrode array is not a simple procedure; it often is unknown whether the electrode array has been stationed in a place that most selectively stimulates the auditory nerve cells. Stimulation of ABI electrodes can produce non-auditory side effects due to activation of the inferior cerebellar peduncle (ICP), the flocculus of the cerebellum, and the IXth and Xth cranial nerves. Young children cannot differentiate the novel auditory sensations from nonauditory sensations and

must be monitored carefully for nonauditory effects during the initial fitting process. Stimulation of the ICP can produce mild tingling sensations along the ipsilateral side of the body to the ABI. Sensations are typically felt along the side of the head, in the shoulder or in the torso. These sensations are usually not painful or unpleasant but are undesirable. If the child indicates nonauditory sensations by touching a location along the ipsilateral body, stimulation on that electrode should be discontinued. A physician should be present during initial stimulation to monitor heart rate and blood pressure to check for activation of the IXth and Xth cranial nerves. If such activation occurs these electrodes should be removed from the stimulation map.

Programming the ABI processor is much more complex than programming a CI processor. Often, not all electrodes on the array are programmed into the processor because of nonauditory effects. Moreover, several electrodes may provide the same pitch percept. Those electrodes that are eventually programmed into the processor typically require individualized fitting characteristics (i.e., pulse duration, frequency allocation). Accordingly, extra time needs to be allocated for mapping. In general, a reasonable stimulation strategy is to start with electrodes that appear to provide purely auditory sensations using evidence from electrophysiology and behavioral observation. Purely auditory sensation, however, is not always evident when programming very young children. Similar to CIs, young children with ABIs may not show overt responses on initial stimulation but, rather, may exhibit subtle responses such as eye widening or blinking, eye rubbing, clinging to a parent, and perhaps even crying. Thus, it may not be obvious that a supposedly "adverse" reaction is a result of nonauditory versus auditory stimulation. Because of the concern that nonauditory responses with an ABI could signal stimulation of other cranial nerves, any suspicion of a nonauditory response must be cautiously monitored. After several weeks when the child has adapted to stimulation, more electrodes can be added to the map. At this point it is hoped that the child will have adequate experience with the ABI to differentiate auditory from nonauditory stimulation, and that differences in their behavioral reaction are apparent to trained observers.

During the first 6 months of device use the ABI child should be seen at regular intervals to monitor auditory progress and nonauditory side effects. Administering a comprehensive assessment battery in areas of speech perception, speech and language, cognition, adaptive behavior, development, and psychosocial performance is advocated (Eisenberg et al., 2008).

Conclusions

Pediatric ABI programs are expanding at a rapid rate. At the time of this writing, all surgeries have been performed outside the United States. ABIs have been demonstrated to provide auditory and cognitive development in deaf children who are not suitable for cochlear implants. The complications observed in the hands of experienced implant teams are minimal and are comparable with those observed in CIs. Most children show limited but beneficial auditory performance and a few children show substantial open-set speech recognition. Further research is necessary to define the etiologies most suitable for an ABI and to document the long-term outcomes in communication skill development.

References

Archbold, S., Lutman, M. E., & Marshall, D. H. (1995). Categories of auditory performance. *Annals of Otology, Rhinology, and Laryngology, 104*(Suppl. 166), 312–314.

Baser, M. E., Evans, D. G., & Gutmann, D. H. (2003). Neurofibromatosis 2. *Current Opinion in Neurology, 16*, 27–33.

Brackmann, D. E., Hitselberger, W. E., Nelson, R. A., Moore, J., Waring, M. D., Portillo, F., et al. (1993). Auditory brainstem implant. I: Issues in surgical implantation. *Otolaryngology-Head and Neck Surgery, 108*, 624–634.

Colletti, L. (2007). Beneficial auditory and cognitive effects of auditory brainstem implantation in children. *Acta Oto-Laryngologica, 127*, 943–946.

Colletti, L., Colletti, V., Carner, M., Veronese, S., & Shannon, R. V. (Manuscript submitted for publication). *The development of auditory perception in children following auditory brainstem implantation.*

Colletti, L., & Zoccante, L. (2008). Non-verbal cognitive abilities and auditory performance in children fitted with ABI: Preliminary report. *Laryngoscope, 118*, 1443–1448.

Colletti, V., Carner, M., Miorelli, V., Guida, M., Colletti, L., & Fiorino, F. (2005a). Auditory brainstem implant (ABI): New frontiers in adults and children. *Otolaryngology-Head Neck Surgery, 133*, 126–138.

Colletti, V., Carner, M., Miorelli, V., Guida, M., Colletti, L., & Fiorino, F. G. (2005b). Cochlear Implantation at under 12 months: Report on 10 patients. *Laryngoscope, 115*, 445–449.

Colletti, V., Fiorino, F., Sacchetto, L., Miorelli, & Carner, M. (2001). Hearing habilitation with auditory brainstem implantation in two children with cochlear nerve aplasia. *International Journal of Pediatric Otorhinolaryngology, 60*, 99–111.

Colletti, V., & Shannon, R. V. (2005). Open set speech perception with auditory brainstem implant? *Laryngoscope, 115*, 1974–1978.

Colletti, V., Shannon, R. V., Carner, M., Veronese, S., & Colletti, L. (2008, April). *Complications in auditory brainstem implant surgery*. Paper presented at the 10th International Conference on Cochlear Implants and Other Implantable Auditory Technologies, San Diego, CA.

Eisenberg, L. S., Johnson, K. C., Martinez, A. S., DesJardin, J. L., Stika, C. J., Dzubak, D., et al. (2008). Comprehensive evaluation of a child with an auditory brainstem implant. *Otology and Neurotology, 29,* 251–257.

Evans, D. G. R., Huson, S. M., Donnai, D., Neary, W., Blair, V., Newton, V., et al. (1992b). A genetic study of type 2 neurofibromatosis in the United Kingdom: II. Guidelines for genetic counseling. *Journal of Medical Genetics, 29,* 847–852.

Evans, D. G. R., Huson, S. M., Donnai, D., Neary, W., Blair, V., Teare, D., et al. (1992a). A genetic study of type 2 neurofibromatosis in the United Kingdom: I. Prevalence, mutation rate, fitness, and confirmation of maternal transmission effect on severity. *Journal of Medical Genetics, 29,* 841–846.

Manrique, M., Cevera-Paz, F. J., Huarte, A., & Molina, M. (2004). Advantages of cochlear implantation in prelingual deaf children before 2 years of age when compared to later implantation. *Laryngoscope, 114,* 1462–1469.

McConkey Robbins, K. M., Koch, D. B., Osberger, M. J., Zimmerman-Phillips, S., & Kishon-Rabin, L. (2004). The effect of age at cochlear implantation on auditory skill development in infants and toddlers. *Archives of Otolaryngology-Head and Neck Surgery, 130,* 570–574.

Nevison, B., Laszig, R., Sollmann, W. P., Lenarz, T., Sterkers, O., Ramsden, R., et al (2002). Results from a European clinical investigation of the Nucleus multichannel auditory brainstem implant. *Ear and Hearing, 23,* 170–183.

Otto, S. R., Brackmann, D. E., Hitselberger, W. E., Shannon, R. V., & Kuchta, J. (2002). The multichannel auditory brainstem implant: Update performance in 61 patients. *Journal of Neurosurgery, 96,* 1063–1071.

Ponton, C. W., Don, M., Eggermont, J. J., Waring, M. D., & Masuda, A. (1996). Maturation of human cortical auditory function: Differences between normal-hearing children and children with cochlear implants. *Ear and Hearing, 17,* 430–437.

Sennaroglu, L., Atas, A., Sennaroglu, G., Yucel, E., Sevinc, S., Ekin, M. C., et al. (2008, May). *Preliminary results of auditory brainstem implantation in prelingual children with severe inner ear malformations*. Paper presented at the meeting of the American Neurotology Society, Orlando, FL.

Shannon, R. V., Fayad, J., Moore, J., Lo, W. W., Otto, S., Nelson, R. A., et al. (1993). Auditory brainstem implant. II: Post-surgical issues and performance. *Otolaryngology-Head and Neck Surgery, 108,* 634–642.

Shannon, R. V., & Otto, S. R. (1990). Psychophysical measures from electrical stimulation of the human cochlear nucleus. *Hearing Research, 47,* 159–168.

Sharma, A., Dorman, M. F., & Spahr, A. J. (2002). A sensitive period for the development of the central auditory system in children with cochlear implants: Implications for age of implantation. *Ear and Hearing, 23,* 532–539.

Spahr, A. J., & Dorman, M. F. (2006). Performance of subjects fit with the Advanced Bionics CII and Nucleus 3G cochlear implant devices. *Archives of Otolaryngology-Head and Neck Surgery, 130,* 624–628.

Svirsky, M. A., Robbins, A. M., Kirk, K. I., Pisoni, D. B., & Miyamoto, R. T. (2000). Language development in profoundly deaf children with cochlear implants. *Psychological Science, 11,* 153–158.

Vongpaisal, T., Trehub, S. E., & Schellenberg, E. G. (2006). Song recognition by children and adolescents with cochlear implants. *Journal of Speech, Language, and Hearing Research, 49,* 1091–1103.

Index